BARRON'S

NEW
MCAT
MEDICAL COLLEGE
ADMISSION TEST

12TH EDITION

Hugo R. Seibel, Ph.D.
Professor Emeritus of Anatomy
School of Medicine
Virginia Commonwealth University
Richmond, Virginia

Kenneth E. Guyer, Ph.D.
Associate Professor of Biochemistry
School of Medicine, Marshall University
Huntington, West Virginia

A. Bryant Mangum, Ph.D.
Professor of English
Virginia Commonwealth University

Carolyn M. Conway, Ph.D.
Assistant Professor of Biology
Virginia Commonwealth University

Arthur F. Conway, Ph.D.
Professor of Biology
Randolph-Macon College
Ashland, Virginia

Wesley L. Shanholtzer, Ph.D.
Professor
Department of Physics and
    Physical Sciences
Marshall University

Melissa B. Cichowicz, Ph.D.
Director of Pre-Medical Programs
West Chester University

Jeffrey W. Schubert
Research Assistant
Villanova University

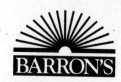

BARRON'S

All inquiries should be addressed to:
Barron's Educational Series, Inc.
250 Wireless Boulevard
Hauppauge, New York 11788
www.barronseduc.com

Library of Congress Control Number: 2008920535

ISBN-13: 978-0-7641-3801-0
ISBN-10: 0-7641-3801-4

ISBN-13: 978-0-7641-9399-6 (book w/CD-ROM)
ISBN-10: 0-7641-9399-6 (book w/CD-ROM)

PRINTED IN THE UNITED STATES OF AMERICA
9 8 7

Contents

Preface

You may be wondering, can I really *prepare* for the Medical College Admission Test (MCAT)?

The simple answer is *YES*! Some students are hesitant to use a book of this sort to assist in preparation for the MCAT, perhaps believing there is something dishonest about this method of preparation. Other students may believe that they can utilize this book or a similar one just before the test to prepare themselves. In our estimation, both of these viewpoints are incorrect. The information in this book will provide you with experience taking timed MCATs and point out your areas of weakness that will require additional study. Through proper and careful preparation, you will be presenting your true potential for the study of medicine when you sit for the actual MCAT. For maximum benefit, we would suggest that students begin their preparation two or three months before the examination. This will allow time to take the practice examinations, review the areas of weakness, and retake some of the practice examinations without having the pressure of time to produce undue frustration.

Obtaining admission to medical school is a very difficult task today. We hope that, in preparing this volume, we have been able to offer you a greater chance of success. Good luck!

We wish to acknowledge the help we have received from many of our colleagues; a special thank-you should be extended to H. Meetz; G. D. Meetz; J. Gregorek; J. D. Reynolds; W. M. Reams; C. Kirksey; R. J. Krieg; J. H. Johnson; S. S. Craig; J. D. Povlishock; W. Seibel; L. Crane; L. P. Gartner; L. M. Sawyer; G. J. Somori; W. J. McIntyre; J. Washburn; J. L. Poland; S. L. Quattropani; M. P. Golka; F. M. Bush; R. L. Salisbury; M. M. Sholley; G. Miller; C. H. Fowlkes; R. B. Brandt; P. L. Szabo; N. Whisner; J. Wood; J. P. Guyer; J. Kass; Lester Schlumpf; B. P. Dezzutti; S. Falzone; I. K. Schneider; L. S. Costanzo; S. C. Dudley; J. Pettit; W. M. Grogan; S. G. Bradley; A. N. Avakian; C. P. Ruch; S. M. Ayers; J. J. McGovern; W. J. Borowy; J. Astruc, Jr.; J. F. Snyder; J. I. Townsend; J. Perlin; W. L. Banks; W. E. Blake, Jr.; L. Padilla; S. E. Kennedy; J. M. Messmer; S. A. Messmer; J. A. Rosecrans; M. N. De Pillars; B. Owen; R. G. Bass; R. S. Vacca; J. Mundie; E. Pollard; D. James; P. F. H. Campbell; T. Fleet; H. Tuttle; M. Ripley; R. Perry; R. Dale; S. V. Doud; L. Graham; D. J. Vick; Robert Lehrman; N. Sharp; E. Hodges; L. Carleton; and A. Arnold. Particular gratitude is extended to Marilyn P. Bertrand for her cheerful and spirited assistance and the typing of the manuscript. We are indebted to Dr. Edith E. Seibel for her contributions and the proofreading of the book. Dr. Erwin E. Seibel deserves a special commendation since he contributed the bulk of the physics review for the first edition.

For recent editions, we received extraordinary help and wish to extend our special gratitude to Karl S. Roth, Charles H. O'Neil, David G. Simpson, J. Dennis Hoban, Donald G. Roebuck, Ruth L. Dennis-Phillips, John W. Bigbee, Caroline G. Jackson, Phyllis J. Jett, Thomas L. Tucker, Emily Mistr, and William L. Banks, Jr.

Introduction

The new MCAT is a solely computer-based exam that attempts to evaluate (1) the student's knowledge and ability to solve problems in the areas of biology, chemistry, and physics, (2) the student's skill in analysis of paragraphs, tabular material, graphs, etc., and (3) the ability to write two first draft compositions in proper English. Separate scores will be reported for Verbal Reasoning, Physical Sciences, Writing Sample, and Biological Sciences.

It is expected that those taking the test will have the equivalent of one year of college study in each of the following scientific areas: biology, general and/or inorganic chemistry, organic chemistry, and physics. Although advanced study in one or more of these disciplines may give a better understanding of concepts, it is not intended that the questions will require a knowledge of concepts not taught in basic courses.

A mathematics background including one year of college mathematics should suffice for the science questions; calculus is not required. Indeed, it has been suggested that high school courses, which included the following, would represent adequate preparation in mathematics: two years of algebra; use of trigonometric functions; memorization of sine and cosine of 0°, 90°, and 180°; facility in use of metric and English units and conversion from one set of units to another (when conversion factors are given); experimental error; statistics to include the concepts of arithmetic mean, range, variability, and significant figures; and vector addition and subtraction.

It is our suggestion that you begin preparation by studying the review sections of this book. Areas that are particularly difficult for you may require some review of your college texts. When you begin taking the practice tests, try to pace yourself to allow completion of each section within the allotted time. (If it is necessary to omit some questions because of time limitations, you may wish to go back after you have scored the test and try to answer them without the pressure of time.)

After taking your first practice test and checking the answers, you should score your test as it will be done after the actual test. First count the number of your correct answers in each section. The number of correct answers is your raw score which must then be converted into a 15-point scaled score *approximated* by the following tables. *Please note that the score approximations below are "best guesses." Since the newly revised MCAT CBT was not administered until January 2007, specific data along these lines is not available as of press time.

Physical Sciences		Verbal Reasoning		Biological Sciences	
Raw Score	*Scaled Score	Raw Score	*Scaled Score	Raw Score	*Scaled Score
0–2	1	1–2	1	0–2	1
3–5	2	3–4	2	3–5	2
6–9	3	5–7	3	6–9	3
10–13	4	8–10	4	10–13	4
14–17	5	11–13	5	14–17	5
18–21	6	14–16	6	18–21	6
22–25	7	17–19	7	22–25	7
26–29	8	20–22	8	26–29	8
30–33	9	23–25	9	30–33	9
34–37	10	26–28	10	34–37	10
38–41	11	29–31	11	38–41	11
42–45	12	32–34	12	42–45	12
46–49	13	35–37	13	46–49	13
50–51	14	38–39	14	50–51	14
52	15	40	15	52	15

*IMPORTANT NOTE: These scaled scores are approximations. For an explanation of how raw and scaled scores are calculated for the Writing Sample, refer to page 363.

THE NEW MCAT

Since its inception, the MCAT had been a "pencil and paper test." However, beginning in January 2007, the paper test was eliminated and replaced by computer-based (CBT) testing. Among other advantages, this updated format will allow the MCAT to be administered much more frequently throughout the year. In fact, there were 22 test dates scheduled in 2007 alone. Additional information about the CBT can be obtained through the AAMC web site (*www.aamc.org/mcat*).

Although individual medical schools will vary with respect to the scores they require, a standard score of 11 or greater will probably be considered to be quite competitive. A standard score of 7 or less would indicate an area requiring substantial additional preparation. Before taking the next practice test, you should concentrate on areas of low score.

The Science area may be remediated by additional study and working problems. The area of Verbal Reasoning, however, may require a slightly different approach. Try going back over this part of the examination, reading carefully, and answering the questions again without a time limit. Read the paragraph again and try to determine why you missed certain questions. Be sure to use only the information in the paragraph. Then go on to additional practice examinations. One additional suggestion: Read the questions carefully before answering. Sometimes students answer the question they *expected* rather than the question that was asked. Try to avoid this pitfall.

As you progress through the other practice tests, you should develop facility in working faster to allow completion of each section. Since there is no penalty for wrong answers, it is to your advantage to guess on questions you are unsure of, especially if you have ruled out some answers.

Remember that we cannot hope to present everything you should have learned in years of study. We can only help you to identify areas of weakness, give some review of important concepts, and provide experience and confidence in taking a test having the format of the Medical College Admission Test. We hope that this will allow you to reach your own potential on this test.

INFORMATION ON THE NEW MCAT
Timetable for the Exam

*Note: The new MCAT testing schedule does *not* allow for a lunch hour.

Physical Sciences	70 minutes (52 questions)
Break (optional)	10 minutes
Verbal Reasoning	60 minutes (40 questions)
Break (optional)	10 minutes
Writing Sample	60 minutes (2 essays)
Break (optional)	10 minutes
Biological Sciences	70 minutes (52 questions)
SURVEY	5 minutes
Total content time (not including breaks)	4 hours, 20 minutes
Total "seat" time	5 hours, 5 minutes

The following four sections constitute the MCAT examination: Biological Sciences, Physical Sciences, Verbal Reasoning, and Writing Sample.

The Biological Sciences test will concentrate on basic biology and biologically related chemistry, whereas the Physical Sciences examination will focus on physics and physically related chemistry areas. The Verbal Reasoning passages will be taken from the social sciences, from the humanities, and from areas of the natural sciences not tested in the Biological and Physical Sciences section of the MCAT. Topics for the Writing Sample are not taken from the content of physics, biology, or chemistry, nor will they ask for personal reasons why the student has chosen medicine as a career.

The Revised Sections

PHYSICAL SCIENCES (52 MULTIPLE-CHOICE QUESTIONS)

Typically this section consists of a series of passages upon which the subsequent multiple-choice questions are based. There are usually 8 or 9 problem sets that are followed by 4–8 questions each and 10 or so questions that are not based on passages.

VERBAL REASONING (40 MULTIPLE-CHOICE QUESTIONS)

This section is typically composed of 7–9 passages from the humanities, social sciences, and natural sciences. Each passage is followed by 5–7 questions, which are based on the information presented.

WRITING SAMPLE (2 ESSAYS)

This section requires you to write two essays; 30 minutes is allowed for each. You will be asked to develop a central thesis, synthesize material, separate major from minor issues, propose alternative solutions, present ideas in a logical and coherent manner, and form your essays in standard English, which includes proper grammar and syntax.

BIOLOGICAL SCIENCES (52 MULTIPLE-CHOICE QUESTIONS)

This section contains 8 or 9 passages that are followed by 4–8 questions each, and 8 or so "stand-alone" questions not based on passages.

OVERALL ROLE OF THE MCAT

The MCAT, in combination with college grades (overall and science GPA), types and quality of courses, letters of recommendation, extracurricular activities, major undergraduate institution attended, the interview, SAT, etc., is a screening device. The test is an objective measure of your ability to apply your knowledge, and high scores should help an individual with average grades. Average or slightly lower MCAT scores probably do not significantly affect a superior college record. Most literature points to a positive correlation between high MCAT scores (especially within science subtests) and future success in the basic medical sciences (preclinical phase) and National Board of Medical Examiners Part I examination scores.

TOOLS FOR LEARNING AND TEST-TAKING STRATEGIES

Principles of Studying

INTRODUCTION

TIP
Failure to prepare is preparation for failure.

The authors have been involved in the training of thousands of medical students and have explored and discussed with these students their test preparation and test-taking strategies. These students have developed into efficient, skillful test takers in order to cope with the volumes of detailed material on which they are tested. They learned to recognize key elements of course content and to train themselves to successfully answer thousands of test questions.

It is not just our observations of medical students, however, that we rely on to give you advice. There is a growing body of scientific literature emerging from psychology and the neurosciences that provides useful information about how to study for tests. These studies have identified the following very important test preparation topics.

- *Study time*: HOW much you use; HOW you use it
- *Study location*: WHERE and WHEN you study
- *Input*: HOW you ENTER knowledge into memory
- *Storage*: HOW you SAVE knowledge in memory
- *Retrieval*: HOW you GET knowledge from memory

All these topics offer something to help you study and prepare for any type of examination you could encounter in the future.

STUDY TIME

Preparation time is a *necessary* element for successful performance on tests but is found to be insufficient when used alone. Students have told us that they must set aside *regular time* periods for studying, which increases their efficiency. It is not just setting aside time, however, that allows learning to take place. Rather, it is what happens during the regular study periods. We all know people who spend large amounts of time looking at textbooks or notes but still have poor grades because they lack effective study strategies. The most important strategy is for you to *concentrate* on what you are learning and to have *learning* as your *sole purpose for studying*. The goal of every study period should be to learn something new or relearn something that you have partially forgotten.

Here is a hint to help you concentrate or *pay attention*: If you find that your eyes are crossing a page of text but nothing is registering in your mind, and you are having trouble paying attention, you need to read faster. So fast that you will finally pay attention but not so fast that you aren't actually reading. *Speed helps you concentrate.* Suppose you are driving along a winding, country road at 20 mph. What are you likely to be doing? Perhaps you are enjoying the scenery—taking in the trees, the horses in the pasture, or the ducks flying overhead. Now push down on the accelerator until you are going 55 mph. What will you do? You either are paying attention to your driving or are likely to find yourself in serious trouble. The point is that speed forces you to focus on what you are doing. Reading rapidly helps you pay attention to what you are reading.

STUDY LOCATION

Research tells us *where and when* to study. If you learn something in a certain environment, you are more likely to remember this information when you are again in that environment; therefore, study in a place similar to that in which you will be tested.

Even your mood is thought to play a role in memory. Although the effect is not thought to be a powerful one, researchers do believe it influences memory in two ways:

1. Recall is better for pleasant than for unpleasant material.
2. Recall is better when you are in the same mood at retrieval time as you were when you encoded the knowledge.

You will want to *study in spurts*. Spread out practice over time with rest intervals spaced between. This is called *distributed study or spaced practice*. The amount of study material and the distribution of practice sessions affects your ability to retrieve the things you have learned. *Massed practice* refers to long study periods and produces the poorest learning outcome. For most academic subjects it is best to work in a series of shorter study sessions distributed over several days. If, however, you are cramming for a test, then long study sessions are better. The problem with cramming is that you do all right on an exam but don't remember much two weeks later.

PUTTING KNOWLEDGE INTO SHORT-TERM MEMORY

Putting information into memory involves the encoding of incoming sensory information into a form that the brain can understand. In other words, our senses take in information from the environment, and our brain makes sense of it. A key to storing information in long-term memory so that you can easily retrieve it is *organization*.

Short-term memory (STM), also known as *working memory*, has a capacity limited to 5 to 9 items. Unrehearsed material stays in STM for 15 to 20 seconds.

What is the usual length of a telephone number? Count the digits in 555-4567. Interestingly, most phone numbers have 7 digits (the ideal number of items to be remembered in working memory). Fortunately, there are ways that your brain can manipulate the limitation of remembering just 5 to 9 items. One way is called *chunking,* in which you arrange pieces of information into meaningful clusters and increase your capacity to remember. Take, for example, the following numbers: 76823318289190827103135466542594214. You can't even hold this 35-digit number in your working memory. Maybe you could remember the first 3 or 4 or last 3 or 4 numbers but you're not going to hold all 35 numbers in your working memory. Now look at the same number chunked into 5 telephone numbers.

768-2331
828-9190
827-1031
354-6654
259-4214

Interesting, isn't it? Do you think you could use chunking to learn material just as apparently overwhelming and meaningless as the 35-digit number you just chunked? What is the key to chunking? You're right—*organization.* It is a key to storing information in your long-term memory.

STORING KNOWLEDGE IN LONG-TERM MEMORY

Strategies that encode information in a meaningful manner help you retrieve easily information from long-term memory (LTM). There are two ways to increase retention of what you are learning. Both require you to practice what you are learning. The first, *overlearning,* involves practicing with the material over and above what is needed to just learn it and is particularly good for learning basic facts and skills. When you learned the multiplication tables, you overlearned them by practicing them over and over again. Furnish yourself with opportunities for overlearning of key concepts and skills. Make up flash cards and use them over and over until you have the facts locked in memory. Repeat until you "know it cold." Most people don't have the time, patience, or determination for this approach, and it's not very efficient when you have a lot to learn in a short period of time.

Because of these deficiencies, an approach called *elaboration* is often recommended. When you elaborate, you reorganize information and make it meaningful by relating it to something already in your memory. In order for you to engage in elaborative activities, you need to connect new information to something you already know. An organizational plan that is useful for school subjects utilizes logical schemes: places, dates, hierarchies, etc. Semantic categories allow you to organize by any meaningful strategy that you prefer. For example, you can categorize alphabetically, by body part, by size, by function, or by structure. Still other ways of organizing information are sounds, pictures, and colors. You should use personally meaningful categories to organize the knowledge you are attempting to store in long-term memory.

Mnemonics are schemes designed to assist you in remembering. "Fall back, spring forward" is a way of remembering to set your clock forward in the spring and back in the fall. "Every good boy does fine" and "FACE" help us remember the lines and spaces of the musical staff. "Please Excuse My Dear Aunt Sally" stands for the order of the following mathematical operations: Parentheses, Exponents, Multiplication, Division, Addition, and Subtraction. You remember these mnemonics, don't you? They are unforgettable acronyms or sentences used to recall a set of already existing strong associations. Other mnemonic schemes include methods of associating things you are trying to remember with words (peg word method) and with locations (loci method).

Peg Word Method

With the peg word method, you begin by using the sequence of numbers 1 to 10 to memorize a word that is concrete and rhymes with the number beside it. For each number, you memorize the word that rhymes with it. Here are 10 numbers and words.

1. bun
2. shoe
3. tree
4. door
5. hive
6. stick
7. heaven
8. gate
9. line
10. hen

These words make up a peg list. You use it to memorize new, unrelated sets of items. Place each item to be remembered in an image with a peg word. For example, if you wanted to memorize a list of words that begins *muscle, tissue, cell, energy* . . . , you could imagine a muscle burger bulging through a bun, Mother Hubbard's shoe house covered with toilet tissue as a result of your high school's big victory, a tree growing through a jail cell, and a door swirling in the sky captured by the energy of a tornado. Try this method with lists that you need to memorize. It could be fun to use the peg word method.

Loci Method

The loci method lets you use knowledge of the spatial arrangement and contents of some familiar place, like your own home or neighborhood. When trying to remember a list of words, take an imagined walk through your location, placing each item in, on, or near some familiar, easily remembered object. To return to the sample words above, your muscles would be seen in the mirror in the bathroom, tissues would be on the nightstand in your bedroom, the cell phone would be on the kitchen table where you left it, and the energy would come from the furnace in the garage. To retrieve these items you recreate the stroll and retrieve each item as you come to it. To remember these words, you imagine driving into the garage and seeing that the furnace is aglow with energy. You open the door inside the garage and enter the kitchen, where you immediately notice your cell phone on the kitchen table. While picking up the phone, you knock over the pepper shaker and start sneezing. You run to your bedroom, where you pick up tissues from the nightstand so you can blow your nose. Then you decide to take a shower. While entering the bathroom, you can't help but stop and admire your muscles in the mirror on the bathroom door.

These methods may seem silly, but you really ought to try them.

RETRIEVING KNOWLEDGE

Retrieval is difficult if the information you are trying to remember is not encoded appropriately. Remember, organization is the key to storing information in long-term memory so that you can easily retrieve it. Also, do you remember the importance of studying in an environment similar to the one in which you will be tested? Retrieval tends to be best when the *context* in which it takes place matches the *context* present at encoding. Two things that you have control over and that affect your ability to retrieve knowledge from memory are the *amount of time* you spend practicing and how you *distribute your practice*. What is the best way to distribute practice? That's right—study in spurts, take breaks, and study over time.

There are two ways in which you are asked to remember on tests. One is to *recall* information without cues, as with fill-in-the-blank and essay questions. These are considered the hardest questions, because recall tasks provide few cues to the answers. The other way you are asked to remember is called *recognition*, which requires you to identify material previously learned. Multiple-choice and matching items are typically aimed at asking you to recognize word associations. Both recall and recognition require retrieval of data stored in long-term memory.

Forgetting

It appears that there is no practical limit to how much information we can put into long-term memory. Many psychologists believe that information is permanently stored in various places in our brain. For them, forgetting is failure in retrieval. Other psychologists theorize that aging, lack of use, and disease decay memory and cause our brain to forget. Still other psychologists think that the ability to remember is linked to the use of the same cues for encoding and retrieving items in long-term memory.

A basic problem with retrieving information from memory is that there are lots of things that interfere. So being forewarned may help you overcome some of the things that will interfere with your ability to remember for recall and recognition tasks.

There are two classic interference effects that we all face when trying to put new knowledge into memory: the recency/primacy effect and the retroactive and proactive interference effect. *Retroactive interference* refers to the new memories impairing the memory of something that you previously stored in memory. *Proactive interference* refers to the effect that old memories have on your ability to remember new material. For example, you memorized the names of the muscles and bones of the leg last week. This week you are trying to learn the names of the muscles and bones of the arm. What will happen? You will have a tendency to forget the parts of the leg as you learn the arm parts (retroactive interference), as well as a tendency to forget some of the arm parts because you learned the leg first (proactive interference). You should avoid studying similar things in consecutive time periods.

Remember that long list of 35 numbers you saw earlier? We told you that virtually no one would remember that list. But we did say that you might remember the first couple or the last couple of numbers, which is an example of the *recency/primacy effect*. You tend to remember the beginning and end of any list much more easily than you remember what is in the middle. When you go to a restaurant and the waitress names 8 or 10 salad dressings, you tend to ask for either the first or last one she mentioned. Or you ask her to repeat the list because you can't remember the fifth one she mentioned. The moral of this story is to make *short lists*.

SUMMARY

Factors that enhance learning and memory are:

1. Study time and place.
2. Characteristics of what must be remembered.
3. Strategies for storing knowledge and remembering.
4. Context characteristics of practice and test situations.

Test Taking

Here are some common suggestions for taking tests. Note that most of them involve common sense, but we don't always think about or use many of these suggestions.

BEFORE THE TEST

To prepare for tests, follow these guidelines:

1. Identify the subject matter that you need to prepare and prioritize it in terms of how much study time you need for difficult, moderate, and easy material.
2. Use review books but have comprehensive textbooks handy to fill in any gaps you discover in your reviewing.
3. Use old examinations. By going over old exams, you are relearning material in the context in which you will be tested and you begin to see how test makers think about a subject. The more old test questions you go over, the better.

4. Remember to use lots of short study periods.
5. It is not "old-fashioned" to use flashcards to help you memorize terms, processes, formulas, etc.
6. Seek help from professors when you hit a roadblock.
7. Reduce your stress through exercise, reading, music, etc.
8. Get plenty of rest.
9. Follow a nutritious diet.
10. The night before the examination, relax and get a good night's sleep.

DURING THE TEST

On the day of a test, keep in mind the following guidelines.

1. Read the directions carefully! Follow the directions!
2. Preview the test to see how much time you need to allot for each section.
3. Pace yourself during the examination so that you do not panic at the end.
4. Save time at the end of the exam to review your test and make sure you haven't left any questions unanswered.
5. Answer the question being asked. Do not change the question to fit your way of thinking.
6. You can change answers during the exam, but do so only if you are at least 90 percent sure that you are changing to the correct answer.
7. Stay calm. If you find yourself getting frustrated or annoyed, stop. Take a deep breath. Think of something pleasant and start again.
8. Stay focused on why it is important to do your best. Remind yourself that good performance on tests provides you with opportunities that otherwise will not be available to you.
9. Don't let your mind or eyes wander. Work efficiently and concentrate on speed and accuracy.
10. Remember that standardized tests are designed to be very difficult. Virtually no one gets all the questions correct, so don't worry when you see a bunch of questions for which you don't know the answer.

Strategies for Success

A. TIME MANAGEMENT

1. Time management is an essential element and an effective tool for test preparation.
2. There are many time management strategies to help you effectively and productively use your time to study within an established time frame.
3. Become aware of the importance of time management, because time is an investment. It is unrelenting and irreplaceable. Once wasted, it is gone forever. If you lack the ability to control your time, you basically are not controlling your life. Experts feel that using time in a controlled, deliberate fashion is far more beneficial than doing everything efficiently. Efficiency is important but time management is key. Of course, the ideal is a structured, solid balance.
4. Only you can determine how much return you want on your investment.
5. You must realistically allocate enough study hours daily to perform meaningful tasks yet balance all your other daily activities. You need not become an obsessed clock watcher.
6. Weigh the importance of each task to be accomplished, then make a decision on what to do. You must critically assess what you are doing; plan the activity but be flexible to change when necessary. Today's priority number one might become tomorrow's priority number three as the situation warrants.

7. When making conscious decisions, utilize the basic principle of time management:

Work smarter, not harder. One way to use this basic principle is a simple, yet effective time management formula:

> **PMS = W**
> **Plan, Make a Molehill Out of a Mountain, and**
> **Safeguard (then you can) = Work Your "A" Off**

Plan

- Plan an effective study schedule by prioritizing and concentrating on one task or subject at a time. Astute planning while focusing on the future puts the future in the present; you are doing something about the situation now, not when chance lets you.
- Prioritize what needs to be accomplished in your life. This is not an easy task unless you understand the broader picture and you have conceptualized established goals. Prioritizing is especially important when studying for an examination some time from now. Your daily school commitments have a certain definite priority, and therefore you must be able to adjust your schedule as necessary. Resolve your conflicts promptly and thoughtfully.
- Prioritize your tasks by establishing a to-do list. This is an extremely powerful tool because it is a method to organize yourself and reduce stress in your life. Write down tasks that need to be done within 24 hours or less (short-range goals, or your A list). Then, write down tasks that need to be done within one week (intermediate-range goals, or your B list). Now write down tasks that need to be accomplished within one month or more (long-range goals, or your C list). This is not a static world and goals can and should be revised periodically. In order to achieve your long-term goals, short-term planning is key. A priority list is essential, but above all realize it is subject to change.
- Determine which things are important to you and which things can be dropped from your list. You must eliminate low-priority items as they crop up.
- Your critical thinking skills will surface as you decide when to implement and how to execute tasks.
- Use the basic guidelines: *Be aware of all that needs to be done.*
- Never be too rigid in your planning. "Flexibility" is the key to a successful plan.
- You should revise and evaluate your plan weekly to analyze whether it is working or if it is taking too long to execute and complete tasks.
- Tailor the plan to fit your needs and know how you will spend your time.
- Allow sufficient time for studying each task by placing blocks of time in your schedule.

Do Not Make an Excuse for Planning

- Many of us fall into the time trap and use the excuse "I am too busy to take time out to plan." Think of it in these terms: If you feel that you have no spare time to plan, most certainly you need a plan.
- Every football team has a game plan, so do not look for a surprise victory.
- The best time to plan is open to debate. You are the best judge and determining factor—stay loose.
- Remember that a guide helps you operate more smoothly and less strenuously. It eliminates anxiety and fosters a positive self-image.

Make a Molehill Out of a Mountain

- Make your plan work for you by reversing the cliché. "Make a molehill out of a mountain." You can break the mountain down for any major and difficult assignment if you have established a to-do list and have estimated the time it will take to complete each task.
- Estimate the amount of time you think it takes to complete each task on your to-do list. At first your guess may be wrong. Eventually, with practice, you will increase your accuracy regarding each task.
- If you spend 30 minutes each day on a major assignment, the assignment will become less intimidating as well as easier to complete by the end of one week. You will see instant results and be amazed at how much you have accomplished on this task.
- Always introduce a "safety net" with each task to be completed on your list. The safety net will assist you with the unexpected events in your plan such as sickness, surprise visitors, fatigue, interruptions, and family demands. You will need to use good judgment and be realistic about the length of time for these activities.
- Don't forget to include time for yourself. During this time you can relax and enjoy things you want to do for at least an hour—such as talk on the telephone, go shopping, or go to the gym.
- A break in the schedule creates a good balance and a healthier attitude.
- Sometimes you get more accomplished doing nothing. The moral is to work hard and play hard.
- Planned relaxing and having fun clears the way to more productivity. How you study is more relevant than how long you study. A clear, focused mind can process more information quickly.
- Utilize your commuting time. One of the authors usually had an hour's subway ride. This was his time to read a novel or magazine, and to set aside schoolwork. You might decide on the exact opposite.

Safeguard Your Time

- Safeguard your valuable time by placing it in a safety deposit box. (Isn't that where valuables are kept?) You are the safety deposit box!
- You must learn to say no to others who don't understand your purpose and goals.
- Strictly speaking in order to follow set priorities, you must learn when to say yes, and when to say no. Too many of us take the easy way out and rationalize; this method is not compatible with an effective plan. An effective plan has availability hours integrated into it. If your motivation waivers at times, do not be discouraged but give yourself credit for your accomplishments.
- Sometimes after succeeding in some very difficult tasks it is beneficial to slow down, refocus, and reward yourself. Whatever you do, do not use escape routes to justify procrastination.
- Do your best always; consider your successes and try and try again. If you do not, you will encounter problems.
- If you do your utmost you have a chance, even though you can never eliminate the possibility of failure. That is being honest and realistic.
- Avoid ploys that others use to break into your safety deposit box and steal your valuables (time and your to-do list.)
- When you open your safety deposit box, remove all external distractions (television and music) or distractions on your desk.
- Study difficult and boring information first.
- Be aware of when your energy and concentration level is high and plan your study periods around this time of the day. We all have our patterns.

- Find a better place to study when your productivity or level of energy decreases. Remember that your study area should provide the least distractions.
- Be critical of your study breaks; space them appropriately.
- Controlling your time gives you the luxury to adapt and to be spontaneous.

Work Your "A"

David Ellis, author of *Becoming a Master Student,* recommends a powerful technique to help students accomplish their goals and efficiently manage their time. To master this technique, stick with completing the "A," or the short-range goals that are on your to-do list.

- Start and finish one task at a time. Don't jump around to other items on the list.
- After each completed task, reward yourself.
- It is more efficient to work on one task no longer than three hours; at that point take an hour break.
- Take more breaks (10 minutes at a time) if you are under a lot of pressure, because you need time to digest and process the material. Also, more breaks will relieve your stress and sustain your motivation.

B. MEMORY AND ASSOCIATION TECHNIQUES

1. Memory is the total storehouse of mentally retained impressions and knowledge.
2. You need total concentration (initial attention) to store information into your long-term memory.
3. There are three main strategies for aiding memory and giving a subject your initial attention. Try each one and see which idea or combination of ideas works for you.

   R = repetition
   A = association
   P = pictures or symbols

4. Repetition is time-consuming to most students but it is an effective way to recall information. The more you see the information, the more you will recall it.
5. Association techniques are mnemonic devices—tricks to help you retain information for long-term use.
6. Mnemonic devices make learning faster and more efficient by linking the information to something familiar. Mnemonic devices are not a substitute for overall comprehension of the material. They provide a way to link difficult information to the main information learned.
7. There are limitations to mnemonic devices. The trick itself may be hard to remember and difficult to retain; the device can be forgotten if it is never stored into long-term memory; and no device can help you digest or understand the information.
8. Types of mnemonic devices are:

   - Acronyms, words formed from the initial letters of a series of words
   - Acrostics, series of words that form creative sentences
   - Songs and rhymes
   - Stories (created)

9. Create pictures and symbols as associations for difficult information you must remember.
10. Visualize the material by creating a story, and have fun with the material to be learned. The more unusual the story, the more likely the information will stick with you.
11. Make up a song with your favorite tune or create a rhyme to retain the information.
12. Take an active role in your learning by paying attention and using association techniques.

C. MEMORY PRINCIPLES

1. Be interested in the material; show excitement at mastering the subject matter. There is pleasure in knowledge. As a physician, you will have to become a lifelong learner.
2. A positive attitude and approach will increase learning and remembering. It will add meaning to your work. Be cognizant of the fact that reasoning, analysis, and persistence will lead to positive conclusions.
3. Remember that the more solid your basic knowledge is, the more easily new building blocks are mastered and added. Accept your strengths and weaknesses.
4. Develop associations between facts and concepts.
5. Visualize, conceptualize, and recite; be active on all fronts.
6. Give yourself a chance to consolidate your knowledge base; remember that everything takes time.
7. Set aside regular time periods for this specific task; do not squeeze it in here and there! Regular time periods increase efficiency and delineate purpose.
8. Skip superfluous material and adjust to repetitious material.
9. If you detect major gaps in your knowledge, fill these in. Otherwise, they will bother you and distract you from your effort. It's easier to remember a story than to remember isolated facts.
10. Study, if you can, in chronological order. You will feel more comfortable because of the sequence, and you will enhance your recall.
11. During your studying, vary your attack as required.

   - Read the material.
   - Speak out the material.
   - Write out the material.
   - Sketch some of the material.
   - Underline some of the material.
   - Outline some of the material.
   - Resort, if necessary, to mnemonic devices.

12. Understand the material before you commit it to memory.
13. Organize the material, and learn it in parts rather than in isolated, single details. Try to build a framework of facts.
14. Note and focus on similar ideas from different subject areas. Put them meaningfully together, and keep them in association. Integrate your material.

D. REVIEW: GENERAL

Most students that we consulted did a thorough preliminary review of the material they expected to master before they undertook intensive, well-planned study. The purpose of a review is to create a sense of familiarity with the material to be studied so that when the period of intensive study begins, none of the material will appear new. It also points out areas that will need more attention for comprehension and understanding. The review helps students avoid the sense that they are cramming for the examination. Remember that the MCAT examination requires understanding, reasoning, and deduction. Once the period of intensive study has begun, students will benefit from the guidelines below.

Guides to Success

1. In order to be successful and competitive, you must not only work harder but smarter. Facts and concepts must be organized and integrated; associations and differences must be looked for. You must develop the skill to draw inferences and utilize presented information effectively on standardized tests.

2. In reviewing, try to integrate and synthesize material that you have learned over the years in a course-by-course manner. Study as if you were preparing for an essay exam; it will help summarize and make your facts more coherent.

3. Despite the fact that the examination stresses reasoning, commit "the basics" to memory. They are the building blocks for reasoning.

4. Test-wise students think deductively; general principles applied wisely usually lead to specific conclusions. The integrated learner has the ability to make associations and to use information better.

5. Standardized tests require you to manipulate related concepts to reach the answer; this is a learned skill. Memorization of facts will serve you well, but thinking in an integrated fashion enhances understanding. What you know will never hurt you.

6. Question analysis requires you to identify the topic and to understand both the right and wrong answers. Understanding the wrong answers often leads to a better comprehension of the right answer.

7. Observe, note, and use all the relevant facts provided. Be systematic and do not jump to conclusions. Do not be sloppy; you cannot answer a question on the basis of superficial considerations or impressions.

8. Do not read too rapidly and skip words and facts. Reread difficult material.

9. Be consistent in your interpretation of words.

10. Break complex problems into parts and draw upon prior knowledge. Actively look for the main ideas; this helps understanding and reasoning.

11. Answer all questions in sequence, even if you have to guess sometimes (there is no penalty for guessing). You can "mark" with your cursor answers that you are not sure of and go back to them if time permits.

12. Pace yourself and train yourself to answer one question per minute. Make a note of any question you were not sure of, since a subsequent question might provide you with the proper answer.

13. Be sure to read the entire question before you consider a quick answer. Highlight your key words and be cognizant of the fact that multiple-choice examinations quite often contain one answer that is ridiculous. The examination is not designed to mislead you. Most questions are quite straightforward. Just as you should rule out ridiculous options, so you should carefully examine options that are the same, since only one answer is the correct one. Always use your knowledge base before you eliminate a statement. After you have eliminated a choice, use the cursor to strike through that statement. Even partial familiarity and hunches are better than outright guessing.

14. Before you change an answer, you should have a very compelling reason.

E. REVIEW: SPECIFIC PRINCIPLES

Be Goal Directed

An old saying proposes: "If we have goals, we tend to do things that move us toward those goals."

1. Your goal is to transfer facts to your long-term memory, and the mechanism for accomplishing that is review. Memorization is a daily task, not just a cramming before an examination.

2. Reflect on what you want to accomplish and be. Stay in touch with your dreams. Frequently challenge yourself to live up to high standards academically and personally.

3. Acknowledge your accomplishments and be proud of yourself. Consistency and hard work got you this far and can help you realize your goals.

4. Remain motivated and realistic. There is no study system that is right for everyone. Find what works best for you and stick with it.

Plan

Planning is the unmistakable road map to success and has been proven to save hours and hours of misdirected, unproductive work.

1. Make a study plan and stick to it. Better students always have an effective study plan. Decide before you begin how many weeks and months you will require to review the material. If you have to deviate, immediately schedule when you will make up the work; compensatory study time is part of every plan.
2. Be cognizant of the fact that certain areas are more prone to be forgotten, so extra time to relearn material needs to be factored into your schedule.
3. Identify and allot more time to subject matter for which you feel the least prepared. There is no point in studying material you already know well.
4. Keep your efforts in proper perspective. You cannot know it all, but a well-rounded knowledge base and the intelligent use of that knowledge will serve you well both on the MCAT and in your future study. Keep the expression "Use it or lose it" in mind. You must focus on learning the material as you plan to use it and test yourself regularly to improve remembering.
5. As you lay out your study plan, take into account other responsibilities and commitments: present courses and exams, holidays, vacations, family occasions, sports commitments, etc.
6. Leaving things to the last minute is bad planning. It robs you of extended memory time and usually leads to quick forgetting. A systematic, orderly, and properly paced and spaced procedure will "pay off in the end."

Strategies

Remember the adage "We forget much of what we learn over the long run." Forgetting is a normal and natural process, but the process can be slowed and lessened. The more organized your original study and review process, the more you will recall.

1. Utilize a regular work area and establish a routine; keep your workspace, books, and notes organized.
2. Spend about 30 minutes each day reviewing the material you studied yesterday.
3. Review material you are least prepared for first; however, beware of the trap of studying material you already know. We sometimes have a subconscious tendency to gravitate to our comfort zones, and that can lead to a false sense of security.
4. You will remember more if both your material and review are organized.

    *   Take advantage of summaries, tables, graphs, schematics, and review books. Draw out pathways and learn similarities and differences between them. Make flow charts for integration.
    *   Be active in your review. Stop periodically and check your memory by jotting down abbreviated notes on what you just learned.
    *   Remain alert and interactive. Guard against slipping into a passive mode. Underline, write, chart, draw—whatever. Be focused, ask questions, and utilize all your auditory and visual senses. Learn it so you can teach it.

5. Choose your sources carefully. Your own learning style should be a determining factor. Your previous class notes and summaries might greatly facilitate your recall and understanding again. Some books are just outlines, others are full-length prose, and most are a combination. Select what fits your needs and learning style.
6. Keep in mind that a review book cannot meet all your needs; therefore, you may have to refer to a comprehensive text with which you are familiar in order to fill in some of the gaps.

7. Divide your material into small units to sustain attention and a sense of accomplishment.

8. Actively tie what you learn or relearn to what you know already. The cornerstone of learning is linking new concepts (facts) to the familiar.

9. Memorization is critical to learning and must be done every day. Keep in mind that memorization requires repetition and that repetition is the mother of all learning.

10. Just because you have reviewed and memorized subject matter, you have no guarantee that you are in a position to solve problems. Use practice exams at least once a week to evaluate your proficiency and to identify your weaknesses.

11. Examine the detailed answers provided with practice questions. This will reinforce what you have learned, refresh your knowledge, and act as one more general guard against forgetting.

12. Vary your memorization methods. Mnemonic devices can get you through dry and boring material. "ACE" can add flavor and fun: Weave difficult lists into an Active, Colorful, Exaggerated story for recall later. Alliteration, flashcards, and acronyms can all be helpful.

F. STRESS MANAGEMENT

1. One of the best stress management techniques is to take control of your life. Realize that you are responsible for your actions and destiny. Accept yourself—your strengths and weaknesses. Feel good about yourself as a person.

2. Do not shun activities that you enjoy. Include entertainment in your schedule so you remain charged and motivated. Treat yourself to anything that brings you pleasure.

3. Keep your study and living area clean and organized. Don't ignore other aspects of your daily responsibilities, such as paying bills. Feeling and being organized is a correlate motivation.

4. Don't study when you are overly tired. It adds to your frustration and translates to low productivity. Take a short nap but set an alarm clock.

5. Use exercise, a hot shower, music, or a chat with a friend to relax and regenerate.

6. Do not expect perfection. You cannot know it all and none of us is perfect.

7. Seek help when you hit roadblocks. Fellow students and professors are excellent resources for discussion. Asking for help is not a weakness but rather a symbol of strength.

8. Reward yourself for your weekly accomplishments. Catch a movie or a play or perhaps go to a sporting event.

9. There is no magic formula. Accept that study is an ongoing challenge; remain persistent and you will be successful. Knowing that you know your material is a wonderful experience. Remember that success begets success!

10. Stay in touch with your dream! Visualize having completed the test successfully. Visualize being a medical student, becoming a physician, and having the kind of satisfying life you want for yourself.

G. EXAMINATION DAY

1. Try to get a good night's rest before the examination. Be cautious about using sleep aids. They often leave you with residual dulling effects the next day.

2. Avoid changing daily habits. Eat foods that agree with you so that gastrointestinal discomfort is avoided. Follow your normal exercise routine but don't overdo it. A sore body is very distracting.

3. Know the location of the testing center and arrive early to avoid being rushed and anxious. Be prepared. Wear comfortable clothes, anticipate a hot or cold room, and

have available your registration materials. Do not bring pencils and scratch paper to use during the exam. These will be provided at the test site.

4. Attitude is critical. Approach the examination with the conviction that you have diligently prepared, and are ready and confident! A positive internal dialogue often translates to positive results, so always maintain a sense of pride and accomplishment.

5. Sometimes a quick scan of the complete test is helpful. Avoid scanning questions at this point. If scanning escalates your anxiety, it is probably best to eliminate it.

6. Read, listen to, and follow all directions and be sure you understand them. Do not assume anything.

7. You are not allowed to bring your own timekeeping devices; the time will be displayed on your computer screen. Proportion your time but avoid being a compulsive clock watcher.

8. Ignore others and your surroundings so your concentration remains undisturbed.

9. Be careful about giving the impression that you are dishonest. Avoid keeping "one eye" on the proctor and the other on your material.

10. You don't have to finish first! Pace yourself. Stay the allotted time. Leave time for checking at the end. Think that the first students finished were probably not prepared.

11. Maintain your pace; standardized tests require that you progress quickly to the end. Skip questions that require time and return to them later. Guess when you are quite unsure and keep moving. Change answers only when you are sure you were wrong initially.

12. If you become frustrated and your concentration lapses, sit back, close your eyes, relax, and regroup.

13. If your frustration persists, scan material you have already completed. It may help you get back on track.

14. Expect "off the wall" questions. Note them, guess if you have to, and keep moving.

15. Avoid premature closure and rushing to judgment. Read the whole question and all answer choices before making a selection.

16. Accept questions at face value and avoid thinking too much or reading too much into questions. Most questions are straightforward and simple. They are not a trick.

17. Break complex questions into parts, then begin with the part you understand and work from there.

18. There is no penalty for guessing; be a gambler. If you can eliminate some choices, you will drastically improve your chances of guessing the correct answer.

A POSITIVE APPROACH TO ANSWERING QUESTIONS

A positive, competitive approach and attitude are qualities of a successful individual. Hand in hand, however, goes a fund in knowledge. Nothing succeeds like knowledge of the subject matter for test taking. Indeed, the suggestions on test taking are all built on knowledge, which is strongly reinforced by your confidence. In turn, your confidence is supported by an understanding of the process involved in the successful answering of questions.

In this section, several specific questions will be selected from the Model Tests and will be examined not only for content but also for the process involved in the selection of the correct answer.

General Key Rules for Answering Questions

1. Are there specific disclaimers? *Best, all, none,* or some variety of negatives that separate the correct answer from the multiplicity of possible answers are the types of disclaimers to look for.

2. Are there specific qualifying words or topics that can be noted? Sometimes these are the same as the disclaimers in item 1.

3. Are there similarities of choices in the answers? These similarities may allow elimination of choices.
4. Can some choices, such as the choice *all of the above,* be eliminated? Sometimes opposite choices help in the selection and in the narrowing down of the answers to one out of two possibilities.
5. Sometimes making a quick drawing or writing a formula on scratch paper will clarify the questions and initiate and aid in recall.
6. Remember, and keep in mind at all times, that all multiple-choice questions are really TRUE or FALSE decisions on a statement. Sometimes, in some cases, when in a quandary, they can best be answered by "I don't know" and "I'll proceed to the next question and not disturb my pace and concentration."
7. *Be positive!* If you have no good answers for several questions in a row, you positively *must forget them.* Do not dwell on failure, but have confidence in how much you know!

Application of Test-Taking Hints

We will use specific examples and apply our principles.

EXAMPLE

6. Glucose is NOT a(an):

   (A) aldose.
   (B) reducing sugar.
   (C) disaccharide.
   (D) monosaccharide.

ITEM 1: Note the specific disclaimer *NOT.* This is an obvious and common one in test questions. You should *highlight* this word.

ITEM 2: Glucose is the topic of the question and should be *highlighted.*

ITEM 3: Similarity or dissimilarity of choices! There is a strong *dissimilarity* between choice (C): *di*saccharide and choice (D): *mono*saccharide. In fact, at this point, the answer is obvious to the knowledgeable individual. Since glucose is a *mono*saccharide, it cannot be a *di*saccharide; for the purpose of analyzation and this review, let us continue.

ITEM 4: Can choices be eliminated? Since both (C) and (D) cannot be true, *one* must be eliminated.

ITEM 5: A quick drawing to stimulate and help recall:

$$H-C(=O)$$

H   O
 \\ //
  C
  |
H—C—OH
  |
 etc.,
  |
 CH_2OH

ITEM 6:   All multiple-choice questions are TRUE or FALSE statements!
For statement (A): "Glucose is NOT an aldose."
FACT: An aldose is an aldehyde carbohydrate. Look at the structure in item 5!
This is indeed an aldehyde:

$$\begin{array}{c} H \diagdown \quad \diagup O \\ C \\ | \end{array}$$

So, the choice is apparently true, but remember the disclaimer *NOT*. In this context, the answer for (A) is FALSE.

For statement (B): "Glucose is NOT a reducing sugar."
FACT: A reducing sugar is one that must be oxidized while reducing a metal ion $(Cu^{2+} \rightarrow Cu^{+})$(a gain of electrons is reduction). Remember the disclaimer *NOT*. In this context, the answer for (B) is FALSE.

For statement (C): "Glucose is NOT a disaccharide."
FACT: A disaccharide is a carbohydrate that may be hydrolyzed to a simpler carbohydrate. Carefully examine the sketch. Can this compound be hydrolyzed (split by water) into a smaller carbohydrate? Remember the disclaimer *NOT*. In this context, the answer for (C) is TRUE. During an examination with stress on speed and limited time, you would not wish to continue working on this question. Here, however, to continue the analyzation of the process, please go on to the next statement.

For statement (D): "Glucose is NOT a monosaccharide." Note the formula and the opposite of choice (C). Remember the disclaimer *NOT*. In this context, the answer for (D) is FALSE.

In summary, we arrive at:

(A)	FALSE
(B)	FALSE
(C)	TRUE
(D)	FALSE

So, the answer is (C). Wow! That's easy if you know all the facts, but what if you don't? Suppose your array of answers was:

(A)	FALSE
(B)	I DON'T KNOW.
(C)	TRUE
(D)	FALSE

or a variation such as:

(A)	I DON'T KNOW.
(B)	I DON'T KNOW.
(C)	TRUE
(D)	I DON'T KNOW.

or:

(A)	FALSE
(B)	FALSE
(C)	I DON'T KNOW.
(D)	FALSE

The answer (C) is obvious in all three sets of answers above. However, what about:

(A)   FALSE
(B)   I DON'T KNOW.
(C)   I DON'T KNOW.
(D)   FALSE

Without additional information or a hunch or a gut feeling (which is a subliminal input), our advice would be to *let it go!* Pick one of the two, (B) or (C), and move on. You have a 50–50% chance of being right. The more "I don't know" answers for possible choices, the lower the probability of being right. So, for a particular examination, without additional information, decide to *always select* the first "I don't know" answer. This will cut through the random answer position on examinations. Remember that the answers on the key are randomly distributed. By adopting the above system, you put a degree of constancy into your pattern, and you don't float likewise. Your chances are drastically enhanced.

We will look at one more question from the chemistry section of the first part of Model Examination B, using the same analytical techniques but in a less detailed way.

EXAMPLE

9. Alcohols have higher boiling points than do alkyl halides of the same chain lengths because:

(A) alcohols are more polar.
(B) alcohols have higher molecular weights.
(C) alcohols form ethers.
(D) alcohols form intermolecular hydrogen bonds.

KEY WORDS: Alcohols, higher boiling points, alkyl halides, and same chain lengths.

(A) false. Alkyl halides are more polar.
(B) false. Halides have higher molecular weights than do alcohols.
(C) false. The statement is true, but this is a chemical property not dealing with the physical property of a boiling point.
(D) true. Compare CH_3OH to CH_3Cl

In summary, we arrive at:

(A)   FALSE
(B)   FALSE
(C)   FALSE
(D)   TRUE

PART 1

MCAT
SCIENCE REVIEW

Review Outline

The purpose of this section is to help the student review some key material quickly, to place some of his or her information in perspective, and to help identify areas of weakness and strength. No attempt has been made to cover all of the material in the subject matter; but it is hoped that after the student has worked through the practice examinations and has studied the explanations to the questions, this section will amplify for him or her the highlights and essentials. The biology section contains a more detailed treatment of anatomy and physiology than will be required for most recall questions on the MCAT. However, familiarity with these areas will probably be useful in analyzing the reading passages and associated questions. The individual who is well prepared will sometimes recognize compromises that must be made for the sake of brevity. This section should not be used as a substitute for a good general text in the areas but it should be used as a guide and in conjunction with a text so that the student may efficiently prepare for the MCAT. Again, we urge the student to begin preparation for the examination early and to be conscientious and thorough.

BIOLOGY

1. The Cell—Its Structure and Function
   - Size
   - Composition of Protoplasm
   - General Structure of Membranes in Cells
   - Mechanisms Moving Molecules Across Membranes of Cells
   - Prokaryotic Versus Eukaryotic Cell Structure
   - Cell Division—Mitosis
   - Methods of Examining the Cell

2. Structure and Function of Viruses
   - Viral Life Cycles

3. Nucleic Acids and Nucleotides
   - Nucleotide Structure
   - Nucleotide Functions
   - Nucleotide Functions in Cells
   - RNA (Ribonucleic Acid) Structure
   - RNA Functions
   - DNA (Deoxyribonucleic Acid) Structure
   - Genetic Information Flow in Cells
   - Protein Structure
   - Protein Function
   - Control of Use of Genetic Information
   - Overview of Genetic Regulation in Prokaryotes and Eukaryotes

12. Respiratory System
    - Removal of Inhaled Particles
    - Pulmonary Ventilation
    - Inspiration and Expiration
    - Positive and Negative Pressure Breathing
    - Neuronal Control and Integration of Breathing
    - Gas Exchange in the Alveoli
    - Oxygen Transport
    - Carbon Dioxide Transport
    - Chemical Regulation of Respiration

13. Urinary System
    - Structure of the Kidney
    - Tubular Passageways
    - Functions of the Kidney and Uriniferous Tubules
    - Hormonal Control of Secretion and Resorption

14. Integumentary (Skin) System
    - Skin
    - Glands
    - Hair
    - Nails

15. Digestive System and Nutrition
    - Nutrition
    - The Digestive System
    - The Major Digestive Glands
    - General Functional Schema of the Digestive Tube (ingestion, digestion, egestion)
    - Intestinal Motility
    - Innervation of the Intestinal Tract
    - Summary of Digestive Juices
    - Hormones of the Digestive Tract
    - General Digestion of the Major Food Groups

16. Nervous System
    - Nervous Tissue
    - The Neuron
    - Classification of Neurons
    - Groups of Neurons
    - Supportive Elements
    - Supportive Elements of the Peripheral Nervous System
    - The Central Nervous System
    - The Peripheral Nervous System
    - Reflex Arc

17. Organs of Special Sense
    - The Eye
    - The Ear
    - The Olfactory System
    - The Gustatory System

18. Endocrine System
    - The Pituitary Gland (Hypophysis)
    - The Thyroid Gland

24. The Animal Kingdom
    - Distribution of Living Organisms
    - Interrelationships of Animals
    - Population Dynamics
    - Major Environment—Habitats
    - Learning, Conditioning, Rhythms

25. Evolution
    - Key People and Concepts
    - Mechanisms of Evolution on a Small Scale (Microevolution)
    - Mechanisms of Evolution on a Large Scale (Macroevolution)
    - Speciation
    - Other Patterns of Macroevolution
    - The Rate of Evolution
    - Artificial Selection

CHEMISTRY

1. General Chemistry
   - The Atom
   - Components of the Atom
   - Placement of Electrons—Energy Levels
   - Periodic Table
   - Gases
   - Liquids and Solids
   - Phase Changes
   - Chemical Compounds
   - Balanced Chemical Equations
   - Solutions
   - Acids and Bases, pH, and Buffers
   - Electrochemistry
   - Thermodynamics
   - Rate Processes in Chemical Reactions

2. General Principles
   - Characteristics of Mixtures and Compounds
   - Reactions
   - Role of Enzymes in a Reaction
   - Temperature of Conversion Factors
   - Formulas and Laws

3. Organic Chemistry
   - General Considerations
   - The Alkanes
   - The Cycloalkanes
   - The Alkenes
   - The Alkynes
   - Aromatic Compounds
   - The Grignard Reagent
   - Alcohols
   - Amines
   - Amides
   - Aldehydes and Ketones

Biology

CHAPTER 2

THE CELL—ITS STRUCTURE AND FUNCTION

The cell is the basic unit of structure and function and basis of all life; all cells come from preexisting cells.

Size

Most eukaryotic cells are between 10 and 100 μm (micrometers) in diameter. Measurements are made utilizing the following units:

$$1 \text{ cm} = 10 \text{ mm}$$
$$1 \text{ mm} = 1000 \text{ μm}$$
$$1 \text{ μm} = 10,000 \text{ Å (angstrom units)}$$

Average sizes of structures may be listed as follows:

eukaryotic cells about	10 μm	(100,000 Å)
mitochondria about	1 μm	(10,000 Å)
bacteria about	1 μm	(10,000 Å)
viruses about	0.1 μm	(1,000 Å)
macromolecules about	0.01 μm	(100 Å)
molecules about	0.001 μm	(10 Å)
hydrogen ion about	0.0001 μm	(1 Å)

Resolution is commonly defined as the ability to discriminate two points and visualize them as two points, even though they are extremely close together. With the unaided eye these points might appear as one point, but the microscope can aid in resolving them as two. The resolution is dependent on the wavelength of the light source and can be calculated to be about one-half the wavelength. Examples of resolving power are:

human eye about 0.1 mm (100 μm)
light microscope about 0.2 μm (2,000 Å)
transmission electron microscope about 2–5 Å

Composition of Protoplasm (Contents of Living Cells)

Protoplasm is made up mainly of proteins, carbohydrates, fats, salts, and water; its average elemental composition is

Oxygen 75+%

Carbon 10+%

Hydrogen 10%

Nitrogen 2+%

Sulfur about 0.2%

Phosphorus about 0.3%

Potassium about 0.3%

Chlorine about 0.1%

less than 0.1%—sodium,
    calcium,
    magnesium,
    iron, etc.

General Structure of Membranes in Cells

Every living cell has a *plasma membrane,* or plasmalemma, which serves as the permeability barrier between the cell and its environment. A eukaryotic cell also contains other membranes that separate different compartments within the cell. All of these membranes consist of *lipid* (primarily phospholipid) *bilayers* with associated *proteins.* Some proteins are associated with the surface of the membrane, whereas other proteins extend across the lipid bilayer. Membrane surfaces that face away from the cytoplasm in eukaryotic cells may have numerous *oligosaccharide groups* (polymers of sugars) attached to proteins and lipids. The oligosaccharide-bearing components are especially numerous on the external surface of the plasma membrane.

When viewed at high magnification by routine transmission electron microscopy, most membranes in a cell appear as two dark lines separated by a light zone. The complex is approximately 10 nm (100 Å) in thickness.

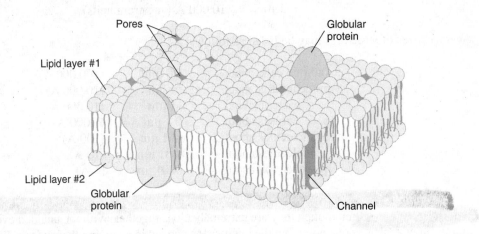

The fluid mosaic model of the plasma membrane at the cell border. The membrane consists of two phospholipid layers in which globular proteins float about.

LIPID BILAYERS IN MEMBRANES

When mixed with water, phospholipids (both glycerophospholipids and sphingolipids) and glycolipids spontaneously form bilayer structures as a result of the strongly polar phosphate-containing or sugar-containing "head" of each molecule associating with the water and the non-polar alkyl "tails" of the fatty acyl groups aggregating by hydrophobic interactions.

Glycerophospholipids contain a glycerol linked to two fatty acyl groups and one phosphate group. The phosphate group may in turn be linked to further groups such as ethanolamine (in phosphatidyl ethanolamine), choline (in phosphatidyl choline), serine (in phosphatidyl serine), or inositol (in phosphatidyl inositol).

Sphingolipids contain a sphingosine linked to one fatty acyl group and are usually linked to a phosphate plus a choline (sphingomyelin), a sugar (ceramides), or to a complex oligosaccharide (gangliosides). Sphingolipids are absent from most prokaryotes and occur primarily in the outer face of the plasma membrane in eukaryotes.

Lysophospholipids have one fatty acyl group removed, cutting the ratio of nonpolar to polar structure in half. Conversion of phospholipids to lysophospholipids promotes conversion of phospholipid bilayers into micelles and may destabilize membranes.

Substitution of *cis-unsaturated fatty acids* for *saturated fatty acids* decreases the closeness of the packing in the nonpolar layer, increasing fluidity in the layer and increasing movement of small polar molecules across the layer.

unsaturated F.A.'s = more fluid.

The addition of *cholesterol* to a lipid bilayer reduces fluidity of the lipids and reduces penetration of small polar molecules across the bilayer.

Add cholesterol = ↓ fluidity

MEMBRANE PROTEINS

Peripheral membrane proteins are attached to integral membrane components (lipids or proteins) by noncovalent bonds. Peripheral proteins may be removed from a membrane by milder treatments than are required to remove integral membrane proteins.

Integral membrane proteins cannot be released from a membrane without breaking covalent bonds or disrupting the lipid bilayer.

Some integral membrane proteins are anchored to the lipid bilayer by covalent linkage to a lipid, usually a fatty acyl group (frequently a myristyl group), a prenyl group (frequently a farnesyl group), or a phospholipid (usually a glycosylphosphatidylinositol [GPI] anchor).

Transmembrane integral membrane proteins contain one or more protein domains that extend across the lipid bilayer. Most transmembrane domains appear to adopt alpha helical secondary structure and consist primarily of amino acids with hydrophobic side chains. Some transmembrane integral membrane proteins form ion channels across the membrane, others are active transport or facilitated diffusion carriers, and still others are receptors for growth factors or hormones. The functions of many membrane proteins are unknown.

Some membrane proteins appear to be free to diffuse in the plane of the membrane, whereas other membrane proteins (particularly receptors) have restricted mobility or can be clustered in response to stimuli, usually by interaction with cytoskeletal elements. The current model of membrane organization is called the fluid mosaic model because of the freedom of movement of lipids and some proteins in the membrane.

MEMBRANE FUNCTION

The primary function of a membrane in a cell is to control movement of materials from one compartment to another. Several processes are involved in these movements. Simple diffusion occurs in any fluid, whereas carrier-mediated processes are peculiar to biological membranes.

Simple Diffusion (Passive Movements) in Fluids

Concentration gradients consisting of differences in concentration of a component in a fluid can drive a net movement of that component. Each component in any fluid will diffuse from regions of high concentrations of that component toward regions of low concentration of that component. This movement, called simple diffusion, is the result of random movements of each particle in the fluid, and occurs whether the component is charged or not.

Electrostatic gradients (potential fields) can drive net movements of charged particles such as ions in a fluid. Charged components in a fluid will be attracted to opposite charges and repelled by similar charges. Therefore, if a potential field is present, positively charged particles will move toward the negative pole and negatively charged particles will move toward the positive pole.

Because both concentration gradients and electrostatic forces act on charged components, the sum of the forces acting on a charged component can be described as an *electrochemical gradient*.

Simple Diffusion Across Lipid Bilayers

Because a biological membrane is composed of a lipid bilayer containing associated proteins, the movement of materials across the membrane is determined by the properties of the lipid bilayer unless movement occurs through a channel or by means of a carrier molecule.

Very small molecules that carry no net charge (water, oxygen, carbon dioxide) cross lipid bilayers relatively easily by simple diffusion, regardless of the polarity of the molecules. These molecules do not require carriers or channels to cross membranes.

Moderate-sized nonpolar molecules with no net charges (benzene, steroids) cross bilayers readily. These molecules have much more trouble moving through the water to get to the membrane than they have crossing the membrane. Small nonpolar molecules move relatively easily in water, but large nonpolar molecules such as fatty acids or triglycerides may primarily move through blood or tissue fluid complexed with a lipoprotein and may be taken up by cells through a receptor-mediated endocytosis mechanism that recognizes the protein component of the lipoprotein and takes up the lipid along with the protein.

Polar molecules up through three carbons in size and with no net charges cross bilayers moderately rapidly. These molecules usually cross membranes without requiring channels or carriers.

Polar molecules in the size range of biological monomers (five and six carbon sugars) and with no net charges cross lipid bilayers very slowly, usually too slowly to support metabolic processes. These molecules must therefore cross membranes by way of a channel or by way of a carrier-mediated mechanism.

Ions and polar macromolecules cross lipid bilayers very slowly, if at all. These ions or molecules must therefore cross membranes by way of a channel or by way of a carrier-mediated mechanism. Many types of macromolecules may initially be taken into cells through receptor-mediated endocytosis, then cross the membrane of the vesicle formed during endocytosis after alteration of the macromolecule.

Mechanisms Moving Molecules Across Membranes of Cells

1. SIMPLE DIFFUSION

Materials that cross lipid bilayers rapidly enough to meet the needs of cells usually cross cellular membranes by simple diffusion. These materials always move down their electrochemical gradient and the rate of movement increases as the electrochemical gradient increases over the full range of reasonable concentrations. Water, oxygen, and carbon dioxide usually cross membranes by simple diffusion.

Osmosis is a special case of simple diffusion. Because of the extensive interactions between solutes and water, the presence of solutes in water reduces the effective concentration of free water. Water will therefore diffuse from areas of lower solute concentration (*hypotonic* = lower solute concentration, therefore higher water concentration) to areas of higher solute concentration (*hypertonic* = higher solute concentration, therefore lower water concentration) When this occurs across a membrane that allows water to cross more easily than most solutes, substantial changes in volume occur. Multicellular animal cells normally operate in *isotonic* body fluids (same total solute concentration as inside the cells). Placing most animal cells in a hypertonic environment causes the cells to shrink. Placing the cells in a hypotonic environment causes the cells to swell and burst.

Mechanisms Moving Molecules Across Cell Membranes

I. *Passive transport* (does not require energy expenditure)	1. Concentration gradients cause each component in a fluid to diffuse from regions of higher concentrations toward regions of lower concentrations.
	2. Electrostatic gradients cause charged particles to be attracted to opposite charges and repelled by similar charges.
Simple diffusion	Water, oxygen, carbon dioxide (dissolved gases), and lipid soluble molecules cross easily through the phospholipid bilayer of a membrane.
Osmosis (a special case of simple diffusion)	Water diffuses from areas of lower solute concentration (hypotonic) to areas of higher solute concentration (hypertonic).
Facilitated diffusion	A channel or uniporter carrier is used; the movement is down the component's electrochemical gradient and shows saturation kinetics.
II. *Energy-requiring transport*	Materials are moved (usually up their electrochemical gradient) using cellular energy.
Active transport	A protein carrier moves the particle independently of its electrochemical gradient; the carrier consumes energy (usually ATP).
Endocytosis	Process whereby the cell membrane engulfs extracellular material, moves it into the cell, and forms membrane-bound vesicles.
Exocytosis	Manufactured and modified materials are secreted by this process and eliminated from the cell.

2. FACILITATED DIFFUSION

Materials that cross lipid bilayers too slowly to meet cellular needs but that are being moved down their electrochemical gradient are usually moved by facilitated diffusion. This process may use either a channel or a uniporter carrier (both usually proteins). In either case, however, the movement is down the component's electrochemical gradient and shows saturation kinetics (increasing the gradient beyond a point causes no further increase in transport).

3. ACTIVE TRANSPORT

Materials that cross lipid bilayers too slowly to meet cellular needs but that are occasionally or frequently being moved up their electrochemical gradient are moved by active transport. This process uses a protein carrier that moves the component independently of its electrochemical gradient because the carrier consumes energy (usually adenosine triphosphate, or ATP) to make its conformational changes directional. Like facilitated diffusion, active transport shows saturation kinetics (increasing the component concentration beyond a point causes no further increase in transport). Unlike facilitated diffusion, active transport is (a) sensitive to the concentration of the component on only one side of the membrane (the "loading" side), (b) insensitive to the concentration of the component on the other side of the membrane, and (c) usually saturates at relatively low component concentrations.

Once a reliable concentration gradient of one component has been established by active transport, its concentration gradient may in turn be used to drive additional coupled active transport mechanisms (sometimes called secondary active transport). If the coupled component moves in the same direction as the gradient component, the process is a *symport* process. If they move in opposite directions, the process is an *antiport* process.

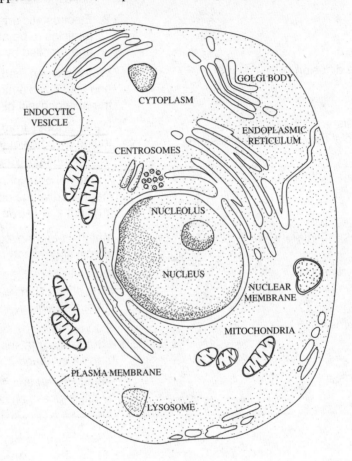

Diagram of eukaryotic cell.

Prokaryotic Versus Eukaryotic Cell Structure

All living cells can be categorized as prokaryotic or eukaryotic on the basis of their structural organization.

Prokaryotic cells have no nuclear envelope separating the nuclear material from the cytoplasm. Organisms with prokaryotic cellular structure are unicellular, so each cell is an organism. Prokaryotic organisms frequently occur in loosely organized colonies.

Eukaryotic cells contain a nuclear envelope that separates their nuclear compartment from their cytoplasmic compartment. Organisms with eukaryotic cellular structure may be unicellular (protistans) or multicellular (fungi, plants, and animals). Multicellular eukaryotes contain multiple cell types in organized patterns.

PROKARYOTIC CELL STRUCTURE

A typical prokaryotic cell consists of a *nuclear area* or *nucleoid* surrounded by *cytoplasm*. The cytoplasm is bounded by a *plasma membrane,* which is in turn typically surrounded by a *cell wall complex.*

NUCLEAR AREA

The nuclear area contains a chromosome consisting of a circular DNA molecule anchored at one location to the plasma membrane, but which is otherwise free in the cytoplasm. The DNA is usually complexed with proteins and other molecules, but is not organized into the nucleosomal histone-DNA complexes typical of eukaryotic nuclear DNA. In routine transmission electron micrographs, the nuclear area is usually lighter staining than the adjacent cytoplasm. The DNA in the nuclear area contains most of the genetic information in a prokaryotic cell, although smaller episomes or plasmids may also be present in the cell. Plasmids frequently contain genes conferring resistance to antibiotics.

CYTOPLASM

The cytoplasm in a prokaryotic cell consists primarily of moderately dark-staining cytosol containing proteins, other macromolecules, small molecules, ions, and water. Most of the metabolism occurs in the cytosol in prokaryotes.

Free ribosomes appear scattered in the cytoplasm as more darkly stained granules of approximately 25 nm (250 Å) diameter. All of the proteins made in prokaryotic cells are made on free ribosomes.

Membranous structures are normally absent from the cytoplasm of most prokaryotic cells. Internal membranes derived from the plasma membrane occur in cyanobacteria and some other photosynthetic bacteria. These membranes, sometimes called chromatophores, contain the photosynthetic pigments and function like the thylakoid membranes in chloroplasts. Cytoplasmic infoldings from the plasma membrane also occur in nitrifying bacteria. A few types of bacteria have cytoplasmic vesicles lined by a single layer of phospholipids.

The *plasma membrane* of a prokaryotic cell consists of a typical phospholipid bilayer with embedded and surface-associated proteins. The plasma membrane of a prokaryotic cell lacks glycolipids and cholesterol, which are typically found in eukaryotic plasma membranes. The plasma membrane appears to be the major structure controlling movement of molecules in and out of prokaryotic cells, but transport mechanisms located in the cell wall are also important in Gram-negative bacteria.

A *cell wall complex* is usually present outside the plasma membrane in most prokaryotic cells. The cell wall complex differs strikingly between Gram-positive and Gram-negative bacteria, and may differ from these two patterns in other prokaryotes.

Gram-positive bacteria have a cell wall consisting of a thick layer of *peptidoglycans,* which consist of sugars and amino acids. This cell wall supports and protects the individual cell that it surrounds.

Gram-negative bacteria are surrounded by a more complex wall structure consisting of a thin layer of peptidoglycans surrounded by an *"outer membrane"* of lipopolysaccharide and protein. Channel-forming proteins called porins allow selected molecules to cross the outer membrane. A fluid-filled *periplasmic space* containing enzymes lies between the peptidoglycan layer and the plasma membrane and between the peptidoglycan layer and the outer membrane. The lipopolysaccharides of the outer membrane cause it to resist passage of water-soluble molecules, which are not transported through the porins. As a result, the outer membrane of the cell wall in Gram-negative plays a greater role in controlling passage of materials than the cell wall in Gram-positive bacteria.

Prokaryotic cells may have structures extending outward from the cell wall complex. *Flagella* consist of a protein rod (about ¹⁄₁₀ as thick as a eukaryotic flagellum and lacking microtubules in its core) attached to the cell by a hook (bent structure) and a swivel (basal rotational mechanism). Flagella are responsible for movement of the cell.

Pili are hollow protein tubes that attach bacteria to surfaces and transfer DNA between cells during conjugation (mating).

Many prokaryotic cells have a *capsule* or *slime layer* consisting of a loose polysaccharide gel located outside the cell wall complex. This layer protects parasitic bacteria against host defense mechanisms.

EUKARYOTIC CELL STRUCTURE

A typical eukaryotic cell consists of a nucleus surrounded by cytoplasm containing ribosomes, a cytoskeleton, and numerous membranous organelles. The cytoplasm is bounded by a plasma membrane that may, in turn, be surrounded by a cell wall complex in plants, fungi, and some protistans or by extracellular matrix materials in animals.

EUKARYOTIC NUCLEAR STRUCTURES

The nuclear compartment (nucleus) is separated from the cytoplasmic compartment by a *nuclear envelope* consisting of two layers of membrane and perforated by nuclear pores. The outer membrane of the nuclear envelope complex is chemically similar to endoplasmic reticulum, whereas the inner nuclear membrane has inserted proteins that connect with the nuclear lamina (containing intermediate filament-like lamin proteins), which in turn connects to the nuclear matrix.

The nuclear contents (nucleoplasm) can exchange materials with the cytoplasmic contents (cytosol) by diffusion and selective transport through *nuclear pores*. Small molecules (diameter <9 nm) move through nuclear pores by simple diffusion. Proteins move from the cytosol into the nucleus by active transport through nuclear pores. Targeting is by short amino acid sequences which are in different locations in different proteins. Transfer RNA molecules are directionally transported from the nucleus into the cytosol, probably through nuclear pores and probably by active transport. Messenger RNA molecules are directionally transported from the nucleus into the cytosol through nuclear pores, probably by active transport. Efficient export requires a 5' methylated guanine cap and release from the spliceosome complexes (normally when splicing out of introns is complete). Ribosomal subunits are directionally transported from the nucleus into the cytosol, probably through nuclear pores and probably by active transport.

The *nucleolus,* which is visible in most eukaryotic cell nuclei during interphase, contains small amounts of DNA (most of the rRNA genes) and larger amounts of RNA (mostly rRNA) and proteins (rRNA processing proteins and ribosomal proteins). The nucleolus is the location of rRNA synthesis and assembly of ribosomal subunits from rRNA and from proteins imported from the cytoplasm.

EUKARYOTIC CHROMOSOME STRUCTURE

Nuclear DNA in eukaryotes is organized into *chromosomes*. Chromosome number, shape of the condensed chromosomes during mitosis and meiosis, and DNA content of each chromosome are consistent among the normal members of a species. Chromosome number, shape, and DNA content may vary widely between species and even between some closely related species. Each unreplicated chromosome appears to contain a single linear DNA molecule.

Functional eukaryotic chromosomes appear to contain three essential components. These three components have been assembled and shown to constitute a functional artificial chromosome in yeast cells.

1. A *centromere sequence* is necessary to integrate the chromosome into the spindle during either mitosis or meiosis. A normal chromosome would contain a single functional centromere.

2. At least one *replication initiation sequence* is needed to initiate DNA replication in the chromosome. Isolated replication initiation sequences are referred to as *autonomously replicating sequences*. Most natural eukaryotic chromosomes contain multiple replication initiation sequences.

3. A *telomere sequence* is needed at each end of the chromosome to allow replication without loss of genetically critical sequences. Telomeres consist of simple repeated sequences added by telomerase enzymes in actively dividing cells.

CHROMATIN STRUCTURE

Each unreplicated eukaryotic chromosome contains a single linear DNA molecule which is complexed with proteins to form *chromatin,* consisting of protein and DNA in an approximately 2:1 ratio by weight.

Histones are the most numerous category of proteins in chromatin, comprising approximately half of the chromatin protein and occurring in approximately a 1:1 ratio to DNA by weight. Histones contain numerous amino acids with side chains containing basic functional groups, resulting in a net positive surface charge which binds ionically to the negatively charged phosphate groups in DNA.

Histone classes H2A, H2B, H3, and H4 aggregate with DNA to form *nucleosomes*. Each nucleosome contains two molecules of each histone class comprising a protein core and has two "turns" of DNA (approximately 146 nucleotide pairs) wound around the outside.

Nucleosomes appear to form at close spacing on most chromosomal DNA regions unless nucleosome assembly is inhibited by regulatory proteins bound to the DNA. As a result, regions of DNA that are transcriptionally active (being used as a template for RNA synthesis) usually contain extensive regions of DNA between nucleosomes and appear as lighter-staining *euchromatin* when viewed by light and electron microscopy. Histones of class H1 (or H5 in some cells) bind to the DNA between closely spaced nucleosomes to aggregate the DNA into 30 nm diameter chromatic fibers, which predominate in darker-staining *heterochromatin*.

Condensed chromosomes, which form during mitosis and meiosis, contain a poorly characterized *scaffolding* that further compacts the 30 nm diameter condensed nucleosome aggregates. The composition of the scaffolding is unclear, but Topoisomerase II enzymes occur bound to DNA at intervals. The topoisomerase functions as an enzyme that reduces DNA coiling during replication, but labeled antibody staining shows that topoisomerase remains in the scaffolding when histones are removed, which suggests that topoisomerase may be part of the scaffolding structure.

EUKARYOTIC CYTOPLASM

1. **Cytosol.** The largest functional compartment in eukaryotic animal cells is the *cytosol* or fluid cytoplasm between recognizable cytoplasmic organelles. The cytosol consists primarily of moderately dark-staining material containing proteins, other macromolecules, small molecules, ions, and water. Glycolysis and many other general metabolic processes occur in the cytosol.

2. **Free ribosomes.** These organelles appear scattered in the cytosol as more darkly stained granules of approximately 25 nm (250 Å) diameter. All of the proteins that will function in the cytosol, nucleus, and peroxisomes are made on free ribosomes. Proteins that will be imported from the cytosol into mitochondria and chloroplasts are also made on free ribosomes. Free ribosomes that are engaged in protein synthesis are organized into *polyribosomes (polysomes),* which may appear as clusters, linear arrays, or rosettes in routine electron micrographs.

3. **Smooth endoplasmic reticulum (sER).** This organelle consists of irregular tubes and flattened sacs or cisterni of cytoplasmic membrane and has no ribosomes on its cytoplasmic surfaces. Endoplasmic reticulum (both sER and rER) provides the surfaces on

which synthesis of phospholipids and part of the synthesis of steroids occurs. Enzymes associated with sER are also involved in detoxifying many foreign molecules such as drugs.

4. **Secretion and Endocytosis Apparatus.** Rough endoplasmic reticulum, Golgi bodies, lysosomes, secretory vesicles, and numerous types of transport vesicles may be viewed as an integrated functional system that manufactures, modifies, and moves proteins and other molecules that may be secreted by exocytosis or taken into the cell by endocytosis.

a. *Rough Endoplasmic Reticulum (rER).* This consists of flattened sacs of cytoplasmic membrane with ribosomes associated with the cytoplasmic surface. The ribosomes on rER are the site of synthesis of proteins that will be "packaged" by the Golgi bodies. These proteins include lysosomal enzymes and proteins that will be secreted by the cell. The ribosomes on the rER do not appear to be permanently attached, but a ribosome attaches to rER if the polypeptide currently being synthesized by the ribosome carries a signal sequence of amino acids near its amino terminal end that triggers uptake of the polypeptide into the rER. After the polypeptide is taken into the rER, the initial oligosaccharide groups are added to glycoproteins prior to their transfer to Golgi bodies.

b. *Golgi bodies.* They consist of stacks of flattened sacs of smooth cytoplasmic membranes. The stack of membrane sacs in a Golgi body is polarized. One surface receives vesicles from the rER and is called the cis face. The other surface buds off vesicles that carry materials to lysosomes, secretory vesicles, and the plasma membrane and is called the trans face. Golgi bodies are called dictyosomes in plant cells. In animal cells with a single large Golgi body, the Golgi body is usually located near the pair of centrioles that are found next to the nucleus.

Proteins synthesized on ribosomes associated with rER enter the Golgi by transfer of membrane vesicles from the rER to the cis face of the Golgi apparatus. Endoplasmic reticulum-resident proteins are retrieved by receptors that recognize their signal sequence and are routed back to the rER.

While in the Golgi body, oligosaccharides on glycoproteins are modified by removal and substitution of sugars and by addition of sialic acid. Lysosomal enzymes are selected by recognition of their signal peptide and tagged with mannose-6-phosphate residues added to their oligosaccharides. Glycosaminoglycans are assembled onto core proteins to form proteoglycans. In addition, ceramides in the lipid bilayers of membrane vesicles that fused with the Golgi body are modified into sphingomyelin or into gangliosides.

Lysosomal enzymes are recognized by receptors for mannose-6-phosphate and are transferred in vesicles from the trans Golgi face to lysosomes. Secretory granule components are recognized through mechanisms that are unclear and are transferred in vesicles from the trans Golgi face to secretory granules. Once in secretory granules, the components are concentrated and proteins may be processed by proteolytic enzymes. Many other components are transferred in vesicles from the Golgi trans face to the plasma membrane and released in the process of constitutive secretion.

c. *Secretory vesicles.* These are spherical sacs of membrane containing materials that will be secreted from the cell by exocytosis.

d. *Lysosomes.* These are spherical sacs of membrane-containing hydrolytic enzymes (digestive enzymes) that function in acidic environments (usually about pH 4.5 to 5.0). Lysosomal enzymes usually function in digestion of material brought into the cell by phagocytosis or in digestion of damaged organelles.

5. **Mitochondria.** These organelles are approximately 0.5 µm in diameter and contain two layers of membrane. The outer membrane is smooth, whereas the inner membrane

is folded into finger-like or shelf-like cristae. The fluid space inside the inner membrane is called the matrix. Most of the ATP synthesis during aerobic cellular respiration occurs in mitochondria. The Krebs cycle occurs in the matrix. Electrons collected by flavin adenine dinucleotide (FAD) or nicotinamide adenine dinucleotide (NAD) are passed along the electron transport system, many of whose enzymes are integral membrane proteins in the inner membrane, and generate a proton (hydrogen ion) gradient across the inner membrane which is used as an energy source to convert ADP into ATP. Mitochondria are also involved in several parts of steroid synthesis and interconversion.

Mitochondria are partially genetically autonomous and appear to arise by division of existing mitochondria. Mitochondria contain circular DNA molecules and prokaryote-like ribosomes which are involved in synthesis of a subset of the proteins which are present in the mitochondria. Most of the mitochondrial proteins are encoded by nuclear DNA and are synthesized on free ribosomes in the cytoplasm. Mitochondrial proteins are imported from the cytosol into the intermembrane space and the matrix in mitochondria by transmembrane transport complexes. Proteins are targeted to mitochondria by recognition of signal peptide sequences within the polypeptide chain of the protein.

6. **Cytoskeleton.** The cytoskeleton consists of the components that alter cell shape and that anchor and move organelles in cells. The cytoskeleton includes microfilaments, microtubules, intermediate filaments, and related structures.

   a. *Microfilaments.* These contain actin protein subunits assembled into very thin filaments (5 nm diameter). Microfilaments are usually associated with myosin and other proteins. Microfilaments are bundled into much larger stress fibers in some cell types. Microfilaments are capable of contraction, usually by sliding past each other due to interaction with myosin or some other "motor" protein.

   b. *Microtubules.* These contain alpha and beta tubulin protein subunits assembled into very small tubules (25 nm diameter). Microtubules are rigid tubes that can support cell shape or serve as a surface along which to move organelles inside the cell. Microtubules are rearranged to form the mitotic spindle during mitotic cell division. Microtubules appear to be organized and oriented by microtubule organizing centers associated with centrioles and several other cellular structures.

   c. *Intermediate filaments.* These contain one of a family of intermediate filament proteins assembled into fibers with a diameter of approximately 10 nm. Five major classes of intermediate filaments have been identified based on protein composition. Intermediate filaments may contain desmin, cytokeratin, vimentin, neurofilament, or glial fibrillary acidic protein. Each type of intermediate filament protein occurs in a different set of cell types. Intermediate filament fibers can be bent but resist stretching. They mechanically link desmosomal (macula adherens) cell–cell junctions across cells and may have additional functions.

   d. *Centrioles.* Each centriole is a cylinder of 9 triplets of microtubules. Centrioles occur in the center of the *centrosome* region next to the nucleus in animal cells and from which most of the microtubules in the cytoskeleton originate. The centrioles are duplicated and are associated with the ends of the mitotic spindle during mitosis. Basal bodies of eukaryotic cilia and flagella have the same structure as centrioles and appear to be the organizing structures for the axoneme in the cilium or flagellum.

   However, centrioles may have no function of their own. Centrioles are always associated with pericentriolar *microtubule organizing centers* in the cytoskeleton. The microtubule organizing centers appear to be essential to formation and spatial organization of microtubules. Because fully functional microtubule organizing centers without associated centrioles have been well documented in plant cells and in early mouse embryos, the function of the centrioles themselves is in question.

7. **Cytoskeleton-Associated Cell Surface Appendages.** Cilia, flagella, and microvilli are cell surface appendages with core structures containing cytoskeletal components.

   a. *Cilia and flagella.* Both have a core axial structure (the axoneme), which contains a cylinder of nine doublets of microtubules with an additional pair of single microtubules in the center. This "nine doublets plus two" pattern of microtubules makes these organelles easy to recognize when viewed in cross section by transmission electron microscopy. Both cilia and flagella have an outer covering of plasma membrane. Many flagella have dense-staining axial structures between the axoneme and the plasma membrane. Both cilia and flagella are motile. The flagellum in a sperm cell moves the cell through its environment. The cilia on epithelial cells of the trachea move the mucus layer, which forms the cell's environment past the cell.

   b. *Microvilli.* These are small finger-like projections of the cell surface. Typical microvilli are usually less than 2 μm long and less than 0.5 μm in diameter. Microvilli contain only microfilaments (no microtubules) and cytosol and have an outer covering of plasma membrane. Microvilli are frequently an adaptation to increase surface area for absorption of solutes.

8. **Peroxisomes.** The organelles are membrane-lined vesicles that typically contain catalase, which generates hydrogen peroxide used to detoxify various organic molecules. Peroxisomes are also involved in beta oxidation of fatty acids, and are involved in photorespiration and the glyoxylate cycle in plant cells. Peroxisomes import all of their enzymes from the cytosol by recognition of a short recognition peptide sequence. The translocation complex, which moves the enzymes across the peroxisome membrane, has not been described.

9. **Inclusions.** Inclusions in eukaryotic animal cells may include lipid droplets, glycogen granules, and melanin granules.

   a. *Lipid droplets.* These are spherical aggregates of lipid. Although the outer layer of the lipid droplet may contain phospholipids, a typical membrane structure does not appear to separate the lipid droplet from the cytoplasm. Lipid droplets appear as dark spheres when viewed by transmission electron microscopy and appear as empty spheres in routine light microscopic (LM) preparations.

   b. *Glycogen granules.* They occur as clusters in cytoplasm. Glycogen granules are easily visible by transmission electron microscopy and are usually very darkly stained and larger than ribosomes in routine preparations. Glycogen granules are not visible by LM, but glycogen can be demonstrated by LM using periodic acid Schiff (PAS) staining.

   c. *Melanin granules.* They are membrane-bound vesicles containing melanin. Melanin granules occur in cells near the basal layer in epidermis of skin and the pigmented cells at the rear of the retina of the eye. Melanin granules in epidermal cells are made in melanocytes and transferred into the epidermal cells.

10. **Plasma Membrane.** The plasma membrane (or plasmalemma) in a eukaryotic cell is a typical cellular membrane consisting of a lipid bilayer with integral and peripheral proteins. Many animal cell plasma membranes have the following additional features.

    a. The *outer face* of the plasma membrane is enriched in *glycolipids,* some of which are gangliosides with extensive oligosaccharide groups.

    b. Many of the transmembrane proteins, lipid-anchored proteins, and peripheral proteins associated with the outer face of the plasma membrane are *glycoproteins* with attached oligosaccharide groups.

    c. The oligosaccharides of the glycoproteins and lipids from the "fuzzy coat" or *glycocalyx* associated with the outer face of the plasma membrane. Although all of the functions of the glycocalyx are not known, glycocalyx oligosaccharides are the ligands for the lectin-like P-selectin receptors involved in initial binding of neutrophils to endothelial cells as the neutrophils leave blood vessels during inflammatory reactions. Likewise, the sialic acid units (which do not occur on bacteria) on the oligosaccharides help prevent complement-mediated damage to body cells during destruction of bacteria by complement. The glycocalyx on absorptive cells in the small intestine contains digestive enzymes that hydrolyze small fragments of molecules.

11. **Cell–Cell Junctions.** These are structures that join adjacent cells in multicellular animals. Junctional structures can be categorized as occluding junctions, attachment junctions, or communicating junctions.

   a. *Occluding junctions* or *zonula occludens*. These are regions in which the outer layers of the plasma membranes of associated cells appear fused (no extracellular space). A zonula occludens complex usually occurs as a band around the apical ends of epithelial cells in a sheet epithelium. Zonula occludens complexes prevent passage of materials through the extracellular space between cells and allow an epithelium to serve as a barrier.

   b. *Attachment junctions*. These may include several types of junctions. *Zonula adherens* typically occur adjacent to zonula occludens junctions. Associated cells appear to be attached by a band of dense material in the intercellular space, which is associated with dense material on the cytoplasmic surface of each membrane. The cytoplasmic dense material is in turn associated with microfilaments of the cytoskeleton. Zonula adherens junctions form a mechanical attachment between cells, which protects the zonula occludens junctions in epithelial cells.

   Macula adherens may occur as *desmosomes* joining two adjacent cells or as *hemidesmosomes* joining a cell to its basal lamina. In a macula adherens junction, a spot of dense material in the intercellular space between attached cells (desmosome) or between a cell and its basal lamina (hemidesmosome) is associated with a spot of dense material on the cytoplasmic surface of the plasma membrane of each cell involved. The cytoplasmic dense material is attached to intermediate filaments of the cytoskeleton of the attached cells. Macula adherens junctions form mechanical attachments between the connected structures (cell–cell or cell–basal lamina).

   c. *Communicating junctions*. These allow ions to move from the cytoplasm of one cell to the cytoplasm of an adjacent cell. A *nexus* or *gap junction* is a region (usually spot-like) in which the plasma membranes of opposed cells maintain a precise apparent gap (about 2 nm), which actually contains protein channels that cross both membranes. Nexus junctions allow rapid ionic communication between the connected cells.

EUKARYOTIC EXTRACELLULAR MATERIALS

1. *Cell Walls*. These structures consist of layers of extracellular material (cellulose, pectins, etc. in higher plants and chitin in fungi) that surround individual cells. A cell wall supports the individual cell it surrounds and helps support the body of the higher plants and fungi.

2. *Extracellular Matrix*. The material located around and between cells in multicellular animals is referred to as extracellular matrix. Unlike a cell wall, extracellular matrix does not usually appear as a series of layers around individual cells. Animal extracellular matrix usually contains fibrous proteins or glycoproteins such as collagen and elastin plus complex polysaccharides such as glycosaminoglycans. Extracellular matrix in bone is hardened by adding calcium and phosphate ions. Extracellular matrix is the major structural component in the connective tissues that give shape to the bodies of most higher animals.

Comparison of Prokaryotic and Eukaryotic Cell Structure

Structure	Prokaryotic Cell	Eukaryotic Cell Animal	Plant
Cell wall complex	+	−	+
Plasma membrane	+	+	+
Nuclear area (nucleoid)	+	−	−
Nucleus	−	+	+
Ribosomes	+	+	+
Endoplasmic reticula (sER and rER)	−	+	+
Golgi bodies	−	+	+
Secretory vesicles	−	+	+
Lysosomes	−	+	+
Mitochondria	−	+	+
Cytoskeleton			
• microfilaments	−	+	+
• microtubules	−	+	+
• intermediate filaments	−	+	+
• centrioles	−	+	−
Cilia and flagella	−*	+	−
Microvilli	−	+	−
Peroxisomes	−	+	+
Chloroplasts	−	−	+

* Many bacteria have flagella, but they are protein rods unrelated to the membrane-covered flagella containing microtubules that occur in eukaryotic cells.

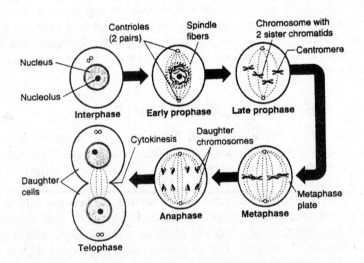

Mitosis in human cells. The four phases of mitosis are shown, with the major structures noted. The chromatids appear in prophase, then line up in the cell center in metaphase. One set of 46 chromosomes move to each daughter cell in anaphase, and the splitting of the cell in telophase completes the process.

Cell Division—Mitosis

For purposes of convenience, mitosis is divided into prophase, metaphase, anaphase, and telophase; the process, however, is a continuous one. The major events during the phases are:

1. *Prophase.* Chromosomes become distinct and nucleolus (nucleoli) disappear(s); centriole(s) and asters and spindle appear; nuclear membrane disappears.
2. *Metaphase.* Chromosomes move to the equator of the cell and duplicate.
3. *Anaphase.* The two chromatids split apart and start migration toward the poles of the spindle; the spindle loses its definition.
4. *Telophase.* Chromosomes lengthen and become less distinct; nucleoli reappear. The next period of growth and rest is known as *interphase.*
5. *Interphase.* Cell growth; protein synthesis; DNA synthesis; chromosome duplication.

Methods of Examining the Cell

1. MICROSCOPY

Microscopes are usually classified as either light or electron microscopes according to the type of energy source.

2. METHOD OF PREPARATION

1. *Fixation:* a piece of tissue is placed in a fixative solution, which kills and preserves the cells in the tissue with as few structural changes as possible;
2. *Dehydration:* water is usually removed from the tissues by passing it through a series of increasing strengths of alcohol solutions;
3. *Embedding:* embedding places the tissues in a solid medium, usually paraffin or plastic;
4. *Sectioning:* tissue is cut into sections with a thickness of 5 microns or 5000 nm for light, and about 60 nm for electron microscopic evaluation;
5. *Staining:* sections are stained with colored dyes for light microscopy and heavy metals for electron microscopy to enhance visualization.

QUICK RECALL TEST QUESTIONS AND ANSWERS

Choose the Best Answer

1. If a cell were put into a hypertonic solution (a solution of greater osmotic pressure than its protoplasm):

    (A) water would pass out through the plasma membrane faster than in.
    (B) water would pass in through the plasma membrane faster than out.
    (C) the cell would swell.
    (D) no unequal rates would be experienced.

2. Messenger RNA is coded by:

    (A) ribosomes.
    (B) endoplasmic reticulum.
    (C) DNA in the nucleus.
    (D) cytoplasm.

3. During metaphase of mitosis:

    (A) there is a dissolution of the chromosomal material.
    (B) the centrioles with asters are at the opposite poles and the centromeres are at the equator.
    (C) the cell membrane starts to reappear.
    (D) the nuclear membrane disappears.

4. The process by which a cell takes up dissolved material into membrane bound vesicles is known as:

    (A) phagocytosis.
    (B) active transport.
    (C) exocytosis.
    (D) endocytosis.

5. Microvilli would most likely be located on the surface of a cell that carries out which of the following processes?

    (A) secretion
    (B) protection
    (C) motility
    (D) absorption

6. Unlike facilitated diffusion, active transport is:

    (A) sensitive to the concentration of the component on only one side of the membrane (the "loading side").
    (B) insensitive to the concentration of the component on the other side of the membrane.
    (C) known to saturate at relatively low component concentrations.
    (D) all of the above.

7. The fluid-mosaic cell model of the cell membrane depicts it as:

    (A) a bilayer of lipid between two layers of protein.
    (B) a bilayer of lipid with integral and peripheral proteins.
    (C) a bilayer of protein between two layers of lipid.
    (D) alternating layers of protein and lipid (jelly roll).

8. Which of the following cell organelles or structures produces chemical energy via the electron transport chain?

    (A) mitochondria
    (B) rough endoplasmic reticulum (rER)
    (C) smooth endoplasmic reticulum (sER)
    (D) peroxisomes

9. The process by which a cell can move a substance from a point of lower concentration to a point of higher concentration (against the concentration gradient) is called:

    (A) osmosis.
    (B) plasmolysis.
    (C) turgor pressure.
    (D) active transport.

10. Which of the following structures is/are NOT considered a modification of the cell membrane?

    (A) basement membrane
    (B) gap junctions
    (C) desmosomes
    (D) occluding junctions

11. The internal structure of a eukaryotic cilium or flagellum, no matter what the organism, has the same arrangement, consisting of _____ microtubules.

    (A) 7 outer doublets and 2 inner
    (B) 9 outer doublets and 2 inner
    (C) 11 outer doublets and 2 inner
    (D) 9 outer doublets and 1 inner

12. Cellular "digestive" or "suicide" packages is a common description for:

    (A) mitochondria.
    (B) Golgi zones or Golgi bodies.
    (C) lysosomes.
    (D) centrosomes.

13. Of the following, which is not considered a membranous organelle?

    (A) ribosome
    (B) endoplasmic reticulum
    (C) Golgi body
    (D) mitochondrion

14. The smallest unit possessing the capability to maintain life and to reproduce is:

    (A) an organ.
    (B) a cell.
    (C) DNA.
    (D) RNA.

15. All of the following are characteristic of prokaryotic cells EXCEPT:

    (A) cell wall complex.
    (B) plasma membrane.
    (C) nuclear area.
    (D) rough endoplasmic reticulum.

16. Mitochondrion

    (A) possesses hydrolytic enzymes
    (B) functions in protein synthesis
    (C) condenses (packages) secretory products
    (D) functions in energy production

17. Lysosome

    (A) possesses hydrolytic enzymes
    (B) functions in protein synthesis
    (C) condenses (packages) secretory products
    (D) functions in energy production

18. Golgi apparatus

    (A) possesses hydrolytic enzymes
    (B) functions in protein synthesis
    (C) condenses (packages) secretory products
    (D) functions in energy production

19. Rough endoplasmic reticulum

    (A) possesses hydrolytic enzymes
    (B) functions in protein synthesis
    (C) condenses (packages) secretory products
    (D) functions in energy production

20. Which of the following is highly developed in a cell that is metabolically very active and has a high energy (ATP) requirement?

    (A) lysosomes
    (B) rough endoplasmic reticulum
    (C) Golgi apparatus
    (D) mitochondria

21. In mitosis the chromosomes are located on the equator of the cell during:

    (A) prophase.
    (B) metaphase.
    (C) anaphase.
    (D) telophase.

Answers

1. **(A)** If a cell is placed in a hypertonic solution, water from within it will cross the semipermeable membrane and leave the cell, and the cell will shrink. If a cell is placed in a hypotonic solution, water from without will enter the cell and it will swell. In an isotonic solution, as many molecules of water will enter as will leave the cell and the cell will remain the same.

2. **(C)** The whole activity is controlled by its genetic components, which are located in the nucleus.

3. **(B)** During metaphase of mitosis the centrioles with asters are at the opposite poles; the chromosomes move to the equator of the cell.

4. **(D)** Proteins and similar dissolved macromolecules are taken into cells by membrane vesicles by endocytosis (pinocytosis).

5. **(D)** Microvilli are small, finger-like projections of the cell surface. Typical microvilli are usually less that 2 μm long and less than 0.5 μm in diameter. Microvilli contain only microfilaments (no microtubules) and cytosol, and have an outer covering of plasma membrane. Microvilli are frequently an adaptation to increase the surface area for absorption of solutes.

6. **(D)** The characteristics of active transport are delineated.

7. **(B)** All membranes consist of lipid (primarily phospholipid) bilayers with associated proteins. Some proteins are associated with the surface of the membrane, whereas other proteins extend across the lipid bilayer. Membrane surfaces which face away from the cytoplasm in eukaryotic cells may have numerous oligosaccharide groups (polymers and sugars) attached to proteins and lipids.

8. **(A)** Most of the ATP synthesis during aerobic cellular respiration occurs in mitochondria. The Krebs cycle occurs in the matrix. Electrons collected by flavinadenine dinucleotide (FAD) or nicotinamide adenine dinucleotide (NAD) are passed along the electron transport system, many of whose enzymes are integral membrane proteins in the inner membrane, and generate a proton (hydrogen ion) gradient across the inner membrane which is used as an energy source to convert ADP into ATP.

9. **(D)** Active transport requires energy and allows a cell to move material from a point of lower concentration to a point of higher concentration.

10. **(A)** Directly underlying epithelium is found a homogeneous, noncellular material, composed of reticular fibers and protein polysaccharides, which serves to bind down the tissue; this structure is the basement membrane.

11. **(B)** The internal structure of a cilium or flagellum is composed of 9 outer doublets and 2 inner microtubules.

12. **(C)** Lysosomes contain hydrolytic enzymes and are also known as digestive bags, etc.

13. **(A)** Ribosomes can be free floating or they may be attached to the endoplasmic reticulum which is then called rough endoplasmic reticulum (RER).

14. **(B)** The cell is the basic unit of structure and function and the basis of all life; all cells come from preexisting cells.

15. **(D)** Prokaryotic cells have no rough endoplasmic reticulum. (See table on p. 22.)

16. **(D)** Mitochondria are the biochemical powerplants of the cell. They recover energy from foodstuffs (via the Krebs cycle and respiratory chain) and convert it (via phosphorylation) into ATP (adenosine triphosphate). In this manner they produce the energy necessary for the metabolic processes. Mitochondria synthesize some of their own proteins, but this is not their major function.

17. **(A)** Lysosomes contain acid phosphatase and other hydrolytic enzymes. These enzymes are enclosed by a membrane and are released when needed into phagocytic vesicles, etc.

18. **(C)** The Golgi complex is prominent in glandular cells and is thought to function in the production, concentration, packaging, and transportation of secretory material.

19. **(B)** Ribosomes are attached to the membranes of the endoplasmic reticulum, which is designated as rough ER. Ribosomes are responsible for synthesis of proteins. Proteins synthesized on ribosomes attached to rough endoplasmic reticulum usually are used in membranes, used in lysosomes, or secreted.

20. **(D)** Most of the ATP synthesis during aerobic cellular respiration occurs in mitochondria. The Krebs cycle occurs in the matrix. Electrons collected by flavin adenine dinucleotide (FAD) or nicotinamide adenine dinucleotide (NAD) are passed along the electron transport system, many of whose enzymes are integral membrane proteins in the inner mem-

brane, and generate a proton (hydrogen ion) gradient across the inner membrane that is used as an energy source to convert ADP into ATP. Mitochondria are also involved in several parts of steroid synthesis and interconversion.

21. **(B)** For purposes of convenience, mitosis is divided into prophase, metaphase, anaphase, and telophase; the process, however, is a continuous one. In metaphase, chromosomes move to the equator of the cell. The major events during the phases are:

1. *Prophase.* Chromosomes become distinct and nucleolus (nucleoli) disappear(s); centriole(s) and asters and spindle appear; nuclear membrane disappears.

2. *Metaphase.* Chromosomes move to the equator of the cell.

3. *Anaphase.* The two chromatids split apart and start migration toward the poles of the spindle; the spindle loses its definition.

4. *Telophase.* Chromosomes lengthen and become less distinct; nucleoli and the nuclear envelope reappear. The next period of growth and rest is known as interphase.

5. *Interphase.* Cell growth; protein synthesis; DNA synthesis; chromosome duplication.

STRUCTURE AND FUNCTION OF VIRUSES

All typical viruses contain *nucleic acid* encoding the genetic information carried by the virus. The type of nucleic acid used by a particular category of virus will be consistent but varies widely among categories of viruses. The nucleic acid may be DNA or RNA and may be linear or circular. DNA and RNA may be either single- or double-stranded in viruses.

Viruses that require unusual replication enzymes such as RNA replicase or reverse transcriptase frequently carry copies of those enzymes bound to the nucleic acid in the virus particles.

Typical viruses contain a protein *capsid* or *capsule*, usually surrounding the nucleic acid. The protein subunits in the capsid are usually arranged to form either a polyhedron or a helix. The capsid may contain a single type of subunit or several types. Likewise, the capsid may contain a single layer of protein subunits or multiple layers.

Many viruses contain accessory structures attached to the capsid or additional layers outside the capsid. Bacteriophages may have a "stalk-like" apparatus at one end of the polyhedral capsid which is involved in passing the nucleic acid across the bacterial cell wall.

Eukaryotic animal cell viruses frequently contain a lipid bilayer structure outside of the capsid. This lipid bilayer is derived from the host cell plasma membrane and envelops the virus as the virus is budded off from the host cell surface. The lipid bilayer usually contains viral proteins which were encoded by viral nucleic acid, synthesized on host cell ribosomes, and inserted into the host cell plasma membrane prior to budding off the viruses.

Viral Life Cycles

A virus is capable of reproduction only while in a suitable host cell. Numerous reproductive patterns have been described in different viruses.

Bacteriophages (viruses infecting bacteria) typically follow one of two strategies or pathways, since release of viruses from the host bacterial cell is constrained by the bacterial cell wall. In a *lytic* replication strategy or pathway, the virus rapidly replicates after entering a host cell, then triggers lysis of the host cell to release the assembled viruses. In a *lysogenic* strategy or pathway, a DNA copy of the viral nucleic acid (the provirus) becomes incorporated into the host cell chromosome where it is replicated along with the adjacent host DNA. The integrated virus may cause little alteration in host cell phenotype or may cause detectable changes in host phenotype. A virus following a lysogenic strategy must shift to a lytic strategy in order to replicate new virus particles and release them from the host cell. In many of the bacteriophages studied so far, environmental insults that damage the bacterial host trigger the integrated *provirus* to exit the host DNA and follow a lytic reproductive strategy.

Animal cell viruses may follow similar patterns of rapid replication leading to death of the host cell or of incorporation into a host chromosome. Incorporated viral DNA may cause no detectable phenotypic changes or may cause changes as fundamental as loss of growth regulation resulting in cancer. In animal cell hosts, an intermediate strategy is also possible because the viruses can be budded from the host cell surface without killing the cell. As a result, viral replication can occur at moderate rates in infected cells for extended periods. As an example, macrophages infected with HIV-1 may survive for extended periods and serve as sources of viruses to infect nearby CD4$^+$ T lymphocytes in lymphoid organs.

Retroviruses are single-stranded RNA viruses that infect animal cells. These viruses use reverse transcriptase to make DNA copies of the viral RNA, after which the DNA copies become incorporated into host chromosomes. Because the viral DNA is somewhat transcriptionally active, these viruses frequently alter the phenotype of infected cells. At one point, some retroviruses (including HIV-1) were thought to be capable of remaining incorporated for 10 years or more, but more recent observations indicate that HIV-1 is replicating actively in lymphoid organs during the period between infection and development of clinical AIDS. This raises the possibility that some incorporated retroviruses may not remain incorporated for as long as was previously assumed. Retroviruses are important as inducers of a number of cancers in experimental animals and a rare form of T-cell leukemia in humans. In addition, HIV-1 and HIV-2 are responsible for essentially all cases of acquired immunodeficiency syndrome (AIDS).

QUICK RECALL TEST QUESTIONS AND ANSWERS

Choose the Best Answer

1. The genome of a typical virus may be either DNA or RNA, each of which may be single-stranded or double-stranded.

   (A) TRUE
   (B) FALSE

2. Typical viruses contain a protein capsid that surrounds the viral nucleic acid. The polypeptide subunits in the capsid may be arranged in a helical or polyhedral pattern.

   (A) TRUE
   (B) FALSE

3. Many eukaryotic animal cell viruses have a lipid bilayer surrounding the protein capsid. The lipids in the bilayer are synthesized by viral enzymes before the virus leaves the host cell.

   (A) TRUE
   (B) FALSE

4. Although typical viruses normally replicate inside a host cell, many viruses can replicate themselves outside of their normal host cell if they are provided with an external source of ATP.

   (A) TRUE
   (B) FALSE

5. A typical bacteriophage following a lytic type of reproductive strategy will insert its DNA into the host cell chromosome before turning on viral replication leading to lysis of the host cell.

   (A) TRUE
   (B) FALSE

6. The enzyme that catalyzes the initial replication of the viral genome during infection of a eukaryotic cell by a typical retrovirus is:

   (A) RNA polymerase.
   (B) reverse transcriptase.
   (C) DNA polymerase I.
   (D) DNA polymerase II.

7. Bacteriophages are:

   (A) quite dangerous to humans.
   (B) grown by innoculation of sterile broth.
   (C) reproduced only in living bacterial cells.
   (D) used as a source of vaccine against many bacterial diseases.

Answers

1. **(A)** Although a single type of virus will have a single type of nucleic acid, examples of viruses with any possible type and configuration of nucleic acid exist.

2. **(A)** Although a virus may contain additional coats derived from the plasma membrane of the host, the nucleic acid is typically surrounded by a polyhedral (or more rarely a helical) protein capsid.

3. **(B)** The first sentence in this statement is true, but the second sentence is false. Although proteins in viral lipid layers typically include proteins coded by viral genes, the lipids are typically derived from the plasma membrane of the host cell and are therefore synthesized by host cell enzymes in the rough endoplasmic reticulum and Golgi apparatus.

4. **(B)** This statement is false because viral replication requires numerous host cell enzymes, host cell ribosomes, and other host cell components. Therefore replication of viruses can occur only inside host cells.

5. **(B)** This statement is false because in a lytic cycle the viral DNA is not typically inserted into the host cell chromosome. Insertion into the host cell chromosome is typical of a lysogenic strategy or process.

6. **(B)** The correct answer is reverse transcriptase, which catalyzes assembly of DNA using an RNA template (RNA genome of the retrovirus in this case). RNA polymerase catalyzes assembly of RNA using a DNA template. DNA polymerase III catalyzes replication of DNA in prokaryotes. DNA polymerases I and II catalyze DNA synthesis during DNA repair in prokaryotes.

7. **(C)** A bacteriophage is a virus that is a parasite of bacteria; sometimes lysis of the bacteria cell is a result.

NUCLEIC ACIDS AND NUCLEOTIDES

DNA (deoxyribonucleic acid) and *RNA* (ribonucleic acid) are nucleic acids that are polymers of nucleotides. Electron carriers such as *FAD, NAD,* and *NADP* are dinucleotides. High energy phosphate carriers such as *ATP, CTP, GTP,* and *UTP* are single nucleotides.

Nucleotide Structure

Nucleotides are the monomers that are assembled to produce more complex nucleic acids. Each nucleotide consists of three components.

1. *Pentose Sugar.* Each nucleotide contains one five-carbon sugar that is either ribose (ATP, FAD, NAD, NADP, and RNA) or deoxyribose (DNA).
2. *Nitrogenous Base.* Each nucleotide contains one nitrogenous base that may be either a purine or a pyrimidine. Pyrimidines consist of a 6-membered ring containing carbon and nitrogen atoms. Pyrimidines include cytosine (C), uracil (U), and thymine (T). Purines consist of a similar 6-membered ring fused to a 5-membered ring. Purines include adenine (A) and guanine (G).
3. *Phosphate.* Each nucleotide contains one (MP), two (DP), or three (TP) phosphate groups. The letter code for the nitrogenous base plus the letter code for the number of phosphates can be used to designate a nucleotide. For example, a nucleotide with adenine and one phosphate is AMP.

ENERGY TRANSFER BY NUCLEOTIDES

If more than one phosphate group is present on a nucleotide, the bonds attaching the extra (second or third) phosphates to the nucleotide are less stable and can be easily hydrolyzed to release the energy used to make those bonds and make that energy available to other processes in the cell. As a result, nucleotide triphosphates are the primary energy source used to supply energy-consuming reactions in cells. ATP is the most widely used nucleotide triphosphate and is used for a wide variety of reactions. UTP is used in biosynthetic reactions involving additions of sugars. GTP is used to provide energy for protein shape changes by G proteins involved in receptor-triggered reaction sequences and protein synthesis.

POSITIONAL NOMENCLATURE

Locations of atoms on nucleotides are specified relative to the carbon atoms in the ribose or deoxyribose ring.

1. The purine or pyrimidine is attached to the *1' carbon* on the sugar.
2. The phosphate group is attached to the *5' carbon* on the sugar.
3. The hydroxyl group on the *3' carbon* on the sugar is reacted with the phosphate group on the adjacent nucleotide when a nucleotide is added to a DNA or RNA chain.

Nucleotide Functions

Nucleotides may be polymerized into *linear chains* of any length by covalently attaching (by a modified dehydration synthesis) the 3' carbon (using its attached hydroxyl) of the sugar of one nucleotide to the phosphate on the 5' carbon of the adjacent nucleotide. This arrangement creates polarity in chains of nucleotides.

The end of the chain with a free (unreacted) hydroxyl on the 3' carbon of the terminal nucleotide is called the *3' end* of the chain. Most reactions that add nucleotides to a DNA or RNA chain can react only with the 3' end of the existing chain. DNA synthesis catalyzed by DNA polymerase enzymes and RNA synthesis catalyzed by RNA polymerase enzymes follow this pattern.

The end of the chain with a free (unreacted) phosphate on the 5' carbon of the terminal nucleotide is called the *5' end* of the chain. The 5' end (or a structure near the 5' end) of a messenger RNA molecule must be recognized by a ribosome before the ribosome can assemble on the messenger RNA during initiation of protein synthesis (translation).

BASE PAIRING BY NUCLEOTIDES

Nucleotides may base pair with complementary nucleotides by forming hydrogen bonds between their nitrogenous bases. Stable base pairs consist of a purine paired with a pyrimidine. Two patterns of base pairing occur normally.

1. Adenine base pairs with uracil or thymine by forming two hydrogen bonds.
2. Guanine base pairs with cytosine by forming three hydrogen bonds.

NUCLEOTIDE FUNCTIONS IN CELLS

1. Nucleotide triphosphates transport energy from energy-generating chemical reactions to energy-consuming reactions within the same cell.
2. Nucleotide triphosphates serve as monomers for the synthesis of RNA and DNA.
3. Nucleotides may be modified into chemical signals for use within a cell. Cyclic AMP is an example.

RNA (Ribonucleic Acid) Structure

RNA is a polymer of *ribonucleotides* (*ribose* is the 5⁻ carbon sugar). The purine bases in RNA are adenine and guanine. The pyrimidine bases in RNA are cytosine and *uracil*. (Ribose is replaced by deoxyribose and uracil is replaced by thymine in DNA. Adenine, guanine, and cytosine occur in both RNA and DNA.)

RNA usually consists of a *single linear* chain of nucleotides. However, RNA chains may fold and form base pairs between regions of the same chain where complementary sequences occur, resulting in "hairpin" loops. Double-stranded RNA occurs as the genetic material in some viruses.

RNA Functions

Messenger RNA (mRNA) codes for the amino acid sequence (primary structure) of polypeptide chains in proteins.

Transfer RNA (tRNA) carries amino acids (as aminoacyl groups on the tRNA) into protein synthesis and uses the nucleotide sequence in a mRNA to determine where to insert the amino acid carried by the tRNA into the forming polypeptide chain. The amino acid–RNA linkage in the aminoacyl tRNA is formed using energy from nucleotide triphosphates and contains the energy needed to form the peptide bond joining the amino acid to the peptide.

Ribosomal RNAs (rRNA) form the structural framework of the ribosomal subunits, and a loop of one of the rRNA molecules appears to be capable of catalyzing the formation of peptide bonds.

Several *ribonucleoprotein (RNP) particles* containing small RNA molecules are involved in RNA and protein processing. Small nuclear ribonucleoproteins (snRNPs) that contain small RNA molecules remove introns from mRNA in eukaryotes. The signal recognition particle that recognizes membrane and secretory polypeptides forming on ribosomes is a cytoplasmic ribonucleoprotein containing a small RNA.

DNA (Deoxyribonucleic Acid) Structure

DNA is made of *deoxyribonucleotides* (*deoxyribose* is the 5-carbon sugar). The purine bases in DNA are adenine and guanine. The pyrimidine bases in DNA are cytosine and thymine.

The nucleotides within a single DNA chain or strand are joined by *covalent bonds* linking the 3' carbon on one nucleotide with the phosphate on the 5' carbon of the adjacent nucleotide.

A DNA molecule usually consists of *two linear chains* of nucleotides and is referred to as *double-stranded,* although single-stranded DNA occurs in some viruses. The two strands in a DNA molecule run in opposite directions (have opposite polarity), so the 3' end of one strand is next to the 5' end of the other strand. The two strands in a DNA molecule are most frequently twisted into a right-handed *helix*. Other possible twisting patterns such as Z form DNA appear to occur less frequently.

The two chains or strands in a DNA molecule are paired by *hydrogen bonds* between complementary base pairs (A-T, G-C). Because the hydrogen bonds between the base pairs are much weaker than the covalent bonds that join the nucleotides within a single strand, the two strands can be separated without breaking the strands. This feature is used during DNA replication and during RNA synthesis.

Genetic Information Flow in Cells

Genetic information *(genotype)* is stored in cells in the form of the sequence of deoxyribonucleotides in DNA. The double-stranded nature of DNA allows repair of damage as long as both strands are not damaged in the same location.

Genetic information is transmitted accurately from cell to cell during mitosis and from parent to offspring during reproduction because the deoxyribonucleotide sequence in the parental DNA molecules determines the deoxyribonucleotide sequence in newly formed DNA molecules during *DNA replication* (except when mutations occur).

Point mutations result from unrepaired mistakes in DNA replication or misrepaired damage in nonreplicating DNA. A point mutation is a change in the sequence of deoxyribonucleotides in DNA.

Conversion of genetic information into a cellular phenotype requires a sequence of events.

Transcription (RNA Synthesis). The deoxyribonucleotide sequence in regions of DNA (genes) codes for (serves as a template for) the ribonucleotide sequence in mRNAs. The bases in RNA can hydrogen bond to the bases in DNA, so one base in DNA specifies one base (complementary to it) in RNA.

Translation (Protein Synthesis). The ribonucleotide sequence in regions of DNA (genes) codes for (serves as a template for) the ribonucleotide sequence in mRNAs codes for the amino acid sequence in proteins (polypeptides). A three nucleotide codon in the mRNA base pairs with the complementary three nucleotide anticodon on an aminoacyl tRNA to allow the aminoacyl group (one amino acid) on the aminoacyl tRNA to be added to the polypeptide (protein) being synthesized. Therefore, a three nucleotide unit in mRNA functions as one codon to specify one amino acid in a polypeptide. A polypeptide in turn forms all or part of a protein.

The proteins form cellular structures and/or perform or catalyze cell functions. Proteins directly or indirectly produce the *phenotype* of a cell.

The phenotype of a cell consists of the structures and functions of the cell. Cell structures consist of proteins plus other molecules whose synthesis is catalyzed by proteins. Cell functions are either performed by proteins, by molecules whose synthesis was catalyzed by proteins, or are catalyzed by proteins (enzymes). Because most chemical reactions in cells do not occur unless they are catalyzed by enzymes, every function in a cell is either directly or indirectly dependent on the protein composition of the cell. The proteins in the cell therefore directly or indirectly interact with the environment of the cell to produce the phenotype of the cell.

Protein Structure

Proteins are made of 20 different types of amino acids that share a common "backbone" structure consisting of an *amino group* covalently bonded to a carbon atom (the alpha carbon), which is in turn covalently bonded to a *carboxylic acid (carboxyl) group*. Each of the 20 different types of amino acids differs in the "side chain" structure attached to the alpha carbon.

One amino acid in a polypeptide chain in a protein is specified by a sequence of three nucleotides in a *messenger RNA (mRNA)*. This three nucleotide *codon* is translated through the mediation of a *transfer RNA (tRNA)*.

The *amino acid sequence* of each polypeptide chain (its primary structure) interacts with the polypeptide's environment and with other functional components in the cell in which the polypeptide was made to determine further modifications and eventual assembly of a functional protein.

1. Many if not most polypeptides must be altered by removal of one or more amino acids from the amino-terminal end, because the functional polypeptide in a protein does not have a methionine in the amino-terminal position. Methionine is the first amino acid (N-terminal) in all newly synthesized polypeptides because the methionine codon is also the initiation codon for protein synthesis.
2. Many polypeptides require addition of prosthetic groups (such as the heme groups in hemoglobin) before the polypeptide becomes functional.
3. A polypeptide must fold into a functional shape during or after its synthesis. Chaperone proteins are required for correct folding of many polypeptides.
4. Altered forms of many polypeptides and proteins are selectively degraded by proteosomes, frequently in response to ubiquitin attachment to the polypeptide or protein.
5. A functional protein may consist of a single polypeptide chain or may contain two or more polypeptides.
6. Many proteins are activated or inactivated by phosphorylation catalyzed by protein kinases.
7. Many proteins can interconvert between two or more shapes in response to allosteric interactions. An allosteric interaction causes a shape change in a protein in response to the binding of a molecule to a location outside the normal active site of the protein.

Protein Function

Proteins serve many types of functions in cells. *Structural proteins* form all or parts of cell structures such as ribosomes, chromosomes, mitotic spindles, and cell membranes. *Enzymes* are almost all proteins and are required to catalyze most chemical reactions in cells, including DNA synthesis, RNA synthesis, protein synthesis, carbohydrate synthesis, and lipid synthesis. Most cellular reactions will not occur under normal intracellular conditions without access to the appropriate enzyme. *Transport proteins* serve as carriers or channels to allow molecules to move across cell membranes to enter cells, leave cells, or move from one part of a cell to another. *Signal* or *regulatory proteins* respond to changes in a cell by changing their interactions with critical components such as DNA, thereby altering cell functions.

Control of Use of Genetic Information

Prokaryotic cells do not use all of their genetic information all of the time, and most eukaryotic cells in complex organisms never use more than a small part of their genetic information. Therefore, use of genetic information in a cell is normally restricted and may change over time.

Cells in a complex organism all contain the same genetic information (because they were all produced from the fertilized egg by mitosis), but may have thousands of different phenotypes. Those phenotypes occur in a well-defined pattern that makes up the body of the organism. Therefore, cells can selectively use parts of their genetic information during development.

In many cases, use of regions of DNA is regulated by regulatory proteins which are produced or activated in response to signals from the cell's environment. Some regulatory proteins make DNA available for coding for RNA, others may make DNA inaccessible for coding for RNA, and some control use of mRNA after it has been produced.

Overview of Genetic Regulation in Prokaryotes and Eukaryotes

1. *Transcriptional regulation* (regulation of RNA synthesis) is the primary regulatory mechanism in prokaryotes and developing eukaryotes and is a major mechanism in adult eukaryotic cells, but post-transcriptional mechanisms can alter or modify the resulting phenotype.

2. Regulation through *differential RNA processing* is not a major mechanism in prokaryotes but has been documented in several eukaryotic systems.

3. Regulation through *differential mRNA transport* is impossible in prokaryotes but may occur in some adult eukaryotic cells and is probably a major mechanism leading to cytoplasmic localization of mRNA in developing eukaryotes.

4. Regulation through *differential mRNA degradation* probably occurs in both prokaryotes and eukaryotes, but the effects of poly-A tail length and 3' untranslated sequences on this process in eukaryotes are well documented.

5. Regulation through *differential translation* of different mRNAs occurs in prokaryotes, but the most spectacular cases have been documented in developing eukaryotes.

6. Regulation through post-translational modification of proteins occurs in both prokaryotes and eukaryotes.

QUICK RECALL TEST QUESTIONS AND ANSWERS

Choose the Best Answer

1. ATP is a:

   (A) polysaccharide.
   (B) fat.
   (C) nucleotide.
   (D) protein.

2. A molecule containing ribose, phosphate, purines, and pyrimidines is a:

   (A) protein.
   (B) phospholipid.
   (C) carbohydrate.
   (D) nucleic acid.

3. Energy is routinely released from ATP (in cells) by:

   (A) converting the entire molecule to CO_2 and water.
   (B) hydrolyzing the adenine from the ribose.
   (C) hydrolyzing one or two phosphates from the molecule.
   (D) converting ATP into NADH.

4. If one strand of a DNA molecule contains the sequence 3'A-C-G-T-A5', the other strand of the DNA molecule could contain the sequence ____ at the same location.

   (A) 3'A-C-G-T-A5'
   (B) 3'A-C-G-U-A5'
   (C) 5'T-G-C-A-T3'
   (D) 5'U-G-C-A-U3'

5. Amino acids are joined to each other to form polypeptides by condensation (dehydration synthesis) of the ____ functional group on the amino acid at the growing end of the polypeptide with the ____ functional group on the next amino acid to be added to the chain.

   (A) carboxyl, hydroxyl
   (B) hydroxyl, carboxyl
   (C) carboxyl, amino
   (D) hydroxyl, hydroxyl

6. In the primary structure of a protein, amino acids are joined together by:

   (A) peptide bonds.
   (B) phosphodiester bonds.
   (C) glycosidic bonds.
   (D) hydrophobic bonds.

7. The sequence of amino acids in a polypeptide chain is the ____ structure of the protein.

   (A) primary
   (B) secondary
   (C) tertiary
   (D) quaternary

8. Enzymes are composed mainly of:

   (A) polysaccharides.
   (B) lipids.
   (C) proteins.
   (D) nucleic acids.

9. During protein synthesis, transfer RNA:

   (A) transfers genetic information from the nucleus to the cytoplasm.
   (B) binds to codons on a mRNA to determine where the amino acid carried on the tRNA belongs in the protein.
   (C) transfers completed proteins from the nucleus to the cytoplasm.
   (D) binds to DNA to pick up genetic information which is then used by ribosomes in the cytoplasm to assemble proteins.

10. Transfer RNA carries ____ to the site of ____ synthesis.

    (A) nucleotides, DNA
    (B) nucleotides, RNA
    (C) amino acids, protein
    (D) amino acids, DNA

11. Most amino acids are specified by codons containing ____ in mRNA.

    (A) a single nucleotide
    (B) pairs of nucleotides
    (C) triplets (sets of three) of nucleotides
    (D) sets of 4 nucleotides

12. The codons that specify the sequence of amino acids in a protein occur in:

    (A) rRNA.
    (B) mRNA.
    (C) tRNA.
    (D) ribosomes.

Answers

1. **(C)** ATP has the typical structure of a nucleotide, consisting of a nitrogenous base (adenine), a 5-carbon sugar (ribose), and one or more phosphate groups (three in the case of ATP).

2. **(D)** Ribose, phosphate, purines, and pyrimidines occur in RNA, which is a nucleic acid.

3. **(C)** Converting the molecule to CO_2 and water releases energy but destroys the energy carrier, so this process is not used routinely. Hydrolyzing the adenine from the ribose does not release useful energy in most circumstances. Hydrolyzing the third or second phosphate releases useful energy and the remaining part of the molecule may be re-phosphorylated by many energy-releasing reactions.

4. **(C)** A DNA strand contains T (thymine) instead of U (uracil), which occurs in RNA, so choices **B** and **D** can be eliminated. A correct DNA strand must have the opposite orientation (since the strands in DNA are antiparallel) and must contain the complementary sequence to the strand in the question (T to pair with A, G to pair with C, C to pair with G, and A to pair with T). Only choice **C** meets these criteria.

5. **(C)** The carboxyl and amino groups are reacted to form a peptide bond through a series of steps which attach the amino acid to a transfer RNA and then eventually transfer the amino acid to the polypeptide.

6. **(A)** Phosphodiester bonds join nucleotides in RNA or DNA, glycosidic bonds join sugars in oligosaccharides or polysaccharides, and hydrophobic "bonds" are involved in protein folding and lipid-lipid attraction.

7. **(A)** Secondary structure involves the local shape of the polypeptide (alpha helix, etc.), tertiary structure involves the overall shape of the polypeptide (globular, etc.), and quaternary structure involves joining two or more polypeptides to form a functional protein.

8. **(C)** Most catalytic macromolecules (enzymes) are proteins, although a few catalytic macromolecules are RNA (nucleic acid).

9. **(B)** tRNA serves as the temporary link between mRNA and an amino acid so that the amino acid carried by the tRNA is inserted into the correct place in a growing polypeptide chain.

10. **(C)** See the answer to question 9.

11. **(C)** Each amino acid is specified by one or more codons. Each codon contains three nucleotides and base-pairs (by hydrogen bonds) with the anticodon on the tRNA carrying the amino acid.

12. **(B)** The codons in mRNA base-pair with anticodons in tRNA.

DNA REPLICATION

DNA Replication in Prokaryotes *(E. coli)*

Synthesis of new DNA strands during DNA replication is catalyzed by *DNA polymerase III*. The nucleotide sequence of the new strand is determined by base pairing with a *template strand of DNA*. The energy to form the bonds is derived from hydrolysis of two of the three phosphates attached to the *deoxyribonucleotide*, which is being added to the DNA strand. DNA polymerase can use only a single-stranded DNA template, can "read" the template strand only in the 3' → 5' direction, can assemble a new strand only in the 5' → 3' direction, and can add nucleotides only to the 3' end of an existing strand of nucleotides.

In addition to catalyzing assembly of DNA strands, DNA polymerase also checks each deoxyribonucleotide after inserting it and removes it if the base pairing is incorrect.

Two additional types of DNA polymerase (I and II) in *E. coli* cells are used in DNA repair.

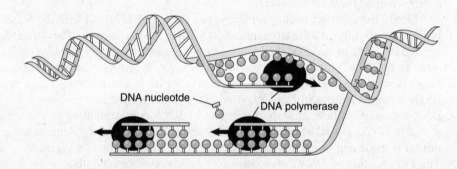

DNA replication. The DNA strands unwind, and the enzyme DNA polymerase unites nucleotides in each chain according to bases present on the old chain. The new strand then unites with an old strand to form two new double helixes.

INITIATION OF DNA REPLICATION IN PROKARYOTES

Initiation of DNA synthesis is not totally understood, but appears to occur at specific points on the DNA called replication initiation sites. A special set of proteins apparently separate the two DNA strands at the replication initiation site, allowing the components of the replication complex to assemble. An RNA primer generated by DNA Primase associated with the initiation complex is also necessary to allow initiation of synthesis of the "leading" strand.

CONTINUATION OF DNA REPLICATION (ELONGATION) IN PROKARYOTES

Once begun, DNA replication is catalyzed by a large complex of associated enzymes called a *replisome* or *replication complex*. A replication complex consists of a minimum of six enzymes, most of which are not physically associated except during DNA replication. Much of this complexity is made necessary by the characteristics of DNA polymerase.

1. *DNA Helicase* separates the two strands of the DNA molecule that will be replicated so that each strand can serve as a template for the synthesis of a new strand. ATP is hydrolyzed as the helicase moves along the DNA.

2. One *DNA Polymerase III* moves along the separated DNA strand which has a 3' "free end" and uses that strand as a template. This DNA polymerase synthesizes a continuous new strand complementary to the template strand and follows closely behind the helicase. This new strand is called the *leading strand*, and the DNA polymerase that catalyzes its formation is called the *Leading Strand DNA Polymerase*.

The other original DNA strand runs in the wrong direction to be used continuously as a template by DNA polymerase since the "free end" of the strand is the 5' end. As a result, the DNA polymerase copies this strand in a series of short (about 200 nucleotides) strands, each formed while the DNA polymerase is moving in the opposite direction from the helicase. Each of the segments must be initiated by forming an RNA primer to create a new strand with a free 3' end to which DNA polymerase III may add nucleotides, after which the RNA primer must be removed and the ends of the adjacent new segments ligated (joined). From the time that the segments are synthesized until the ligase catalyzes their joining, experimental dissociation of the hydrogen bonds holding the new strand to the template strand releases the segments as *"Okazaki fragments,"* named for their discoverer.

Due to the complex events, replication of the template strand with the 5' free end is delayed slightly relative to replication of the leading strand. The strand being formed in segments is called the *lagging strand* because its replication lags behind the other strand. The following enzymes are involved in lagging strand replication.

3. *Single-strand DNA Binding Protein* (ssb protein in *E. coli*) binds to and protects single-stranded regions of DNA exposed in the lagging strand.

4. *DNA Primase* synthesizes a short segment of RNA complementary to the template strand of DNA. The RNA primer is usually about 10 nucleotides in length, and a new primer is made approximately 200 nucleotides after the last primer segment.

5. The *Lagging Strand DNA Polymerase III* adds deoxyribonucleotides to the 3' end of the RNA primer, moving along the template strand until it contacts the 5' end of the next RNA primer. The DNA polymerase then releases the DNA and somehow "leapfrogs" back up the DNA template to the next RNA primer.

6. A *DNA Repair Complex* (containing DNA Polymerase I) then treats the RNA primer segments in the same way that the repair complex treats any other structurally abnormal segment of DNA. The abnormal part (the ribonucleotides) are removed and replaced with normal components (deoxyribonucleotides).

7. *DNA Ligase* then joins the free ends of adjacent segments of the new DNA strand to form a continuous strand.

TERMINATION OF DNA REPLICATION IN PROKARYOTES

Termination of DNA replication, like initiation of DNA replication, is not completely understood. In some prokaryotes, termination apparently occurs at precise points on the DNA, possibly due to a protein bound to the DNA. In other systems, termination appears to occur when two replication complexes moving in opposite directions along the DNA collide.

DNA Replication in Eukaryotes

Synthesis of new DNA strands during DNA replication in eukaryotic cells is similar to the process in prokaryotes, but several differences have been reported. Synthesis of the new DNA strands is catalyzed by *DNA polymerase alpha* (lagging strand) and *DNA polymerase delta* (leading strand). This represents a major difference from prokaryotes in which two molecules of the same type of polymerase are involved. DNA repair uses a separate enzyme (DNA polymerase beta) as is the case in prokaryotes. DNA replication in mitochondria uses a single type of polymerase (DNA polymerase gamma) that is distinct from the nuclear enzymes and apparently functions in a prokaryotic pattern.

The rest of the mechanism appears similar to the process in prokaryotes. The nucleotide sequence of the new strand is determined by base pairing with a template strand of DNA. The energy to form the bonds is derived from hydrolysis of two of the three phosphates attached to the deoxyribonucleotide which is being added to the DNA strand. Both DNA polymerases can use only a single-stranded DNA template, can "read" the template strand only in the $3' \rightarrow 5'$ direction, can assemble a new strand only in the $5' \rightarrow 3'$ direction, and can add nucleotides only to the 3' end of an existing strand of nucleotides. Error checking of inserted nucleotides appears to occur in eukaryotic DNA replication, but the isolated nuclear DNA polymerases lack the exonuclease activity responsible for error checking in prokaryotes.

When a nucleic acid sequence is written out, it is assumed that the 5' end is first and the 3' end last unless otherwise noted. Therefore, ATGTGCA is 5'-ATGTGCA-3' and the Watson-Crick complementary sequence is TGCACAT (5'-TGCACAT-3' or 3'-TACACGT-5')—not TACACGT, which would be the wrong polarity. This is true of all nucleic acid pairings, including DNA-DNA, DNA-RNA and codon-anticodon interactions.

Chromosomal Replication Patterns in Eukaryotes

Initiation of replication occurs at numerous points within each region of a eukaryotic chromosome. Different parts of the same chromosome are replicated at different points in the S (DNA synthesis) phase of the cell cycle. A cluster of simultaneously active replication origins is called a *replication unit*.

In mature body cells, initiation appears to occur at specific points on the DNA called *replication initiation sites* or *replication origins* (called *autonomous replicating sequences* in yeast). In oocytes and some early embryonic cells, initiation appears to occur at much larger than normal numbers of sites on each chromosome, and injected bacterial DNA is replicated at the same time as chromosomal DNA is replicated, thus indicating that initiation is apparently occurring irrespective of the nucleotide sequence in the DNA. The proteins involved in either case have not been clearly identified.

Termination of DNA replication, like initiation of DNA replication, is not well understood in eukaryotes. Some mechanism of precise termination is essential because of the multiple initiation points which do not operate simultaneously and which could easily lead to excess replication.

Nonsimultaneous replication of the DNA molecule extending from end to end in a chromosome requires a mechanism to prevent repeated replication of any parts of the DNA during any one S phase. Mammalian cells appear to achieve this through an unknown inhibitor of DNA replication which is associated with replicated regions of chromosomes from the time of their replication during S phase until the cell divides. The evidence for this is that fusing a cell in S phase with a cell in G2 fails to trigger DNA replication in the G2 nucleus. However, fusing a cell in S phase with a cell in G1 triggers DNA replication in the G1 nucleus.

Tangle Prevention During DNA Replication in Prokaryotes and Eukaryotes

Excessive twisting of DNA or interlocked loops of DNA are prevented by *topoisomerase* enzymes, which fall into the same categories in prokaryotes and eukaryotes.

Type I topoisomerases occur in both prokaryotes and eukaryotes. Although the detailed mechanisms differ, these enzymes all temporarily clip one strand of a double-stranded DNA to allow untwisting.

Type II topoisomerases also occur in both prokaryotes and eukaryotes. These enzymes cut both strands of one DNA double-stranded helix to allow a second double-stranded helix to pass through. This is used to separate interlocked loops in prokaryotes and in mitochondria. Topoisomerase II is bound to nuclear DNA at intervals and may attach DNA to the chromosomal scaffolding as well as to reduce tangling during replication.

DNA Repair in Prokaryotes and Eukaryotes

Repair of damage to DNA can occur by at least three fundamentally different pathways in *E. coli* (and presumably other prokaryotes) and in some eukaryotes. Two of these three mechanisms occur in other eukaryotes.

1. **Photoreactivation. Pyrimidine dimers** produced by ultraviolet light can be repaired by *photoreactivation* without excision of components. The enzyme that catalyzes the repair is called DNA photolyase or *photoreactivating enzyme* and is the product of a single gene. The enzyme uses visible light energy to remove the covalent bonds generated by the UV light. This system is active in many prokaryotes and plants, but is absent in many animals, including humans.

2. **Base Excision Repair.** Some single damaged nitrogenous bases (especially uracil) can be removed from their deoxyribose by a glycosylase enzyme, after which one or more nucleotides in the damaged area are removed and replaced. This process is called *base excision repair* and occurs in both prokaryotes and eukaryotes.

3. **Nucleotide Excision Repair.** This more generalized process can remove almost any type of damage as long as one of the two DNA strands is undamaged. In this case, a stretch of nucleotides is removed, then replaced by a new strand whose assembly is catalyzed by a DNA polymerase. Methylation of the older DNA strand in the molecule is apparently used to decide which is the preferable template strand when a mismatch occurs without obvious damage. This process occurs in both prokaryotes and eukaryotes, but the size of the region that is excised differs in different organisms.

QUICK RECALL TEST QUESTIONS AND ANSWERS

Choose the Best Answer

1. In most prokaryotes, initiation of DNA replication appears to occur:

    (A) at specific sites on the DNA that are used in each replication cycle.
    (B) at random locations on the DNA that change from one replication cycle to the next.

2. Initiation of replication in prokaryotes and eukaryotes appears to use a similar mechanism in which protein factors (different in each case) bind to the initiation sequences on the DNA and separate the strands to allow replication.

    (A) TRUE
    (B) FALSE

3. The enzyme (catalyst) for DNA replication is:

    (A) DNA.
    (B) mRNA.
    (C) DNA polymerase.
    (D) RNA polymerase.

4. The template (information source) for DNA replication is:

    (A) DNA.
    (B) mRNA.
    (C) DNA polymerase.
    (D) RNA polymerase.

5. The raw material (reactant) for DNA replication is:

    (A) DNA.
    (B) deoxyribonucleotide monophosphate.
    (C) deoxyribonucleotide triphosphate.
    (D) ribonucleotide monophosphate.

6. DNA replication in prokaryotes:

    (A) produces both new strands continuously by adding nucleotides to the end of the strands.
    (B) polymerizes nucleotides into short segments, then joins the segments using a ligase enzyme to form both new strands.
    (C) produces one new strand continuously by adding nucleotides to the end of the strand. Replication of the other strand polymerizes nucleotides into short segments, then joins the segments using a ligase enzyme to form the other new strand.

7. The enzyme that catalyzes the replication of the leading strand during DNA replication in *E. coli* is:

    (A) RNA polymerase.
    (B) DNA polymerase I.
    (C) DNA polymerase II.
    (D) DNA polymerase III.

8. The enzyme that catalyzes the replication of the lagging strand during DNA replication in *E. coli* is:

    (A) RNA polymerase.
    (B) DNA polymerase I.
    (C) DNA polymerase II.
    (D) DNA polymerase III.

9. Initiation of synthesis of a new DNA segment complementary to the lagging strand template requires synthesis of ____ before the Okazaki fragment of DNA can be extended from its 3' end.

    (A) an RNA primer
    (B) a DNA primer
    (C) a protein primer
    (D) a new DNA polymerase

10. The function of DNA ligase in DNA replication in prokaryotes is to:

    (A) join adjacent Okazaki fragments on the lagging strand.
    (B) fill in the gaps created by primer removal on the lagging strand.
    (C) synthesize RNA primers on the lagging strand.
    (D) add deoxyribonucleotides to the new leading strand.

11. The function of topoisomerases I and II in DNA replication in prokaryotes is to:

    (A) join adjacent Okazaki fragments on the lagging strand.
    (B) fill in the gaps created by primer removal on the lagging strand.
    (C) synthesize RNA primers on the lagging strand.
    (D) remove excess twisting of the DNA molecules.

12. A mutation that caused loss of the 3'→5' exonuclease proofreading activity from *E. coli* DNA polymerase III but had no effect on the catalysis of phosphodiester bond formation would ____ the rate of DNA replication and would ____ the mutation rate in the bacteria.

    (A) have no effect on, have no effect on
    (B) slightly increase, increase
    (C) slightly reduce, decrease
    (D) slightly increase, decrease

13. Photoreactivation-type DNA repair involves:

    (A) chemical reversal of the damage without removal of bases or nucleotides.
    (B) removal of a single base followed by excision and replacement of a segment of nucleotides.
    (C) removal and replacement of a segment of nucleotides.

14. Base excision-type DNA repair involves:

    (A) chemical reversal of the damage without removal of bases or nucleotides.
    (B) removal of a single base followed by excision and replacement of a segment of nucleotides.
    (C) removal and replacement of a segment of nucleotides.

15. Nucleotide excision-type DNA repair involves:

    (A) chemical reversal of the damage without removal of bases or nucleotides.
    (B) removal of a single base followed by excision and replacement of a segment of nucleotides.
    (C) removal and replacement of a segment of nucleotides.

Answers

1. **(A)** Initiation occurs at specific sites, typically one per chromosome in prokaryotes.

2. **(A)** Although the specific proteins involved probably differ, the processes involved in initiation appear to use similar mechanisms.

3. **(C)** DNA polymerase enzymes of different types catalyze chromosomal replication and DNA replication during DNA repair processes.

4. **(A)** Each existing DNA strand in a DNA molecule serves as a template for assembly of a new strand of DNA (catalyzed by DNA polymerase) during DNA replication.

5. **(C)** DNA contains deoxyribonucleotides, not ribonucleotides (that is why it's called DNA instead of RNA). The extra two phosphates on each deoxyribonucleotide are removed when the nucleotide is added to the new DNA strand and provide the energy to form the new phosphodiester bond.

6. **(C)** The continuously formed strand is the leading strand, and the strand made in segments is the lagging strand. The discontinuous replication of the lagging strand is caused by the lack of a form of DNA polymerase that can add to the 5' end of a growing DNA strand, so only the existing strand with the correct orientation is replicated continuously.

7. **(D)** Separate molecules of DNA polymerase III catalyze replication of the leading strand and the lagging strand in *E. coli*.

8. **(D)** Separate molecules of DNA polymerase III catalyze replication of the leading strand and the lagging strand in *E. coli*.

9. **(A)** Remember that DNA polymerase can add nucleotides only to existing strands, but RNA polymerase enzymes (like the primase) can initiate new strands.

10. **(A)** DNA ligase is needed to join the DNA fragments (called Okazaki fragments, after their discoverer) resulting from the lagging strand replication.

11. **(D)** Type I topoisomerases primarily reduce twisting. Type II topoisomerases may also allow separation of interlocked loops of DNA.

12. **(B)** This mutation should slightly speed up replication, because the enzyme would not be degrading any mispaired bases in the newly synthesized DNA strand. As a result, however, the frequency of new mutations would be greatly increased.

13. **(A)** Photoreactivation usually achieves repair without excision of entire nucleotides.

14. **(B)** Base excision repair begins with removal of one or more damaged bases, usually followed by excision of the rest of the nucleotides associated with the damaged bases.

15. **(C)** Nucleotide excision usually involves removal of a patch of nucleotides surrounding the damaged region in the DNA.

OVERALL GENETIC ORGANIZATION OF PROKARYOTIC CELLS

The DNA in prokaryotic cells is located in the cytoplasm, so DNA replication, RNA synthesis (transcription), and protein synthesis (translation) occur in the same cellular compartment.

In some cases a single structural gene (DNA coding an mRNA, which codes for one polypeptide) is controlled as a single unit. In most cases, a single promoter (binding site for RNA polymerase to initiate RNA synthesis) controls a series of structural genes that are transcribed as a single mRNA with a series of translation initiation and termination points. The mRNA is translated to form all or some of the enzymes for a biochemical pathway. A cluster of structural genes controlled by a single promoter is called an *operon*.

Translation of a mRNA molecule typically begins before transcription of the mRNA is complete. This allows very rapid changes in cellular phenotype through transcriptional control mechanisms.

In most cases of both single gene units and operons, access to the promoter by RNA polymerase is controlled by one or more regulatory proteins that respond to conditions in the cell.

Cytoplasmic proteins have rapid access to DNA because the DNA is not separated from the cytoplasm by a nuclear membrane. Therefore, proteins that alter transcription can act very quickly after they are altered by cytoplasmic conditions.

Transcription in Prokaryotes

RNA synthesis (transcription) in prokaryotes follows the general pattern typical of all RNA synthesis in normal cells. The template or sequence information source is one of the two nucleotide strands in a DNA molecule, the enzyme that catalyzes the process is RNA polymerase, and the reactants that combine to form the new RNA strand are ribonucleotide triphosphates containing adenine, guanine, cytosine, or uracil. Release of two of the three phosphates from each nucleotide as it is bonded to the chain provides the energy for bond formation. The process of transcription may be subdivided into initiation, elongation, and termination phases. Locations on the DNA are described relative to the RNA polymerase movement during transcription. The polymerase moves toward downstream locations and away from upstream locations.

INITIATION OF TRANSCRIPTION IN PROKARYOTES

Prokaryotes typically use a single type of *RNA polymerase* (the core enzyme) in combination with multiple *sigma factors* for initiation of RNA synthesis. RNA polymerase complexed with one of the sigma factors binds to a *promoter sequence* on the DNA just upstream of the starting point for RNA synthesis. The position and orientation of the DNA sequence in the promoter regions determines the position and orientation of the RNA polymerase, which in turn determines the location of the starting point for RNA synthesis and determines which DNA strand serves as a template. Because each sigma factor recognizes a different promoter sequence, a prokaryote can use availability of different sigma factors to switch large-scale processes such as nitrogen metabolism, heat shock responses, or sporulation on or off.

CONTROL OF INITIATION OF TRANSCRIPTION IN PROKARYOTES

In an actively growing prokaryote, most of the operons that are used are transcribed by RNA polymerase, which initiates RNA synthesis complexed to a single type of sigma factor (sigma 70 in *E. coli*). Two types of control systems control initiation of RNA synthesis in these operons.

1. *Activator Proteins.* Many promoters do not bind the RNA polymerase-sigma factor complex effectively unless an *activator protein* is bound upstream of the promoter. These operons are not fully active unless the activator protein is available in a form that can bind to the activator site on the DNA. Availability of functional activator

protein is controlled by interactions between the protein and critical molecules in the cytoplasm.

As an example, the lac operon (like several other metabolic operons) in *E. coli* requires binding of the catabolite activator protein (CAP) to a site just upstream of the promoter. Active metabolism due to abundant glucose results in low cyclic AMP levels in the cytoplasm. Because CAP requires cyclic AMP for activity, CAP is inactive under these conditions. As a result, turning on the other transcription control system in the lac operon results in very little transcription as long as glucose is readily available. Starvation increases cyclic AMP levels, resulting in active CAP. Under these conditions, the activator site is usually complexed with CAP, so turning on the other control system results in very rapid transcription.

2. *Repressor Proteins.* Many operons have a protein-binding sequence called an *operator sequence* located downstream of and overlapping the promoter. The operator sequence binds a *repressor protein* which prevents transcription of the operon. Availability of functional repressor protein is controlled by interactions between the protein and critical molecules in the cytoplasm.

In the case of the lac operon in *E. coli,* the unaltered repressor protein binds to the operator sequence. Therefore, the lac operon is normally totally turned off regardless of the status of CAP. However, when lactose is available in the cell's environment, binding of lactose or related molecules inactivates the repressor protein. In the absence of active CAP, this results in a low rate of transcription of the genes in the lac operon. In the presence of active CAP, the result is active transcription of the genes in the operon.

At the beginning of the initiation process, the complex of the RNA polymerase core enzyme plus the appropriate sigma factor initially binds to the double-stranded DNA to form a closed complex in which the two DNA strands are still held together by base-pair hydrogen bonding. The closed complex becomes an open complex when the polymerase binds more tightly to the DNA and forces the two DNA strands apart along a short region. Synthesis of the new RNA strand begins in the open complex. Only the DNA strand oriented in the correct direction (3' → 5') is used as a template.

THE ELONGATION PHASE OF TRANSCRIPTION IN PROKARYOTES

As each ribonucleotide triphosphate base-pairs with the exposed bases on the DNA template, the 3' hydroxyl on the previously added nucleotide binds to the proximal (next to the sugar) phosphate on the newly base-paired ribonucleotide, forming the new phosphodiester bond and releasing the terminal two phosphates (which provides the energy to form the bond).

At about the point that the new RNA chain reaches ten nucleotides in length, the sigma factor is released from the RNA polymerase, the core enzyme becomes more compact, and one or more elongation factors may bind to the RNA polymerase. Elongation continues from the time the RNA polymerase leaves the initiation site just downstream of the promoter until the RNA polymerase encounters a termination sequence. As the RNA polymerase moves along the DNA, the newly formed RNA strand is separated from the DNA template strand and the two DNA strands reassociate.

TERMINATION OF TRANSCRIPTION IN PROKARYOTES

Sites at which transcription terminates in prokaryotes frequently contain nucleotide sequences in the RNA that allow base-pairing to form a hairpin loop. In many cases the loop is enriched in guanine and cytosine and the RNA just downstream of the loop is rich in uridine. Sites of this type appear to cause termination without intervention of protein termination factors and are called *rho-independent termination sites*. Termination sites that lack the guanine and cytosine-rich region in the hairpin loop and lack the adjacent uridine-rich region typically require a protein termination factor called *rho* for efficient termination. These sites are called *rho-dependent termination sites*. In either case, when termination occurs, the RNA polymerase detaches from the DNA and releases the RNA strand.

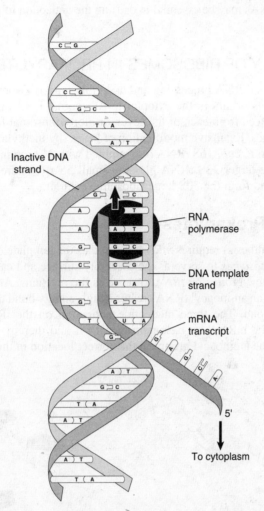

Inactive DNA strand

RNA polymerase

DNA template strand

mRNA transcript

5'

To cytoplasm

Transcription in protein synthesis. A strand of mRNA forms according to the complementary base sequence in one strand of the DNA molecule. This synthesis transcribes the DNA message to an RNA molecule. The mRNA molecule then carries the genetic message to the cytoplasm for protein synthesis.

Post-Transcriptional Processing of RNA in Prokaryotes

mRNA PROCESSING IN PROKARYOTES

Messenger RNA in prokaryotes is usually translated without modification, in most cases with translation beginning before transcription has been completed.

rRNA AND tRNA PROCESSING IN PROKARYOTES

Ribosomal RNAs and tRNAs are typically transcribed as large RNA molecules, which are then cut apart by ribonucleases to release the functional RNAs. Ribosomal RNA genes in *E. coli* occur in at least six transcriptional units, each containing one 16S, one 23S, and one 5S rRNA gene separated by intervening spacer RNA regions. Most of these transcriptional units also contain one or two tRNA sequences. The remaining tRNAs are transcribed singly or in clustered units that must be cut apart.

Both rRNAs and tRNAs also require modification of numerous bases on the nucleotides prior to becoming functional. The functions of base modification in rRNAs are unclear, but modified bases in some tRNAs may be essential in causing the anticodon to pair with the correct set of codons.

INITIAL ASSEMBLY OF RIBOSOMES IN PROKARYOTES

In prokaryotes, ribosomal RNA processing and assembly with ribosomal proteins to form the large and small subunits occurs in the cytoplasm. Ribosomal RNAs are cut out of the large initial transcripts produced from each of the seven or more ribosomal RNA transcription units by ribonuclease enzymes. Extensive modification of bases (by methylation) occurs in all three size classes of rRNA. In *E. coli,* 16S rRNA is assembled with 21 proteins to form the 30S small ribosomal subunit. The larger 23S rRNA plus the small 5S rRNA are assembled along with more than 30 proteins to form the 50S large ribosomal subunit.

Translation in Prokaryotes

Translation (protein synthesis) requires *mRNA* to serve as the template or amino acid sequence information source, *ribosomes* to serve as the assembly surface and catalyst for peptide bond formation, and *aminoacyl groups on tRNA* to serve as the reactants. Attachment of the amino acid to a tRNA to form an aminoacyl tRNA creates a high-energy bond that provides the energy to form the peptide bond. The three nucleotide anticodon on the tRNA "reads" the three nucleotide codon on the mRNA by base-pairing with it and thereby places the amino acid carried by the tRNA (the aminoacyl group) in the correct location in the growing polypeptide.

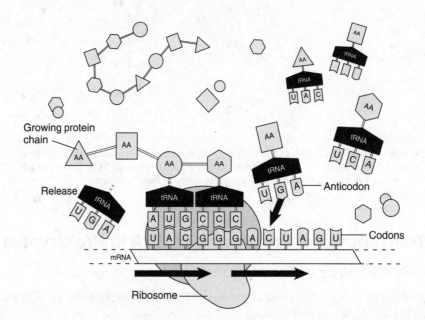

Translation in protein synthesis. A strand of mRNA arrives at the ribosome, where it is met by molecules of tRNA carrying amino acids. The tRNA molecules have three-base sequences (anticodons) that complement three-base sequences (codons) on the mRNA. This matching places the amino acids in a certain position: then they are attached to the growing protein chain. In this manner, the genetic code is translated to an amino acid sequence of a protein.

AMINOACYLATION OF tRNAS

Aminoacyl groups are attached to tRNAs by *aminoacyl synthetase* enzymes. Each amino acid appears to be attached to its tRNAs by a single type of aminoacyl synthetase that distinguishes that amino acid from the other 19, some of which may be very similar chemically. The aminoacyl synthesase must also clearly distinguish the one or more tRNAs which carry that amino acid from all other tRNAs. All aminoacyl synthesase enzymes appear to use the same reaction mechanism to attach the aminoacyl group to the tRNA. The linkage between the aminoacyl group and the tRNA contains sufficient energy to drive the formation of a peptide bond when the aminoacyl group is transferred during translation.

INITIATION OF TRANSLATION

In *E. coli,* three protein *initiation factors* and a special *formylmethionyltRNA initiator tRNA* (fMet-tRNAi) are required for initiation of translation. The small ribosomal subunit recognizes the 5' end of the mRNA and the fMet-tRNAi binds to the AUG *initiation codon* on the mRNA positioned in the P site on the ribosome. The larger ribosomal subunit then binds to the small subunit-mRNA-fMet-tRNAi complex, completing initiation.

THE ELONGATION PHASE OF TRANSLATION

Elongation requires the aminoacyl-tRNA whose anticodon will base-pair to the next codon in the mRNA and three elongation factors. An elongation factor carries the next aminoacyl-tRNA into the A site on the ribosome, and a rRNA loop on the ribosome catalyzes formation of the new peptide bond.

TERMINATION OF TRANSLATION

Termination in *E. coli* requires one of two closely related *protein termination factors* that recognize the termination codons. The result of termination is release of the polypeptide from the tRNA to which it is attached, release of the ribosome from the mRNA, and dissociation of the small and large ribosomal subunits.

QUICK RECALL TEST QUESTIONS AND ANSWERS

Choose the Best Answer

1. Most of the genes in prokaryotes are organized into operons containing a regulatory complex that controls a series of DNA regions which code for mRNAs or rRNAs and tRNAs.

   (A) TRUE
   (B) FALSE

2. The primary chromosome in a typical prokaryote:

   (A) is a series of interlocked DNA circles.
   (B) is a single circular DNA molecule.
   (C) is a single linear DNA molecule with two free ends.
   (D) is a series of linear DNA molecules, each with a pair of free ends.

3. The enzyme (catalyst) for RNA synthesis in prokaryotes is:

   (A) DNA.
   (B) mRNA.
   (C) RNA polymerase.
   (D) part of the structure of the ribosome.

4. The template (information source) for RNA synthesis is:

   (A) DNA.
   (B) mRNA.
   (C) RNA polymerase.
   (D) part of the structure of the ribosome.

5. The raw material (reactant) for RNA synthesis is:

   (A) deoxyribonucleotide monophosphate.
   (B) deoxyribonucleotide triphosphate.
   (C) ribonucleotide monophosphate.
   (D) ribonucleotide triphosphate.

6. When mRNA is synthesized by an RNA polymerase:

   (A) both DNA strands serve as templates to produce two types of RNA.
   (B) one of the DNA strands serves as a template and the other strand is not used.
   (C) both DNA strands are averaged to determine the RNA sequence.

7. RNA polymerase in *E. coli*:

   (A) can initiate new RNA strands and add nucleotides to the 5' end of existing RNA strands.
   (B) can initiate new RNA strands and add nucleotides to the 3' end of existing RNA strands.
   (C) can initiate new RNA strands and add nucleotides to either the 3' end or the 5' end of existing RNA strands.
   (D) cannot initiate new RNA strands but can add nucleotides to the 5' end of existing RNA strands.

8. RNA polymerase attaches to the ___ region of a prokaryote operon to begin RNA synthesis.

   (A) operator
   (B) promoter
   (C) repressor
   (D) structural gene

9. An appropriate sigma factor is required for ____ in prokaryotes.

   (A) initiation of transcription
   (B) initiation of translation
   (C) elongation during transcription
   (D) elongation during translation

10. The functions of the promotor region in a prokaryotic operon include:

    (A) serving as a template for the synthesis of messenger RNA.
    (B) serving as an attachment site for RNA polymerase.
    (C) serving as a binding site for repressor proteins.
    (D) coding for the amino acid sequence of one or more enzymes.

11. In an inducible operon (i.e., the lac operon in *E. coli*), the repressor protein coded by the regulator gene binds to the ____ to inactivate the operon.

    (A) promotor
    (B) operator sequence
    (C) regulator gene
    (D) first structural gene in the operon

12. The enzyme (catalyst) for protein synthesis in prokaryotes is:

    (A) mRNA.
    (B) DNA polymerase.
    (C) RNA polymerase.
    (D) part of the structure of the ribosome.

13. The template (information source) for protein synthesis in prokaryotes is:

    (A) mRNA.
    (B) DNA polymerase.
    (C) RNA polymerase.
    (D) part of the structure of the ribosome.

14. The raw material (reactant) for protein synthesis in prokaryotes is:

    (A) mRNA.
    (B) part of the structure of the ribosome.
    (C) free amino acid.
    (D) aminoacyl tRNA.

15. In prokaryotes, most amino acids are specified by ____ in mRNA.

    (A) a single type of codon
    (B) several different types of codons

16. Initiation of translation in *E. coli* (a prokaryote) involves all of the following EXCEPT:

    (A) recognition of the mRNA by the small ribosomal subunit.
    (B) fMet-tRNA.
    (C) attachment of the small ribosomal subunit to the large ribosomal subunit.
    (D) two releasing factors.

17. Attachment of the aminoacyl groups to tRNA molecules in prokaryotes is catalyzed by:

    (A) a single form of enzyme which can attach any amino acid to any tRNA.
    (B) a single form of enzyme for each amino acid which can attach that amino acid to any tRNA which recognizes a codon for that amino acid.
    (C) a single form of enzyme for each tRNA which can attach the amino acid for which the tRNA recognizes a codon.
    (D) multiple forms of enzymes for each tRNA which can attach the amino acid for which the tRNA recognizes a codon.

18. Initiation of protein synthesis on a prokaryotic mRNA occurs:

    (A) wherever a ribosome attaches to the mRNA (randomly along the molecule).
    (B) at the first AUG codon in the mRNA molecule after each ribosome attachment point.
    (C) at the poly-A tail on the mRNA.
    (D) at the first nonsense (termination) codon on the mRNA.

Answers

1. **(A)** Operon organization appears to be typical of most prokaryotic genes.

2. **(B)** The primary or main chromosome and the episomes or plasmids in prokaryotes are typically circular.

3. **(C)** RNA polymerase is the catalyst for all genome-encoded RNA synthesis. Most prokaryotes contain a single type of RNA polymerase, whereas eukaryotes typically contain three nuclear RNA polymerases.

4. **(A)** The nucleotide sequence in most RNA (except poly-A "tails") is coded by DNA.

5. **(D)** RNA contains ribonucleotides, not deoxyribonucleotides (that is why it's called RNA instead of DNA). The extra two phosphates on each ribonucleotide are removed when the nucleotide is added to the new RNA strand and provide the energy to form the new phosphodiester bond.

6. **(B)** A single strand of the DNA serves as a template for RNA synthesis. If promoters are located appropriately to initiate RNA synthesis using both strands of DNA in a given region (e.g., in the DNA of some viruses), only one strand can be used by one RNA polymerase at a time.

7. **(B)** RNA polymerase can add to the 3' end of existing strands (as can DNA polymerase), but unlike DNA polymerase, RNA polymerase can initiate new strands.

8. **(B)** The promoter is the region of DNA recognized by RNA polymerase (in prokaryotes) or by a cluster of transcription initiation factors (in eukaryotes), leading to initiation of RNA synthesis (transcription).

9. **(A)** The sigma factor is required for initiation and is then released, so it is not needed for elongation or termination.

10. **(B)** Repressor protein binding sites in some operons may overlap the promoter region, but the promoter region is defined by RNA polymerase binding.

11. **(B)** The operator sequence is defined by repressor protein binding. The operator sequence may partially overlap the promoter and/or the first structural gene in some operons.

12. **(D)** A loop of rRNA appears to catalyze peptide bond formation.

13. **(A)** The sequence of nucleotides in mRNA (read in groups of three as codons) determines the sequence of amino acids in the polypeptide being synthesized.

14. **(D)** The aminoacyl group on tRNA is ready to participate in protein synthesis. A free amino acid would have to be activated and attached to tRNA as an aminoacyl group before it could be used in protein synthesis.

15. **(B)** Almost all amino acids are specified by two or more codons.

16. **(D)** Releasing factors are involved in termination of translation instead of initiation. All of the other choices are involved in initiation.

17. **(B)** In both prokaryotes and eukaryotes, a single enzyme appears to load a particular amino acid onto all tRNAs which can carry that amino acid.

18. **(B)** The AUG codon is the codon for methionine. In prokaryotes, the first methionine codon after each ribosome attachment point on an mRNA serves as the initiation codon and binds initiator tRNA carrying N-formylmethionine.

OVERALL GENETIC ORGANIZATION OF EUKARYOTIC CELLS

Because the nuclear DNA in eukaryotic cells is separated from the cytoplasm by the nuclear envelope, DNA replication and RNA synthesis (transcription) occur in a different compartment (the nucleus) from protein synthesis (translation), which occurs in the cytoplasm. In addition, nuclear DNA exists in complex chromatin structures and extensive processing of most RNA types occurs between their transcription and their function. Additional complexity results from large amounts of nuclear DNA for which the functions are unknown and the presence of DNA-based genetic systems in mitochondria and chloroplasts which function in an integrated fashion with the nuclear genetic system.

Several functionally distinct categories of DNA can be described in eukaryotes.

1. Protein-coding DNA. Some DNA regions code for functional amino acid sequence-coding regions of mRNA molecules. In most eukaryotic cells, each structural gene coding for the mRNA which is translated into a single polypeptide typically has its own promoter and associated genetic control regions. This differs strikingly from the operon organization typical of most genes in prokaryotes.

About 50% of apparent protein-coding genes occur as single copies per haploid genome and have no closely related protein-coding genes in the genome.

About 50% of apparent protein-coding genes occur as families containing 2 to 1,000 closely related but nonidentical versions per haploid genome. In very closely related genes, the proteins have very similar properties; in less closely related gene families, however, the proteins may have evolved into very different functional roles while retaining recognizable sequence homology.

Histone genes are apparently unique among protein-coding genes in that histone genes occur as a cluster which is tandemly repeated 20 to 50 times.

2. RNA-coding DNA. Genes that code for structural RNAs typically occur in tandemly repeated units in eukaryotes. Large rRNA molecules are coded by 250 copies of a tandemly repeated cluster. 5S rRNA genes occur in about 2,000 copies and are located separately from other rRNA genes. Transfer RNA genes vary, with most types occurring in 10 to 100 copies.

3. Noncoding DNA. More than 70% of the DNA sequences in a multicellular eukaryote are not represented in functional mRNA, rRNA, or tRNA molecules in the cytoplasm.

Some of this DNA has known functions. *Regulatory protein-binding sequences* may or may not be transcribed, depending on their location relative to the structural gene sequence. This DNA has clear functions, however, independent of its transcription because it is involved in regulation of transcription of nearby structural genes. *Intron* and *spacer DNA* sequences are transcribed but they are removed during processing and do not appear in the cytoplasm as parts of functional RNAs. The functions of most of these sequences are not understood. Some spacer DNA regions may serve simple mechanical connection functions.

Other categories of DNA lack obvious functions. *Mobile (transposable) element DNA* has no known functions that benefit the cells that contain it. The Alu sequence in humans comprises 6% of the nuclear DNA, but appears to be defective copies of the 7SL gene that now function as *retroposons* (transposable elements which utilize RNA copies in the same way as retroviruses). The normal copies of this gene encode the RNA component of the signal recognition particle in protein synthesis. The L1 transposable element comprises about 4% of the nuclear DNA and codes for a reverse transcriptase. This transposable element also is a retroposon. Numerous other mobile elements occur in much lower numbers of copies per cell.

Simple sequence DNA has some identified functions (telomeres) but many regions have no known function. Satellite DNA located near centromeres is puzzling because it occurs in large numbers of copies (suggesting some important function), but shows rapid changes (indicating that mutations have no harmful effects).

Transcription in Eukaryotes

RNA synthesis in eukaryotes is mechanistically similar to the process in prokaryotes. The *template* or sequence information source is one of the two nucleotide strands in a *DNA molecule*; the enzyme, which catalyzes the process, is one of the three types of *RNA polymerase* in eukaryotes (each type catalyzes synthesis of a different class of RNA); and the *reactants*, which combine to form the new RNA strand, are *ribonucleotide triphosphates* containing adenine, guanine, cytosine, or uracil. The process of transcription may be subdivided into initiation, elongation, and termination phases.

EUKARYOTIC RNA POLYMERASE ENZYMES

Eukaryotic cells typically contain three distinct RNA polymerase core enzymes (Pol I, Pol II, and Pol III). Each core enzyme transcribes a distinct class of genes and responds to a distinct set of transcription factors. The core structure of all three RNA polymerases is much more complex than in prokaryotic RNA polymerase.

Enzyme	RNA Pol I	RNA Pol II	RNA Pol III
Genes transcribed	Class I	Class II	Class III
Gene products (after processing)	rRNA	mRNA U1–U5 snRNP	tRNA, 5S rRNA, U6 snRNP

INITIATION OF TRANSCRIPTION IN EUKARYOTES

The promoter sequences in Class I and Class II genes are primarily upstream of the starting point for transcription. The promoter sequences in most Class III genes are downstream of the starting point for transcription.

TATA binding protein is involved in initiation of at least some genes in all three classes, but the other transcription initiation factors appear to be distinct for each class of genes.

Multiple proteins are required for initiation of transcription of genes in all three classes. These transcription initiation factors bind to the DNA in the promoter region, after which RNA polymerase of the appropriate type binds to the DNA-protein complex.

REGULATION OF INITIATION OF TRANSCRIPTION IN INDIVIDUAL CLASS II GENES

Regulatory sequences for class II genes may be located near the upstream end of the promoter region, far upstream of the promoter, downstream of the promoter within introns in the structural gene, or downstream of the structural gene.

Regulatory DNA sequences that bind proteins that increase transcription of the associated genes are called *enhancers* and the proteins that bind to the enhancers are called *gene activator proteins*. Many gene activator proteins act by directly interacting with the complex of general transcription factors, apparently as a result of loop formation by the intervening DNA.

Regulatory DNA sequences that bind proteins that decrease transcription of the associated genes are called *repressor binding sites*, and the proteins that bind to the enhancers are called *gene repressor proteins*. Repressor proteins may act by blocking enhancer functions or by inhibiting general transcription factor complex formation at the promoter.

A single structural gene may be associated with large numbers of regulatory sequences, each of which leads to activation or inhibition of transcription of the gene under a particular set of conditions.

THE ELONGATION PHASE OF TRANSCRIPTION IN EUKARYOTES

The elongation phase of transcription appears identical in prokaryotes and eukaryotes. As each ribonucleotide triphosphate base-pairs with the exposed bases on the DNA template, the 3' hydroxyl on the previously added nucleotide binds to the proximal (next to the sugar) phosphate on the newly base-paired ribonucleotide, forming the new phosphodiester bond and releasing the terminal two phosphates (which provides the energy to form the bond). As the RNA polymerase moves along the DNA template, the DNA strands are separated just ahead of the active site for RNA synthesis. Just behind the active site, the RNA strand is separated from the DNA template and the DNA strands are allowed to re-form complementary base pairs. Elongation continues from the time the RNA polymerase leaves the initiation site until termination occurs.

TERMINATION OF TRANSCRIPTION IN EUKARYOTES

Termination of transcription of class I genes appears to depend on sequences located downstream from the termination site. The mode of action of these sequences is unclear, but at least one soluble protein is needed.

Termination patterns in class II genes are unclear due to the very rapid processing of the transcripts, which removes the 3' end in preparation for poly-A addition. Some class II genes appear to contain adenine and thymine-rich regions just downstream of the termination point. These structures resemble the rho-dependent termination signals in *E. coli*.

Termination of transcription of the 5S rRNA gene (a class III gene) occurs within a series of uridines following a guanine- and cytosine-rich region. This resembles the rho-independent termination sequences in bacteria, but in the eukaryotic 5S gene, mutations that prevent hairpin loop formation in the G-C region do not alter termination. The mechanism is unclear, but at least in vitro no additional protein factors appear to be essential and the interaction must therefore be between the transcribed RNA and the RNA polymerase III itself.

Post-Transcriptional Processing of RNA in Eukaryotes

POST-TRANSCRIPTIONAL ALTERATION OF rRNA (CLASS I GENES)

Large ribosomal RNAs (5.8S, 18S, 28S) are transcribed as a single large (45S) RNA molecule, which is the cut apart by nucleases to release the functional RNAs. Ribosomal RNA genes occur as tandemly repeated transcription units, with clusters of tandem repeated units on 10 chromosomes in diploid human cells. Each transcription unit contains one 18S, one 5.8S, and one 28S rRNA gene separated by intervening spacer RNA regions. Introns are not present within the 18S, 5.8S, or 28S structural genes in most eukaryotes, but some unicellular eukaryotes have introns in their large rRNA sequences and these introns are capable of removal by self-splicing. rRNAs undergo methylation and other modifications to numerous bases on the nucleotides prior to entry into the cytoplasm as part of a ribosome. The functions of base modification in rRNAs are unclear.

ASSEMBLY OF RIBOSOMAL SUBUNITS

In eukaryotes, ribosomal RNA processing and assembly with ribosomal proteins to form the large and small subunits occurs in the nucleolus. Ribosomal RNAs are cut out of the large initial transcripts produced from each of the ribosomal RNA transcription units by ribonuclease enzymes. Extensive modification of bases (by methylation) occurs in all three size classes of larger rRNAs.

More than 100 different polypeptides synthesized in the cytoplasm move into the nucleus and into the nucleolus and complex with the 45S rRNA transcript before it is processed. These protein components include most, if not all, of the proteins that will be present in mature ribosomes, proteins involved in rRNA processing, and generalized RNA-binding proteins.

Approximately 30 min after synthesis of a 45S rRNA precursor, the 18S rRNA processed from the transcript has been assembled with approximately 33 proteins to form the 40S small ribosomal subunit and has been transported through a nuclear pore and into the cytoplasm where it becomes active.

Approximately 60 min after synthesis of a 45S rRNA precursor, the 5.8S and 28S rRNA from the transcript plus 5S rRNA synthesized elsewhere in the nucleus have been assembled with approximately 49 proteins to form a 60S large ribosome subunit and have been transported through a nuclear pore and into the cytoplasm where it becomes active.

POST-TRANSCRIPTIONAL ALTERATION OF mRNA (CLASS II GENES)

Processing of the RNA transcribed from a class II gene into a functional mRNA occurs within the nucleus and requires a series of modifications to the RNA.

1. *Capping*

   Almost immediately after initiation of transcription, one of the three phosphates on the 5' nucleotide on the RNA is removed and a GMP (derived from a GTP) is attached using a 5'–5' linkage. Methyl groups are then added to the guanine in the terminal position and to the base (usually A or G) on the original 5' terminal nucleotide.

2. *Polyadenylation*

   Just after the RNA polymerase II passes the poly-A addition signal on the DNA, the RNA transcript is cleaved at the signal. Poly-A polymerase then adds 100 to 200 adenosine nucleotides to the 3' end of the transcript to form the poly-A "tail." Different patterns of 3' cleavage and poly-A addition may produce different carboxy-terminal ends on the protein and different life spans for the mRNAs in the cytoplasm.

3. *Intron Removal*

   The snRNPs U1, U2, U5, and U4/U6 plus other components assemble on the recognition sequences on each intron to form a spliceosome. The intron is excised in a loop or lariat form and the adjacent exons are ligated together. In many genes, intron removal may destroy over half of the original transcript. Different patterns of intron removal in different cells types lead to different protein coding sequences in mRNAs produced from identical transcripts.

4. *Editing*

   mRNA nucleotide sequence can be changed by editing enzymes that change or delete nucleotides. Conversion of single bases has been documented for several human mRNAs, and extensive editing using guide RNAs has been demonstrated in trypanosomes. The full effect and extent of this process is not fully understood.

TRANSPORT OF mRNA TO THE CYTOPLASM

Transport of mRNA to the cytoplasm is delayed until splicing has removed all introns. As the mRNA then moves through a nuclear pore, spliceosomes and other nuclear proteins are removed and cytoplasmic RNA-binding proteins bind to the mRNA. Different mRNAs may be transported into different regions of the cytoplasm. In at least some cases, correct transport of mRNA depends on sequences in the 3' UTR (untranslated region between polypeptide termination and the poly-A tail).

POST-TRANSCRIPTIONAL ALTERATION OF 5S rRNA
AND tRNA (CLASS III GENES)

5S rRNA transcripts are the same length as the functional RNA in ribosomes and therefore undergo no length processing.

Transfer RNAs are formed from transcripts with excess nucleotides on both the 5' and 3' ends, and some eukaryotic tRNA transcripts contain an intron. Some tRNAs appear to form their typical hairpin loop structures and fold at least partially into the L-shaped tertiary structure prior to excision from the original transcript by a ribonuclease. Extensive modification of bases on the nucleotides may occur before or after excision. The 3' end created by excision requires addition of a CCA unit catalyzed by tRNA nucleotidyl transferase to provide the attachment point for the aminoacyl group.

In addition, modification of numerous bases occurs in most tRNAs after transcription. The timing of modification relative to excision is not clear. After processing, tRNA is apparently transported into the cytoplasm through nuclear pores.

Translation in Eukaryotes

AMINOACYLATION OF tRNAS

This process in eukaryotes closely resembles aminoacylation of tRNAs in prokaryotes. Aminoacyl groups are attached to tRNAs by *aminoacyl synthetase enzymes*. Each amino acid appears to be attached by a single type of amino acyl synthetase that distinguishes that amino acid from the other 19, some of which may be very similar chemically. The aminoacyl synthetase must also clearly distinguish the one or more tRNAs that carry that amino acid from all other tRNAs.

INITIATION OF TRANSLATION

Initiation of translation in eukaryotes is more complex than in prokaryotes. In eukaryotes, at least 9 *initiation factors* are required, and the methionine on the initiator tRNA is not formylated. The initiation factors are proteins present in the cytoplasm.

The *initiator Met-tRNA (met-tRNA$_i$)* in both prokaryotes and eukaryotes is a tRNA distinct from the met-tRNA which is used to translate AUG codons in the interior of the mRNA. Methionine is attached to eukaryotic Met-tRNA$_i$ in the same way as any other aminoacyl group is attached, but Met-tRNA$_i$ is the only tRNA that can enter a ribosome at the P site to initiate translation.

THE ELONGATION PHASE OF TRANSLATION

Each elongation reaction in eukaryotes is similar to the same event in prokaryotes in that it requires the *aminoacyl-tRNA* to fit the next codon in the mRNA and *elongation factors*. Several elongation factors are GTP-binding proteins that hydrolyze GTP to GDP during elongation.

TERMINATION OF TRANSLATION

Termination in eukaryotes uses a single *release factor*. The result of termination is release of the polypeptide from the tRNA to which it is attached, release of the ribosome from the mRNA, and eventual dissociation of the small and large ribosomal subunits.

TECHNIQUES USED TO IDENTIFY DNA, RNA, AND PROTEIN SEQUENCES

Techniques available for isolation and characterization of DNA, RNA, and protein include "blots," which involve electrophoretic separation followed by transfer to nitrocellulose sheets and testing for complementary sequences or immunological binding.

1. The Southern Blot consists of restriction enzyme digests of DNA separated by gel electrophoresis, transferred (blotted) on to nitrocellulose sheets or similar material, and tested against a specific, labeled DNA probe for complementary sequences.
2. The Northern Blot consists of electrophoretically separated RNA molecules transferred on to nitrocellulose sheets and tested against labeled DNA probes. It is widely used to estimate the amount of a specific mRNA in a cell at different points in development.
3. The Western Blot involves the separation of proteins by gel electrophoresis, transfer to nitrocellulose sheets, and probing with labeled antibodies directed against specific proteins. The present confirmatory test for HIV infection is a Western Blot analysis directed against specific viral proteins in blood.

QUICK RECALL TEST QUESTIONS AND ANSWERS

Choose the Best Answer

1. During interphase in a typical eukaryotic cell, the DNA coding for ribosomal RNAs is:

   (A) in a single location on a single chromosome in the center of the nucleolus.
   (B) in multiple locations on multiple chromosomes around the perimeter of the nucleolus.
   (C) in multiple locations on multiple chromosomes in the heterochromatin along the inner surface of the nuclear envelope.
   (D) in multiple locations on multiple chromosomes scattered throughout the euchromatin in the nucleus.

2. Introns are found:

   (A) primarily in prokaryotic genes.
   (B) primarily in eukaryotic genes.
   (C) commonly in both eukaryotic and prokaryotic genes.

3. The DNA of eukaryotic cells is wrapped around histones to form structures called:

   (A) nucleoli.
   (B) nuclear matrix.
   (C) nucleosomes.
   (D) centromeres.

4. Eukaryotic genes that code for mRNA and tRNA are similar in that:

   (A) they are transcribed by the same RNA polymerase.
   (B) the promoter sequences are upstream of the transcription initiation point.
   (C) multiple proteins must bind to the DNA before the RNA polymerase binds.

5. Compared with DNA binding proteins that activate or inactivate eukaryotic class II genes, DNA binding proteins that activate or inactivate bacterial operons typically bind to DNA that is:

   (A) closer to the promoter.
   (B) farther from the promoter.
   (C) at a similar distance from the promoter.

6. The enzyme (catalyst) for protein synthesis in eukaryotes is:

   (A) mRNA.
   (B) DNA polymerase.
   (C) RNA polymerase.
   (D) part of the structure of the ribosome.

7. The template (information source) for protein synthesis in eukaryotes is:

   (A) mRNA.
   (B) DNA polymerase.
   (C) RNA polymerase.
   (D) part of the structure of the ribosome.

8. The raw material (reactant) for protein synthesis in eukaryotes is:

   (A) mRNA.
   (B) free amino acid.
   (C) aminoacyl tRNA.
   (D) part of the structure of the ribosome.

9. Ribosomes in eukaryotes contain:

   (A) a single subunit.
   (B) two identical subunits.
   (C) one large and one small subunit.

10. In comparison with ribosomes in prokaryotes, ribosomes in eukaryotes contain:

    (A) larger rRNAs and more proteins.
    (B) smaller rRNAs and more proteins.
    (C) larger rRNAs and fewer proteins.
    (D) smaller rRNAs and fewer proteins.

11. In eukaryotes, most amino acids are specified by _____ in mRNA.

    (A) a single type of codon
    (B) several different types of codons

12. The release of the completed polypeptide chain from the ribosome occurs:

    (A) wherever a ribosome bumps into another ribosome along the mRNA (randomly along the molecule).
    (B) at the first AUG codon in the mRNA molecule.
    (C) at the poly-A tail on the mRNA.
    (D) at the first nonsense (termination) codon on the mRNA.

Answers

1. **(B)** The rRNA-coding regions of the chromosomes (usually on multiple chromosomes) are associated with the outer region of the nucleolus, while the center is occupied by partially assembled ribosomes.

2. **(B)** Introns occur primarily in genes in eukaryotes.

3. **(C)** The DNA-histone complexes called nucleosomes form "string of beads" structures that occupy most locations in dispersed euchromatin and which occur in packed "solenoid" arrays in heterochromatin and condensed chromatin.

4. **(C)** Although multiple proteins bind to the DNA prior to RNA polymerase binding in both cases, mRNA is produced by RNA polymerase II and tRNA is produced by RNA polymerase III. The promoter sequences in Class II genes (coding for mRNA) are upstream of (located 5' relative to) the starting point of RNA synthesis, whereas the promoter sequences of Class III genes (coding for tRNA) are downstream of (located 3' relative to) the starting point for RNA synthesis.

5. **(A)** Prokaryotic regulatory proteins typically bind just downstream or just upstream of the promoter, but eukaryotic regulatory proteins typically utilize much more distant sites, many of which are believed to interact with the promoter by looping out the intervening DNA.

6. **(D)** A loop of rRNA appears to catalyze peptide bond formation.

7. **(A)** The sequence of nucleotides in mRNA (read in groups of three as codons) determines the sequence of amino acids in the polypeptide being synthesized.

8. **(C)** The aminoacyl group on a tRNA is ready to participate in protein synthesis. A free amino acid would have to be activated and attached to tRNA as an aminoacyl group before it could be used in protein synthesis.

9. **(C)** The subunits in eukaryotic ribosomes are larger than the corresponding subunits in prokaryotic ribosomes, but prokaryotes and eukaryotes each contain ribosomes composed of large and small subunits.

10. **(A)** The larger ribosomes in eukaryotes contain larger rRNAs and more different proteins than the ribosomes in prokaryotes.

11. **(B)** Almost all amino acids are specified by two or more codons.

12. **(D)** Nonsense codons trigger releasing factors to terminate translation.

CLASSIFICATION OF LIVING ORGANISMS

Taxonomy is the classification of living organisms based on characteristics and ancestry. Two *kingdoms*—animal and plant—are easily distinguished. In general, members of the former consume food and are mobile, whereas those of the latter are stationary and produce their own nutrients.

Several systems have evolved to classify the great variety of living organisms. One such system divides living things into five kingdoms based on: (1) the presence (eukaryotic) or absence (prokaryotic) of membrane-bound nuclei in the cells; (2) the number of cells forming the organism; and (3) the mechanism for nutrition. This five-kingdom classification system is shown in the following table.

Five-Kingdom Classification System

Kingdom	Characteristics	Examples
Monera	unicellular without organized nuclei; absorb or produce their own nutrients	bacteria, blue-green algae
Protista	unicellular with membrane-bound nuclei; ingest, absorb, or produce nutrients via photosynthesis	protozoans, algae
Fungi	multicellular with membrane-bound nuclei; absorb nutrients	mushrooms, molds
Plantae	multicellular with membrane-bound nuclei and a cell wall; possess chlorophyll and undergo photosynthesis	flowering plants and trees; evergreens
Animalia	multicellular with membrane-bound nuclei; ingest nutrients	mammals, birds, amphibians, fish, reptiles, insects, crustaceans, etc.

These kingdoms can be divided into three main groups based on the mode of nutrition—photosynthetic organisms (plants and algae), organisms that absorb their nutrients (bacteria and fungi), and organisms that engulf or ingest their nutrients (protozoa and animals).

Each kingdom is further divided into phyla (sing. phylum), which are subdivided as follows: phyla → into classes → into families → into genera → into species. Each of these groups may be divided into six additional subgroups.

All living organisms are given a scientific name using the combination of genus and species. Under this binomial naming system, the scientific name for a human is *Homo sapiens*. To illustrate the classification system a demonstration of how one classifies a human is given below:

Classification of the Human

Classification	Group	Distinguishing Features
Kingdom	Animalia	Consume food by ingestion and are multicellular and usually mobile.
Phylum	Chordata	Notochord, hollow nervous system (neural tube) dorsally positioned, gill slits in pharyngeal wall, heart ventral to digestive system.
Subphylum	Vertebrata	Segmental vertebral column.
Class	Mammalia	Mammary glands for nourishment of young; hair or fur; warm-blooded; diaphragm.
Order	Primates	Large cerebral hemispheres; opposable digits; nails; highly developed sense of sight—eyes directed forward; teeth specialized for different functions.
Family	Hominidae	Walk with two limbs (bipedal locomotion); binocular color vision.
Genus	*Homo*	Ability to speak and most highly developed and largest brain.
Species	*sapiens*	Large skull, high forehead, reduced size of brow (supraorbital) ridges, prominent chin; decreased amount of body hair.

QUICK RECALL TEST QUESTIONS AND ANSWERS

Choose the Best Answer

1. All are distinguishing features of the phylum Chordata EXCEPT:

   (A) notochord.
   (B) neural tube dorsally positioned.
   (C) gill slits.
   (D) mammary glands.

2. Phyla may be subdivided into:

   (A) classes.
   (B) families.
   (C) genera.
   (D) all of the above.

Answers

1. **(D)** The characteristics of the phylum Chordata are listed in A, B, and C. Choice D is only in mammals.

2. **(D)** Each kingdom is further divided into phyla, which are subdivided into classes, families, genera, and species. Each of these groups may be divided into subgroups.

ORGANIZATION OF THE HUMAN BODY

A multicellular organism is composed of millions of cells organized into functional units (organs and systems) that are formed by various groups of similar cells organized into tissues. These cells are embedded in an extracellular matrix and tissue fluids. A *tissue* consists of a group of cells performing a similar function. Four basic tissues compose the human (mammalian) body: epithelial, connective, muscle, and nervous tissues. The four basic tissues may be organized to form functional units known as *organs*. Each organ has a definite function that results from the combined functions of the various tissue components. Organs that function together as a unit for a specified purpose make up an organ *system*. The animal *organism* is composed of several interrelated organ systems.

Organ Systems

The human body is composed of the systems listed in the following table.

Organ Systems in the Human

System	Functions
Muscular	Produces motion of body parts and viscera.
Skeletal	Supports the body, protects organs, and produces blood cells.
Circulatory	Transports nutrients, wastes, gases (oxygen and carbon dioxide), hormones, blood cells throughout body; also protects body against foreign organisms.
Nervous	Responds to internal and external stimuli; regulates and coordinates body activities and movements.
Integumentary	Limits and protects the body as a whole; prevents excess loss of water and functions in regulating body temperature.
Digestive	Enzymatically breaks down food materials into usable and absorbable nutrients.
Respiratory	Functions in the exchange of gases (oxygen and carbon dioxide).
Urinary	Removes body wastes from bloodstream and helps regulate homeostasis of internal environment.
Reproductive	Perpetuates the living organism by the production of sex cells (gametes) and future offspring.
Endocrine	Regulates body growth and function via hormones.

Four Basic Tissues

1. MUSCLE TISSUE

Muscle tissue is composed of cells (muscle cells or myocytes) that are contractile in nature. Muscle tissue functions to move the skeletal system and body viscera.

Types of Muscle

Type	Characteristics	Location
Skeletal	Striated, voluntary	Skeletal muscles of the body
Smooth	Nonstriated, involuntary	Walls of digestive tract and blood vessels, uterus, urinary bladder
Cardiac	Striated, involuntary	Heart

2. NERVOUS TISSUE

Nervous tissue is composed of cells *(neurons)* that respond to external and internal stimuli and have the capability to transmit a message *(impulse)* from one area of the body to another. This tissue thus induces a response of distant muscles or glands, as well as regulating body processes such as respiration, circulation, and digestion. Nervous tissue composes the central (brain and spinal cord) and peripheral (peripheral nerves, ganglia, and receptors) nervous systems and the special sensory receptors (eye, ear, taste buds, and olfactory region).

3. EPITHELIAL TISSUE

Epithelial tissue covers the external surfaces of the body and lines the internal tubes and cavities. It also forms the glands of the body. Characteristics of epithelial tissue (epithelium) are that it

1. has compactly aggregated cells;
2. has limited intercellular spaces and substance;
3. is avascular (no blood vessels);
4. has a basally located basal lamina usually attached to underlying connective tissue;
5. has cells that form sheets and are polarized (have distinct apical and basal surfaces);
6. is derived from all three germ layers.

Types of Epithelium

Classification	Location(s)	Function(s)
Simple squamous epithelium	Endothelium of blood and lymphatic vessels; Bowman's capsule and thin loop of Henle in kidney; mesothelium lining pericardial, peritoneal and pleural body cavities; lung alveoli; smallest excretory ducts of glands.	Lubrication of body cavities (permits free movement of organs); pinocytotic transport across cells.
Stratified squamous keratinized epithelium	Epidermis of skin.	Prevents loss of water; protection.
Stratified squamous nonkeratinized epithelium (moist)	Mucosa of oral cavity, esophagus, anal canal; vagina; cornea of eye and part of conjunctiva.	Secretion; protection; prevents loss of water.
Simple cuboidal epithelium	Kidney tubules; choroid plexus; thyroid gland; rete testis; surface of ovary.	Secretion; absorption; lines surface.
Stratified cuboidal epithelium	Ducts of sweat glands; developing follicles of ovary.	Secretion; protection.
Simple columnar epithelium	Cells lining lumen of digestive tract (stomach to rectum); gall bladder; many glands (secretory units and ducts); uterus; uterine tube (ciliated).	Secretion; absorption; protection; lubrication.
Pseudostratified columnar epithelium	Lines lumen of respiratory tract (nasal cavity, trachea, and bronchi) (ciliated); ducts of epididymis (stereocilia); ductus deferens; male urethra.	Secretion; protection; facilitates transport of substances on surface of cells.
Stratified columnar epithelium	Male urethra; conjunctiva	Protection.
Transitional epithelium	Urinary tract (renal calyces and pelvis, ureter and urinary bladder).	Protection.

Epithelial cells may also have specializations at the cell surface. For example,

microvilli—fingerlike projections from the cell surface, covered by plasma membranes and containing a core of microfilaments. Mainly located at luminal surfaces of absorptive cells (brush border of proximal convoluted tubules and striated border of intestinal epithelium).

cilia—motile organelles extending into the lumen, consisting of a covering of plasma membrane and a core of specifically arranged microtubules. Mainly located in respiratory epithelium and part of female reproductive tract.

flagella—similar to cilia. Primary examples are on spermatozoa.

stereocilia—are actually very elongated microvilli.

4. CONNECTIVE TISSUE

Connective tissue is the packing and supporting material of the body tissues and organs. It develops from mesoderm (mesenchyme). All connective tissues consist of three distinct components: ground substance, cells, and fibers.

a. *Ground substance.* Ground substance is located between the cells and fibers, both of which are embedded in it. It forms an amorphous intercellar material. In the fresh state, it appears as a transparent and homogenous gel. It acts as a route for the passage of nutrients and wastes to and from the cells within or adjacent to the connective tissue. The ground substance is composed of mucopolysaccharides *(glycosaminoglycans),* proteins, lipids, and water. The primary glycosaminoglycans found in the ground substance are chondroitin sulfate and hyaluronic acid, the latter present in greater quantity.

b. *Fibers.* The fiber components of connective tissue add support and strength. Three types of fibers are present: *collagenous, elastic,* and *reticular.*

Collagen fibers (white fibers) are the most numerous fiber type and are present in all types of connective tissue in varying amount. Collagen bundles are strong and resist stretching. They are found in structures such as tendons, ligaments, aponeuroses, and fascia, which are subjected to pull or stretching activities.

Elastic fibers (yellow fibers) are refractile fibers, which are thinner (0.2 to 1 μm diameter) than collagen fibers. They are extremely elastic and are located in structures with a degree of elasticity, such as the walls of blood vessels (elastic arteries), true vocal cords, and trachea.

Reticular fibers are thinner (0.2 to 1 μm diameter) than collagenous fibers. They are arranged in an intermeshing network (reticulum), which supports the organ. Reticular fibers are inelastic. They are found in the walls of blood vessels, lymphoid tissues (spleen and lymph nodes), red bone marrow, basal laminae, and glands (liver and kidney).

c. *Cells.* The *cells* of connective tissue are primarily attached and nonmotile *(fixed cells),* but some have the ability to move *(wandering or free cells).* The typical cells found in connective tissue are:

Fibroblasts constitute the largest number of cells present in connective tissue. In an actively secreting state, they are flattened stellate-shaped cells with an oval nucleus and basophilic cytoplasm due to the numerous rough endoplasmic reticulum. In the inactive state, they appear as elongated spindles with a more basophilic oval or elongated nucleus. In this state, they are referred to as *fibrocytes.* The latter are the main cellular constituents of connective tissue structures such as tendons and ligaments. Only the nuclei of fibrocytes are observed between the fibers since the cytoplasm is indistinct. The terms fibrocyte and fibroblast are often used interchangeably.

Mesenchymal cells are undifferentiated connective tissue cells that have the potential to differentiate into other types of connective tissue cells. They are primarily found in embryonic and fetal tissues; some are thought to be present in the adult abutting the walls of capillaries. They are smaller than fibroblasts and are stellate in shape. They are capable of moving by extending their cell processes into the gel-like ground substance.

Macrophages (histiocytes) may be fixed or free. Free macrophages may wander through the connective tissue by extending their cell processes. Fixed macrophages are very numerous in loose connective tissue. They are polymorphic in shape and contain an oval nucleus. They have the ability to engulf extracellular material (foreign matter or necrotic cells). Macrophages are difficult to distinguish except when they are actively phagocytosing material and thus contain many vacuoles.

Adipocytes (fat cells) are found in most connective tissue, either singly or in groups. If the connective tissue layer is primarily composed of fat cells, it is referred to as adipose tissue. An adipocyte is a round, large cell with a distinct, dense nucleus usually located at the periphery of the cytoplasm. The majority of the cytoplasmic (cell) volume is taken up by a large lipid droplet. Due to the clear appearing cytoplasm and dark nucleus at one pole, the cell has a signet ring appearance. Fat cells do not undergo mitosis.

Mast cells are ovoid cells with small round nuclei. The cytoplasm contains numerous coarse basophilic granules which also stain metachromatically and are soluble in water. The mast cell granules are composed of *histamine* and an anticoagulant known as *heparin*. Histamine dilates blood vessels and increases the permeability of capillaries, thus increasing interstitial fluid. Mast cells take part in the allergic response of the body. Mast cells are found in most connective tissue and are numerous in the respiratory tract and near small blood vessels.

Plasma cells have a characteristic eccentric nucleus that contains chromatin arranged in a definite pattern near the nuclear envelope. This pattern gives a "cartwheel or spoke wheel" appearance. The juxtanuclear cytoplasm appears clear and less basophilic due to the Golgi complex located in this area. Plasma cells are found in the lamina propira of the gastrointestinal tract. They function in protecting the body against bacterial invasion by secreting antibodies [immunoglobulins (IgG)] into the circulating blood.

Reticular cells are star-shaped cells that join via their processes to form a cellular network. They are found abutting reticular fibers in certain glands and lymphoid tissues.

Pericytes are located in the adventitia (outer layer) of blood vessels. They are believed to be multi-potential cells that may differentiate into various connective tissue cells as well as into smooth muscle cells.

Certain white blood cells or leukocytes migrate out of the blood into the extracellular ground substance. The main leukocytes found in the connective tissue are lymphocytes, monocytes, eosinophils, basophils, and neutrophils. The leukocytes in connective tissue are similar in structure and function to those in the blood. The agranular leukocytes migrate in large numbers under normal conditions. Lymphocytes accumulate in areas in response to chronic inflammation. Neutrophils also migrate in large numbers into the interstitium during an inflammatory response. Eosinophils occur in areas involved in allergic reaction, such as the respiratory tract.

QUICK RECALL TEST QUESTIONS AND ANSWERS

Choose the Best Answer

1. Simple squamous epithelium is found in all of the following EXCEPT:

   (A) lung.
   (B) kidney.
   (C) skin.
   (D) blood vessels.

2. Which of the following is NOT considered a basic tissue that makes up the human body?

   (A) epithelium
   (B) connective tissue
   (C) bone
   (D) muscle

3. Which of the following cells are multipotent and can differentiate into other types of cells?

   (A) fibroblasts
   (B) chondroblasts
   (C) adipocytes
   (D) mesenchymal cells

4. Ground substance found in connective tissue is composed of all of the following EXCEPT:

   (A) chondroitin sulfate.
   (B) hyaluronic acid.
   (C) actinomyosin.
   (D) mucopolysaccharides.

5. Epithelial cells may have specializations at the cell surface such as:

   (A) microvilli.
   (B) cilia and stereocilia.
   (C) flagella.
   (D) all of the above.

6. Epithelial tissue:

   (A) is derived from all three germ layers.
   (B) is avascular.
   (C) lies on a connective tissue layer—the basal lamina.
   (D) is characterized by all of the above.

7. A group of cells subserving the same general function and bound together or united by varying amounts of intercellular substance and tissue fluids is called a (an):

   (A) organ.
   (B) tissue.
   (C) system.
   (D) organ system.

8. Epithelial tissues may be characterized by:

   (A) protection.
   (B) secretion.
   (C) absorption.
   (D) all of the above.

9. The outstanding features of connective tissue include:

   (A) an orderly arrangement of cells into sheets.
   (B) possessing a fairly large amount of intercellular material.
   (C) making up the majority of the ducts of secretory organs.
   (D) all of the above.

10. The function of mast cells is related to the:

    (A) secretion of immunoglobulins (IgG).
    (B) phagocytic activity.
    (C) allergic response of the body.
    (D) secretion and storage of coagulants.

11. The adult tissue that lines the lumen of the human digestive and respiratory passageways is:

    (A) epithelium.
    (B) nervous tissue.
    (C) blood.
    (D) connective tissue.

12. The adult tissue that covers the surface of the human body is:

    (A) epithelium.
    (B) nervous tissue.
    (C) blood.
    (D) connective tissue.

13. The adult tissue that is capable of rapid transmission of signals among parts of the human body is:

    (A) epithelium.
    (B) nervous tissue.
    (C) blood.
    (D) connective tissue.

14. The adult tissue that supports the shape of the human body is:

    (A) epithelium.
    (B) nervous tissue.
    (C) blood.
    (D) connective tissue.

15. The adult tissue whose mechanical properties are due to the extracellular material in the tissue is:

    (A) epithelium.
    (B) connective tissue.
    (C) nervous tissue.
    (D) muscle.

16. The adult tissue that forms most glands is:

    (A) epithelium.
    (B) connective tissue.
    (C) nervous tissue.
    (D) muscle.

17. The adult tissue responsible for contraction during the heartbeat is:

    (A) epithelium.
    (B) connective tissue.
    (C) nervous tissue.
    (D) muscle.

18. The adult tissue that can generate the most mechanical force by contraction is:

    (A) epithelium.
    (B) nervous tissue.
    (C) connective tissue.
    (D) muscle

Answers

1. **(C)** The epidermis of skin is composed of stratified squamous epithelium.

2. **(C)** The four basic tissues that compose the human body are epithelium, connective tissue, muscle, and nervous tissue. Bone is a member of the connective tissues.

3. **(D)** Mesenchymal cells are undifferentiated connective tissue cells that have the potential to differentiate into other types of connective tissue cells. They are primarily found in embryonic and fetal tissues; some are thought to be present in the adult, abutting the walls of capillaries. They are smaller than fibroblasts and are stellate in shape. They are capable of moving by extending their cell processes into the gel-like ground substance.

4. **(C)** Ground substance is located between the cells and fibers, both of which are embedded in it. It forms an amorphous intercellular material. In the fresh state, it appears as a transparent and homogenous gel. It acts as a route for the passage of nutrients and wastes to and from the cells within or adjacent to the connective tissue. The ground substance is composed of mucopolysaccharides (glycosaminoglycans), proteins, lipids, and water. The primary glycosaminoglycans found in the ground substance are chondroitin sulfate and hyaluronic acid; the latter is present in greater quantity.

5. **(D)** Epithelial cell specializations at the cell surface may include microvilli, cilia and stereocilia, and flagella.

6. **(D)** Besides the four characteristics listed, epithelial tissue has compactly aggregated cells, and has cells that form sheets and are polarized.

7. **(B)** A tissue consists of a group of cells performing a similar function. The cells are embedded in intercellular substances and tissue fluids. Four basic tissues compose the human body: epithelium, connective tissue, muscle, and nervous tissue. The four basic tissues may be organized to form functional units known as organs.

8. **(D)** Epithelium is a group of cells forming a tissue. Epithelium lines the gut, the respiratory system, and the genitourinary system, and forms the epidermis. It therefore can protect, secrete, and absorb.

9. **(B)** Connective tissue, cartilage, and bone are basically supporting tissues. An abundance of non-living-formed substance is the feature that is common to the group as a whole. Cells are interspersed in the intercellular substance, and fibers are a constituent of the formed substance. Fibers and ground substance are called matrix.

10. **(C)** The mast cell granules contain *histamine* and an anticoagulant known as *heparin.* Histamine dilates blood vessels and increases the permeability of capillaries, thus increasing interstitial fluid. Mast cells take part in the allergic response of the body. Mast cells are found in most connective tissue and are numerous in the respiratory tract and near small blood vessels. Plasma cells are found in the lamina propria of the gastrointestinal tract. They function in protecting the body against bacterial invasion by secreting antibodies (immunoglobulins, or IgG) into the circulating blood.

11. **(A)** Epithelial tissue lines most naturally occurring spaces in the human body, including the spaces in the digestive and respiratory systems.

12. **(A)** Epithelial tissue (the stratified squamous epithelium of the epidermis) lines naturally occurring surfaces on the human body.

13. **(B)** Nervous tissue is responsible for transmitting rapid signals among body parts. Muscle tissue (cardiac or smooth types) may transmit rapid signals over smaller distances, and epithelial tissue in endocrine glands can transmit somewhat slower signals over long distances within the body.

14. **(D)** Connective tissue in the form of bone and cartilage forms most of the skeleton, which supports the overall shape of the human body, and fibrous connective tissues in the walls of organs support the shapes of the organs within the body.

15. **(B)** Mechanical properties of connective tissues are almost totally due to extracellular matrix. Mechanical properties of epithelia, muscle tissues, and nervous tissues are primarily due to cytoskeletal components inside the cells in the tissues.

16. **(A)** All exocrine glands are composed of epithelial tissues, as are some endocrine tissues. Some endocrine structures are modified nervous tissue structures (posterior pituitary, pineal).

17. **(D)** Cardiac muscle contracts to produce the heartbeat, and modified cardiac muscle cells in the pacemaker region (sino-atrial node) initiate the contraction. Nervous tissue in the sympathetic and parasympathetic branches of the nervous system may modify the rate of the heartbeat but cannot initiate it.

18. **(D)** Muscle tissue is specialized for contraction. Cells in some epithelia and some connective tissues may also contract, but generate much less force at the tissue level.

Anatomical Terms Used for Planes and Positions

For descriptive purposes a standard body position, "the anatomic position," has been adopted. The anatomic position is the position of a person standing erect, feet together and parallel, face forward, arms at the sides, and palms forward (supinated).

Terms of Planes

Plane	Definition
Midsagittal or median	A vertical plane in the antero-posterior direction that divides the body into equal right and left halves.
Sagittal	A vertical plane parallel to the midsagittal plane; it allows longitudinal slices that are parallel to the median plane.
Frontal or coronal	A vertical plane that passes from side to side; it is at right angles to the midsagittal plane and cuts the specimen into anterior and posterior components.
Transverse, horizontal, or cross	A horizontal plane at right angles to both the sagittal and frontal plane; it cuts the specimen into superior (upper or cephalad) and inferior (lower or caudad) portions. Cross sections of the specimen are obtained.

Terms of Positions

Position	Definition
Anterior or ventral	Toward the front of the body or belly side; (volar or palmar side are used in referring to the hand).
Posterior or dorsal	Toward the back (the dorsum) of the body.
Superior, craniad, or cephalad	In the direction of the head; nearer the head.
Inferior or caudad	In the direction of the feet; away from the head.
Superficial or external	Nearer the surface; without or nearer the outside of the body.
Deep or internal	Away from the surface; within or toward the inside or interior.
Medial	Nearer the midline of the body; toward the midsagittal plane or center.
Lateral	Farther from the midline; toward the side of the body or away from the midsagittal plane; to the side.
Proximal	Nearest a point of origin in general or nearest the trunk as far as the extremities are concerned; nearer the attachment to the body. Nearer the midline axis.
Distal	Farther from the point of origin of a structure or farther from the reference point or the midline axis.
Central	Toward the center of the body; toward the inside.
Peripheral	Away from the center of the body; toward the outside.
Plantar	The sole of the foot.

SKELETAL SYSTEM

The skeletal system of vertebrates is an *endoskeleton*—that is, it is within the body—as compared to an *exoskeleton* characteristic of arthropods. The human skeletal system provides:

(1) support;
(2) protection of vital organs;
(3) sites for muscle attachment;
(4) storage sites of body calcium and phosphates; and
(5) sites for blood cell formation.

The *human skeleton* consists of bone and cartilage. The bones form the main rigid structure of the skeleton. The human skeleton consists of about 206 bones, some of which are fused, whereas others are joined together at sites that permit various degrees of movement. The sites of junction, or articulation, whether movable or immovable, are known as *joints*.

The human skeleton is divided into an *axial skeleton* and an *appendicular skeleton*.

Axial Skeleton

The axial skeleton consists of 80 bones forming the trunk (spine and thorax) and skull.

Vertebral Column: The main trunk of the body is supported by the spine, or vertebral column, which is composed of 26 bones, some of which are formed by the fusion of a few bones. The vertebral column from superior to inferior consists of 7 cervical (neck), 12 thoracic, and 5 lumbar vertebrae, as well as a sacrum, formed by fusion of 5 sacral vertebrae, and a coccyx, formed by fusion of 4 coccygeal vertebrae. Each vertebra consists of a body anteriorly and an arched posterior region circumscribing an inner central canal, the *vertebral canal,* which extends from the foramen magnum at the base of the skull through the sacrum. The vertebral column functions to support the trunk of the body and to protect the spinal cord located in the vertebral canal. The vertebrae of the cervical, thoracic, and lumbar regions are separated from each other by round fibro-cartilaginous articular discs known as *intervertebral discs*. The entire vertebral column is held together by ligaments.

Ribs and Sternum: The axial skeleton also contains 12 pairs of *ribs* attached posteriorly to the thoracic vertebrae and anteriorly either directly or via cartilage to the *sternum* (breastbone). The ribs and sternum form the *thoracic cage,* which protects the heart and lungs. Seven pairs of ribs articulate with the sternum *(fixed ribs)* directly, and three do so via cartilage; the two most inferior pairs do not attach anteriorly and are referred to as *floating ribs*.

Skull: The *skull* consists of 22 bones fused together to form a rigid structure that houses and protects organs such as the brain, auditory apparatus, and eyes. The bones of the skull form the *face* and *cranium* (brain case) and consist of 6 single bones *(occipital, frontal, ethmoid, sphenoid, vomer,* and *mandible)* and 8 paired bones *(parietal, temporal, maxillary, palatine, zygomatic, lacrimal, inferior concha,* and *nasal)*. The *lower jaw* or *mandible* is the only movable bone of the skull (head); it articulates with the temporal bones.

Other Parts: Other bones considered part of the axial skeleton are the *middle ear bones (ossicles)* and the small U-shaped *hyoid bone* that is suspended in a portion of the neck by muscles and ligaments.

Appendicular Skeleton

The *appendicular skeleton* forms the major internal support of the appendages—the *upper* and *lower extremities* (limbs).

Pectoral Girdle and Upper Extremities: The arms are attached to and suspended from the axial skeleton via the *shoulder (pectoral)* girdle. The latter is composed of two *clavicles (collarbones)* and two *scapulae (shoulder blades)*. The clavicles articulate with the sternum; the two *sternoclavicular joints* are the only sites of articulation between the trunk and upper extremity.

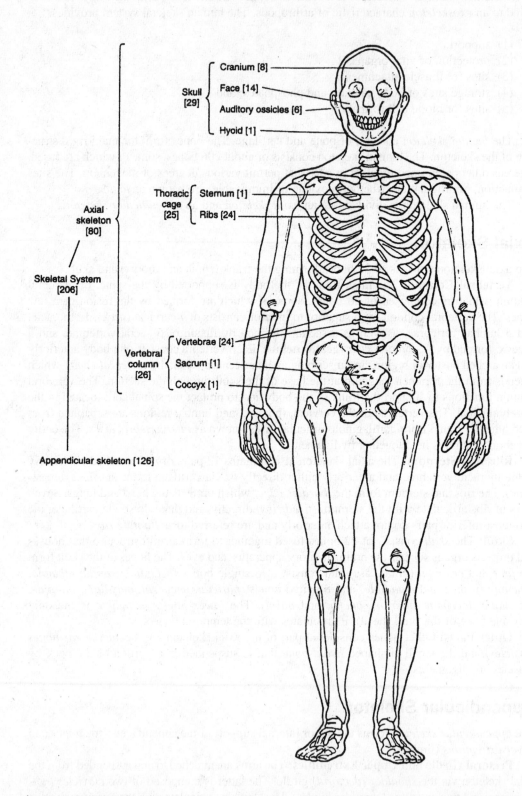

The axial skeleton. Eighty bones make up this portion of the skeleton. Numbers in square brackets indicate number of bones for each item.

The Human Skeletal System

Part of the Skeleton	Number of Bones
Axial Skeleton	**80**
Skull	22
Ossicles (malleus, incus, and stapes)	6
Vertebral column	26
Ribs	24
Sternum	1
Hyoid	1
Appendicular Skeleton	**126**
Upper extremities	64
Lower extremities	62

Appendicular Skeleton

Upper Extremity	Bones
Shoulder girdle	Clavicle and scapula
Arm	Humerus
Forearm	Radius (lateral) and ulna (medial)
Wrist	Eight carpal bones (proximal row: scaphoid, lunate, triquetrium, pisiform) (distal row: trapezium, trapezoid, capitate, hamate)
Palm	Five metacarpal bones
Digits	Thumb—two phalanges; fingers—three phalanges

Lower Extremity	Bones
Pelvic girdle	Pubic, ileum, and ischium (innominate bone)
Thigh	Femur
Leg	Tibia (medial) and fibula (lateral)
Foot	Seven tarsal bones (talus, calcaneus, navicular, cuboid, and three cuneiform bones)
Digits	Big toe—two phalanges; other toes—three phalanges

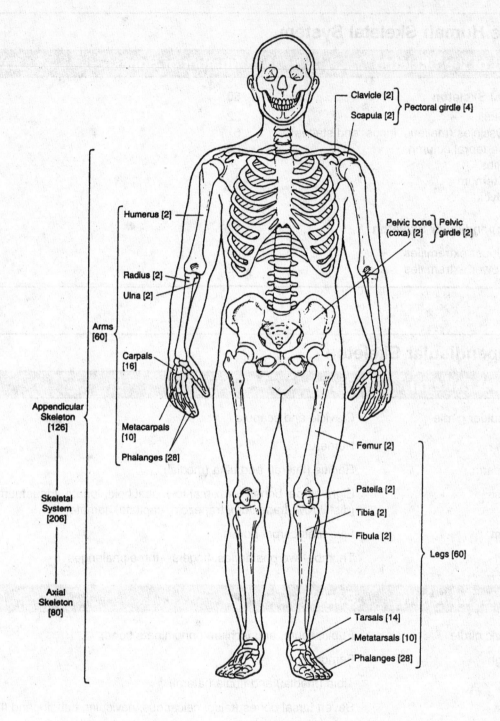

The appendicular skeleton. One hundred twenty-six bones make up this portion of the skeleton. Numbers in square brackets indicate number of bones for each item.

Each upper limb from distal to proximal (closest to the body) consists of hand, wrist, forearm, and arm (upper arm). The *hand* consists of 5 *digits* (fingers) and 5 *metacarpal* bones. Each digit is comprised of three bones known as *phalanges,* except the thumb, which has only two bones. The *wrist* consists of eight *carpal* bones that articulate with metacarpals. The *forearm* consists of two bones, the *ulna* on the side of the fifth digit (little finger), and the *radius* on the thumb side. The articulation between radius and ulna at the wrist permits rotation of the radius over the ulna during pronation (palm facing backward) and supination (palm turned forward). The ulna articulates at the elbow joint with the *humerus* creating a hinge joint. The humerus, in turn, is connected to the shoulder girdle at the *glenoid cavity* of the scapula.

Pelvic Girdle and Lower Extremities: The lower *extremities,* or legs, are attached to the axial skeleton via the *pelvic* or *hip girdle.* Each of the two coxal, or *hip,* bones that make up the pelvic girdle is formed by the fusion of three bones—*ilium, pubis,* and *ischium.* The coxal bones attach the lower limbs to the trunk by articulating with the sacrum.

From distal to proximal the lower limb consists of foot, ankle, shank, and thigh. The *foot* consists of 5 digits *(toes)* and 5 *metatarsals.* The digits contain 3 *phalanges* each, except for the big toe, which has two. The lower leg contains the *tibia* and *fibula.* The tibia is larger, is located medially, forms the shin, and articulates at the knee joint with the *femur (thigh bone).* The knee joint is protected anteriorly by the kneecap, or *patella.* The femur articulates with the *acetabular fossa* of the coxal bone.

Characteristics of Bone

Bone is a specialized type of connective tissue consisting of cells *(osteocytes)* embedded in a calcified matrix that gives bone its characteristic hard and rigid nature. Bones are encased by a *periosteum,* a connective tissue sheath. All bone has a central marrow cavity. *Bone marrow* fills the marrow cavity or smaller marrow spaces, depending on the type of bone.

Types of Bone: There are two types of bone in the skeleton: *compact bone* and *spongy* (cancellous) *bone.*

Compact Bone. *Compact bone* lies within the periosteum, forms the outer region of bones, and appears dense due to its compact organization. The living osteocytes and calcified matrix are arranged in layers, or *lamellae.* Lamellae may be circularly arranged surrounding a central canal, the *Haversian canal,* which contains small blood vessels. This unit of a Haversian canal circumscribed by Haversian lamellae is known as an *Haversian system,* or *osteon.* Osteons are oriented along the longitudinal axis of the bone and communicate with each other, the periosteum, and the marrow cavity via oblique or transverse canals known as *Volkmann's canals.* Blood vessels enter and leave and are distributed throughout bone via the Haversian and Volkmann's canals. Irregular lamellae structures, the *interstitial lamellae,* are present between the Haversian systems. They are remnants of resorbed lamellar systems resulting from the remodeling of bone. The inner (next to marrow cavity) and outer (next to periosteum) limits of compact bone are formed by lamellar structures, the *inner (endosteal)* and *outer (periosteal) circumferential lamellae,* respectively. The Haversian systems are the major component of compact bone and lie between these two circumferential lamellae. The marrow cavity and Haversian canals are lined by *endosteum,* a thin layer of connective tissue. Both the endosteum and periosteum contain *osteogenic cells,* which can transform into bone-forming cells, or *osteoblasts.*

Spongy bone. Spongy bone consists of *bars, spicules,* or *trabeculae,* which form a lattice meshwork. Spongy bone is found at the ends of long bones and the inner layer of flat, irregular, and short bones. The trabeculae consist of osteocytes embedded in calcified matrix, which in definitive bone has a lamellar nature. The spaces between the trabeculae contain bone marrow.

Bone Cells: The cells of bone are osteocytes, osteoblasts, and osteoclasts. *Osteocytes* are found singly in *lacunae* (spaces) within the calcified matrix and communicate with each other via small canals in the bone known as *canaliculi.* The latter contain osteocyte cell processes. The osteocytes in compact and spongy bone are similar in structure and function.

Osteoblasts are cells that form bone matrix, surrounding themselves with it, and thus are transformed into osteocytes. They arise from undifferentiated cells, such as mesenchymal cells. They are cuboidal cells which line the trabeculae of immature or developing spongy bone.

Osteoclasts are found during bone development and remodeling. They are multinucleated cells lying in cavities, *Howship's lacunae,* on the surface of the bone tissue being resorbed. Osteoclasts remove the existing calcified matrix releasing the inorganic or organic components.

Bone Matrix: *Matrix* of compact and spongy bone consists of collagenous fibers and ground substance which constitute the organic component of bone. Matrix also consists of inorganic material which is about 65% of the dry weight of bone. Approximately 85% of the inorganic component consists of calcium phosphate in a crystalline form (hydroxyapatite crystals). Glycoproteins are the main components of the ground substance.

Joints

The bones of the skeleton articulate with each other at *joints,* which are variable in structure and function. Some joints are immovable, such as the *sutures* between the bones of the cranium. Others are *slightly movable joints;* examples are the *intervertebral joints* and the *pubic symphysis* (joint between the two pubic bones of the coxal bones). These contain fibrocartilage plates separating the articulating bones and have a slight gliding motion. The most common joints are *freely movable joints.* They are also referred to as *synovial joints* since their joint capsules are lined by a serous *synovial membrane* which produces a lubricating fluid—*synovial fluid*—between the articulating bones. The *capsule* is a fibrous connective tissue sheath which encases the joint. Another feature of synovial joints is that a thin layer of *hyaline cartilage* lines the articular surfaces of the abutting bones. The synovial joints can be classified according to the type of motion permitted by the structure of the joint.

Adjacent bones at a joint are connected by fibrous connective tissue bands known as *ligaments.* They are strong bands that support the joint and may also act to limit the degree of motion occurring at a joint.

QUICK RECALL TEST QUESTIONS AND ANSWERS

Choose the Best Answer

1. The skeletal system of vertebrates is an:

   (A) axial skeleton.
   (B) appendicular skeleton.
   (C) endoskeleton.
   (D) exoskeleton.

2. Each statement concerning osteoclasts is correct EXCEPT that they:

   (A) are multinucleated.
   (B) lie in cavities known as Howship's lacunae.
   (C) remove existing calcified matrix.
   (D) are stimulated by thyro-calcitonin.

3. The appendicular skeleton is composed of bones of the:

   (A) cranium.
   (B) vertebral column.
   (C) pelvis.
   (D) upper and lower extremities.

4. The principal cells that form bone matrix are known as:

   (A) osteoblasts.
   (B) osteocytes.
   (C) osteoclasts.
   (D) interstitial lamella.

5. Cells that are active in bone removal during remodeling are:

   (A) osteoblasts.
   (B) osteocytes.
   (C) osteoclasts.
   (D) Haversian systems.

6. The main trunk of the body is supported by the spine or vertebral column. Concerning that structure, all of the following are true statements EXCEPT:

   (A) The vertebrae are separated from each other by a fibro-cartilaginous disc.
   (B) There are seven cervical vertebrae.
   (C) The sacrum is made up of five fused vertebrae.
   (D) The vertebral body is located posterior to the vertebral canal.

7. _____ give(s) origin to most of the skeletal system.

   (A) Ectoderm
   (B) Mesoderm
   (C) Endoderm
   (D) Ectoderm and mesoderm

8. The human skeletal system provides:

   (A) support and protection.
   (B) sites for muscle attachment.
   (C) storage sites for calcium and phosphates.
   (D) all of the above.

9. One of the functions of human bone tissue is to:

   (A) provide metabolic energy for movement.
   (B) store calcium and phosphate.
   (C) store potassium and chloride.
   (D) form slippery surfaces at joints in the skeleton.

10. Compact bone tissue:

    (A) is composed primarily of cells (little extracellular matrix).
    (B) is composed primarily of extracellular matrix (with cells scattered throughout the matrix).
    (C) contains only extracellular matrix (no living cells).

11. Cartilage:

    (A) makes up most of the skeleton of adult mammals.
    (B) forms the joint surfaces of many bones in the human skeleton.
    (C) does not occur in the skeleton of adult humans.

Answers

1. **(C)** The skeleton system of vertebrates is an endoskeleton—that is, it is within the body—in contrast to an exoskeleton characteristic of arthropods.

2. **(D)** Osteoclasts are stimulated by parathyroid hormone and inhibited by thyro-calcitonin. Osteoclasts are found during bone development and remodeling. They are multinucleated cells lying in cavities, Howship's lacunae, on the surface of the bone tissue being resorbed. Osteoclasts remove the existing calcified matrix releasing the inorganic or organic components.

3. **(D)** The appendicular skeleton forms the major internal support of the appendages—the upper and lower extremities (limbs).

4. **(A)** The cells of bone are osteocytes, osteoblasts, and osteoclasts. Osteoblasts are cells that form bone matrix, surrounding themselves with it, and thus are transformed into osteocytes. Osteoclasts are bone resorption cells which are most numerous during bone development and remodeling.

5. **(C)** Osteoclasts are cells involved in bone development and remodeling. Osteoclasts remove existing calcified matrix and release inorganic (calcium) or organic components to the system.

6. **(D)** The main trunk of the body is supported by the spine, or vertebral column. Each vertebra consists of a body anteriorly and an arched posterior region circumscribing an inner central canal.

7. **(B)** Mesoderm is the germ layer of origin of most of the skeletal system.

8. **(D)** The human skeletal system provides support, protection of vital organs, sites for muscle attachment, storage sites of body calcium and phosphates, and sites for blood cell formation.

9. **(B)** In addition to providing mechanical support for the body, the calcium and phosphate used to solidify the extracellular matrix in bone are used as metabolic reserves. Bone matrix is continually remodeled by resorption and deposition, allowing removal of calcium and phosphate from bone when they are needed and deposition of excess calcium and phosphate into bone matrix.

10. **(B)** Compact bone consists of layers of extracellular matrix interspersed with scattered layers of spider-shaped osteocytes (bone cells).

11. **(B)** Cartilage forms the articular surfaces of movable joints. Its slippery surface prevents excess wear in healthy joints. Cartilage also forms the supporting structures in the nose and ear and parts of the lower ribs.

MUSCULAR SYSTEM

Classification

A muscle cell not only has the ability to propagate an action potential along its cell membrane, as does a nerve cell, but also has the internal machinery to give it the unique ability to contract.

Most muscles in the body can be classified as striated muscles in reference to the fact that when observed under a light microscope the muscular tissue has light and dark bands or striations running across it. Although both skeletal and cardiac muscles are striated and therefore have similar structural organizations, they do possess some characteristic functional differences. Individual skeletal muscle cells are typically relatively large in diameter and extremely long, containing hundreds of nuclei. Skeletal muscle cells are not interconnected by gap junctions and are therefore not electrically coupled. Each skeletal muscle cell is innervated by axons from motor neurons in the central nervous system. Skeletal muscle cells normally contract only in response to synaptic transmission (usually acetyl choline) released by the motor axon synapses with the muscle cell. A single motor neuron typically makes synapses with multiple skeletal muscle cells. A motor unit consists of a single motor neuron coming from the spinal cord of the central nervous system and all the muscle fibers it innervates (a few to 2,000). Because each motor unit responds as a unit, the number and size of motor units determine many of the characteristics of a muscle. A muscle containing many small motor units is capable of finely graded responses (caused by triggering different numbers of motor units) and may be capable of sustained partial contraction achieved by triggering different motor units in sequence so no one unit is contracting frequently enough to cause fatigue. Conversely, a muscle containing a few large motor units would be easier to contract fully very quickly (because the activity of fewer units would need to be coordinated and controlled by the nervous system) but would not be capable of finely graded or sustained responses.

In contrast to skeletal muscle, cardiac muscle is a functional syncytium. Cardiac muscle cells are mechanically and electrically connected at their ends by their intercalated disks. The gap junction-like components of the intercalated disks allow the ionic changes involved in an action potential to spread from cell to cell in a layer of cardiac muscle. As a result, excitation of any point on the heart will spread through the interconnected cardiac muscle cells in the myocardium (muscle layer) throughout the adjacent chambers and then across the atrioventricular node to the other chambers of the heart.

Cardiac muscle cells undergo spontaneous depolarization, so isolated cardiac muscle cells trigger their own contractions. Because the modified cardiac muscle cells at the sinoatrial node region of the atria of the heart have the most rapid rate of self-depolarization, they serve as the pacemaker region and drive the contraction of the rest of the heart. Autonomic nerve endings alter the inherent rate of the pacemaker, but the initiation of contraction is intrinsic to cardiac muscle.

Smooth muscle is made up of spindle-shaped uninucleated cells in which the myosin is not organized into typical thick filaments, resulting in the absence of visible cross striations when viewed by light or electron microscopy. Some types of smooth muscle cells appear to be interconnected by modified gap junctions that allow ionic changes involved in excitation to pass from cell to cell, resulting in a wave of contraction passing along the muscle layer. Different types of smooth muscle differ in the type and extent of nervous control, but in most cases the nerve endings appear to be neurosecretory rather than synaptic and alter the activity level of the muscle rather than directly triggering contractions. Smooth muscle is part of the urinary bladder, uterus, spleen, gallbladder, and numerous other internal organs. It is also the muscle of blood vessels, most of the respiratory tract, and the iris of the eye.

The basic contractile mechanism is probably the same in all muscle types, although the structural organization of smooth muscle is very different from that of striated muscle. We will concentrate on skeletal muscle, knowing that what we discuss can be applied to cardiac muscle and to some extent to smooth muscle.

Skeletal Muscles

In order for the human being to carry out the many intricate movements that must be performed, approximately 650 skeletal muscles of various lengths, shapes, and strength play a part. Each muscle consists of many muscle cells or fibers held together and surrounded by connective tissue that gives functional integrity to the system. Three definite units are commonly referred to:

1. endomysium—extracellular matrix and very sparse, loose connective tissue layer enveloping a single fiber;
2. perimysium—connective tissue layer enveloping a bundle of fibers; and
3. epimysium—connective tissue layer enveloping the entire muscle.

Muscle Attachment and Function

For coordinated movement to occur, the muscle must attach to either bone or cartilage or, as in the case of the muscles of facial expression, to skin. The portion of a muscle attaching to bone is the tendon. A muscle has two extremities, its origin and its insertion; the origin is the relatively fixed attachment site, whereas the insertion is the end attached to a structure that will be moved when the muscle contracts. A pair of muscles usually control the movement of a joint; they are opposing or antagonistic muscles. For example, a flexor muscle is opposed by an extensor.

Terms to Describe Movement

Flexion is bending, most often ventrally to decrease the angle between two parts of the body; it is usually an action at an articulation or joint.

Extension is straightening, or increasing the angle between two parts of the body; a stretching out or making the flexed part straight.

Abduction is a movement away from the midsagittal plane (midline); to abduct is to move laterally.

Adduction is a movement toward the midsagittal plane (midline); to adduct is to move medially and bring a part back to the mid-axis.

Circumduction is a circular movement at a ball and socket (shoulder or hip) joint, utilizing the movements of flexion, extension, abduction, and adduction.

Rotation is a movement of a part of the body around its long axis.

Examples: a.   The atlas (1st cervical vertebra) rotates on the axis (2nd cervical vertebra).
           b.   The thigh may be rotated medially or internally; it may also be rotated laterally or externally.

Supination refers only to the movement of the radius around the ulna. In supination the palm of the hand is oriented anteriorly; turning the palm dorsally puts it into pronation. The body on its back is in the supine position.

Pronation refers to the palm of the hand being oriented posteriorly. The body on its belly is the prone position.

Inversion refers only to the lower extremity, specifically the ankle joint. When the foot (plantar surface) is turned inward, so that the sole is pointing and directed toward the midline of the body and is parallel with the median plane, we speak of inversion. Its opposite is eversion.

Eversion refers to the foot (plantar surface) being turned outward so that the sole is pointing laterally.

Opposition is one of the most critical movements in humans; it allows us to have pulp-to-pulp opposition, which gives us the great dexterity of our hands. In this movement the thumb pad is brought to a finger pad. A median nerve injury negates this action.

Muscle Names

The names of some muscles may appear strange; the naming, however, is based essentially on anatomical position, function, shape, or other feature. Here are some examples:

1. Position and Location:

a. Pectoralis major and minor	pectoral region of thorax; the major is larger
b. Temporalis	temporal region of head
c. Infra- and supraspinatus	below and above spine of scapula
d. External and internal intercostals	refers to their location in the intercostal spaces

2. Principal Action:

a. Pronators (e.g., pronator quadratus) and supinators	pronation refers to palm down and supination to palm up; quadratus refers to the shape
b. Flexors and extensors (e.g., flexor and extensor digitorum)	flexors and extensors of digits
c. Levator scapulae	elevator of the scapula (shoulder)

3. Shape:

a. Trapezius	trapezoid in shape
b. Rhomboid major and minor	rhomboid in shape

4. Number of Divisions (Heads) and Position:

a. Biceps brachii	two-headed muscle in anterior brachium (arm)
b. Triceps brachii	three-headed muscle in posterior brachium (arm)

5. Size, Length, and Shape:

a. Flexor pollicis longus and brevis	long and short flexors of the thumb
b. Rhomboid major and minor	major is larger in size; rhomboid in shape.

6. Attachment Sites:

a. Sternocleidomastoid	extends from sternum and clavicle (cleido) to mastoid process
b. Sternohyoid	extends from sternum to hyoid bone

Structural Organization of a Muscle Fiber

A muscle fiber is a single muscle cell. If we look at a section of a fiber we see that it is complete with a plasma membrane called the sarcolemma and has several nuclei located just under the sarcolemma—it is multinucleated. Each fiber is composed of numerous cylindrical fibrils running the entire length of the fiber.

The fibril exhibits light and dark bands—the "I" and "A" bands, respectively. The "I" band is bisected by the "Z" line and the "A" band by the "M" line. There is a somewhat lighter band within the "A" band that is called the "H" band. An even lighter area in the middle of the "H" zone on either side of the "M" line is called the "pseudo-H" band.

These striations are produced by the arrangement within the fibril of myofilaments which comprise the contractile machinery. A sarcomere, the area between two "Z" bands, is the functional unit of muscle; it is the region between two "Z" lines and consists of an "A" band and half of two abutting "I" bands. Refer to the illustration of the relaxed myofibril (page 82) for the positions of these lines and bands.

Myofilaments

1. The thick and thin myofilaments form the contractile machinery of muscle and are made up of proteins. Approximately 54% of all the contractile proteins (by weight) is myosin. The thick myofilament is composed of many myosin molecules oriented tail-end to tail-end. The head domains are oriented outward.

2. The second major contractile protein is actin, a globular protein. The thin myofilament contains two chains of F-actin arranged in a twisted fashion. This configuration gives the thin myofilament a certain periodicity. Associated with the thin myofilament along its entire length is the globular protein troponin. The presence of troponin along with tropomyosin-B inhibits myosin-actin interaction—it represses actomyosin formation. Calcium ions released following an action potential in the fiber membrane and T-tubules bind with troponin. Calcium-troponin binding removes the inhibition of actomyosin formation.

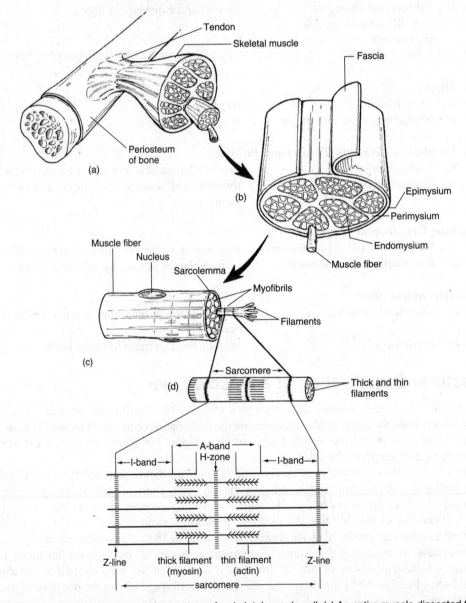

The microscopic and submicroscopic structure of a skeletal muscle cell. (a) An entire muscle dissected through its belly. (b) A cross section through the entire muscle to show numerous fibers (cells) organized into bundles. (c) A single muscle fiber (cell) displaying three nuclei, the sarcolemma, and a number of sarcomeres at the end of the fiber. (d) A sarcomere expanded to show the thick and thin filaments of the various bands and zones. Muscle activity takes place at the sarcomere.

Sarcoplasm

The sarcoplasm (cytoplasm of the muscle cell) contains Golgi complexes near the nuclei. Mitochondria are found between the myofibrils and just below the sarcolemma. The myofibrils are surrounded by smooth endoplasmic reticulum *(sarcoplasmic reticulum)* composed of a longitudinally arranged tubular network *(sarcotubules)*. The sarcotubules are continuous with dilated sacs called terminal cisternae. In skeletal muscle the terminal cisternae lie over the I–A junction of the sacromeres. The terminal cisternae of cardiac muscle are less well developed and are located adjacent to the Z discs. The terminal cisternae are in association with invaginations of the sarcolemma T-tubules.

The complex (terminal cistern-T-tubule-terminal cistern) formed at this position is known as a *triad*. The T-tubules function to bring a wave of depolarization of the sarcolemma into the fiber and thus into an intimate relationship with the terminal cisternae. The sarcoplasmic reticulum concentrates calcium ions (Ca^{2+}) within its lumen, but depolarization of the T-tubule membrane induces the nearby terminal cisternae of the sarcoplasmic reticulum to release this Ca^{2+} into the sarcoplasma among the myofilaments. The Ca^{2+} becomes associated with the troponin of the thin myofilament, bringing about contraction as on page 74.

Excitation

Contraction in a skeletal muscle is triggered by the generation of an action potential in the muscle membrane. Each axon from a motor neuron upon entering a skeletal muscle loses its myelin sheath and divides into branches with each branch innervating a single muscle fiber, forming a *neuromuscular junction*. Each muscle fiber normally has one neuromuscular junction (typically consisting of multiple endings), which is located near the center of the fiber. A *motor unit* consists of a single motor neuron and all the muscle fibers innervated by it. The *motor end plate* is the specialized part of the muscle fiber's membrane lying under the axon ending.

The impulse arriving at the end of the motor axon causes liberation of *acetylcholine* from vesicles in the axon terminal. The acetylcholine acts at specific sites normally found only on the motor end plate section of the fiber membrane and increases the permeability of the motor end plate. The resulting Na^+ influx produces a depolarizing potential called the end-plate potential. This in turn depolarizes adjacent areas of the fiber membrane, triggering an action potential which is propagated in both directions from the central neuromuscular junction toward the fiber ends. Normally the magnitude of the end-plate potential is sufficient to discharge the muscle membrane, so that each impulse in the nerve ending produces a response in the muscle. The acetylcholine is rapidly destroyed by the enzyme *acetylcholinesterase* which is found in high concentrations at the neuromuscular junction.

Contraction

According to the sliding filament theory (Huxley) the sarcomere response to excitation involves the sliding of thin and thick myofilaments past one another making and breaking chemical bonds with each other as they go. Neither the thick nor thin myofilaments change in length. If we could imagine observing this contraction under a light microscope we would see the narrowing of the "H" and "I" bands during contraction while the width of the "A" band would remain constant.

The word *contraction* refers to those processes which are manifested externally by either a *shortening* of a muscle or by *tension development* in a muscle. If the muscle length is held constant, the contraction is referred to as an *isometric contraction*. In an isometric contraction the passive tension remains constant with the *active tension* being added to it to produce the *total tension* of the muscle.

If the muscle shortens during contraction, it is called an *isotonic contraction* and the total tension remains constant.

EVENTS LEADING TO MUSCLE CONTRACTION

1. Action potential of the axon of the motoneuron.
2. Depolarization of axon terminal.
3. Ca^{2+} enters axon terminal.
4. Acetylcholine (ACh) released into synaptic cleft.
5. ACh diffuses across synapse.
6. ACh binds to receptors on muscle end plate; degradation of ACh by acetylcholinesterase.
7. Depolarization of muscle end plate (end plate potential).
8. Action potential in muscle.
9. Action potential invades transverse (T) tubule.
10. Ca^{2+} released from sarcoplasmic reticulum (SR).
11. Increased intracellular $[Ca^{2+}]$.
12. Ca^{2+} binds to troponin C on the thin filaments.
13. Action and myosin bind, forming cross bridges.
14. Cross bridges pivot.
15. Thick and thin filaments slide, producing muscle tension.
16. Ca^{2+} reuptake into sarcoplasmic reticulum by (Ca^{2+} ATPase).
17. Decreased intracellular $[Ca^{2+}]$.
18. Relaxation.

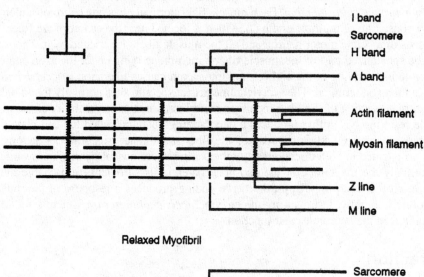

Relaxed Myofibril

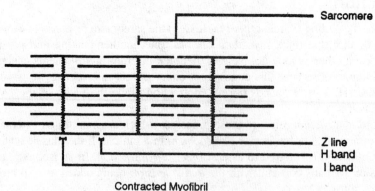

Contracted Myofibril

SCHEMATIC OF SKELETAL (STRIATED) MUSCLE

Muscle Twitch

A muscle's response to a single maximal stimulus is a *muscle twitch*. The beginning of muscular activity is signalled by the record of the *electrical activity* in the sarcolemma. The *latent period* is the delay between imposition of the stimulus and the development of tension.

Tetanus

When a volley of stimuli is applied to a muscle, each succeeding stimulus may arrive before the muscle can completely relax from the contraction caused by the preceding stimulus. The result is *summation,* an increased strength of contraction. If the frequency of stimulation is very fast, individual contractions fuse and the muscle smoothly and fully contracts. This is a *tetanus*.

Energy Sources

In any phenomenon including muscular contraction the energy input to the system and the energy output from the system are equal. The immediate energy source for contraction is ATP, which can be hydrolyzed by actomyosin to give ADP, P_i, and the energy which is in some way associated with cross-bridge motion.

The ultimate source of this ATP is the ATP produced by the intermediary metabolism of carbohydrates and lipids. Skeletal muscle has the biochemical machinery to utilize both. With mild exercise, oxygen availability after an initial period of adjustment is sufficient so that the aerobic pathways for ATP production can keep pace with the ATP utilization during the exercise—a new equilibrium is reached. During short-term, violent exertion, however, aerobic energy production cannot keep pace with energy utilization and even during the onset of mild exercise aerobic energy production initially lags behind energy utilization. Yet the ATP concentration remains constant. The reason is that there are stores of CP (creatine phosphate) in muscles and ATP levels can be maintained at the expense of CP levels. In these cases of insufficient oxygen availability ("oxygen debt"), anaerobic pathways can produce enough additional ATP to permit those short-term bursts of exercise but lactic acid is generated. This incomplete oxidation produces substantially less energy than the complete aerobic oxidation to carbon dioxide and water. Physiological muscle fatigue apparently involves lactic acid accumulation rather than depletion of ATP.

Type of Muscle Fibers

Skeletal muscle fibers can be described, on the bases of structure and function, as follows:

1. *White (fast) fibers*—contract rapidly; fatigue quickly; energy production is mainly via anaerobic glycolysis; contain relatively few mitochondria; examples are the muscles of the eye.
2. *Red (slow) fibers*—contract slowly; fatigue slowly; energy production mainly via oxidative phosphorylation (aerobic); contain relatively many mitochondria; examples are postural muscles.
3. *Intermediate fibers*—have structural and functional qualities between those of white and of red fibers.

QUICK RECALL TEST QUESTIONS AND ANSWERS

Choose the Best Answer

1. Of the elements listed, which is most essential for muscular contraction?

    (A) sodium
    (B) potassium
    (C) magnesium
    (D) calcium

2. Sustained muscle activity leads to fatigue, which is accompanied by the accumulation of:

    (A) ATP.
    (B) ADP.
    (C) Troponin.
    (D) Lactic acid.

3. Muscle contraction results when actin unites with:

    (A) calcium ions.
    (B) troponin.
    (C) myosin.
    (D) ATP.

4. According to the sliding filament theory (Huxley), when a contraction is observed under the light microscope, the following occurs:

    (A) there is a narrowing of the H band.
    (B) there is a widening of the I band.
    (C) there is a narrowing of the A band.
    (D) there is a widening of the Z line.

5. A Triad, in relation to skeletal muscles, refers to:

    (A) the A and I bands and T-tubule collectively.
    (B) one T-tubule and two adjacent terminal cisternae together.
    (C) three Z bands in very close approximation.
    (D) a sarcotubule, a T-tubule, and a terminal cisternae collectively.

6. A sustained contraction is called:

    (A) tonus.
    (B) a recovery period.
    (C) tetanus.
    (D) a contraction period.

7. Vigorous exercise will cause muscle fatigue, which is primarily due to:

    (A) the utilization and exhaustion of ATP.
    (B) the accumulation of ADP.
    (C) the accumulation of lactic acid.
    (D) the accumulation of carbon dioxide.

8. The state of a continuously mild or partial contraction of a muscle is denoted as:

    (A) tetanus.
    (B) tonus.
    (C) an "all or none" contraction.
    (D) a twitch.

9. Which of the following muscle types is not under the control of the autonomic (involuntary) nervous system?

    (A) heart (cardiac)
    (B) smooth
    (C) skeletal (striated)
    (D) arrector pili

10. If we examine the three types of muscles in respect to their characteristics, which of the series below is false?

	Characteristic	Cardiac	Skeletal	Smooth
(A)	No. of nuclei per cell	One	Several	One
(B)	Position of nuclei	Central	Central	Central
(C)	Striations	Present	Present	Absent
(D)	Control	Autonomic	Voluntary	Autonomic

11. The functional unit of a striated muscle is known as the sarcomere. A sarcomere on an electron micrograph is the region between:

    (A) two A bands.
    (B) two I bands.
    (C) two H bands.
    (D) two Z bands.

12. A fiber of striated (skeletal) muscle:

    (A) possesses only one nucleus.
    (B) possesses no clear Z bands.
    (C) possesses more than one nucleus.
    (D) has the same characteristics as smooth muscle.

13. Which of the following is NOT true of normally functioning human skeletal muscle?

    (A) Contraction occurs only in response to a nerve impulse.
    (B) The plasma membrane of the muscle cells can conduct action potentials.
    (C) Cells maintain a state of partial contraction (due to spontaneous contractions) which is then adjusted to a state of greater or lesser contraction in response to nerve impulses from motor neurons.

14. A normal vertebrate skeletal muscle fiber (cell) is:

    (A) uninucleate and striated.
    (B) multinucleate and striated.
    (C) uninucleate and unstriated.
    (D) multinucleate and unstriated.

15. A normal vertebrate skeletal muscle fiber (cell):

    (A) produces rapid, brief contractions under direct somatic nervous system control (contracts only in direct response to a nerve impulse).
    (B) produces rapid, brief contractions under autonomic nervous system rate control (contracts spontaneously at a rate which may be altered by autonomic nervous system activity).
    (C) produces slow, long-lasting contractions under direct somatic nervous system control (contracts only in direct response to a nerve impulse).
    (D) produces slow, long-lasting contractions under autonomic nervous system rate control (contracts spontaneously at a rate which may be altered by autonomic nervous system activity).

16. Prior to the contraction of a vertebrate fast-twitch skeletal muscle cell, the action potential passes along the motor axon and results in the release of _____ from the presynaptic ending when it reaches the synapse with the muscle cell.

    (A) adrenalin
    (B) sodium
    (C) acetyl choline
    (D) electricity

17. The sliding of the thick and thin myofilaments during the contraction of a vertebrate skeletal muscle cell is triggered by the _____ the sarcoplasmic reticulum.

    (A) release of calcium from
    (B) uptake of calcium by
    (C) release of sodium from
    (D) uptake of sodium by

18. The sliding of the thick and thin myofilaments during the contraction of a vertebrate fast-twitch skeletal muscle cell is powered by the _____ by the filaments.

    (A) synthesis of ATP
    (B) hydrolysis of ATP
    (C) synthesis of protein
    (D) hydrolysis of protein

Answers

1. **(D)** The sarcoplasmic reticulum concentrates calcium ions (Ca^{2+}). The Ca^{2+} becomes associated with the troponin of the thin myofilament, bringing about contraction. Although Na^+ is required for the action potential that triggers the contraction, it is not involved in the contraction itself.

2. **(D)** In cases of insufficient oxygen availability ("oxygen debt") anaerobic pathways can produce enough additional ATP to permit short-term bursts of exercise but lactic acid is generated.

3. **(C)** In muscle contraction, first the actomyosin complex must be established; at that point ATP is hydrolyzed and the energy necessary is provided.

4. **(A)** According to the sliding filament theory (Huxley) the sarcomere response to excitation involves the sliding of thin and thick myofilaments past one another. We see the narrowing of the "H" and "I" bands during contraction while the width of the "A" band would remain constant.

5. **(B)** The complex (terminal cistern-T-tubule-terminal cistern) formed is known as a *triad*. The T-tubules function to bring a wave of depolarization of the sarcolemma into the fiber and thus into intimate relationship with the terminal cisternae.

6. **(C)** If more than two stimuli are given to a muscle in rapid succession, a partial fusion of all contractions results. The contractions occur before relaxation can take place or is completed. If a contraction is steadily maintained and no relaxation occurs between separate stimuli, the contraction is known as tetanus.

7. **(C)** The cause of muscle fatigue is said to be the accumulated anaerobically produced lactic acid. Lactic acid may later be broken down into carbon dioxide and water for elimination, or it may be converted into glycogen and stored for future use.

8. **(B)** Tonus refers to muscular activity in which a shortened condition is maintained for a prolonged period. Visceral muscle is the outstanding example of tonus. The word can be applied to any sustained process which is the result of probable regularly repeated excitation.

9. **(C)** Skeletal (striated) muscle is under voluntary control. The autonomic nervous system innervates cardiac muscle, smooth muscle, and glands. Arrector pili musculature is associated with skin and is smooth musculature.

10. **(B)** In skeletal muscle the nuclei are found peripherally. To complete the chart, the speed of contraction should also be mentioned. Skeletal muscle is the fastest working, smooth muscle is the slowest, and cardiac muscle occupies an intermediate position.

11. **(D)** A sarcomere is the region between two Z bands. In simple terms, we are dealing with this unit: ZIAHAIZ. Contraction of the sarcomere is due to the fine filaments (actin) sliding between the thick filaments (myosin), pulling the Z bands to which they are attached with them. This pulls the Z bands closer together, and so the sarcomeres are shortened.

12. **(C)** The striated muscle fiber is multinucleated.

13. **(C)** Normally functioning skeletal muscle does not spontaneously contract. Contraction occurs only in response to somatic nervous system nerve impulses (action potentials).

14. **(B)** Skeletal muscle cells are large and heavily multinucleated owing to their origin by fusion of myoblasts in the embryo. A typical skeletal muscle cell may contain hundreds of nuclei. These cells are also strongly striated as a result of the precise arrangement of the thick and thin myofilaments within each cell.

15. **(A)** Skeletal muscle cells vary in the speed and force of their contractions, but produce faster and more forceful contractions than cardiac and smooth muscle. Skeletal muscle contractions occur in response to nerve impulses in the motor neuron controlling the particular muscle cell and are of brief duration.

16. **(C)** In mammals, acetyl choline is the transmitter used in neuromuscular synapses.

17. **(A)** Depolarization resulting from influx of sodium across the plasma membrane and transverse tubules of the muscle cell activates the sarcoplasmic reticulum (endoplasmic reticulum of the muscle cell) to release calcium ions. The calcium ions trigger the thin myofilaments to interact with the thick myofilaments.

18. **(B)** Hydrolysis of ATP drives a conformational change in myosin that in turn drives sliding of the thick and thin myofilaments past each other.

CIRCULATORY SYSTEM

Functions

The circulatory system serves to:

(1) transport nutrients and oxygen to the tissues;
(2) remove waste materials by transporting nitrogenous compounds to the kidneys and carbon dioxide to the lungs;
(3) transport chemical messengers (hormones) to target organs and modulate and integrate the internal milieu of the body;
(4) transport agents which serve the body in allergic, immune, and infectious responses;
(5) initiate clotting and thereby prevent blood loss;
(6) maintain body temperature;
(7) produce, carry, and contain blood;
(8) transfer body reserves, specifically mineral salts, to areas of need.

General Components and Structure

The circulatory system consists of the heart, blood vessels, blood, and lymphatics. It is a network of tubular structures through which blood travels to and from all the parts of the body. In vertebrates this is a completely closed circuit system, as William Harvey (1628) demonstrated. The heart is a modified, specialized, powerful pumping blood vessel. Arteries, eventually becoming arterioles, conduct blood to capillaries (essentially endothelial tubes), and venules, eventually becoming veins, return blood from the capillary bed to the heart. (Malpighi [1661] demonstrated the capillary system.) The system is lined entirely by endothelium. Fluids (mostly water) that leave capillaries return as lymph to the bloodstream via lymphatic channels. The spleen, liver, and bone marrow function in the formation, destruction, and replacement of blood cells.

Systemic arteries originating from the left side of the heart (via the aorta) distribute oxygenated and nutrient-rich blood to the body. The systemic venous system returns deoxygenated blood to the heart. The pulmonary arterial circuit delivers this blood from the right side of the heart to the lungs and the pulmonary venous component returns oxygenated blood to the left side of the heart. Arteries travel away from the heart; veins come to it.

The Heart

The heart is a highly specialized blood vessel that pumps 72 times per minute and propels about 4,000 gallons (about 15,000 liters) of blood daily to the tissues. It is composed of:

> endocardium (lining coat; epithelium)
> myocardium (middle coat; cardiac muscle)
> epicardium (external coat or visceral layer of pericardium; epithelium and mostly connective tissue)
> impulse conducting system

Mammals possess modified cardiac muscle fibers specialized for conduction (Purkinje system). The heart has an automatic rhythmic beat. Cardiac (autonomic) nerves exert an influence on heartbeat but serve only to change the force and frequency of the contractions in accordance with the physiologic needs of the organism.

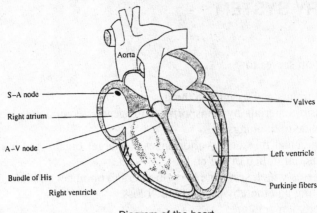

S–A node

Right atrium

A–V node

Bundle of His

Right ventricle

Aorta

Valves

Left ventricle

Purkinje fibers

Diagram of the heart.

Cardiac Nerves: Modification of the intrinsic rhythmicity of the heart muscle is produced by cardiac nerves of the sympathetic and parasympathetic nervous system. Stimulation of the sympathetic system increases the rate and force of the heartbeat and dilates the coronary arteries. Stimulation of the parasympathetic (vagus nerve) reduces the rate and force of the heartbeat and constricts the coronary circulation. Visceral afferent (sensory) fibers from the heart end almost wholly in the first four segments of the thoracic spinal cord.

Cardiac Cycle: Alternating contraction and relaxation is repeated about 75 times per minute; the duration of one cycle is about 0.8 sec. Three phases succeed one another during the cycle:

(a) atrial systole: 0.1 sec
(b) ventricular systole: 0.3 sec
(c) diastole: 0.4 sec

The actual period of rest for each chamber is 0.7 sec for the atria and 0.5 sec for the ventricles, so, in spite of its activity, the heart is at rest longer than at work.

Course of Circulation

The circulatory system is organized as two anatomically and functionally distinct subdivisions: the blood vascular subdivision and the lymph vascular subdivision. The blood vascular subdivision distributes blood containing nutrients, gases, hormones, and so on, to all parts of the body. The lymph vascular subdivision collects tissue fluid from tissues for return to the blood vascular subdivision.

Blood Vascular Subdivision: Functionally, this subdivision of the circulatory system consists of two different circulatory routes: the systemic route and the pulmonary route. Systemic arteries originating from the left side of the heart (via the aorta) distribute oxygen-rich and nutrient-rich blood to all parts of the body. Systemic veins return oxygen-poor and nutrient-poor blood back to the right side of the heart (via the vena cavae). Pulmonary arteries deliver this blood from the right side of the heart to the lungs, and pulmonary veins return oxygen-rich blood back to the left side of the heart. The pathway of blood flow through the heart and associated blood vessels is depicted in the following box.

> venous blood returns to heart via inferior/superior vena cavae →
> right atrium → tricuspid valve → right ventricle → pulmonary semilunar
> valve → pulmonary arteries → lungs (i.e., smaller arteries, capillary beds,
> smaller veins) → pulmonary veins → left atrium → bicuspid valve → left
> ventricle → aortic semilunar valve → aorta

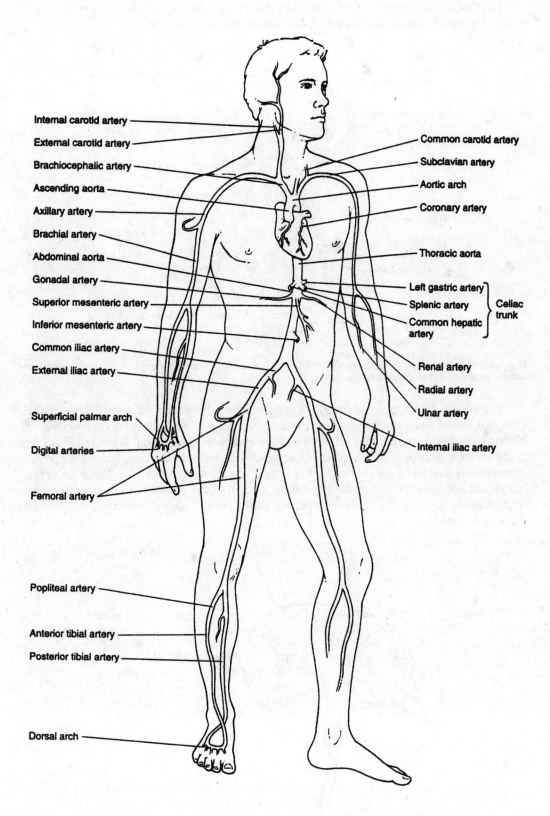

Internal carotid artery

External carotid artery

Brachiocephalic artery

Ascending aorta

Axillary artery

Brachial artery

Abdominal aorta

Gonadal artery

Superior mesenteric artery

Inferior mesenteric artery

Common iliac artery

External iliac artery

Superficial palmar arch

Digital arteries

Femoral artery

Popliteal artery

Anterior tibial artery

Posterior tibial artery

Dorsal arch

Common carotid artery

Subclavian artery

Aortic arch

Coronary artery

Thoracic aorta

Left gastric artery
Splenic artery
Common hepatic artery

Celiac trunk

Renal artery

Radial artery

Ulnar artery

Internal iliac artery

The major arteries of the human body, excluding the pulmonary arteries.

Because of these two different circulatory routes, the heart is often referred to as a double pump. The circulatory system is often said to have double circulation.

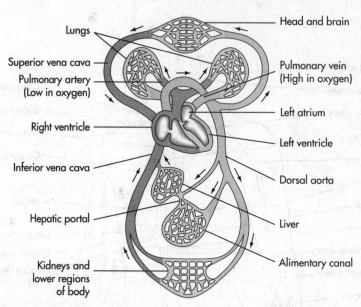

Distribution of blood in a complete double circulation. The relation of the capillaries to the arteries and veins cannot be shown in this diagram but is implied.

Lymphatic Drainage: A network of lymphatic capillaries permeates the body tissues. Lymph is a fluid similar in composition to blood plasma, and tissue fluids not reabsorbed into blood capillaries are transported via the lymphatic system eventually to join the venous system at the junction of the left internal jugular and subclavian veins. Like veins, lymphatics possess valves. Interposed along the course of some lymph vessels are lymph nodes. These nodes filter lymph and add lymphocytes to the circulation. Lymph nodes possess an outer cortex and an inner medulla. Lymphoid follicles are present in the cortex; irregular cords of lymphocytes make up the medulla.

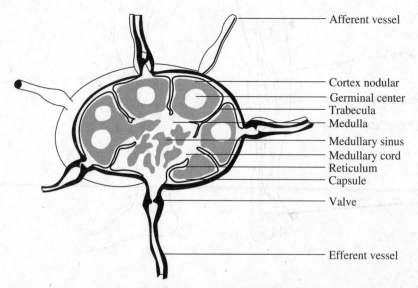

Schematic of Lymph Node. Afferent vessels bring material to the nodes; this material passes through the reticulum of the nodes and is processed (foreign material is filtered out by phagocytic cells); lymphocytes (manufactured in germinal centers) and immunologic material are added and lymph leaves via efferent vessels (at the hilus) eventually to gain access to the venous system.

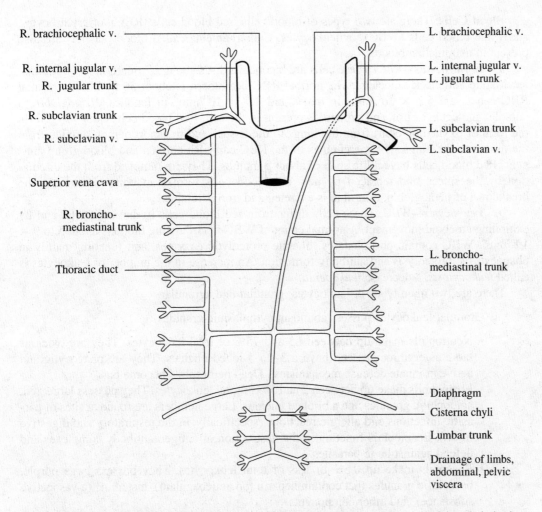

R. brachiocephalic v.

R. internal jugular v.

R. jugular trunk

R. subclavian trunk

R. subclavian v.

Superior vena cava

R. broncho-
mediastinal trunk

Thoracic duct

L. brachiocephalic v.

L. internal jugular v.
L. jugular trunk

L. subclavian trunk

L. subclavian v.

L. broncho-
mediastinal trunk

Diaphragm

Cisterna chyli

Lumbar trunk

Drainage of limbs,
abdominal, pelvic
viscera

Schema of Main Lymphatic Pathways. Note that the right jugular lymphatic trunk and the right subclavian lymphatic trunk form the right lymphatic duct. The left jugular lymphatic trunk and the left subclavian lymphatic trunk empty into the thoracic duct. The thoracic duct also receives the drainage from the lower limbs, abdomen, pelvis, perineum, and left thorax. The right head and neck specimen, the right upper extremity, and most of the right thorax drain via the right lymphatic duct. Both sides feed into the venous system at the junction (confluens) of the internal jugular and subclavian veins. Numerous variations exist.

Blood

Blood is composed of cells (corpuscles) and a liquid intercellular material called plasma. The average blood volume is 5 to 6 liters (7% of body weight). Plasma constitutes about 55% of blood volume; cellular elements about 45%.

Plasma: Over 90% of plasma is water; the balance is made up of plasma proteins and dissolved electrolytes, hormones, antibodies, nutrients, and waste products. Plasma is isotonic (0.85% sodium chloride). Plasma plays a vital role in respiration, circulation, coagulation, temperature regulation, buffer activities, and overall fluid balance. The plasma proteins (albumin, globulin, and fibrinogen) are responsible for the viscosity of blood, for carrying immune material, and for controlling osmotic pressure. Fibrinogen, in bleeding, is transformed into fibrin and helps form a clot. Plasma defibrinated by clotting is known as *blood serum*.

Blood Cells: There are two types of blood cells: red blood cells (RBC), or erythrocytes, and white blood cells (WBC), or leukocytes. Cell fragments called blood platelets are also present in mammalian blood.

a. *Erythrocytes—RBC.* These cells are biconcave discs about 7.7 micrometers in diameter. Mature cells lack a nucleus. The normal RBC hematocrit is about 36 to 45. The normal RBC counts are $5.2 \times 10^6/mm^3$ in males and $4.5 \times 10^6/mm^3$ in females. *Hemoglobin,* a complex molecule of iron and protein, is present in the cell. Red blood cells carry oxygen (in the form of oxyhemoglobin) from the lungs to the tissues and transport carbon dioxide from the tissues to the lungs. The membranes of the RBC carry Rh antigen and blood group antigens. Red blood cells have a life span of about 3 months. They are removed from the circulation by the spleen and replaced by new red blood cells formed in bone marrow. In the breakdown of hemoglobin, bilurubin is excreted and iron is retained.

b. *Leukocytes—WBC.* These cells differ from red blood cells by having nuclei and by exhibiting ameboid movement. A normal count of WBC in circulating blood is about 5 to $9 \times 10^3/mm^3$. WBC contain phosphatases, liberate proteolytic enzymes, and function mainly in phagocytosis, proteolysis and antibody formation. An increase in the number of leukocytes is called *leukocytosis,* a decrease *leukopenia.*

There are two main types of leukocytes: granular and agranular.

1. Granular leukocytes possess abundant cytoplasmic granules.

   - Neutrophils make up between 65 and 75% of total leukocytes. They are twice as large as erythrocytes and have a 3- to 5-lobed nucleus. They are phagocytic and active in innate defense mechanisms. Dead neutrophils become pus.
   - Eosinophils make up between 2 and 5% of total leukocytes. They possess large, red, acidophilic granules and a bilobed nucleus. Large numbers are found at sites of parasitic infections and allergic reactions (specifically, in the respiratory and digestive tracts). Eosinophils function in the destruction of antigen-antibody complexes and defend against large parasites.
   - Basophils make up 0.5% or less of total leukocytes. They possess large purple, basophilic granules that contain heparin (an anticoagulant), histamine (a vasoactive substance), and other components.

2. Agranular leukocytes do not possess abundant cytoplasmic granules.

   - Lymphocytes make up between 20 and 25% of total leukocytes. They originate from lymphoid tissue and bone marrow, are prevalent at sites of chronic inflammation, and function in specific immune responses.
   - Monocytes make up between 3 and 8% of total leukocytes. After extravasation and migration into connective tissues, monocytes differentiate into macrophages, which function in both innate defense mechanisms and specific immune responses.

c. *Blood platelets.* These cytoplasmic structures are not true cells but are cell fragments characteristic of mammalian blood. (In lower vertebrates, cells called thrombocytes have a function similar to platelets.) Blood platelets average about 3 microns in diameter. About 250,000 to 350,000/mm^3 are normally present. These structures arise by the fragmentation of cytoplasmic processes of giant bone marrow cells. Platelets agglutinate and adhere to regions of injured vessels; they plug wounds of blood vessels. They help physically in clotting and form thromboplastin (thrombokinase), an integral chemical component of clot formation.

Blood Clotting: Platelets contribute thromboplastin (thrombokinase), an enzymatically active substance. Thromboplastin interacts with calcium ions and prothrombin (a plasma protein). Prothrombin is an inactive precursor of the catalyst thrombin. In the presence of these components prothrombin is converted to thrombin. Subsequently thrombin reacts with the plasma protein fibrinogen, forming fibrin. Fibrin is an insoluble, coagulated protein which clots. A clot also contains blood cells. Diagrammatically we can represent clotting reactions as follows:

$$\text{platelets} \rightarrow \text{thromboplastin}$$

$$\downarrow$$

$$\text{prothrombin} + \text{Ca}^{2+} \rightarrow \text{thrombin}$$

$$\downarrow$$

$$\text{fibrinogen} \rightarrow \text{fibrin}.$$

Anticoagulants. An anticoagulant is a substance that prevents or retards coagulation of blood. Examples are: *heparin,* an acid mucopolysaccharide which occurs most abundantly in the liver; *aspirin* (acetylsalicylic acid), which also acts as an analgesic, antipyretic, antirheumatic compound; and the drug *Dicumarol,* a tradename for bihydroxycoumarin.

Blood Pressure: Blood pressure is usually measured by placing a sphygmomanometer cuff around the arm compressing the brachial artery and vein. Maximum blood pressure is obtained during ventricular contraction (systole) and minimum blood pressure indicates ventricular rest (diastole). The normal blood pressure listed for a young adult is 120 systolic and 80 diastolic (mm Hg).

Composition of Human Blood in Review

Whole Blood

Plasma 55%			Cellular elements 45%		
Water	Metabolites	Electrolytes	Red blood cells		
				Platelets	
					White blood cells
90%	- lipids	Na$^+$			
	- amino acids	K$^+$			
	- carbohydrates	Ca^{++}			- lymphocytes
	- waste products	Mg^{++}			- monocytes
		CL			- neutrophils
		HCO$^-_3$			- eosinophils
		HPO$^{-2}_4$			- basophils
		SO$^{-2}_4$			

QUICK RECALL TEST QUESTIONS AND ANSWERS

Choose the Best Answer

1. Cardiac muscle makes up the greater portion of the:

   (A) pericardium.
   (B) epicaradium.
   (C) myocardium.
   (D) endocardium.

2. The most important function attributed to neutrophils and monocytes is to be active in:

   (A) phagocytosis.
   (B) the immunologic response.
   (C) the allergic response.
   (D) production of heparin.

3. Blood is delivered to the right atrium by the superior and inferior vena cavas. From the right atrium blood passes to the right ventricle; in its passage it traverses the:

   (A) tricuspid valve.
   (B) pulmonary semilunar valve.
   (C) bicuspid valve.
   (D) aortic semilunar valve.

4. Heparin, an anticoagulant, is associated with cytoplasmic granules, which are produced by the:

   (A) lymphocytes.
   (B) monocytes.
   (C) neutrophils.
   (D) basophils.

5. Eosinophils:

   (A) make up between 20% and 25% of the total leukocytes.
   (B) function in the destruction of antigen–antibody complexes.
   (C) are classified as agranular leukocytes.
   (D) possess basophilic granules and a bilobed nucleus.

6. Heartbeat is initiated by the:

   (A) vagus nerve.
   (B) sympathetic nervous system.
   (C) A-V (atrio-ventricular) node.
   (D) S-A (sino-atrial) node.

7. The most numerous leukocytes are the:

   (A) lymphocytes.
   (B) monocytes.
   (C) eosinophils.
   (D) neutrophils.

8. Administration of which of the following compound(s) increases clotting time?

   (A) heparin
   (B) aspirin
   (C) dicumarol
   (D) all of the above

9. When a physician informs a patient that the blood pressure reading is 160/90, the physician refers to the:

   (A) systolic blood pressure of the left ventricle.
   (B) blood pressure in the veins of the arm.
   (C) systolic and diastolic pressures of the brachial artery.
   (D) systolic pressure of the aorta and diastolic pressure in the superior vena cava.

10. Blood in the pulmonary vein is rich in:

    (A) oxyhemoglobin.
    (B) carbaminohemoglobin.
    (C) hemoglobin.
    (D) uric acid.

11. Abnormal blood clots (thrombi) occur more frequently in people with:

    (A) prothrombin deficiency.
    (B) impeded venous blood flow.
    (C) vitamin K deficiency.
    (D) platelet deficiency.

Answers

1. **(C)** The heart is a highly specialized blood vessel that pumps 72 times per minute and propels about 4000 gallons (about 15,000 liters) of blood daily to the tissues. It is composed of:

   endocardium (lining coat; epithelium)
   myocardium (middle coat; cardiac muscle)
   epicardium (external coat or visceral layer of pericardium; epithelium and mostly connective tissue)
   impulse conducting system

2. **(A)** Both neutrophils and monocytes are phagocytic, helping to destroy foreign organisms.

3. **(A) Pulmonary Circuit:** Blood is oxygenated and depleted of metabolic products such as carbon dioxide in the lungs. The pathway is as follows:

   (1) Deoxygenated blood arrives in the right atrium and passes through the tricuspid valve into the right ventricle.
   (2) Blood leaves the right ventricle via the pulmonary (trunk) artery and passes to the lungs; backflow is prevented by the pulmonary semilunar valves.
   (3) In the capillary network of the lung, blood is oxygenated. It then leaves the lung via two pulmonary veins each from the right and left lung and passes to the left atrium.
   (4) Blood passes through the bicuspid valve into the left ventricle and from there is expelled to the rest of the body via the ascending aorta; backflow is prevented by the aortic semilunar valves.

4. **(D)** Basophils make up 0.5% or less of the total blood cell count. They are rarely phagocytic. Basophils contain basophilic granules, are involved in immune phenomena, and produce heparin, which prevents the clotting of blood. Heparin, an anticoagulant, occurs most abundantly in the liver. Other examples of anticoagulants are aspirin and the drug dicumarol.

5. **(B)** Leukocytes (WBC) differ from red blood cells by having nuclei and by exhibiting ameboid movement. A normal count of WBC in circulating blood is about 5 to 9 $\times$ 10^3/mm^3. WBC contain phosphatases, liberate proteolytic enzymes, and function mainly in phagocytosis, proteolysis, and antibody formation. An increase in the number of leukocytes is called *leukocytosis*, a decrease *leukopenia*. There are two main types of leukocytes: nongranular and granular.

   Non- or Agranular Leukocytes:

   (1) *Lymphocytes* make up between 20 and 25% of total leukocytes and are seldom phagocytic. They originate from lymphoid tissue and bone marrow, function in immunologic responses and the detoxificiation of noxious substances, and are prevalent at sites of chronic inflammation. Some live several years.
   (2) *Monocytes* make up between 3 and 8% of total WBC. They are sometimes phagocytic and help in debridement.

   Granular (possess abundant, specific granules) Leukocytes:

   (1) *Neutrophils* make up about 65 to 75% of leukocytes. They are twice as large as a RBC and have a lobulated nucleus. They are the most active and phagocytic, providing the first line of defense against invading organisms. Dead neutrophils become *pus*.
   (2) *Eosinophils* make up about 2 to 5% WBC. They possess large red acidophilic granules and a bilobed nucleus. Large numbers are found at sites of parasitic infections and allergic reactions (specifically, in the respiratory and digestive tracts). Eosinophils function in the destruction of antigen–antibody complexes.
   (3) *Basophils* make up 0.5% or less of the total white blood cell count. They are rarely phagocytic. Basophils contain large quantities of basophilic granules. They are involved in immune phenomena, and produce heparin, which prevents the clotting of blood.

6. **(D)** Heartbeat is initiated by the S-A (sino-atrial) node.

7. **(D)** The most numerous Leukocytes are the neutrophils (65–75%).

8. **(D)** An anticoagulant is a substance that prevents or retards coagulation of blood. Heparin is an acid mucopolysaccharide; it occurs most abundantly in the liver. Aspirin (acetylsalicylic acid) is an analgesic, antipyretic, antirheu-matic compound that possesses anticoagulant properties. Dicumarol is a trademark for bishydroxycoumarin, an excellent anticoagulant.

9. **(C)** Blood pressure is usually measured by placing the sphygmomanometer cuff around the arm to compress the brachial artery and vein. Maximum blood pressure is obtained during ventricular contraction (systole); in our case, 160. Minimum blood pressure indicates ventricular rest (diastole); in our case, 90.

10. **(A)** From the right ventricle blood is sent to the lungs via the pulmonary arteries; this blood is rich in carbaminohemoglobin and the CO_2 will be exchanged for O_2. Blood returns from the lungs to the left auricle via the pulmonary veins; this blood has been oxygenated and is rich in oxyhemoglobin. Blood then passes to the left ventricle and then out via the aorta to supply the tissues of the body.

11. **(B)** Impeded or sluggish venous blood flow, especially of the veins of the lower extremity, can lead to the formation of blood clots. The disease, thrombophlebitis, is characterized by an inflammation of veins with thrombosis.

RESPIRATORY SYSTEM

The respiratory system is composed of a conduit for air and an air-blood interface for gaseous exchange in the alveoli of the lungs. The function of the lung is to facilitate movement of oxygen from the air into the pulmonary circulation and the movement of carbon dioxide from the body out. This is accomplished by simple diffusion from an area of high concentration to one of a low partial pressure.

The respiratory system contains several components:

1. nasal passageways – external/anterior nares, nasal cavities, internal/posterior nares
2. pharynx—nasopharynx and oropharynx
3. larynx—contains false and true vocal cords
4. trachea
5. left and right extrapulmonary bronchi
6. left and right lungs—contains intrapulmonary bronchi, bronchioles (terminal and respiratory), and alveoli organized as alveolar ducts and alveolar sacs

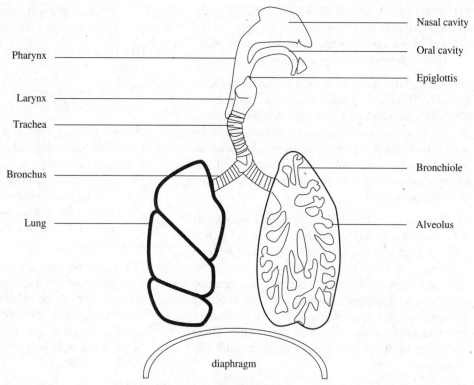

The human air passages.

The tracheobronchial tree (anatomic dead space) consists of about 16 generations of branches, and the respiratory unit is made up of an additional seven generations of respiratory bronchioles, alveolar ducts, and alveolar sacs for a total of 23 generations. The last seven are functional in gas exchange. (The upper parts of the respiratory system function in the removal of inhaled particles.)

Removal of Inhaled Particles

Large particles are filtered by hairs and mucous material in the nose and respiratory tract. Air is also warmed and humidified. Mucus is continually moved by cilia toward the throat and expelled by swallowing, expectoration, or through the nose. No cilia are present in alveoli; macrophages and leukocytes debride this area. Material so gathered is removed via the lymphatic system.

Pulmonary Ventilation

Respiratory refers to the gaseous exchanges that occur between the body as a whole and the environment. It entails:

1. ventilation of the lungs
2. gas exchange between lungs and blood
3. transport of gases in the blood
4. gas exchange between blood and interstitial fluids of the body

Ventilation must be adequate in environments ranging from sea level to high altitude and under degrees of physical activities ranging from sleep to exertion.

Respiratory minute ventilation is the amount of air that one inspires or expires each minute. It is equal to the amount of air inspired with each breath (the *tidal volume*) times the frequency (the number of breaths per minute). With each breath we normally inspire about 500 ml and breathe at a rate of 12 breaths per minute. The resting respiratory minute ventilation under these conditions is 6 1/min. During severe exercise, the respiratory minute ventilation may reach 80 to 100 1/min; this is an indication of the practical upper limit of our respiratory system. Thus a 15-fold increase in ventilation is possible, indicating that the respiratory system has considerable reserve.

Inspiration and Expiration

During inspiration the thoracic cavity expands, its volume increases, and air rushes into the respiratory tract due to the creation of negative pressure; the musculature involved is the diaphragm (innervated by the phrenic nerve) and the external intercostal muscles (innervated by intercostal nerves). During its contraction the diaphragm descends as much as 7 cm; the external intercostal muscles raise the rib cage. Relaxation of these muscles, the stabilization of the thoracic cage by the internal intercostal contraction of the abdominal musculature, plus the elasticity of the lung, return the organ to the pre-inspiratory resting phase. A normal breath involves a volume of about 500 ml. Normal expiration is passive and involves no great muscular contraction. When ventilation exceeds about 40 1/min, expiratory (abdominal) muscles come into play to speed up expiration. By contracting, they push on contents of the abdominal cavity which then push the diaphragm upward, forcing air out of the lungs.

Positive and Negative Pressure Breathing

Gases flow from regions of higher pressure to those of lower pressure. Thus, when the gas pressure in the alveoli is equal to that of the surrounding atmosphere, no movement of gas occurs. For inspiration to occur, the alveolar gas pressure must be less than the atmospheric pressure. There are two ways in which this pressure difference can be produced. The first is by positive pressure breathing as is the case when using a resuscitator. Here the pressure at the nose and mouth (the atmospheric pressure) is made greater than the alveolar gas pressure. The second method is by negative pressure breathing as is the case when using the iron lung. Here the alveolar gas pressure is lowered below atmospheric pressure.

Normal breathing is a form of negative pressure breathing. If we plot intra-alveolar pressure (intrapulmonary pressure) during inspiration and expiration, we see that enlarging the thorax and lungs enables the alveolar gas to expand until its pressure drops below that of the surrounding atmosphere and the inflow of gas then occurs. For expiration to occur, the alveolar gas pressure must be made greater than the atmospheric pressure. This is produced by the natural recoil of the lungs, during which time the alveolar gas is compressed until its pressure is above atmospheric pressure. Gas then flows out of the lungs. Resistance to respiration arises due to the elastic fibers of the lung itself and the surface tension phenomena (forces) present at any liquid-air interface.

Because the inner surface of the lung is lined with a fluid (surfactant, which has a low surface tension), surface tension forces play a role. As a result of this surface tension the alveolus will tend to collapse unless opposed by the inflating pressure. The amount of pressure needed to oppose surface tension and maintain inflation is determined by the Law of Laplace:

$$p = \frac{2T}{\text{radius}}$$

where p = the inflation pressure, T = surface tension forces, and radius means the radius of the alveoli.

With a plasmalike liquid lining the lungs (constant surface tension), as the radius decreases (deflation) the distending pressure increases. Also, smaller alveoli would require a greater distending force than the larger alveoli.

The density of the surfactant molecules at the liquid-air interface is such that at high lung volumes there are few surfactant molecules per unit of area and the surface tension is relatively high (like plasma). As deflation occurs, the surfactant molecules become more concentrated at the liquid air interface, and surface tension becomes relatively low (like surfactant). Thus, during deflation, the alveolar radius is decreasing, tending to increase the needed distending pressure, but the surface tension is becoming less, which tends to decrease the required distending pressure. The lung, therefore, has alveoli which will not collapse until very low pressures are reached (because the surface tension is low), and can have small and large alveoli existing side by side (because the surface tension is area dependent).

Absence of the ability to produce surfactant is a key element in hyaline membrane disease. Infants afflicted die of respiratory distress because their lungs collapse with each breath due to the high surface tension. Extreme muscular efforts are required for reinflation and respiration is very labored in these cases.

Neuronal Control and Integration of Breathing

Normal spontaneous breathing is under control of motor neurons (primarily the phrenic nerves to the diaphragm) which innervate the respiratory muscles. Brain impulses regulate and modulate the process. Voluntary activity originates in the cerebral cortex, automatic (autonomic) control rests in the pons and medulla of the brain.

The respiratory center, located in the medulla, has an inspiratory and an expiratory portion. The ventral portion produces forced and deep inspiration; the dorsal portion produces expiration.

Rhythmicity is spontaneous (12 to 15 times/minute) but is modulated by centers in the pons and medulla and by input from afferent vagal (stretch) receptors located in the lung. Stretching of the lung during inspiration reflexively limits the inspiratory drive.

Smooth muscle in the walls of the airways is innervated by parasympathetic and sympathetic nerves. Parasympathetic stimulation causes bronchoconstriction and an increase in airway resistance. Sympathetic stimulation produces relaxation. (Therefore, during an asthmatic attack it is helpful to inhale an aerosol containing a sympathomimetic drug, a drug that mimics the action of stimulating the sympathetic nervous system.)

Gas Exchange in the Alveoli

Abutting the alveoli (about 150 million/lung) is a large capillary bed providing an enormous diffusion area (about 90 m^2) with an extremely thin barrier (about 5000 Å) for gaseous exchange. Gas exchange occurs only in the alveoli and not in the tracheobronchial tree; the nonfunctional space (anatomic dead space) volume comprises about 150 ml. The alveolar portion, known as the respiratory zone, has a volume of about 2,000 ml. Oxygen passes from the alveolar air spaces into the blood in the capillaries surrounding the alveoli via a specific diffusion pathway.

> air in alveoli → surfactant (lowers surface tension) → alveolar epithelium
> (simple squamous epithelium) → fused basal laminae of alveolar epithelium
> and capillary endothelium → capillary endothelium (simple squamous
> epithelium) → blood plasma → erythrocytes/red blood cells

Oxygen Transport

Oxygen is transported mainly in the form of oxyhemoglobin. Normal hemoglobin (Hb) values are, respectively, 14 g/100 ml for women and 16 g/100 ml for men. Blood then contains an average of 15 g hemoglobin/100 ml blood; each gram of hemoglobin can combine with 1.39 ml of oxygen. Fully oxygenated blood can be calculated thus:

$$(15 \text{ g Hb}/100 \text{ ml blood}) \times (1.39 \text{ ml O}_2/\text{g Hb})$$

to contain 21 ml O_2/ml blood. This is known as the *oxygen capacity* of blood.

If the concentration of oxygen against the PO_2 is plotted, a sigmoid shaped curve, also called the *oxygen dissociation curve,* is obtained.

Four factors affect the affinity of hemoglobin for oxygen:

(1) pH
(2) temperature
(3) concentration of 2,3-diphosphoglycerate (DPG)
(4) carbon dioxide

A decrease in pH, an increase in temperature, or an increase in DPG will facilitate the release of oxygen in the tissue capillaries.

Actively metabolizing tissues have a higher temperature and produce metabolic acids (e.g., lactic acid) and carbonic acid via the reaction of released carbon dioxide and water. An increase in CO_2 and a decrease in affinity of hemoglobin for oxygen with a decrease in pH and an increase in carbamino Hb is called the *Bohr effect.* Most of the oxygen released is due to the decrease in PO_2 in the interstitial fluid but an extra amount is released due to these factors. Chronic hypoxia (lack of oxygen) increases the amount of DPG and thus facilitates oxygen release by this mechanism.

Carbon Dioxide Transport

Although some carbon dioxide remains in plasma, most diffuses into red blood cells. Here, it can be (1) transported in physical solution, (2) bound to the amino groups of hemoglobin as carbamino hemoglobin, or, most importantly, (3) converted to bicarbonate ions via its interaction with water to form carbonic acid, which almost completely dissociates into bicarbonate and hydrogen ions. This reaction occurs rapidly in red blood cells because the cells contain the enzyme carbonic anhydrase, which catalyzes the reaction.

The carbon dioxide in plasma can also be transported (1) in physical solution, (2) bound to the amino groups of plasma proteins (although the amount carried as carbamino compounds in plasma is small compared to the amount carried in red blood cells as carbamino hemoglobin), or (3) as bicarbonate ions. Few bicarbonate ions are produced in the plasma, however, because there is no carbonic anhydrase in plasma.

Bicarbonate ions produced in the red blood cells diffuse into the plasma because of the concentration gradient. However, the red blood cell membrane is not very permeable to cations so no positively charged ion can accompany the bicarbonate ions into the plasma. The result is that the inside of the red blood cell is slightly positive and so attracts negatively charged chloride ions from the plasma. This exchange of chloride for bicarbonate is referred to as the *chloride shift*. Thus, although bicarbonate is produced in red blood cells it is transported in plasma.

The hydrogen ions produced are buffered to a great extent by hemoglobin. The fact that reduced hemoglobin holds hydrogen ions more strongly than oxyhemoglobin means that, as oxygen is released to tissues, hydrogen ions generated by the addition of carbon dioxide can be taken up by the deoxygenated (reduced) hemoglobin. Slightly more hydrogen ions are produced than can be handled by the reduced hemoglobin produced. Thus, the pH of venous blood is slightly lower than that of arterial blood.

Because deoxygenated hemoglobin forms carbamino compounds much more readily than oxygenated hemoglobin does, venous blood can handle more CO_2 than can arterial blood.

The changes in the quantity of oxygen and carbon dioxide in the lungs are as indicated:

	Inspired Air, %	Expired Air, %	Change, %
Oxygen	20.96	16.02	4.94 loss
Carbon dioxide	0.04	4.48	4.44 gain

The carbon dioxide resulting from cellular metabolic activity diffuses into the blood because it is less concentrated there; here it then either combines with hemoglobin or is converted into carbonic acid:

$$CO_2 + H_2O \; H_2CO_3$$

The carbonic acid reacts with sodium in the plasma to form sodium bicarbonate:

$$H_2CO_3 + Na^+ \rightarrow NaHCO_3 + H^+$$

or it can react with potassium in the hemoglobin to form potassium bicarbonate:

$$H_2CO_3 + K^+ \rightarrow KHCO_3 + H^+$$

In the lungs the carbon dioxide is dissociated from the bicarbonate and hemoglobin and diffuses into alveolar space air for exchange.

Chemical Regulation of Respiration

Chemical stimulants of physiological importance that affect respiration are:

(1) increased arterial PCO_2 (hypercapnia),
(2) decreased arterial PO_2 (hypoxia),
(3) an increased arterial hydrogen-ion concentration (acidosis).

Arterial [H^+] and PO_2 are monitored by carotid and aortic bodies which contain nerve endings that are sensitive to arterial pH and PO_2. The carotid bodies lie near the carotid sinus at the bifurcation of the common carotid arteries and send impulses through fibers of the glossopharyngeal nerves. The aortic bodies lie near the arch of the aorta; their neural fibers are part of the vagus nerves.

Increases in arterial PCO_2 are also sensed to some extent by these peripheral chemoreceptors (carotid and aortic bodies) but, more importantly, by a central chemosensitive area on the surface of the medulla overlying the medullary respiratory center. This central chemosensitive area, bathed in cerebrospinal fluid (CSF), is sensitive to changes in [H^+] in the CSF. Although hydrogen ions poorly penetrate the blood-brain barrier which separates arterial blood and CSF, carbon dioxide can rapidly diffuse between the two fluids. Thus, arterial PCO_2 and CSF PCO_2 equilibrate. Once in the CSF, carbon dioxide reacts with water to form carbonic acid, which dissociates into bicarbonate and hydrogen ions. The central chemosensitive area is sensitive to the pH changes thus produced. In a similar manner (but of less importance) arterial PCO_2 alters arterial pH, which is best detected by the carotid and aortic bodies.

Oxygen lack stimulates ventilation solely by its effect on the peripheral chemoreceptors, but alveolar PO_2 must fall to low levels (50 to 60 membrane Hg) before ventilation begins to increase. However, some chemoreceptor discharge is present at normal oxygen tensions. Hypercapnia, which often accompanies hypoxia, will potentiate sensitivity of peripheral chemoreceptors to hypoxia. Hypoxia is the stimulus for increased ventilation observed at high altitudes.

Acidosis stimulates ventilation mainly via peripheral chemoreceptors. Arterial [H^+] may also affect the central chemosensitive area but its influence there is slow in onset and much less pronounced. Hyperventilation driven by acidosis will "blow off" CO_2 and generate alkalosis in the CSF, which tends to depress ventilation. The results of these opposing forces is a lesser increase in ventilation than would occur with a constant arterial PCO_2. The effects of acidosis and either hypoxia or hypercapnia are additive with no complicated potentiation occurring.

Ventilation is much more sensitive to hypercapnia than to either hypoxia or acidosis. Changes in ventilation produced by hypercapnia are only slightly altered when the peripheral chemoreceptors are denervated, indicating the importance of the central chemosensitive area in monitoring CO_2. Hypoxia potentiates this CO_2 sensitivity.

QUICK RECALL TEST QUESTIONS AND ANSWERS

Choose the Best Answer

1. Exchange in the lung of CO_2 and O_2 takes place in the:

   (A) bronchi.
   (B) bronchioles.
   (C) alveoli.
   (D) broncho-pulmonary segment.

2. Blood pH is influenced by respiration; experimental hyperventilation in a physiology laboratory will result in the student's blood pH being:

   (A) lowered.
   B. raised.
   (C) unaffected.
   (D) raised to pH6.

3. An area of the lung involved in gas exchange includes the:

   (A) trachea.
   (B) primary bronchi.
   (C) alveolar ducts.
   (D) pharynx.

4. During exercise, an individual's tidal volume is 2L and her rate of breathing is 20 breaths/minute. Under these exercising conditions the respiratory minute ventilation is:

   (A) 0.4 L/min.
   (B) 1.0 L/min.
   (C) 4.0 L/min.
   (D) 40 L/min.

5. Contraction of the diaphragm:

   (A) decreases the volume of the thoracic cavity.
   (B) makes the intra-alveolar pressure less than atmospheric pressure.
   (C) is responsible for "positive pressure breathing."
   (D) occurs during expiration.

6. Respiratory distress in an infant (hyaline membrane disease) is associated with:

   (A) high surface tension in the lungs.
   (B) lungs that are more compliant than normal lungs (i.e., not as stiff).
   (C) high concentrations of surfactant in the lungs.
   (D) large alveoi collapsing before smaller ones.

7. Of the following, quantitatively the most important for transporting carbon dioxide is:

   (A) carboxyhemoglobin.
   (B) carbaminohemoglobin.
   (C) dissolved carbon dioxide.
   (D) bicarbonate ions.

8. Which of the following will facilitate the release of oxygen from the blood to the tissues?

   (A) an increase in the partial pressure of carbon dioxide
   (B) a decrease in temperature
   (C) an increase in pH
   (D) a decrease in diphosphoglycerate concentration

9. *Most* hydrogen ions produced when carbon dioxide is added to blood:

   (A) are taken up by reduced hemoglobin molecules.
   (B) are buffered by albumin and other plasma proteins.
   (C) remain free and produce a large pH shift to the acid state.
   (D) are buffered by bicarbonate ions in plasma.

10. The increase in ventilation that occurs at high altitude is stimulated by:

    (A) hypercapnia.
    (B) hypoxemia.
    (C) decreased blood pH.
    (D) cerebrospinal fluid acidosis.

Answers

1. **(C)** CO_2 and O_2 exchange takes place in the alveoli of the lung.

2. **(B)** Hyperventilation is abnormally rapid, deep breathing resulting in a loss of CO_2 and an increase in blood pH. A person would be in the state of respiratory alkalosis, since a decreased blood concentration of hydrogen ion is the result of pulmonary CO_2 elimination.

3. **(C)** Gas exchange occurs only in the alveoli and not in the tracheobronchial tree. The alveolar portion, known as the respiratory zone, has a volume of about 2000 ml. Alveolar ducts have numerous alveoli extending from their walls.

4. **(D)** Respiratory minute ventilation, or the amount of air that we inspire or expire each minute, is equal to the amount of air inspired with each breath (the tidal volume) times the frequency (the number of breaths per minute). With each breath we normally inspire about 500 ml and breathe at a rate of 12 breaths per minute. The resting respiration minute ventilation under these conditions is 6 L/min.

5. **(B)** During inspiration the thoracic cavity expands, its volume increases, and air rushes into the respiratory tract because of the creation of negative pressure; the musculature involved is the diaphragm (innervated by the phrenic nerve) and the external intercostal muscles (innervated by intercostal nerves).

6. **(A)** Because the inner surface of the lung is lined with a fluid (surfactant, which has a low surface tension), surface tension forces play a role. As a result of this surface tension the alveolus will tend to collapse unless opposed by the inflating pressure. Immature lungs contain less surfactant and tend to collapse more readily.

7. **(D)** Although some carbon dioxide remains in plasma, most diffuses into red blood cells. Here, it can be (1) transported in physical solution, (2) bound to the amino groups of hemoglobin as carbaminohemoglobin, or, most importantly, (3) converted to bicarbonate ions via its interaction with water to form carbonic acid, which almost completely dissociates into bicarbonate and hydrogen ions. This reaction occurs rapidly in red blood cells because the cells contain the enzyme carbonic anhydrase, which catalyzes the reaction.

8. **(A)** A decrease in pH, an increase in temperature, or an increase in DPG will facilitate the release of oxygen in the tissue capillaries. Actively metabolizing tissues have a higher temperature and produce metabolic acids (e.g., lactic acid) and carbonic acid via the reaction of released carbon dioxide and water.

9. **(A)** The hydrogen ions released by bicarbonate formation are largely buffered by hemoglobin, in part because most bicarbonate formation occurs in the hemoglobin-rich interior of red blood corpuscles. The stronger uptake of hydrogen ions by reduced (deoxygenated) hemoglobin aids the process of buffering. The slight excess of hydrogen ions released over the buffering capacity of the hemoglobin produces a small pH decrease.

10. **(C)** Oxygen lack stimulates ventilation solely by its effect on the peripheral chemoreceptors, but alveolar PO_2 must fall to low levels (50 to 60 mm Hg) before ventilation begins to increase. However, some chemoreceptor discharge is present at normal oxygen tensions. Hypercapnia, which often accompanies hypoxia, will potentiate sensitivity of peripheral chemoreceptors to hypoxia. Hypoxia is the stimulus for increased ventilation observed at high altitudes. Acidosis stimulates ventilation mainly via peripheral chemoreceptors. Arterial $[H^+]$ may also affect the central chemosensitive area but its influence there is slow in onset and much less pronounced. Hyperventilation driven by acidosis will "blow off" CO_2 and generate alkalosis in the CSF, which tends to depress ventilation. The results of these opposing forces is a lesser increase in ventilation than would occur with a constant PCO_2. The effects of acidosis and either hypoxia or hypercapnia are additive with no complicated potentiation occurring. Ventilation is much more sensitive to hypercapnia than to either hypoxia or acidosis. Changes in ventilation produced by hypercapnia are only slightly altered when the peripheral chemoreceptors are denervated, indicating the importance of the central chemosensitive area in monitoring CO_2. Hypoxia potentiates this CO_2 sensitivity.

URINARY SYSTEM

The urinary system has been charged by evolution with the protection of the *milieu interieur* of Claude Bernard, the great French physiologist. For organisms living in an aqueous environment, this protection requires a relatively simple mechanism, but for land dwellers such protection is critical for survival. Thus, we must think of excretion by way of the urinary tract as the end result of conservation of all useful circulating materials and simultaneous elimination of waste material. By contrast, excretion via the digestive tract is the end result of ingestion of either indigestible material or nutritional matter which remains unabsorbed. Overall then, the gut provides the nutrients to the blood, which is filtered by the kidney; the nutrients are then returned while waste is lost. Sugars, electrolytes, and amino acids are reclaimed from the filtrate at an efficiency of 95% or better. Given the large daily volume of digestive tract secretions, there is very efficient (almost 99%) water absorption in the gut but slightly lower efficiency of water absorption in the kidney, which must use a minimal volume of loss to solubilize the waste. Indeed, it is the ability to vary this efficiency of fluid absorption which accounts for the remarkable ability of the kidney to defend the osmolarity of the body fluids. The kidney also plays a critical role in adjustment of blood pH through its ability to vary urinary acid excretion and bicarbonate reabsorption. Finally, the kidney is a major factor in the maintenance of skeletal integrity through its ability to vary calcium and phosphate loss into the urine in response to vitamin D. It should not be forgotten that the kidney is the site of production of the 1,25-dihydroxy form of vitamin D, the most biologically active form of the vitamin.

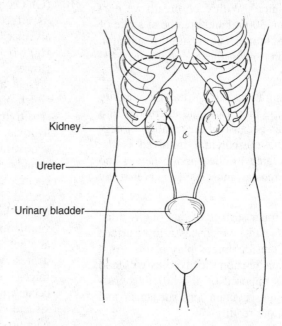

Kidney

Ureter

Urinary bladder

The human urinary system in place in the human body. The dotted line represents the position of the diaphragm.

Structure of the Kidney

The kidney is a bean-shaped organ encased by a fibrous capsule and embedded within a fatty connective tissue and perirenal fascia. The kidney lies deep to the *peritoneum* (i.e., retroperitoneal) which lines the abdomino-pelvic cavity. It is approximately 10 cm long, 5 cm wide, and 3 cm thick. Its medial aspect, which is indented or concave, is known as the *renal hilus (hilum);* it is the location for the renal arteries and veins as well as for the renal pelvis. The hilus leads into a cavity, the *renal sinus,* within the kidney which contains fat, blood vessels, nerves, calyces, and renal pelvis.

The internal aspect of the kidney when bissected in a medial to lateral plane presents two zones; an outer *cortex* and an inner *medulla*. The medulla is adjacent to the renal sinus. The cortex is redder in appearance and has fine striations known as *medullary rays*. These striations are due to medullary structures (collecting tubules) extending into the cortex. The medulla consists of triangular (pyramidal) structures, *the renal pyramids,* separated by columns of cortical material known as *renal columns*. The bases of the renal pyramids face the cortex while the apices or *papillae* extend into the *minor calyces*.

The kidney is divided into functional *lobes,* each defined as one renal pyramid, its abutting cortex and part of the two adjacent renal columns. There are about 6 to 18 lobes. A *lobule* of a kidney is considered to be a medullary ray and the adjacent nephrons draining into the collecting ducts forming the ray.

The functional unit of the kidney is the *uriniferous tubule,* which consists of a *nephron* and a *collecting tubule* (duct) within the kidney. There are 1 to 3 million/kidney. The individual nephron is considered by many as the functional unit and the collecting tubule as a separate entity being part of the internal excretory pathway for urine.

Nephron: Each nephron consists of a glomerulus and an associated epithelial tubule that is 30 to 40 mm in length. The functionally sequential regions of the nephron are the glomerulus, Bowman's capsule, proximal convoluted tubule, loop of Henle (descending and ascending), and distal convoluted tubule. The urine that exits the distal convoluted tubule enters the collecting tubule, which joins the collecting duct system, and empties into the renal pelvis.

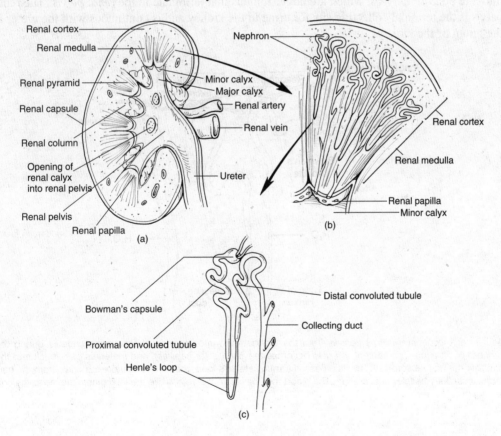

Structure of the kidney and its fine structures. (a) A sagittal section of the kidney showing the entry and exit of the renal artery and renal vein, respectively. Note the minor calyx leading to the major calyx then to the renal calyx and the renal pelvis and ureter for the elimination of urine. (b) The renal cortex and renal medulla are enlarged and the nephron can be seen. The swollen portion is Bowman's capsule. Tubes lead down into the renal medulla then turn up back toward the cortex. Here they join with ducts leading down to the minor calyx. (c) A nephron expanded to show its details. Note the location of Bowman's capsule and how it leads to the proximal tubule, Henle's loop, the distal convoluted tubule, and the collecting duct. The peritubular capillary is not shown.

Bowman's capsule is a cup-shaped structure that is intimately associated with the glomerulus (a capillary tuft). The outer and inner layers of Bowman's capsule are the *parietal* and *visceral* epithelial layers, respectively; the space between these layers is *Bowman's space*. The glomerulus and Bowman's capsule together form a unit referred to as a renal corpuscle (*corpuscle of Malpighi*). The entry and exit point of the arterioles associated with the glomerulus is referred to as the *vascular* pole. The point at which Bowman's capsule is continuous with the proximal convoluted tubule is referred to as the *urinary* pole of the renal corpuscle.

The visceral layer of Bowman's capsule is composed of specialized epithelial cells referred to as *podocytes* that are intimately associated with glomerular capillary endothelium via the *glomerular basal lamina*. Podocytes are characterized by numerous cellular extensions that wrap around and enclose the glomerular capillaries. Each of the larger primary processes is characterized by numerous smaller, secondary processes. Each of the secondary processes has numerous tiny processes referred to as *pedicels* or *foot processes*. The pedicels of adjacent podocytes interdigitate with one another. This arrangement results in slit-like spaces, referred to as filtration slits, between adjacent podocytes.

Urine leaving the distal convoluted tubule enters a collecting tubule that unites with other collecting tubules. These form 10 to 25 larger collecting ducts (papillary ducts of Bellini) that extend into the renal pyramids and terminate at the papillae.

The urine passes from the ends of these large collecting ducts into funnel-shaped collecting vessels, the *minor calyces,* into which the papillae extend. The 7 to 18 minor calyces empty into 2 to 3 *major calyces,* which are larger funnels that terminate in the *renal pelvis*. The renal pelvis is the terminal collecting site for urine in the kidney and is continuous with the ureter at the hilum of the kidney.

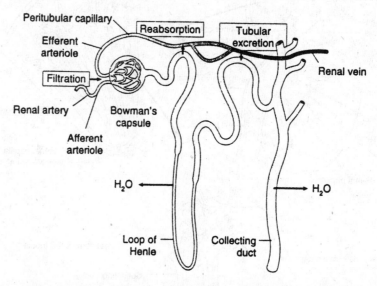

Activity at the nephron. Fluid passes from the bloodstream into the wall of Bowman's capsule during the process of filtration. The efferent arteriole becomes the peritubular capillary, and materials pass back into the capillary during reabsorption. The fluid passes through Henle's loop, then receives more materials from the peritubular capillary by tubular excretion. The blood then passes out a vein, while the fluid (urine) moves to the collecting duct.

The Nephron and Its Function

Structure	Function	Nature of Urine
Renal corpuscle	Deliver blood; make ultrafiltrate.	Same as plasma, contains equivalent electrolytes, is isosmolar, very little albumin.
Proximal convoluted tubule	Active transport reabsorption of sugars, amino acids, bicarbonate and electrolytes, passive water reabsorption, secretion of uric acid and other waste.	Diminished volume, isosmolar with plasma.
Descending loop of Henle	Passive diffusion of water, Na^+ and Cl^- out into medulla; water remains in medulla, while Na^+ and Cl^- diffuse back into loop.	Smaller volume, hypertonic with respect to plasma.
Ascending loop of Henle	Impermeable to water, Cl^- actively pumped to interstitium; Na^+ follows passively.	Little change in volume; becomes hypotonic.
Distal convoluted tubule	Reabsorption of Na^+, secretion of K^+, and H^+; regulated by aldosterone; excretion of fixed acids, net H excretion.	Decreased pH, lower Na^+, and very little bicarbonate, volume can change (see "Collecting ducts").
Collecting ducts	Variably permeable to water; regulated by antidiuretic hormone (ADH).	Both volume and osmolarity vary, depending upon ADH secretion by neurohypophysis.

Tubular Passageways

The *ureter* is a long muscular tube that connects the renal pelvis to the urinary bladder. It passes inferiorly on the posterior abdominal wall, enters the pelvis by crossing the pelvic inlet, and then pierces the wall of the urinary bladder at its posterior-lateral aspect. The smooth muscles that are part of the bladder and surround the oblique path of the ureter through the wall act as a sphincter of the ureter.

The *urinary bladder* is located in the pelvis superior and posterior to the pubic bone, anterior to the uterus in the female, anterior to the rectum in the male. The bladder consists of a thick wall composed of three intermeshing smooth muscle layers known as *detrusor muscles*. The bladder stores urine as well as expels it. The excretory pathways and the bladder are lined by the urinary type of the epithelium known as transitional epithelium.

The *urethra* is a fibromuscular tube that transmits urine to the outside of the body. It is continuous inferiorly with the urinary bladder. It traverses the prostate gland and then exits the pelvic cavity by passing through the pelvic floor (urogenital diaphragm) and terminates at the external urethral orifice of the penis or in the vestibule of the female.

The male urethra (20 cm in length) is longer than the female urethra (2 to 6 cm). The male urethra consists of three regions: prostatic, membranous, and penile. The penile region of the urethra is located with the corpus spongiosum of the penis.

Functions of the Kidney and Uriniferous Tubules

The kidney, during the production of urine,

(a) excretes the waste products of metabolism;
(b) maintains the fluid volume of the extracellular regions of the body;
(c) excretes foreign materials from the body;
(d) regulates the type and concentration of salts retained in the body (maintain electrolyte balance);
(e) regulates the total body water;
(f) regulates the acid–base balance of the body.

The physiological processes occurring during the production of urine are

(a) *filtration*—the production of an ultrafiltrate of plasma within Bowman's space;
(b) *reabsorption*— the selective removal of material from the ultrafiltrate as it passes through the tubular nephron and the return of these substances into peritubular capillaries;
(c) *secretion*—the cells forming the nephron actively secrete material into the filtrate;
(d) *passive diffusion*—diffusion of fluids along the osmotic gradient.

Urine formation involves the filtration of blood (in the renal corpuscle) to form an ultrafiltrate. Water and dissolved solutes from the ultrafiltrate (in the remainder of the nephron) are then selectively reabsorbed. The fluid remaining after completion of this process is urine.

Filtration: As blood flows through the glomerulus, blood plasma components (including water, ions, monosaccharides, amino acids, fatty acids, urea, uric acid, and plasma proteins) pass freely across the endothelium of the glomerular capillaries. Some of these blood plasma components (water, ions, and so on) then pass through the glomerular basal lamina, then through the filtration slits between pedicels of podocytes, and then enter Bowman's space as the ultrafiltrate. The glomerular basal lamina provides a selectively permeable barrier to determine which components will pass through (i.e., most materials smaller than 70,000 daltons) and which components will be retained (i.e., most materials larger than 70,000 daltons). Because the glomerular basal lamina is negatively charged, it repels most proteins and impedes the movement of blood plasma proteins across the glomerular basal lamina. This gives a true sense of the tremendous efficiency of the kidney, which normally clears 25% of the total cardiac output of blood per minute, forming approximately 120–130 ml of filtrate per minute. Thus, in a day the kidneys will receive 5000 L for filtration, form about 170–180 L of ultrafiltrate, and put out approximately 1–2 L of urine—an ultimate efficiency of fluid retention of 99.8%, and clear proof that Claude Bernard was correct!

The factors in formation of the ultrafiltrate are:

(a) *filtration pressure* (about 25 mm Hg), which is the net pressure differential between the driving force within the glomerular arterioles and the total back pressure exerted by osmotic pressure of the blood + pressure within Bowman's space and the proximal tubule. Thus, fluid is driven outward from the capillary against the filtration barrier under pressure, where its contents either pass through the barrier or are selectively absorbed by the podocytes before they can enter the tubule.
(b) *pore size,* which prevents passage of protein with molecular weights > 70,000, as well as red and white blood cells.

The conseqence of these two factors is to produce an ultrafiltrate that is similar to blood plasma (minus plasma proteins) and is isotonic to blood.

Reabsorption: The ultrafiltrate, isotonic with plasma, enters the proximal tubule, which is lined with columnar epithelium; the cell surface (luminal) facing the tubular opening has many microvilli, called the brush border, precisely like the columnar epithelium of the proximal small intestine (jejunum). This surface is the site of the carrier, or transport proteins, which exhibit specificity for particular sugars and amino acids and which subserve active transport. This efficient system results in reabsorption of

    (a) >95% of filtered amino acids
    (b) >98% of filtered glucose
    (c) 85% of the sodium, chloride, and bicarbonate
    (d) calcium, magnesium, and phosphate

There is also a passive diffusion of 80–85% of the filtered water, which follows the concentration gradient established through the active transport of the solutes listed above. In addition, any trace amounts of albumin which escape the filtration barrier and enter the proximal tubule are taken up by pinocytosis, or are hydrolyzed by membrane-bound enzymes into smaller peptide units.

Secretion: The cells of the proximal tubule are also capable of secretion and routinely put out a number of substances into the urine forming in the lumen. These materials include creatinine, uric acid, antibiotics, drug metabolites, and radiopaque dyes. It should be recognized that the majority of these materials derive not from the renal parenchyma, but from the blood, so that secretion depends upon intracellular transport in a direction opposite to that for reabsorption. The secretion of urate becomes an important factor in evaluation of uric acid excretion in patients with gout.

Passive Diffusion: Although the passage of the ultrafiltrate through the proximal convoluted tubule results in dramatic decreases in solute within the lumen, there has also been fluid reabsorption in proportion. Thus, the urine that enters the descending loop of Henle remains isosmotic with plasma, although very much diminished in volume. The function of the loop, overall, is to produce urine which is hypertonic to plasma, a task that is accomplished by a countercurrent multiplier system. The basis for this process is the difference in water permeability between the descending (permeable) and ascending (impermeable) limbs of the loop. Thus, as the urine passes through the descending loop, Na^+, Cl^- and water pass through the wall by passive diffusion down a concentration gradient. Toward the end of the descending loop, the water which has left the tubular lumen continues to diffuse outward into the relatively hypertonic interstitium of the renal medulla, leaving the Na^+ and Cl^- to diffuse back into the loop, following a new concentration gradient. Effectively, the process succeeds in separating water from solute. In the ascending loop, the wall of the tubule is impermeable to water and is capable of actively pumping Cl^- out into the interstitium. Sodium ions follow chloride ions passively, thereby diminishing the tonicity of the urine and increasing the tonicity of the interstitium, since water cannot also passively diffuse. The creation of a hypertonic interstitium in the renal medulla is key to water reabsorption in the collecting duct system, a major regulatory system of the osmolarity of plasma which is under neuroendocrine regulatory control.

Elimination of Fixed Acids and Hydrogen Ions: Fixed acid includes molecules and ions produced by the cells and that cannot be further degraded or eliminated through conversion to CO_2. The largest proportion of fixed acid is generally phosphate, followed by lactate and beta-hydroxybutyrate. In contrast to the major body buffer system of carbonic acid, which can be converted to CO_2 and excreted easily by the lungs, these compounds are not volatile and will rapidly accumulate if not excreted by other means. In the distal tubule, the now-hypotonic urine containing these materials, whose pH is essentially the same as that of the ultrafiltrate, is made acid under normal circumstances. Reabsorption of Na^+ by exchange with K^+ and H^+ allows formation of mono- and dihydrogen potassium phosphates; simultaneously, the distal tubule generates NH_4^+ for production of ammonium phosphate salts and net excretion of hydrogen ions. The rate of exchange between sodium and potassium-hydrogen is regulated by *aldosterone*, a steroid hormone produced in the adrenal cortex.

Control of Water Reabsorption and Osmolarity: The pituitary gland, or neurohypohysis, regulates the plasma osmolarity by exerting control over water reabsorption at the level of the distal and collecting ducts. It does so by secretion of the *antidiuretic hormone* (ADH); since "diuresis" implies urinary fluid excretion, ADH diminishes urinary volume by increasing the permeability of the distal tubule and collecting ducts to water. Because of the hypertonicity of the medullary interstitium, water passes out of these structures into the interstitial space by passive diffusion and leaves concentrated urine behind. The increased water in the interstitium enters the circulation by way of the medullary vascular network (*vasa recta*) and reduces plasma osmolarity, thus inhibiting further ADH secretion. A frequent result of head trauma or severe cerebral hypoxia is the "syndrome of inappropriate ADH secretion," in which urine flow becomes very slow and plasma osmolarity decreases to dangerous levels.

Hormonal Control of Secretion and Resorption

The simple cuboidal epithelium lining the distal convoluted tubule may also increase the Na^+ concentration in the interstitium by reabsorbing Na^+. At the same time, potassium ions (K^+) are excreted into the tubular lumen. The latter processes are regulated by *aldosterone,* a hormone produced by the adrenal cortex. The distal convoluted tubules also participate in maintaining the acid–base balance of the blood by adding hydrogen and ammonium ions into the filtrate.

The permeability of water through the walls of the distal convoluted tubules and collecting tubules is regulated by the *antidiuretic hormone* (ADH) secreted by the posterior lobe of the pituitary gland (neurohypophysis). The presence of this hormone makes these tubules more permeable to water. Because the interstitium of the renal pyramids is more highly concentrated (hypertonic) than the filtrate, water exits the collecting tubules and passes into the interstitium. This process continues along the length of the collecting ducts and results in concentrating the urine which therefore is *hypertonic*. The amount of water resorbed is regulated by ADH production. For example, an increase in ADH increases resorption of water resulting in a more hypertonic urine, whereas a decrease in ADH decreases resorption resulting in the excretion of more water and therefore, a diluted or hypotonic urine. Diuretic drugs counteract the action of ADH, causing less water resorption and increased urine volume. The osmotic gradient in the renal pyramids is also maintained by the *vasa recta* adjacent to the collecting tubules due to flow of water and Na^+ into and out of the vessel lumen. This establishes a countercurrent exchange system between the arterioles and venulae rectae.

QUICK RECALL TEST QUESTIONS AND ANSWERS

Choose the Best Answer

1. Which of the following structure/function relationships is appropriately paired?

    (A) glomerulus—produces ultrafiltrate isotonic to blood.
    (B) proximal tubule—chloride ions are reabsorbed.
    (C) loop of Henle (descending limb)—water diffuses out and urine becomes hypertonic.
    (D) All of the above are correctly paired.

2. Filtration in the kidneys results mainly from:

    (A) blood flow (m/sec).
    (B) reabsorption.
    (C) blood pressure.
    (D) secretion.

3. The functional unit of the kidney that is concerned with urine formation is the nephron; it consists of all of the following EXCEPT:

    (A) Bowman's capsule
    (B) proximal convoluted tubule.
    (C) loop of Henle.
    (D) minor calyx.

4. The kidney-filtered fluid leaving the distal convoluted tubule passes next through structures in which order?

    (A) minor calyx → major calyx → urethra → urinary bladder
    (B) collecting duct → minor calyx → major calyx → pelvis
    (C) pelvis → ureter → urinary bladder → urethra
    (D) descending limb of Henle → collecting duct → ureter → bladder

5. A defining feature of active transport is:

    (A) binding of solute to a carrier molecule.
    (B) sterospecificity of substrate binding.
    (C) existence of membrane pores.
    (D) energy expenditure.

6. Which of the following structure—function relationships is NOT correct?

    (A) glomerulus—produces ultrafiltrate isotonic to blood.
    (B) proximal tubule—active reabsorption of glucose, sodium and potassium.
    (C) descending limb—water diffuses out of lumen, urine becomes hypertonic.
    (D) distal convoluted tubule—primary site of acidification and urine becomes hypertonic to blood plasma.

7. The kidney plays a role in:

    (A) maintaining electrolyte balance.
    (B) regulating acid-base balance.
    (C) maintaining fluid volume of the extracellular regions.
    (D) all of the above.

8. Antidiuretic hormone (ADH) elicits its effect (conserving water) on the:

    (A) proximal tubule.
    (B) descending limb.
    (C) ascending limb.
    (D) distal convoluted and collecting tubules.

9. The _____ is a long muscular tube that connects the renal pelvis to the urinary bladder.

    (A) urethra
    (B) uriniferous tubule
    (C) collecting tubule
    (D) ureter

10. The internal aspect of the kidney when bisected in a medial to lateral plane presents two zones:

    (A) renal hilus and renal sinus.
    (B) major and minor calyx.
    (C) cortex and medulla.
    (D) renal pyramids and columns.

11. Major reabsorption of substances from the ultrafiltrate occurs in the proximal convoluted tubule and results in:

    (A) the active reabsorption of all the glucose.
    (B) the active reabsorption of 85% of the sodium chloride.
    (C) the passive diffusion, due to the osmotic gradient, of 85% of the water from the filtrate.
    (D) all of the above.

12. The ascending limb of the loop of Henle is:

    (A) permeable to water.
    (B) impermeable to water.
    (C) passively permeable to Na$^+$ and Cl$^-$.
    (D) impermeable to Na$^+$ and Cl$^-$.

13. Aldosterone is the most powerful mineralocorticoid. All of the following are true statements EXCEPT:

    (A) It functions in the retention of water.
    (B) It functions in the retention of sodium and chloride.
    (C) It increases urinary loss of potassium and phosphorus.
    (D) It is under pituitary control.

14. The kidney in humans removes most waste products by:

    (A) filtering fluid from blood, then resorbing the useful solutes.
    (B) filtering fluid from the coelom, then resorbing the useful solutes.
    (C) selectively transporting the waste products into the urine.
    (D) selectively transporting the waste products into the feces.

15. The glomeruli of the human kidney are responsible for:

    (A) selective resorption of water from the urine (controlled by antidiuretic hormone).
    (B) resorption of glucose and amino acids from the urine.
    (C) selective resorption of salt from the urine (controlled by aldosterone).
    (D) ultrafiltration of water and solutes from blood plasma into the nephron.

16. The proximal convoluted tubules of the human kidney are responsible for:

    (A) selective resorption of water from the urine (controlled by antidiuretic hormone).
    (B) resorption of glucose and amino acids from the urine.
    (C) selective resorption of salt from the urine (controlled by aldosterone).
    (D) establishment of a high salt concentration in the medulla of the kidney.

17. The loop of Henle of the human kidney is responsible for:

    (A) selective resorption of water from the urine (controlled by antidiuretic hormone).
    (B) resorption of glucose and amino acids from the urine.
    (C) selective resorption of salt from the urine (controlled by aldosterone).
    (D) establishment of a high salt concentration in the medulla of the kidney.

18. The distal convoluted tubules of the human kidney are responsible for:

    (A) selective resorption of water from the urine (controlled by antidiuretic hormone).
    (B) resorption of glucose and amino acids from the urine.
    (C) selective resorption of salt from the urine (controlled by aldosterone).
    (D) establishment of a high salt concentration in the medulla of the kidney.

19. The collecting ducts of the human kidney are responsible for:

    (A) selective resorption of water from the urine (controlled by antidiuretic hormone).
    (B) resorption of glucose and amino acids from the urine.
    (C) selective resorption of salt from the urine (controlled by aldosterone).
    (D) establishment of a high salt concentration in the medulla of the kidney.

Answers

1. **(D)** All the pairings are appropriate. Review the material if you erred.

2. **(C)** The peculiar features of renal circulation, such as the renal arteries originating directly from the aorta, the glomerulo-capillary arrangement, and differences in calibers of the afferent and efferent vessels indicate that blood pressure is of great functional significance for the production of urine. The vascular component probably plays an important role in the filtration process.

3. **(D)** The nephron is a tubular structure about 30–40 mm long and lined by epithelium. It functions in producing an ultrafiltrate and then reabsorbing material from and excreting substances into the filtrate, resulting in an excretory product.

It consists of several morphologically and physiologically different sections forming a continuous tubular unit. The regions of a nephron sequentially are: Bowman's capsule, proximal convoluted tubule, loop of Henle, and distal convoluted tubule. The latter is continuous with the collecting tubule (excretory duct) draining it. The loop of Henle extends into the medullary pyramid while the other three regions are found entirely in the cortex.

Nephrons vary in their level or position in the cortex, with the cortical nephrons abutting the medulla. These vary in that the size of the renal corpuscle and the length of the loop of Henle are larger in the juxtamedullary nephrons.

4. **(B)** The route for the filtrate and excretory product is from Bowman's space through the proximal convoluted tubule, descending thick and thin limbs of the loop of Henle, ascending thin and thick limbs and the distal convoluted tubule, and then moving into the collecting tubule. The latter unite and form 10 to 25 larger collecting ducts (papillary ducts of Bellini) which extend into the renal pyramids and terminate at the papillae.

The urine passes from the ends of these large collecting ducts into funnel-shaped collecting vessels, the minor calyces, into which the papillae extend. The 7 to 18 minor calyces empty into 2 to 3 major calyces, which are larger funnels that terminate in the renal pelvis. The renal pelvis is the terminal collecting site for urine in the kidney and is continuous with the ureter at the hilum of the kidney.

5. **(D)** Active transport makes it possible for a cell to maintain internal concentrations of small molecules that differ from concentrations in the immediate vicinity. The transport is "uphill" against the concentration gradient; the cell must expend energy to accomplish this phenomenon.

6. **(D)** In the distal convuluted tubule, more sodium is lost. It is replaced by potassium, hydrogen, and ammonia. This area is also the primary site of acidification, and water is reabsorbed by osmosis.

7. **(D)** The kidney, during production of urine,
   (a) excretes the waste products of metabolism;
   (b) maintains the fluid volume of the extracellular regions of the body;
   (c) excretes foreign materials from the body;
   (d) regulates the type and concentration of salts retained in the body (maintain electrolyte balance);
   (e) regulates the total body water;
   (f) regulates the acid-base balance of the body.

8. **(D)** The permeability of water through the walls of the distal convoluted tubules and collecting tubules is regulated by the antidiuretic hormone (ADH) secreted by the posterior lobe of the pituitary gland (neurohypophysis). The presence of this hormone makes these tubules more permeable to water. Because the interstitium of the renal pyramids is more highly concentrated (hypertonic) than the filtrate, water exits the collecting tubules and passes into the interstitium. This process continues along the length of the collecting ducts and results in concentrating the urine, which therefore is hypertonic. The amount of water resorbed is regulated by ADH production. For example, an increase in ADH increases resorption of water, resulting in a more hypertonic urine; a decrease in ADH decreases resorption, resulting in the excretion of more water and therefore a diluted or hypotonic urine.

9. **(D)** The ureter is a long muscular tube which connects the renal pelvis to the urinary bladder. It passes inferiorly on the posterior abdominal walls, enters the pelvis by crossing the pelvic inlet, and then pierces the wall of the urinary bladder at its posterior-lateral aspect. The smooth muscles that are part of the bladder and surround the oblique path of the ureter through the wall act as a sphincter of the ureter.

10. **(C)** The internal aspect of the kidney when bissected in a medial to lateral plane presents two zones; and outer cortex and an inner medulla. The medulla is adjacent to the renal sinus. The cortex is redder in appearance and has fine striations known as medullary rays. These striations are due to medullary structures (collecting tubules) extending into the cortex. The medulla consists of triangular (pyramidal) structures, the renal pyramids, separated by columns of cortical material known as renal columns. The bases of the renal pyramids face the cortex while the apices or papillae extend into the minor calyces.

11. **(D)** The functions of the proximal convoluted tubule are stated in responses **A** to **C**.

12. **(B)** The loop of Henle functions by setting up the mechanism (countercurrent multiplier system) in the renal medulla for the production of hypertonic urine. The descending limb of the loop is permeable to water Na^+, and Cl^-. These materials pass through the walls according to osmotic gradients. Water diffuses out of the tubule lumen into the more concentrated (hypertonic) interstitial tissue of the renal pyramids; Na^+, and Cl^- diffuse passively into the tubule.

The ascending limb of the loop differs in that its wall is impermeable to water. Therefore, water remains in the tubule. Also, chloride ions are actively reabsorbed and pumped into the interstitium surrounding the loop of Henle, as well as into the collecting ducts passing through the medullary pyramid. Sodium ions are thought to diffuse passively out of the tubules in conjunction with the Cl⁻. This decrease in sodium chloride concentration of the filtrate results in a hypotonic filtrate at the distal end of the loop of Henle as it enters the distal convoluted tubule. The flow of the sodium chloride out of the tubule also increases its concentration in the surrounding interstitial tissue, which thus becomes hypertonic. This hypertonic interstitium is essential for production of hypertonic urine as the filtrate passes through the collecting ducts of the renal pyramid.

13. **(D)** The zona glomerulosa of the adrenal gland is rich in lipids, especially cholesterol, from which the mineralocorticoids are formed. Aldosterone is the most powerful mineralocorticoid. Mineralocorticoids function in the retention of water, sodium, and chloride, and increase urinary loss of potassium and phosphorus by action on the renal tubules. This regulation of the electrolytes is essential to life. No pituitary control is present.

14. **(A)** Urine is formed by filtering plasma components smaller than proteins from blood across the wall of the glomerulus into the nephron. As the fluid passes down the nephron, useful solutes are resorbed in the proximal and distal convoluted tubules and water is resorbed in the collecting duct.

15. **(D)** The wall of the glomerulus is the filtering surface across which water and solutes smaller than proteins move from blood into the nephron.

16. **(B)** The proximal convoluted tubules normally resorb essentially all of the sugars and amino acids from the urine. These useful solutes are actively transported across the epithelium from the urine to the surrounding connective tissue, where they are taken up into capillaries.

17. **(D)** The loops of Henle establish a high salt environment in the medulla by exporting sodium and chloride ions from the ascending limb of each loop of Henle (which is carrying urine back up toward the cortex) and absorbing sodium and chloride ions into the descending limb of each loop of Henle (which is carrying urine down into the medulla). These processes have the net effect of moving sodium and chloride ions deeper into the medulla, creating a high salt environment through which the collecting ducts pass.

18. **(C)** The distal convoluted tubules are the major site of hormonally controlled salt resorption.

19. **(A)** The epithelium lining the collecting duct changes permeability in response to an antidiuretic hormone. When the permeability is high, as the urine moves down the collecting duct (which passes down through the medulla to the renal pelvis), water leaves the collecting ducts by osmosis (because of the high salt environment established in the medulla by the loops of Henle). As the permeability of the collecting ducts changes, urine may vary from approximately isotonic to blood plasma when the collecting duct epithelium allows little water resorption, to strongly hypertonic to blood plasma when the collecting duct epithelium allows maximum water resorption.

INTEGUMENTARY SYSTEM (SKIN AND ASSOCIATED STRUCTURES)

The skin, the hypodermis, and the specialized structures derived from the skin (hairs, nails, and glands) form the integumentary system.

Skin

The skin covers the external surface of the body. It is continuous with the mucous membranes of (1) the respiratory pathways via the nose; (2) the digestive tract via the mouth and anus; (3) the genitourinary system via urethra and/or vagina.

Functions: The skin protects the body from dehydration as well as from damage by the elements in the external environment. The skin also helps maintain normal body activities. The skin performs the following functions.

(1) Protects the body against dehydration. The skin is impermeable to water, which, therefore, prevents loss of body fluids. This property permits humans, as well as other animals, to live in a nonfluid environment such as land.

(2) Protects the body against abrasive forces. The ability to withstand frictional forces also allows humans to walk and perform manipulatory skills with the hands.

(3) Protects the body against damage from toxic chemicals and extreme heat.

(4) Protects the body from the harmful effects of ultraviolet rays. This is primarily the function of the melanin pigment secreted by the melanocytes in the epidermis.

(5) Acts as a barrier to infectious organisms invading the body.

(6) Takes part in regulating the temperature of the body. The degree of heat loss or retention is regulated by neurovascular processes. The body is cooled by the evaporation of water (sweat) from its surface.

(7) Functions to excrete body wastes and fluids via the production of sweat by the sweat glands.

(8) Acts as a primary sense organ of the body for general somatic sensations, such as touch, pressure, heat, cold, and pain.

(9) Plays a role in the production of vitamin D through the action of ultraviolet light. The latter transforms vitamin D precursors (7-dehydrocholesterol) found in the skin into vitamin D.

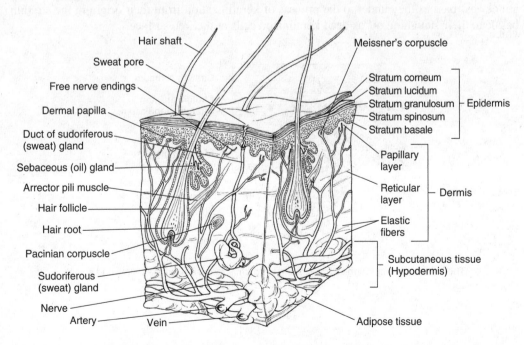

A general overview of the skin and the subcutaneous layer beneath it.

Structure: Skin consists of the *epidermis* and *dermis (corium)*. Deep to the dermis and therefore, the skin, is the *hypodermis*, which is also known as the *subcutaneous* or superficial connective tissue of the body. The latter comprises loose connective tissue with various amounts of adipose cells (tissue).

The epidermis provides the protective permeability barrier at the body surface, and epidermal derivatives do most of the skin-associated secretion. The dermis provides most of the mechanical strength of the skin. The hypodermis allows the skin and underlying structures to move somewhat independently and contains the adipose tissue that provides much of the body surface thermal insulation.

Epidermis: The epidermis is derived from the ectoderm and is composed of a keratinized stratified squamous epithelium. The epidermis varies in thickness depending on the function of the specific region of the body. Its thickness is used to differentiate two types of skin: thick and thin.

Thick skin denotes skin with a thicker epidermis which contains more cell layers when compared to *thin skin*. The epidermis ranges in thickness from 0.07 mm to 1.4 mm. Skin itself (both epidermis and dermis) ranges from 0.5 mm to more than 4 mm. The epidermis, similar to other epithelial layers, is avascular and lies on a basal lamina (basement membrane) to which the basal layer of epidermis cells is anchored.

The epidermis consists of specific cell layers that differ in their morphology and function. The layers of the epidermis of thick skin (sole of foot and palm of hand) from the basal lamina to the free surface are:

(1) stratum basale or germinativum
(2) stratum spinosum
(3) stratum granulosum
(4) stratum lucidum
(5) stratum corneum

The combined layers of the strata basale and spinosum are also referred to as the *stratum malpighi* or *malpighian layer.*

In thin skin the stratum lucidum is absent and the stratum granulosum often appears as a discontinuous layer. The strata spinosum and corneum are always present as distinct layers but are thinner than in thick skin.

The layers of skin represent the different stages through which the epidermal cells (keratinocytes) pass as they undergo the process of keratinization from their origin in the stratum basale to their sloughing off as dead keratinized cells at the free surface.

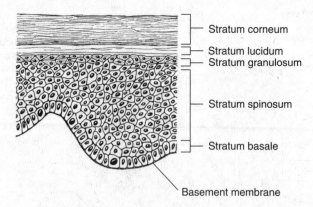

Stratum corneum
Stratum lucidum
Stratum granulosum
Stratum spinosum
Stratum basale
Basement membrane

The layers of the epidermis. The stratum lucidum is found only in the palms and soles.

The five layers of the epidermis of thick skin are characterized as follows:

1. Stratum basale
   a. Simple cuboidal to columnar epithelial cell layer resting on the basal lamina.
   b. Cells with the ability to divide (mitosis) and thus give rise to cells which migrate into the overlying stratum spinosum. This continuous process replenishes the keratinized epithelial cells which are shed from the surface.
   c. *Melanocytes,* which synthesize the brown pigment, *melanin,* in the form of pigment granules *(melanosomes).* Melanocytes have long cell processes which extend among the cells of the strata basale and spinosum. Via these processes they release and transfer melanosomes to the cells of the stratum malpighi. Increased exposure to UV light stimulates an increase in the secretion and release of melanosomes by the melanocytes, which results in the darkening of the skin (tanning). Dark color skin results from melanin, from carotene, a yellowish pigment, and from the degree of vascularity of the area, which adds a reddish-blue tint.
2. Stratum spinosum—consists of several layers of polygonal (polyhedral) cells which adhere to each other via desmosomes.
3. Stratum granulosum
   a. Consists of 3 to 5 layers of flat epithelial cells with pycnotic (dark, condensed) nuclei.
   b. Has a granular appearance due to the accumulation of irregular granules, the *keratohyalin granules,* within the cytoplasm. The granules are basophilic and are not encased by a membrane. The keratohyalin granules are associated with the numerous tonofilaments; both are involved in the production of keratin.
   c. The cells also contain *membrane-coating granules* (lamellated granules) composed of glycolipids which are secreted into the intercellular regions surrounding the cells of the stratum granulosum. This intercellular material appears to block the passage of substances through the epidermis.
   d. The keratinocytes die in this stratum.
4. Stratum lucidum
   a. It is a homogeneous translucent layer separating the strata granulosum and corneum in thick skin.
   b. Consists of 3 to 5 layers of flattened cells whose organelles and nuclei are indistinct or absent.
5. Stratum corneum
   a. Composed of layers of compressed, flat, cornified (keratinized) cells which lack nuclei and organelles. These scalelike cells are often referred to as *horny cells.*
   b. The most superficial horny cells slough off or desquamate constantly.

Dermis: The *corium,* or dermis, is derived from mesoderm and is the connective tissue layer between the epidermis and hypodermis. Depending on the region, its thickness may range from 0.5 mm to 4 mm. The border between these two strata is irregular in contour. This is caused by the irregular pattern of the surface of the dermis, to which the epidermis conforms. In a section perpendicular to the skin's surface, the dermis is seen to project into folds of the epidermis. These connective tissue projections are known as *dermal ridges* (or *papillae*); the epidermal regions between these ridges are the *epidermal* or *interpapillar pegs (ridges).* The dermal ridges are more numerous in thick skin (palm and soles), where greater abrasive forces occur. Because the epidermis follows the contours of the skin, the irregular contour of the dermis is projected onto the surface of the skin as ridges and grooves. The orientation and patterns of these surface grooves differ according to the skin region. They are very evident in the palm and fingers. The pattern is also extremely specific for each individual as is illustrated by the use of fingerprints to identify a person. These fingerprints, therefore, are actually the impressions of the grooves on the surface of the skin that represent the contour of the dermo-epidermal junction.

The dermis consists of two strata: the *papillary* and *reticular* layers.

Papillary layer. The *papillary layer* abuts the epidermis and forms the dermal ridges (papillae). It is thinner than the reticular layer and is composed of loose fibroelastic connective tissue. It consists of fine collagen, reticular, and elastic fibers associated with typical connective tissue cells (mainly fibroblasts and macrophages). The region abutting the basal cell layer is organized into a basement membrane. The processes of the basal cells anchor in the fibers of the membrane. The dermal ridges have extensive capillary networks. The epidermis is nourished by the diffusion of nutrients from this vascular bed. The papillary layer also contains encapsulated sensory receptors.

Reticular layer. The *reticular layer* is thicker and is composed of dense irregular fibroelastic connective tissue. The collagen and elastic fibers are thicker and coarser and form an interlacing network. Most fibers are primarily oriented parallel to the surface forming lines of skin tension called *Langer's lines,* which are important for surgical incisions. Capillaries are sparse. A rich nerve supply as well as encapsulated receptors are present in this layer. The reticular layer is the location of epidermal derivatives such as sweat and sebaceous glands and hair follicles, which extend through the dermis into the hypodermis. It also contains smooth muscles (arrector pili) associated with hair follicles and skeletal muscles in the head and neck (muscles of facial expression).

HYPODERMIS

Below the dermis, and therefore below the skin, is the *hypodermis* or *superficial fascia.* The hypodermis is often referred to as the subcutaneous layer or superficial connective tissue of the body. The hypodermis is composed of variable amounts of loose fibroelastic connective tissue interspersed with adipose tissue.

Glands

Glands are specialized structures containing secretory cells derived from epidermis. There are two basic types: sebaceous and sweat.

Sebaceous Glands: Sebaceous glands are *simple branched alveolar (acinar) glands* with a *holocrine* mode of secretion. They are found in all areas of the body except the palms and soles. The excretory ducts of several glands open into the necks of a hair follicle.

The cells of the gland differentiate and become progressively larger as they accumulate lipid droplets in their cytoplasm. The cells eventually rupture releasing their lipid content and cell remnants into the lumen. The latter comprise the oily secretion of the sebaceous glands called *sebum,* which helps protect the skin from becoming extremely dry.

Sweat Glands: Sweat is a watery fluid containing ammonia, urea, uric acid, and sodium chloride. The production of sweat is important for the excretion of some body wastes and the regulation of body temperature and is under nervous system control.

There are two types of sweat glands: eccrine and apocrine.

Eccrine Sweat Glands: The *eccrine sweat glands* are simple, coiled tubular glands with a merocrine mode of secretion. These glands are the ones that are typically considered when discussing sweat glands. Up to 3 million are found distributed all over the body in humans, except at the margin of the lip, glans penis, and ear drums. The largest number occur in the thick skin of the palms and soles. The *secretory tubular* unit is very coiled and is located in the reticular layer of the dermis near the hypodermis.

Apocrine Sweat Glands: The *apocrine sweat glands* are very large glands which are now (despite their name) thought to have a merocrine mode of secretion. They occur mainly in the hypodermis of the axilla, aerola of breast, labia majora, and scrotum. They are branched tubular glands whose secretory tubule is very dilated. Their secretory product is more viscous. The excretory ducts open into the hair follicles above the openings of this sweat gland.

The *ceruminous glands* of the external auditory canals, which secrete wax, and the *glands of Moll,* in the eyelid margin, are also considered to be apocrine sweat glands.

Hair

Hairs are long, filamentous keratinized structures derived from the epidermis of skin. The process of keratinization is similar to that in skin because cells divide, differentiate, and move toward the surface and become keratinized. Hairs are found covering the whole body except palms, soles, sides of fingers and toes, glans and prepuce of penis, clitoris, and labia minora.

Structure: A hair consists of a *shaft,* which extends above the skin surface, and a *root,* which lies within the skin. The root is encased by a tubular *hair follicle* composed of epidermal and dermal cell layers. At its deeper end, the follicle dilates and forms an invaginated *hair bulb* that is continuous with the root. The invaginated portion of the hair bulb contains a connective tissue papilla, the *dermal papilla,* which has a rich blood supply.

Hairs consist of three concentrically oriented epidermal layers: the *medulla, cortex,* and *cuticle.* The *medulla* forms the center of the hair and consists of two or three layers of cuboidal cells found only in coarse hair; these cornified cells contain soft keratin. The medulla is encased by the *cortex,* which constitutes the largest part of the hair. It consists of several layers of keratinized cells which contain numerous filaments embedded in an amorphous matrix. The latter form the *hard keratin* found in these compactly arranged spindle-shaped cells. Melanin granules are found in the cells of the cortex giving hair its coloration. Air in the intercellular region of these cells also affects the pigmentation of hairs. The *cuticle* surrounds the cortex and consists of a single layer of transparent, enucleated cells which form keratinized scales.

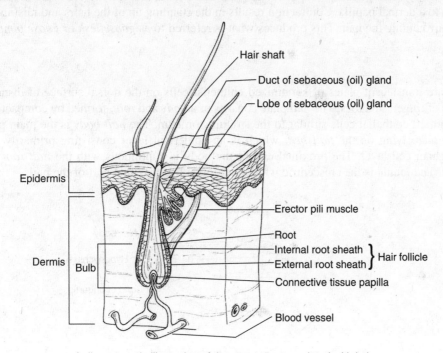

A diagrammatic illustration of the structures associated with hair.

Hair Follicle: The *hair follicle* consists of two sheaths: the *epithelial root sheath* and the *connective tissue root sheath.* The epidermally derived epithelial root sheath abuts the cuticle and is subdivided into the *inner epithelial root sheath* and the *outer (external) epithelial root sheath.* The *inner epithelial root sheath* extends from hair bulb to the level of the excretory duct of the sebaceous glands. It comprises three layers: (1) the *cuticle root sheath,* abutting the cuticle; (2) *Huxley's layer;* and (3) *Henle's layer,* adjacent to the outer epithelial root sheath. These layers are composed of keratinized cells containing soft keratin. The cells of the inner epithelial root sheath arise from the *hair matrix* in the hair bulb and migrate upward from it.

The *outer epithelial root sheath* is continuous with the epidermis of the skin. Close to the hair bulb the outer epithelial root sheath consists of a simple cuboidal layer similar to the stratum germinativum.

The *connective tissue root sheath* (or *dermal root sheath*) is derived from the dermis and consists of three layers: (1) the *glassy membrane,* the innermost layer which is a noncellular translucent membrane that corresponds to the basal lamina deep to the epidermis; (2) the *middle layer,* similar to the papillary layer of the dermis, and consisting of fine connective tissue fibers arranged in a circular pattern; and (3) the *outer layer,* similar to the reticular layer and consisting of longitudinally arranged coarse collagen fibers.

Hair Growth: Growth of a hair depends on the viability of the epidermal cells of the hair matrix which lie adjacent to the dermal papilla in the hair bulb. The matrix cells abutting the dermal papilla proliferate and give rise to cells which move upward to become part of the specific layers of the hair root and the inner epithelial root sheath. The hair matrix, therefore, functions similarly to the malpighian layer of the epidermis in that it gives rise to cells which become cornified as they move toward the surface. Due to this upward movement of the cells arising from the hair matrix, the hair (root and shaft) grows outward. Hairs do not grow continuously but have specific growth and rest periods that vary according to the area of the body. Hair growth is influenced by growth hormone and the sex hormones.

Hair Musculature: Hairs are oriented at a slight angle to the skin surface and are associated with *arrector pili muscles.* These smooth muscle bundles extend from the dermal root sheath to a dermal papilla. Contraction results in the standing up of the hairs and raising of the skin surrounding the hair. This produces what is referred to as *gooseflesh* or *goose pimples.*

Nails

Nails are translucent plates of keratinized epithelial cells on the dorsal surface of distal phalanges of fingers and toes. The nail plate consists of a *body* and *root,* formed by compact layers of cornified epithelial cells similar to the stratum corneum. The *nail body* is the main portion of the plate lying on the *nail bed,* which is an epidermal layer consisting primarily of the malpighian cell layer. The proximal end of the body is continuous with the *nail root* at the *lunula.* The lunula is the crescentric whitish region at the proximal part of the nail.

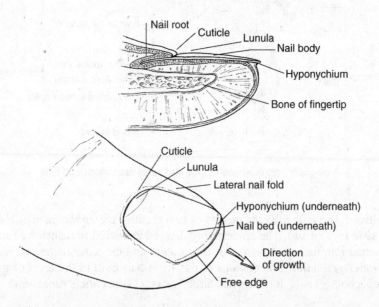

The prominent features associated with a typical fingernail.

Deep to the root and continuous with the proximal end of the nail bed is the *nail matrix*. The latter is a thickened stratum malpighi which gives rise to new cells that migrate upward and become keratinized. The matrix, therefore, functions in producing cornified cells composed of hard keratin which are added to the proximal end of the nail plate (root). This process increases the length of the nail. Nails increase in length at about 0.5 mm per week.

The *cuticle,* or *eponychium,* is a fold of the stratum corneum that extends over the surface of the nail body in the area of the lunula.

A similar fold, the *hyponychium,* occurs deep to the distal free margin of the nail plate. The hyponychium is actually a thickening of the stratum corneum of the skin where the nail bed and epidermis of the skin are continuous.

The Integumentary System

Organ	Major Function
Epidermis	Protection of the body; a barrier mechanism.
Dermis	Nourishes the epidermis by diffusion of nutrients; has sensory receptors.
Hair follicles	Produce hair.
Hair	Secondary sex characteristics; some protection.
Nails	Help in shaping the distal digits; some protection.
Sebaceous glands	Produce oily secretion that helps protect the skin from drying.
Sweat glands	Produce perspiration; control temperature of body.
Ceruminous glands	Secrete wax; protect auditory canals.
Superficial fascia	Stores fat.

QUICK RECALL TEST QUESTIONS AND ANSWERS

Choose the Best Answer

1. Which is the correct sequence of epidermal maturation?

   (A) stratum basale, stratum granulosum, stratum spinosum, stratum lucidum, stratum corneum
   (B) stratum basale, stratum spinosum, stratum granulosum, stratum lucidum, stratum corneum
   (C) stratum basale, stratum spinosum, stratum lucidum, stratum granulosum, stratum corneum
   (D) stratum basale, stratum spinosum, stratum granulosum, stratum corneum, stratum lucidum

2. The reticular layer of the dermis contains all of the following EXCEPT:

   (A) dense irregular connective tissue.
   (B) collagen and elastic fibers.
   (C) erector pili muscles.
   (D) a rich capillary supply.

3. The stratum spinosum consists of several layers of polygonal cells which adhere to each other via:

   (A) dermal ridges.
   (B) gap junctions.
   (C) terminal bars.
   (D) desmosomes.

4. The stratum basale is also called the:

   (A) epidermis.
   (B) dermis.
   (C) stratum corneum.
   (D) stratum germinativum.

5. Certain cells of the skin produce a pigment that provides protection against ultraviolet irradiation. These cells are the:

   (A) keratinocytes.
   (B) fibroblasts.
   (C) macrophages.
   (D) melanocytes.

6. A common feature of sweat glands, salivary glands, and sebaceous glands is that they are:

   (A) endocrine glands.
   (B) exocrine glands.
   (C) apocrine glands.
   (D) merocrine glands.

7. The eccrine sweat glands are classified as _____ glands.

   (A) branched tubular
   (B) simple coiled tubular
   (C) simple branched acinar
   (D) compound acinar

8. The dermis of the skin is derived from the embryonic germ layer known as the:

   (A) neural crest.
   (B) endoderm.
   (C) mesoderm.
   (D) ectoderm.

9. The barrier which prevents bacteria from entering the human body by passing through the skin is the _____ tissue in the _____.

   (A) epithelial, epidermis
   (B) epithelial, dermis
   (C) connective, epidermis
   (D) connective, dermis

10. Most of the mechanical strength of skin is due to the _____ tissue in the _____ .

    (A) epithelial, epidermis
    (B) epithelial, dermis
    (C) connective, epidermis
    (D) connective, dermis

11. When sweat glands are actively secreting, heat loss from the body surface of a human is:

    (A) increased.
    (B) decreased.
    (C) unchanged.

12. All of the cells in keratinocyte lineage (keri-
    tinized cells) in the epidermis are produced by
    mitotic division of cells in the:

    (A) stratum germinativum.
    (B) stratum granulosum.
    (C) stratum lucidum.
    (D) stratum corneum.

13. The papillary layer of the dermis in human skin
    contains:

    (A) loose fibroelastic connective tissue.
    (B) dense irregular fibroelastic connective tissue.
    (C) dense regular collagenous connective tissue.
    (D) dense regular elastic connective tissue.

14. The reticular layer of the dermis in human skin
    contains:

    (A) loose fibroelastic connective tissue.
    (B) dense irregular fibroelastic connective tissue.
    (C) dense regular collagenous connective tissue.
    (D) dense regular elastic connective tissue.

15. Eccrine sweat glands (typical sweat glands)
    usually occur attached:

    (A) directly to the epidermis.
    (B) to sebaceous glands.
    (C) to hair follicles.

16. The hair shaft in a hair follicle contains cells pro-
    duced by the:

    (A) outer epidermal root sheath.
    (B) inner epidermal root sheath.
    (C) dermal root sheath.
    (D) epidermal cells adjacent to the dermal papilla.

17. Sebaceous glands usually occur attached:

    (A) directly to the epidermis.
    (B) to eccrine sweat glands.
    (C) to hair follicles.

18. Sebaceous glands use _____ secretory mechanisms.

    (A) merocrine
    (B) apocrine
    (C) holocrine

Answers

1. **(B)** The epidermis consists of specific cell layers
   which differ in their morphology and function. The
   layers of the epidermis of thick skin (sole of foot
   and palm) from the basal lamina (dermis) to the
   free surface are:

   (1) stratum basale or germinativum
   (2) stratum spinosum
   (3) stratum granulosum
   (4) stratum lucidum
   (5) stratum corneum

2. **(D)** The reticular layer is composed of dense
   irregular connective tissue. Capillaries are sparse.
   The reticular layer is the location of epidermal
   derivatives such as sweat and sebaceous glands
   and hair follicles. It also contains smooth muscle
   (arrector pili) associated with hair follicles and
   skeletal muscles in the head and neck (muscles of
   facial expression).

3. **(D)** The stratum spinosum consists of several
   layers of polygonal (polyhedral) cells which
   adhere to each other via desmosomes.

4. **(D)** The stratum basale is also called the stratum
   germinativum.

5. **(D)** Melanocytes extend among the cells of the
   strata basale and spinosum. They produce pigment
   granules called melanosomes. Melanin is formed
   in the presence of tyrosinase in the melanosome;
   the starting product is carotene.

6. **(B)** Sweat glands, salivary glands, and sebaceous
   glands are all exocrine glands.

7. **(B)** There are two types of sweat glands: eccrine
   and apocrine. The eccrine sweat glands are simple,
   coiled tubular glands with a merocrine mode of
   secretion; they are the typical sweat glands. The
   aporine sweat glands occur mainly in the hypodermis of the axilla, areola of the breast, labia majora,
   and scrotum and are branched tubular glands.

8. **(C)** Whereas the epidermis is derived from ectoderm, the dermis and subcutaneous tissue under
   the skin is of mesodermal origin.

9. **(A)** The epithelium provides the primary barrier to
   bacterial entry, since the cells are tightly joined to
   each other laterally.

10. **(D)** The connective tissue in the dermis provides most of the mechanical strength of the skin. The strength is due to the extensive array of collagen fibers and other extracellular matrix components which make up most of the connective tissue. The dermis is the part of animal skin which is chemically preserved by tanning and used to make leather. The epithelium in the epidermis contributes some mechanical strength, but less than the dermis. The loose connective tissue and adipose tissue in the hypodermis contribute little mechanical strength, but allow the skin to move relative to the underlying structures.

11. **(A)** Evaporation of the water transported to the body surface by the sweat glands removes heat from the body surface, leading to much more rapid heat loss. This process allows moving heat from the body surface into air which on a hot day may be warmer than the body surface.

12. **(A)** Dividing cells in the stratum germinativum produce all of the keratinocyte lineage cells in the more superficial layers.

13. **(A)** The connective tissue in the papillary layer is much less dense than in the deeper (and much thicker) reticular layer of the dermis. Like the reticular layer, it consists of collagen and elastic fibers plus other extracellular matrix components, so it qualifies as loose fibroelastic connective tissue (loose FECT).

14. **(B)** The reticular layer makes up most of the dermis. It contains very large collagen fibers and large elastic fibers, most of which run roughly parallel to the skin surface but which are otherwise irregularly arranged. The cells are primarily fibroblasts. These characteristics are typical of dense irregular fibroelastic connective tissue.

15. **(A)** Eccrine sweat glands usually are attached directly to the epidermis and are not usually associated with sebaceous glands or hair follicles.

16. **(D)** The cells that form the hair shaft are produced by division of epidermal cells adjacent to the dermal papilla. The cells in the epidermal sheath around the hair do not contribute cells to the hair.

17. **(C)** Although solitary sebaceous glands can occur, most sebaceous glands are attached to hair follicles.

18. **(C)** Sebaceous gland cells fill with oily secretion and then are shed along with the secretion, so the mechanism is holocrine.

DIGESTIVE SYSTEM AND NUTRITION
Nutrition

Every living organism is faced with a fundamental dilemma—how to simultaneously maintain its individual integrity while assimilating the essential fuels for life from the surrounding environment. Primitive single-celled organisms living in water literally bathe in their environment, while more complex beings such as we are must draw nutrients from our environment while guarding those which we already have assimilated. Thus, the heterotrophic animal cell has evolved a highly specialized structure known as the cell or plasma membrane which allows selection of those environmental nutrients necessary for metabolism, elimination of metabolic waste products, and physical delineation of the cell as a unit. In the human organism, which is composed of billions of cells that have differentiated into many distinct cell types (e.g., neurons and muscle cells), the function of the plasma membrane has become very specialized. Perhaps nowhere in the body is the relationship of cell function to structure more apparent than in the gastrointestinal tract and the kidney. Nonetheless, every cell must retain its individual integrity and find a nutrient supply, no matter how specialized its processes may become.

Nutrients, once assimilated, must be guarded against loss. Thus, it should not be surprising to find that the cells of the early, or proximal, portion of the intestine are very close in appearance and function to those of the early, or proximal, part of the renal tubule. While the columnar epithelial cells of the jejunum are engaged in absorbing nutrients from within the intestinal passage and passing them into the blood, the columnar cells of the renal proximal tubule are responsible for protecting against loss of these same nutrients as they circulate through the kidney. In this section we will restrict ourselves to discussion of the function of the intestine, occasionally referring to significant similarities in the kidney.

Absorption of most nutrients within the intestine occurs only after *digestion* of the foods eaten. Thus, it is essential that the dinner we see and salivate over be broken down into its component chemical monomers, which can be transported across plasma membranes, before they can become useful to the body. Accordingly, nutrients are classified as *macro, micro,* or *trace* nutritional elements: macro elements include proteins, fats and complex carbohydrates, all of which require *digestion* prior to absorption; micro elements include materials like iron, calcium, and inorganic phosphate, which can be absorbed directly and for which there is a substantial daily need; trace elements include materials such as vitamins and elements like magnesium, selenium, and manganese. What follows is a more detailed examination of the broad issues raised above to provide a functional picture of the dual processes of digestion and absorption in achievement of a good nutritional state.

Unit for Measuring Value of Foods: A fundamental characteristic of all life is the need for energy production from nutrients; in humans this process occurs through oxidative combustion, the same basic process by which energy is released from wood or gasoline. As with wood and gasoline, a common end product is heat energy, which according to thermodynamic theory contributes to the *entropy*, or disorder, of the universe. Although we measure the energy value of wood and gasoline in British thermal units (BTUs), the unit commonly used to measure the energy value of foods is the *kilocalorie* (kcal). One kilocalorie is the amount of energy required to raise 1 kg (1,000 cc) of water one degree Celsius. In common parlance we speak of "calories," each one of which is $\frac{1}{1,000}$ of a kcal, or the energy necessary to raise 1 g (1 cc) of water one degree Celsius. Calories in the diet are derived exclusively from protein, fat, and carbohydrate, or the macronutrients. It is important to understand that, while these nutrient sources contain calories for energy production, the body can utilize their components for synthesis of many other molecules with minimal energy loss. Only when a molecule is completely utilized for energy production is its caloric value nutritionally relevant.

Proteins: These macromolecules are heteropolymers of L-amino acids, and their species-specific structures are rigidly controlled by the genome. Dietary protein in humans derives chiefly from animal and vegetable sources whose genomes differ significantly from that of the human. Accordingly, for humans to synthesize their own species-specific proteins, the dietary molecules must be reduced to their simplest component units (amino acids) and reutilized in human cells for synthesis of structural and enzyme proteins under direction of the human genetic code. There are 21 naturally occurring amino acids, 8 of which humans cannot synthesize *de novo* or by using any molecule of similar structure; these are termed *essential amino acids*. The reason for our inability to construct these amino acids is that our genetic code does not include messages for the synthesis of the requisite enzyme proteins to establish the proper chemical bonds; thus, we must depend upon other organisms for production of these molecules, which are essential to our own lives. The remaining 13 amino acids can be made from other materials in human cells and, for this reason, are called *nonessential amino acids*. The relative amount of essential to nonessential amino acids, both in general and with respect to specific ones, varies widely with each dietary source; some proteins do not contain any of a given essential amino acid.

A final point to touch on in this very brief summary is that protein is the sole source of dietary nitrogen. Even though we exist in an atmosphere comprising about 80% nitrogen, our bodies' only nitrogen source is the food we eat and the protein contained in it. Moreover, nitrogen liberated from dietary protein is in the form of ammonia, a very potent neurotoxin. Since each amino acid comprising the protein we eat contains a minimum of one amino (-NH$_2$) group, the potential for ammonia toxicity with every meal is immense. We are, however, protected by two factors. The first is that most dietary protein is reutilized as intact amino acids, with the amino group acting as a sort of metabolic "lock" which prevents utilization for energy. The second is that the detoxification process in the liver known as the "urea cycle" converts any liberated ammonia to the biologically inert compound called *urea*. Urea is excreted by the kidney into the urine, and a rough measure of kidney function can be obtained by assessing the *blood urea nitrogen*, or BUN. By contrast, if the liver has failed, the BUN will be low while the *blood ammonia* will be high. In each case, however, the abnormalities can be traced back to the breakdown or *catabolism* of amino acids for energy, since these compounds are the sole source of nitrogen.

Carbohydrates: These sugars, or saccharides, are generally present in the diet in single (mono-), dual (di-), or complex (poly-) saccharide form. The common dietary monosaccharides are fructose, glucose and galactose; disaccharides include sucrose (glucose + fructose) and lactose (glucose + galactose); ingested polysaccharides are usually starch and cellulose, both of which are large glucose polymers. The monosaccharides can be absorbed directly by the intestine, but the di- and polysaccharides must be enzymatically hydrolyzed into their monomer units. Nutritionally, the carbohydrates have important roles: The first is as a primary source of energy to offset the use of amino acids; the second is to supply the carbon skeletons for synthesis of nonessential amino acids; and the third is to serve as intrinsic components of many complex molecules called glycoproteins and glycolipids. Glycoproteins are important components of all cell membranes and glycolipids are especially important for normal function of the central nervous system. Regarding their use as a fuel, the caloric value of a gram of glucose is essentially identical to that of a gram of protein, from which one might correctly conclude that a diet which has more carbohydrate by weight than protein will ensure that all amino acids can be utilized for protein synthesis. Finally, the initial cellular steps in the breakdown of glucose result in two 3-carbon compounds which can be used for synthesis of fat (see below) as well as for amino acids. This is the reason that diets higher than normal in carbohydrate and total calories result in obesity.

Fats: The basic building block of dietary fat is the fatty acid, which is generally a straight- or simple-branched chain molecule composed of an even number of 12–18 carbon atoms and terminating in a carboxyl group. There are, of course, similar molecules that are either longer or shorter and are made up of odd as well as even numbers of carbon atoms, but the bulk of dietary fatty acids are as described above, and are called *saturated fatty acids*. Further variation is seen in the C12–C18 compounds by virtue of insertion of one or more double bonds, a change that renders the compounds *unsaturated fatty acids*. Humans are able to synthesize saturated fatty acids starting from the common 2-carbon biochemical intermediate, acetyl-coenzyme A; unlike the situation with nitrogen, the human body has evolved enzymes capable of fixing carbon dioxide, thus permitting it to elongate a carbon chain as necessary. The system has limitations in the creation of double bonds, rendering certain unsaturated fatty acids essential in the diet.

Utilizing the 3-carbon triol fragment produced from glucose, called *glycerol*, the human body is able, by stepwise addition of fatty acids to each alcohol group, to create *triglycerides*. These mono-, di-, or triglycerides are simply one, two, or three fatty acids linked to the glycerol through ester bonding, created by an enzymatically-mediated reaction between the alcohol and carboxyl groups. It is also possible for humans to create, from the fundamental triglyceride structure, very complex macromolecules which are vital to the structure and function of various components of the central nervous system. It is worth noting that the bulk of the weight of the CNS, and specifically the brain, derives from the presence of simple and complex lipids.

In addition to the above, the human organism is capable of synthesis of cholesterol from acetyl-coenzyme A. Cholesterol is a molecule with a complicated ring structure from which many steroid hormones and compounds related to blood coagulation are derived. Cholesterol is also an important component of all cell membranes. This vital body molecule can be produced from almost any dietary macronutrient, so that dietary cholesterol restriction can go only so far in lowering an already elevated blood cholesterol level in prevention or treatment of coronary artery disease.

Nutritionally, fat is present in virtually all animal and plant constituents of the human diet, so that elimination of dietary fat is exceedingly difficult to accomplish. Moreover, the caloric, or energy value of fat is more than twice that of carbohydrate and protein; thus, reduction of fat may produce a diet too low in calories to meet daily energy requirements. In addition, because of the association between protein and fat, there is a risk of protein deficiency with draconian fat-reduction type diets.

Vitamins: Vitamins are a group of organic molecules which are derived from microorganisms and are essential for human nutrition. All vitamins undergo intracellular changes ("activation") which render them *cofactors*, in which form they interact with specific enzyme proteins to participate in the production of "transition states" of reactions. In their native form, as ingested, vitamins are not active and have no biological value *per se*. Once bound to an enzyme protein in the activated form, a vitamin molecule will remain in the body for as long as the integrity of the protein remains. Many vitamins are recycled by the body as well; both of these phenomena account for the very small daily quantities required by humans. Vitamins are essential to many key metabolic reactions, including 1-carbon transfer reactions involved in synthesis of DNA, so that deficiency, though rare in the Western world, can cause some striking diseases. Most authors tend to subgroup vitamins into those which are fat-soluble and those which are water-soluble, a classification that does little to describe their activities. It does have the advantage of explaining various aspects of secondary vitamin deficiencies, however, and we shall therefore follow the same classification.

FAT-SOLUBLE VITAMINS

Fat-Soluble Vitamins and Their Roles

Vitamin	Physiological Role	Deficiency Syndrome
A (Retinol)	Contributes to visual pigments in eye	Night blindness, drying of mucous membranes in body
D (Calciferol)	Absorption of calcium and phosphorus; construction of teeth and bones	Rickets, especially in children
E (Tocopherol)	Protects blood cells from destruction during formation	Lysis of red blood cells, anemia
K	Used in synthesis of prothrombin required for blood clotting	Excessive bleeding, especially in newborns; poor blood clotting

1. **Vitamin A (retinol, retinoic acid, retinal).** The chief function of this compound is in the eye, where it supports dark vision and normal structure of the conjunctiva and cornea. Primary dietary sources of vitamin A are vegetables, fruits (beta-carotene, or two retinal molecules linked through their aldehydic groups) and animal liver (retinol, the storage form found chiefly in liver).

2. **Vitamin D (1,25-dihydroxycholecalciferol).** Although originally described as a vitamin and identified as the antirachitic dietary factor, vitamin D is considered by many authorities to be a hormone. The human skin produces an activated cholesterol molecule utilizing the sun's ultraviolet radiation, from which 25-hydroxycholecalciferol is synthesized in liver. This material is essentially inactive in a biological sense, and must be carried in the blood to the kidney, where the enzyme necessary for 1-alpha-hydroxylation is expressed and the 1,25-dihydroxy compound produced. For this reason, severe kidney disease can result in rickets in children or osteomalacia in adults because of the inability to produce the biologically active metabolite. Thus, it is important in such cases to distinguish between states of dietary deficiency, liver and/or kidney disease, and other disorders which may all resemble simple dietary D deficiency. The chief action of vitamin D is to enhance the synthesis of calcium-binding protein, which increases calcium and phosphate absorption by the intestine. The process enables the bone to produce *hydroxyapatite*, the crystalline material from which bone is constructed.

3. **Vitamin E (tocopherol).** The chief function of vitamin E is as an antioxidant in cells throughout the body, suppressing the oxidation of polyunsaturated fatty acids by free radicals. Since the largest amount of these polyunsaturated fatty acids is found in membrane phospholipids, which in turn are present in large quantities in the central nervous system, vitamin E is now recognized as an important defense in maintenance of CNS integrity. It also acts in the same capacity in the red cell, protecting against excessive hemolysis. Vitamin E is known to increase sperm motility and to prevent second-trimester abortion in a number of animal species, although any such function in humans has yet to be demonstrated.

4. **Vitamin K (phylloquinone).** A key element in the intrinsic coagulation pathway, vitamin K is essential for conversion of glutamate residues to gamma-carboxyglutamate in the prothrombin molecule, which then enables prothrombin to bind calcium, an essential step for its function in the coagulation cascade. Newborns are usually hypoprothrombinemic, resulting in a bleeding tendency; for this reason, it is standard neonatology practice to provide supplemental vitamin K by injection shortly after birth in order to maximize the ability of existing prothrombin to bind calcium.

WATER-SOLUBLE VITAMINS

1. **Thiamine (vitamin B_1).** Thiamine, once activated, is a cofactor for many critical reactions, including those mediated by dehydrogenases; a pivotal step in energy production is the pyruvate dehydrogenase reaction, which converts a 3-carbon fragment of glucose (pyruvate) to acetyl coenzyme A. The acetyl CoA then either enters the tricarboxylic acid cycle or can be utilized for fatty acid synthesis. Another very important reaction in which thiamine participates is the transketolase step of the pentose phosphate shunt, which generates ribose-5-phosphate for nucleic acid synthesis. Thiamine is widely distributed in the normal human diet. Deficiency of thiamine results in the disease known as beriberi.

2. **Riboflavin (vitamin B_2).** Ingested riboflavin, derived predominantly from animal sources in the diet, is converted enzymatically to flavin mononucleotide (FMN) or to flavin adenine dinucleotide (FAD). Both of these cofactors are facile and reversible oxidation-reduction agents and are, therefore, predictably involved in many key mitochondrial reactions. Riboflavin is also a cofactor in production of niacin and pyridoxine to the limited degree possible in humans. The most remarkable fact is that riboflavin deficiency does not have a well-defined clinical state associated with it, as other water soluble vitamins do.

3. **Niacin (vitamin B_3).** Niacin can be produced in limited quantities by humans from the dietary amino acid tryptophan. As already mentioned, riboflavin is a cofactor in this

Water-Soluble Vitamins and Their Roles

Vitamin	Physiological Role	Deficiency Syndrome
Thiamine (B$_1$)	Coenzyme in carbohydrate metabolism	Beriberi, loss of appetite, fatigue
Riboflavin (B$_2$)	Part of FAD, coenzyme in respiration and protein metabolism	Inflammation and breakdown of skin
Pyridoxine (B$_6$)	Coenzyme in amino acid and fat metabolism	Anemia, nerve problems
Cyanocobalamin (B$_{12}$)	Coenzyme in formation of erythrocytes and nucleic acids	Pernicious anemia
Niacin (B$_3$)	Part of NAD, coenzyme in energy metabolism	Pellagra, fatigue
Ascorbic acid (C)	Assists synthesis of collagen in connective tissues	Scurvy, anemia, slow wound healing
Pantothenic acid	Part of coenzyme A, used in carbohydrate and fat mebaolism	Similar to other B vitamins
Biotin	Coenzyme in addition of carboxyl groups	Rare; tiny amounts required
Folic acid	Coenzyme in formation of nucleotides and hemoglobin	Some types of anemia

process. From the basic compound, nicotinic acid, activation produces nicotinamide adenine dinucleotide (NAD), and an additional phosphorylation reaction produces NADP. NAD is an important cofactor in oxidative metabolic pathways, such as the tricarboxylic acid cycle, while NADP is found in reductive pathways, such as the pentose phosphate shunt. Animal tissues are rich in both niacin and tryptophan. Deficiency of niacin causes the disease called pellagra.

4. **Pyridoxine (vitamin B$_6$).** Pyridoxine comprises a pyridine nucleus which is substituted in one of three ways: It occurs in plant foods as pyridoxamine, and in animal foods as either pyridoxal (the aldehyde) or pyridoxol (the alcohol). While the alcohol-substituted form has no biological activity, it can be converted either to the aldehyde or the amine, both of which function as cofactors. Of all the water-soluble vitamins, pyridoxine is the one involved in the most diverse biochemical reactions, including amino acid transamination and decarboxylation, heme biosynthesis, and glycogenolysis. Another critical function is as a cofactor in conversion of L-glutamic acid to gamma-aminobutyric acid, or GABA, which is a key neurotransmitter substance in the brain. Isolated B$_6$ deficiency is almost never seen in a clinical setting—it is usually part of a more global vitamin B complex deficiency.

5. **Cobalamin (vitamin B$_{12}$).** Despite being involved as a cofactor in only two reactions in the human body, vitamin B$_{12}$ is of critical importance. Cobalamin is synthesized exclusively by microorganisms and is, therefore, not present in plants, but can be found in relatively high concentration in animal liver. Unlike the other water-soluble vitamins, B$_{12}$ is bound to a specific transfer protein produced in the stomach and called the *intrinsic factor*. When the bound B$_{12}$ reaches the intestine, the complex is bound to specific cell surface receptors and taken up by pinocytosis. Once absorbed, cobalamin is hydroxylated to form hydroxycobalamin, the form in which it enters cells. Once intracellular in location, this compound enters one of two enzymatic conversion steps: within the cytosol it is converted to methylcobalamin, while in the mitochondrion it becomes adenosylcobalamin. As methylcobalamin, B$_{12}$

is involved in reconversion of homocysteine to methionine, in the process generating tetrahydrofolate, which is a compound critical to methyl-group transfer and DNA synthesis. As adenosylcobalamin, B_{12} is involved in the transformation of methylmalonyl coenzyme A to succinyl CoA, a metabolic conversion required of a multitude of biologic subtrates for complete degradation. Failure to negotiate this enzymatic step results in severe clinical disease manifest as methylmalonic acidemia. Vitamin B_{12} deficiency can be due to many things and is manifested as the condition called pernicious anemia.

6. **Folic Acid.** Folic acid is actually a group of compounds based upon a pteridine ring substituted with glutamic acid, linked through para-aminobenzoic acid. The number of glutamate residues, linked as a polypeptide chain, can be varied and the multiple compounds thus formed are called pteroylglutamates. The most active of the latter group is tetrahydrofolate, converted to 5-methyltetrahydrofolate in the liver and released as the chief circulating form of the vitamin. As mentioned earlier, folic acid is a key component of the 1-carbon transfer system so critical to nucleic acid synthesis. Indeed, it is this critical importance which lies at the bottom of the use of folic acid antagonists in the treatment of leukemias, where the synthetic rate of DNA is extraordinarily accelerated. Foods rich in folic acid include vegetables and fruits. Not only is folate deficiency a serious disorder in adults, causing a severe anemia; folate deficiency during pregnancy can adversely affect the formation of the neural tube of the early embro, resulting in neural tube malformations.

7. **Biotin.** Biotin is the cofactor for CO_2 fixation, or carboxylation reactions. There are four such reactions, each at pivotal metabolic junctures. Fatty acid synthesis depends upon this process, which utilizes acetyl coenzyme A carboxylase to produce the 3-carbon malonyl CoA. A second biotin-dependent enzyme is propionyl coenzyme A carboxylase, which is the reaction producing methylmalonyl CoA (see above, vitamin B_{12}). A third is beta-methylcrotonyl CoA carboxylase, which is a step in leucine catabolism. The fourth is pyruvate carboxylase, a key enzyme in gluconeogenesis. The process by which biotin becomes a cofactor in these relationships is relatively unique and requires a separate enzyme (holocarboxylase synthase) to establish a bond between free biotin and a lysine residue in the carboxylase enzyme protein. Biotin is present in soy flour, yeast, egg yolk, and liver in high concentrations. Biotin deficiency results in loss of appetite, diminished activity, a skin rash and hair loss, and in its extreme form can mimic a genetic disease resulting in absence of the holocarboxylase synthase.

8. **Pantothenic Acid.** Pantothenic acid is an integral part of the coenzyme A molecule and functions as a cofactor in transfer of acyl groups. Acyl-group transfer is a key metabolic reaction in fatty acid synthesis and catabolism, amino acid catabolism and normal function of the tricarboxylic acid cycle. The presence of pantothenate in the coenzyme A molecule permits generation of a highly reactive thiol ester which serves as a thermodynamically favorable carrier for the acyl group. Pantothenic acid is widely distributed in foods. As with riboflavin, isolated pantothenate deficiency has not yet been described in humans.

9. **Ascorbic Acid (vitamin C).** Vitamin C qualifies as perhaps the best-known of the water-soluble vitamin group. However, it is unlike the other vitamins discussed above in that it does not bind chemically to a protein in order to function. Ascorbate has a valuable metabolic role as a mild reducing agent, since it donates hydrogen ions at precisely the proper energy level to maintain the reduced state of vital metal ions, especially copper and iron. In this capacity, vitamin C maintains the integrity of important metalloenzymes involved in collagen synthesis and steroidogenesis, as well as maintenance of cytochromes and intestinal absorption of iron. Ascorbate is found in citrus fruits and green vegetables. Vitamin C deficiency causes scurvy, a disease in which many of the clinical findings—such as gingival hemorrhage and death, hemorrhage into old scars and refracture of old, healed fractures—point to a common effect on collagen metabolism.

Minerals: Upon leaving the ocean, land-dwelling organisms have had to evolve ways in which to carry with them adequate supplies of those minerals which are critical to the function of their enzyme systems. These include iron, calcium, and phosphorus as well as copper, magnesium, and many others. Generally speaking, a normal diet will supply adequate amounts of each essential mineral. Deficiencies result in clinical entities like anemia (iron), tetany (calcium), etc.

The Digestive System

REGIONALIZATION OF THE EMBRYONIC GUT

During embryonic development, the endoderm of the primitive gut gives rise to four regions: pharynx, foregut, midgut, and hindgut (cranial to caudal). Specific components of the digestive tract develop from each of these regions of the embryonic gut.

1. Pharynx: oropharynx and laryngeal pharynx.
2. Foregut: esophagus, stomach, and cranial portion of duodenum from which the primordia of the liver, gallbladder, and pancreas arise.
3. Midgut: caudal duodenum, jejunum, ileum, and ascending colon and two-thirds of transverse colon including the appendages cecum and vermiform appendix.
4. Hindgut: distal third of transverse colon, descending colon, sigmoid colon, and rectum.

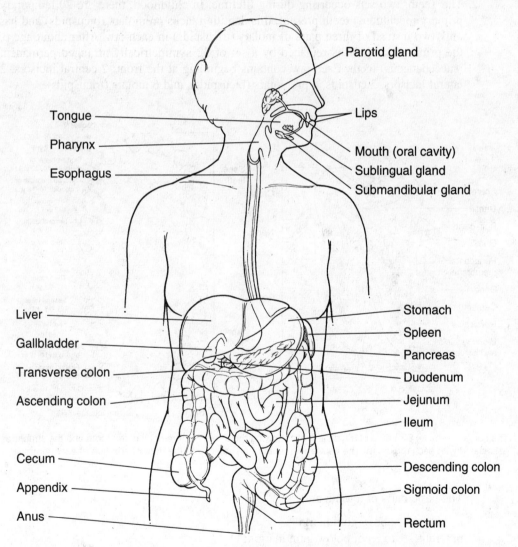

The human digestive tract relative to other structures of the body as seen from the ventral position.

Parts of the Adult Digestive Tract: The adult digestive tract includes the oral cavity; oral and laryngeal pharynx; esophagus; cardiac sphincter; stomach; pyloric sphincter; duodenum; jejunum; ileum; cecum; ascending colon; transverse colon; descending colon; sigmoid colon; rectum; and anal sphincter.

The Oral Cavity. The oral cavity contains the tongue and teeth. It receives the secretions of the salivary glands.

1. The Tongue: composed primarily of a core of skeletal muscle and glands and covered by a mucous membrane. The anterior two-thirds of the upper (oral) portion is separated from the posterior one-third (pharyngeal) portion by the sulcus terminalis.

   Three types of lingual papillae appear as surface projections:

   a. Circumvallate papillae—located along the sulcus terminals and possessing taste buds;
   b. Filiform papillae—the most numerous;
   c. Fungiform papillae—relatively few but possessing taste buds.

2. The Teeth: two sets occurring during lifetime. In childhood, there are 20 temporary primary (deciduous) teeth present; this dentition lacks premolars (bicuspids) and has only two instead of three pairs of molars (tricuspids) in each jaw. After about age 6, the primary dentition is replaced by a set of 32 symmetrically arranged permanent (succedaneous) teeth. Each jaw contains beginning at the front: 2 central incisors, 2 lateral incisors, 2 cuspids, 4 premolars (bicuspids), and 6 molars (tricuspids).

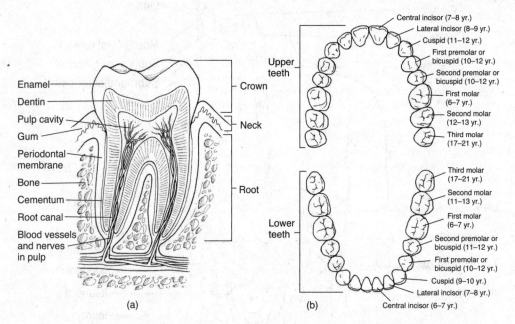

The human teeth. (a) Structure of a typical tooth showing the three major regions of the tooth and the structures associated with each region. (b) The permanent teeth of an adult, with the date of eruption of each tooth.

The basic parts of a tooth are:

a. crown—above gum margin;
b. root—1 to 3 cm below gum margin;
c. alevolus—root socket in jaw bone;
d. neck—junction of root and crown;

     e.   periodontal membrane—attaches the root to the alveolar wall;

     f.   pulp chamber—extends from crown into root canals;

     g.   apical foramen—canal opening at the tip of root;

     h.   dental pulp—soft core of loosely arranged connective tissue occupying the chamber and containing blood vessels and nerves to teeth;

     i.   tooth wall with dentin, which borders pulp; enamel, which covers the crown and thins at the neck; and cementum, which encrusts the root and thins at the neck.

3. Salivary Glands: There are three pairs of major salivary glands.

     a.   Parotid (largest gland)—located in relation to the mandibular ramus below and anterior to the ear. It is a compound tubulo-alveolar, serous gland of the merocrine type. Connective tissue divides the gland into lobes and lobules. The major duct (Stenson's) opens into the vestibule of the oral cavity opposite the second upper (maxillary) molar.

     b.   Submandibular (intermediate in size)—located in relationship to the mylohyoid muscle, medial and inferior to the mandible. It is a tubulo-alveolar, merocrine gland (mixed-mucus and serous). The major duct (Wharton's) opens on the anterolateral margin of the frenulum of the tongue.

     c.   Sublingual (smallest gland)—a collection of glands located under the mucous membrane of the floor of the mouth. It is a tubulo-alveolar merocrine gland with mostly mucous acini. The major duct (Bartholin's) empties on the side of the frenulum of the tongue, having joined the submandibular duct.

Tubular Digestive Tract. The adult tubular digestive tract has a general structural plan of mucosa, submucosa, muscular tunic, and adventitia.

1. Mucosa

     a.   moist surface epithelium (containing organ-specific cell types)

     b.   connective tissue (lamina propria)

     c.   thin muscular layer (muscularis mucosae)

2. Submucosa

     a.   connective tissue

     b.   plexi of peripheral nerves and ganglion cells termed Meissner's plexus

     c.   some areas may contain exocrine glands

     d.   rich in blood vessels

3. Muscular tunic

     a.   inner circular smooth muscle layer

     b.   outer longitudinal smooth muscle layer

     c.   Auerbach's myenteric plexus—between the two muscle layers is located a parasympathetic plexus of nerves associated with numerous ganglion cells

4. Adventitia or serosa

     a.   connective tissue containing blood vessels, nerves, and lymphatics

     b.   peritoneal covering (mesothelium) located in some regions

Esophagus (about 10 to 12 in). The upper third of the esophagus features skeletal muscle (voluntary), the middle third both skeletal and smooth (involuntary) muscle, the lower third only smooth muscle.

The Stomach. The stomach is highly vascular, contains gastric glands, and has smooth muscle fibers extending around the glands. There are two types of gastric glands: cardiac and fundic.

1. Cardiac and pyloric glands secrete mucus
2. Fundic glands:

   a. surface lining/mucous cells—form barrier epithelium and secrete mucus; mucus protects against autodigestion and neutralizes acid to a small degree.
   b. parietal or oxyntic cells—secrete hydrochloric acid (HCl). Acid (pH below 5.5) is necessary to convert pepsinogen into pepsin; at pH 2, this reaction is almost instantaneous. Parietal cells secrete acid under the influence of the hormone gastrin (probably of greatest importance); parasympathetic mediation via acetyl-choline; histamine; and the presence of foodstuffs, such as peptides and amino acids.
   c. chief (zymogenic) cells—secrete pepsinogen, the precursor of pepsin (proteolytic enzyme). These cells also secrete and release the hormone gastrin, as well as the protein called the *intrinsic factor* critical for vitamin B_{12} absorption.
   d. argentaffin or enterochromaffin cells—thought to secrete serotonin, a vasocon-strictor substance.

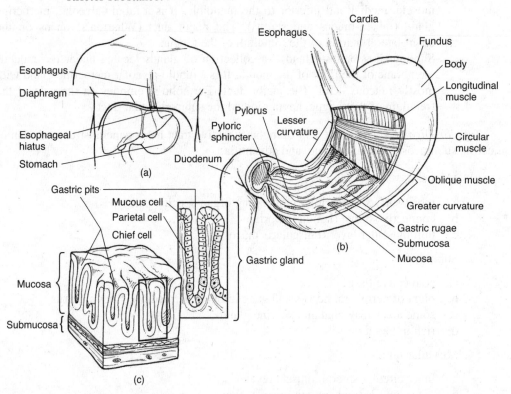

Aspects of the human stomach. (a) The stomach in place in the upper abdominal cavity in the epigastric region. (b) The major anatomical regions and muscle layers of the stomach. Note the inner folds (rugae) that become taut when the stomach is filled. (c) A closeup of the stomach tissue showing the various cells of the gastric wall.

Small Intestine. The small intestine has three major regions:

1. Duodenum (10 in)
2. Jejunum (8.5 ft)
3. Ileum (12.5 ft)

The small intestine has mucosal surface modifications:

a. Villi (projections of mucosa)—covered by simple columnar epithelium and having a core of connective tissue; they are broad in the duodenum, fingerlike in the ileum. In the core of the villus (in the connective tissue layer called the lamina propria) are found lymphocytes, eosinophils, plasma cells, macrophages, capillaries, and *lacteals* (lymphatic capillaries).

   b. Microvilli—cell surface modifications present on absorptive cells of columnar epithelium of villi. The plasmalemma associated with the microvilli contains proteins (transport carriers) with high specificity for binding with sugars and amino acids. Some transport carriers are linked with the action of Na$^+$-K$^+$ ATPase at the opposite surface (pole) of the epithelial cell, and the energy liberated by hydrolysis of ATP powers active transport (against a concentration gradient). A similar process occurs in the proximal renal tubule. The density of some of these intestinal carrier proteins is genetically regulated.

Large Intestine (cecum, ascending, transverse, and descending colon)

Colon and Rectum

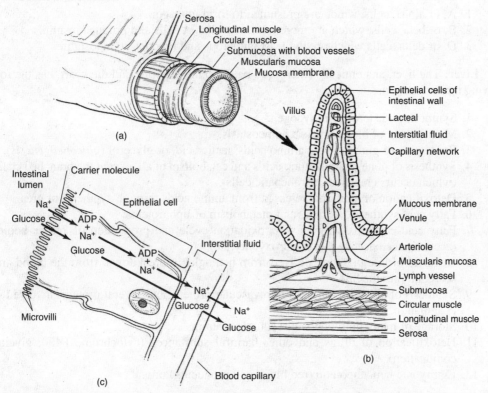

Structure of the small intestine and absorption. (a) The multiple muscle layers of the intestinal wall. (b) A single villus expanded to show its structure. The capillary network receives the products of protein, carbohydrate, and nucleic digestion, while the lacteal receives the breakdown products of lipids. (c) Absoprtion of sodium ions and glucose molecules from the intestinal lumen, then through the epithelial cell, through the intestinal fluid, and into the capillary.

The Major Digestive Glands

Pancreas: The pancreas has both an exocrine and endocrine secretory function. Two excretory ducts are usually present and enter the second part of the duodenum. Exocrine glandular elements are arranged in acini. Acinar cells have a basal zone containing extensive rough endoplasmic reticulum and an apical zone containing zymogen granules which are the precursors of the enzymes in pancreatic juice—namely trypsin, chymotrypsin, amylase, and lipase. Acinar cells secrete

   1. trypsinogen, which will be converted into trypsin.
   2. chymotrypsinogen, which will be converted into chymotrypsin.
   3. procarboxypeptidase, which will be converted into carboxypeptidase.

The above reactions are autocatalyzed (trypsinogen-trypsin). Trypsin, chymotrypsin, and carboxypeptidase attack proteins and polypeptides and eventually render amino acids which can be absorbed.

Pancreatic lipase, amylase, and proteases are controlled by the presence of foodstuffs and hormones. As acid chyme enters the duodenum from the stomach, secretin is released and fluid and bicarbonate are secreted.

Pancreatic juice

1. neutralizes the acid chyme in the duodenum and
2. provides enzymes for the digestion of proteins, carbohydrates, and fats.

Islets of Langerhans are the endocrine portion of the pancreas. The endocrine cell aggregations are interspersed irregularly among the acini. Three cell types can be identified:

1. A, or alpha, cells, which are presumed to form glucagon.
2. B, or beta, cells, which are more numerous than A cells and produce insulin.
3. D, or delta, cells which are the least numerous and produce somatostatin.

Liver: The liver, anatomically interposed between the intestine and the heart, has the following major functions:

1. Synthesis and storage of glycogen.
2. Maintenance of blood glucose homeostasis.
3. Production of glucose from amino acids, lactic acid, or glycerol (*gluconeogenesis*).
4. Synthesis of nonessential amino acids and catabolism of all, except the branched chain (which occurs chiefly in extrahepatic cells).
5. Detoxification of ammonia released from amino acids through synthesis of urea.
6. Fatty acid synthesis, storage, and metabolism of lipoproteins.
7. Fatty acid catabolism by the beta-oxidation cycle and production of ketone bodies (acetone, acetoacetate, beta-hydroxybutyrate).
8. Removal of bile pigment, derived from hemoglobin breakdown, from the blood and secretion into the bile.
9. Synthesis of albumin, the chief intravascular protein, and several proteins involved in coagulation.
10. Storage of many lipid-and water-soluble vitamins.
11. Detoxification of drugs and other harmful substances (cytochrome P450, glycine conjugation).
12. Embryonic hematopoietic (red blood cell producing) organ.

Gallbladder: *Bile*, which is a composite of *bile salts, bile acids*, and *bile pigments,* as well as electrolytes secreted continuously by the hepatocytes, is collected and stored in the gallbladder. The bile salts and acids, synthesized from cholesterol, are critical for normal fat digestion in the intestine, since they enable micelle formation. Certain drugs and their hepatic metabolites are excreted in the bile. The ileum is extremely efficient in the reabsorption of bile salts, so that 95% of the amount excreted per day is returned to the liver via the cyclical path called the *enterohepatic circulation*. Since steroid hormone is made from the cholesterol nucleus, the 5% which is lost is a major excretory pathway for steroid hormone precursors.

General Functional Schema of the Digestive Tube (ingestion, digestion, egestion)

Oral Cavity: The oral cavity
a) Receives food and perceives taste, odor, texture, and temperature.
b) Grinds foodstuffs to facilitate the action of enzymes.
c) Adds salivary enzymes, mucus, and moisture and shapes the bolus for the process of swallowing.

Pharynx and Esophagus: The oral and laryngeal pharynx, and the esophagus are essentially conduits for food to reach the stomach.

Stomach: Food is received, stored, and churned; digestive juices are added; and the digestive process started in the mouth is continued. Intrinsic factor (antipernicious anemia factor) is secreted.

Small Intestines: Digestion is completed and most absorption occurs in jejunum and ileum.

Large Intestines: The following occurs in the large intestines:

1. Water and electrolytes are reabsorbed to preserve that delicate balance in the body.
2. Food is propelled along for elimination (egestion).

Intestinal Motility

Intestinal motility facilitates

1. the mixing of food with secretions and enzymes,
2. the contact of foodstuffs with the intestinal mucosa, and
3. propulsion along the tube (peristalsis).

This process is controlled by the nervous system, hormonal secretions, and intestinal distension and similar phenomena.

Epinephrine (from the adrenal) inhibits contraction; serotonin (from the small intestines) stimulates contractions.

Innervation of the Intestinal Tract

The nerves supplying the intestinal tract affect smooth muscle, glands, endocrine tissue, and control motility and secretion. Motility or *peristalsis* is a wave of compression (contraction) that is followed by a regional relaxation. The gut musculature (smooth) is controlled by the autonomic nervous system.

Sympathetic Innervation: Effects of sympathetic innervation are:

1. some excitation of salivary secretion
2. decrease of motility and secretion in the stomach and small intestines due mainly to the vasoconstrictive action
3. inhibition of muscular contraction and intrinsic ganglion cell activity due to the release of the neurotransmitters epinephrine and norepinephrine

Parasympathetic Innervation: Effects of the parasympathetic innervation are:

1. stimulation of motility and secretion via its supply of the intrinsic plexi and the release of the neurotransmitter acetylcholine
2. release of gastrin

Summary of Digestive Juices

A key concept in understanding the secretions of the digestive tract is the necessity for reduction of most complex dietary molecules to their simplest units. Thus, proteins must be reduced to amino acids, complex carbohydrates to monosaccharides, and complicated lipids to fatty acids and triglycerides. This is necessary for rapid and efficient absorption when nutrients reach the intestine, and subsequently for easy transport via circulation to the liver.

The Sources and Enzymes of Human Digestion

Source	Fluids	Enzyme	Substrate	Product	Site of Action
Salivary glands	Saliva	Salivary amylase	Starches	Maltose	Mouth
Stomach glands	Gastric juice	Pepsin	Proteins	Peptides	Stomach
		Renin	Milk protein	Clotted protein	Stomach
		Hydrochloric acid	Many foods	Smaller units	Stomach
Pancreas	Pancreatic juice	Pancreatic amylase	Starches	Maltose	Small intestine
		Lipase	Fats	Fatty acids, glycerol	Small intestine
		Trypsin	Proteins	Peptides	Small intestine
		Chymotrypsin	Proteins	Peptides	Small intestine
		Carboxypetidase	Proteins	Peptides	Small intestine
Small intestine	Intestinal juice	Maltase	Maltose	Glucose	Small intestine
		Lactase	Lactose	Glucose, galactose	Small intestine
		Sucrase	Sucrose	Glucose, fructose	Small intestine
		Aminopeptidase	Peptides	Amino acids	Small intestine
		Dipeptidase	Dipeptidase	Amino acids	Small intestine
		Nucleases	DNA and RNA	Nucleotides	Small intestine
Liver	Bile	Bile salts	Large fat droplets	Emulsified fats	Small intestine

Hormones of the Digestive Tract

Endocrine cells of the gut originate from the neural crest. Hormones of the gastrointestinal tract are produced by the mucosa of the stomach (gastrin) and by the small intestines (secretin and cholecystokinin).

Primary actions are as follows:

1. Gastrin

    a.   stimulates gastric acid and pepsinogen secretion
    b.   increases the distension of the stomach and gastric motility

2. Secretin

    a.   stimulates the pancreas to secrete pancreatic fluid and bicarbonate
    b.   stimulates biliary fluid secretion and bicarbonate
    c.   potentiates the enzymatic response to cholecystokinin
    d.   slows gastric motility and emptying
    e.   stimulates pepsinogen secretion
    f.   inhibits gastrin release

3. Cholecystokinin

    a. stimulates pancreatic enzyme secretion
    b. increases the pancreatic bicarbonate response to secretin
    c. increases the distensibility of the stomach and inhibits gastric emptying
    d. induces gallbladder contractions and emptying

General Digestion of the Major Food Groups

Carbohydrates: Starch digestion begins in the oral cavity under the influence of α-amylase and ends in the small intestines after exposure to pancreatic amylase. Products resulting from the above processes are further hydrolyzed by enzymes associated with the microvilli of the intestinal cells. For example: (1) maltase acts on maltose and maltotriose to yield glucose units; (2) sucrase acts on sucrose to produce glucose and fructose; and (3) lactase breaks down lactose to yield monosaccharide subunits.

Summary of Carbohydrates Digestion

Organ	Food	Enzyme	End Product	Absorption In
Oral Cavity	Polysaccharides	Amylase	Glucose	All in small intestine
	Disaccharide (maltose)	Disaccharidase (maltase)	Glucose	
Stomach	NO DIGESTION			↑
Small Intestine	Polysaccharides	Intestinal and pancreatic amylase	Glucose	
	Disaccharides	Disaccharidases	Glucose	
	↕	↕		
	Maltose	Maltase	Glucose	
	Sucrose	Sucrase	Glucose and fructose	
	Lactose	Lactase	Glucose and galactose	↓
Large Intestine	CONTINUATION OF THE ABOVE PROCESSES (Essentially digestion is completed before large intestine)		Glucose, Fructose, and Galactose	Large Intestine

    Proteins: Digestion begins in the stomach by the action of pepsin, which has a specificity for peptide bonds; it is inactivated by pancreatic juice. When products are transferred from the stomach to the duodenum, this stimulus results in the release of cholecystokinin (CCK) which is responsible for the release of pancreatic proteolytic enzymes such as (1) endo and exopeptidases, (2) trypsin, (3) chymotrypsin, and (4) elastase.

Summary of Protein Digestion

Organ	Food	Enzyme	End Product	Absorption In
Stomach	Milk protein (Casein)	Rennin (In newborn)	Smaller peptides and a few amino acids	All in small intestine as amino acids
	Proteins (Casein)	Pepsin		
Small Intestine	Proteins	Trypsin, chymotrypsin, carboxypeptidase —all secreted by the pancreas	↕	↕
	Polypeptides, dipeptides	Intestinal amino-peptidase, dipeptidase, enterokinase		

Fats: In the stomach, fat products are acted on by pepsin; when the products are released into the duodenum, cholecystokinin stimulates the pancreas to secrete lipases and the gallbladder to release its contents, which emulsify fat droplets resulting in the formation of micelles. The absorption is completed in the jejunum.

Summary of Fat Digestion

Organ	Food	Enzyme	End Product	Absorption In
Stomach	Fats	Absolute minimal digestion		All in small intestine
Small Intestine	Fats emulsified by bile	Intestinal and pancreatic lipase	Fatty acids and glycerol	↕

QUICK RECALL TEST QUESTIONS AND ANSWERS

Choose the Best Answer

1. The enzyme ptyalin (salivary amylase) is produced mainly by the:

   (A) chief cells of the stomach.
   (B) cardiac glands of the stomach.
   (C) argentaffin cells of the stomach.
   (D) serous cells of salivary glands.

2. All of the following are liver functions EXCEPT:

   (A) gluconeogenesis.
   (B) lipid metabolism.
   (C) glucagon synthesis.
   (D) plasma protein synthesis.

3. A surgeon can find the appendix by locating the:

   (A) jejunum.
   (B) cecum.
   (C) colon (transverse).
   (D) duodenum.

4. Bile, which is important in the digestion of fats, is produced by the:

   (A) stomach.
   (B) liver.
   (C) duodenum.
   (D) gallbladder.

5. The gastric juice in the stomach:

   (A) has a neutral pH.
   (B) is alkaline.
   (C) is acidic.
   (D) contains trypsin.

6. The large intestine functions mainly in:

   (A) absorption of water.
   (B) excretion of water.
   (C) absorption of sodium and potassium.
   (D) finishing the digestive process.

7. One enzyme that is important in protein digestion is:

   (A) ptyalin.
   (B) trypsin.
   (C) maltose.
   (D) pancreatic lipase.

8. _____ is a zymogen or enzyme precursor.

   (A) Pepsin
   (B) Trypsin
   (C) Pancreatic amylase
   (D) Chymotrypsinogen

9. _____ is a proteinase with a pH optimum around 2.

   (A) Pepsin
   (B) Trypsin
   (C) Pancreatic amylase
   (D) Chymotrypsinogen

10. _____ has chloride ion as an activator.

    (A) Pepsin
    (B) Trypsin
    (C) Pancreatic amylase
    (D) Chymotrypsinogen

11. _____ can be activated by trypsin because of splitting of a single peptide bond.

    (A) Pepsin
    (B) Trypsin
    (C) Pancreatic amylase
    (D) Chymotrypsinogen

Match the letter of the nutrient deficiency disease in Column II with the deficient nutrient in Column I. Each letter may be used only once.

Column I	*Column II*
12. _____ vitamin A	(A) Kwashiorkor
13. _____ vitamin B_{12}	(B) night blindness
14. _____ vitamin C	(C) pernicious anemia
15. _____ vitamin D	(D) pellagra
16. _____ iodine	(E) beriberi
17. _____ niacin	(F) rickets
18. _____ protein	(G) scurvy
19. _____ thiamine	(H) goiter

Match the letter of the nutrient in Column II with the function in Column I. Each letter may be used only once.

Column I

20. _____ enhances the absorption of iron

21. _____ necessary for calcium's role in blood clotting

22. _____ needed for the synthesis of the protein that transports vitamin A from the liver

23. _____ part of active cytochromeoxidase

24. _____ needed for the absorption of calcium in the intestine

Column II

(A) vitamin C
(B) vitamin D
(C) vitamin K
(D) copper
(E) zinc

25. A pediatric patient fails to thrive, has most of his dietary nitrogen appearing in the feces, and has (by various tests) a normal small intestine mucosal surface. When a test protein is added directly to the small intestine, it is found that no significant amount of amino acids appears in the intestine or in the blood. However, addition of a trace amount of trypsin directly to the small intestine results in the complete hydrolysis of the protein with the rapid increase of amino acids in the portal blood supply. The problems of this infant are consistent with a deficiency in:

(A) lactase.
(B) enterokinase.
(C) chymotrypsinogen.
(D) trypsin.

26. Which hormone causes contraction and emptying of the gall bladder?

(A) steapsin
(B) gastrin
(C) secretin
(D) cholecystokinin

27. The hormone which plays a key role in the secretion of pancreatic fluid and bicarbonate is:

(A) steapsin.
(B) gastrin.
(C) secretin.
(D) cholecystokinin.

28. The nutritional value of the carotenoid provitamins lies in their conversion to:

(A) Vitamin A.
(B) Vitamin B$_1$.
(C) Vitamin C.
(D) Vitamin D.

Answers

1. **(D)** Ptyalin (salivary amylase), produced mainly by the parotid, submandibular, and sublingual salivary glands, functions in the breakdown of starch into molecules of the disaccharide maltose. Chief cells secrete pepsinogen, the precursor of pepsin. Cardiac glands secrete mucus. Argentaffin cells secrete seretonin. Acinar cells secrete zymogen granules, which are the precursors of the enzymes of pancreatic juice.

2. **(C)** Please see summary of liver function in text (page 136).

3. **(B)** The appendix is a blind sac originating from the cecum of the ascending colon (large intestines).

4. **(B)** Bile is secreted by the liver, stored and concentrated in the gall bladder, and poured into the duodenum. It contains bile salts, cholesterol, lecithin, fat, pigments, and mucin. It aids in the emulsification, digestion, and absorption of fat, and contributes to the alkalinization of the intestines.

5. **(C)** The gastric mucosa secretes hydrochloric acid, mucin, and the enzymes rennin, pepsin, and lipase. An average of 2 to 3 liters is secreted within a 24-hour time period. The pH of gastric juice usually varies from 0.9 to 1.5. This acidity allows pepsin to act while it inhibits ptyalin (salivary amylase). Food usually remains in the stomach for 3 to 4 hours.

6. **(A)** One of the main functions of the large intestine is the reabsorption of water.

7. **(B)** Trypsin is the enzyme that is functional in protein digestion. Ptyalin (salivary amylase) acts on starches while pancreatic lipase (steapsin) acts on fats. Maltose is not an enzyme but a sugar.

8. **(D)** Chymotrypsinogen is the precursor in pancreatic juice of the enzyme chymotrypsin. Trypsin is active in this conversion. Chymotrypsin acts with trypsin to hydrolyze proteins and protein products to polypeptides and amino acids.

9. **(A)** Pepsin is a proteinase of gastric juice (derived from its precursor pepsinogen), which is secreted by the chief cells of the gastric mucosa. The pH of the stomach varies around 1.5.

10. **(C)** Pancreatic juice contains proteolytic, lipolytic, and amylolytic enzymes. Pancreatic amylase is the enzyme which hydrolyzes starch to maltose.

11. **(D)** Chymotrypsinogen is the precursor in pancreatic juice of the enzyme chymotrypsin. Trypsin is active in this conversion. Chymotrypsin acts with trypsin to hydrolyze proteins and protein products to polypeptides and amino acids.

12. **(B)** Vitamin A is formed from the carotenoid provitamins (yellow pigments of most vegetables and fruits). Deficiency causes poor dark vision adaptation, conjunctivitis, and keratinization of the cornea.

13. **(C)** Despite being involved as a cofactor in only two reactions in the human body, vitamin B_{12} is of critical importance. Vitamin B_{12} deficiency can be due to many things and is manifested as the condition called pernicious anemia.

14. **(G)** Vitamin C maintains the integrity of important metalloenzymes involved in collagen synthesis and steroidogenesis, as well as maintenance of cytochromes and intestinal absorption of iron. Vitamin C deficiency causes scurvy, a disease in which many of the clinical findings such as gingival hemorrhage and death, hemorrhage into old scars and refractures of old, healed fractures point to a common effect on collagen metabolism.

15. **(F)** Vitamin D does not occur naturally and is manufactured in the animal body by the utilization of ultraviolet light. Deficiency mainly affects calcification of bones and teeth; rickets in the child and osteomalacia in the adult are consequences. The vitamin enhances the absorption of calcium and phosphorus from the intestinal tract.

16. **(H)** A goiter is an enlargement of the thyroid gland not due to neoplasm or inflammatory disease. Endemic goiters are due to lack of intake of iodine (less than 10 μg/day) caused by deficiency in the soil and water. This interferes with hormone production and results in increased TSH production, thyroid compensatory hypertrophy, and eventual exhaustion of the gland.

17. **(D)** Niacin is the functional group of the coenzymes NAD and NADP. Deficiency results in black tongue in canines and pellagra in humans. Dermatitis and neurological lesions are manifestations of pellagra.

18. **(A)** Kwashiorker is a result of severe protein deficiency. It is characterized by anemia, edema, pot belly, depigmentation of the skin, loss or change in hair color, hypoalbuminemia, and bulky stools containing undigested food.

19. **(E)** Vitamin B_1 is essential for the proper functioning of the nervous system; it is an antagonist to acetylcholine. Deficiency will result in beriberi in humans and polyneuritis in birds.

20. **(A)** Vitamin C maintains the integrity of important metalloenzymes involved in collagen synthesis and steroidogenesis, as well as maintenance of cytochromes and intestinal absorption of iron.

21. **(C)** Vitamin K is necessary for the production of prothrombin and thus for normal clotting to occur. Deficiency causes abnormally long clotting times and hemorrhage.

22. **(E)** Zinc is an essential component of nearly 100 different enzymes. It is a cofactor in dehydrogenase, DNA polymerase, and carbonic anhydrase.

23. **(D)** Copper is a prosthetic group of cytochrome oxidase. Animals that are copper deficient have defective collagen molecules lacking cross links. The collagen and elastin of major arteries weaken and rupture occurs. Copper is also essential for the proper utilization of iron.

24. **(B)** The chief action of vitamin D is to enhance the synthesis of calcium-binding protein which increases calcium and phosphate absorption by the intestine, from which the bone produces hydroxyapatite, the crystalline material from which bone is constructed.

25. **(B)** Trypsinogen is secreted by the pancreas and converted by enterokinase to the active enzyme trypsin. Trypsin's substrates are proteins, but specifically it further disintegrates proteoses and peptones. Chymotrypsin acts with trypsin to hydrolyze proteins and protein products to polypeptides and amino acids.

26. **(D)** Cholecystokinin stimulates pancreatic enzyme secretion, increases the pancreatic bicarbonate response to secretin, increases the distensibility of the stomach and inhibits gastric emptying, and induces gallbladder contractions and emptying.

27. **(C)** Secretin stimulates pepsinogen secretion, pancreatic fluid secretion, and bicarabonate, and biliary fluid secretion and bicarbonate; potentiates the enzymatic response to cholecystokinin; slows gastric motility and emptying; and inhibits gastrin release.

28. **(A)** Vitamin A is formed from carotenoid provitamins (yellow pigments of most vegetables and fruits). Deficiency causes poor dark vision adaptation, conjunctivitis, and keratinization of the cornea.

NERVOUS SYSTEM

The nervous system is usually divided into: (a) central nervous system (brain and spinal cord) and (b) peripheral nervous system (peripheral nerves and ganglia). The peripheral nervous system is divided into a somatic system and visceral (autonomic) system.

Nervous Tissue

Nervous tissue consists of neurons (nerve cells and their processes) and supportive elements. Neuroglia in the central nervous system and Schwann cells in the peripheral nervous system are the supportive elements.

The Neuron

A neuron has a single axon that usually transmits signals to other neurons in the central nervous system, but may transmit sensory signals into the central nervous system or may transmit signals to muscle cells or glandular cells. The axon that extends out of the central nervous system may be as much as a meter long. The cell body of the neuron is attached to the axon by a tapered axon hillock that typically lacks the rough endoplasmic reticulum (Nissl substance) found in most of the neuron cytoplasm. Most neurons have a large euchromatic nucleus with a prominent nucleolus. Most types of neurons contain abundant rough endoplasmic reticulum that makes the cytoplasm basophilic. The cytoskeleton of neurons is highly developed. Most neurons have one or more dendrites extending out from the cell body and supported by cytoskeletal arrays. The axon is the only part of the neuron that can generate an action potential and forms primarily pre-synaptic parts of synapses that communicate with other neurons, muscle cells, or glandular cells. The cell body and dendrites cannot generate an action potential and form post-synaptic parts of synapses that deliver signals from axons of other neurons or from sensory receptors.

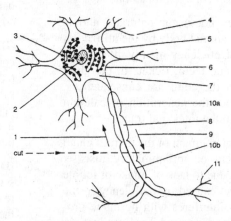

A typical single multipolar neuron. (1) Proximal portion (in a lesion (cut) the process distal from the cell body could completely degenerate; retrograde degeneration would be detected in the proximal portion; however, with time the proximal portion has the capacity to regenerate in the PNS); (2) nucleus with nucleolus, containing the genetic material of the cell and directing the synthetic activity of the cell; (3) Golgi apparatus (zone), the packaging and contrating area of the cell's secretory activity; (4) dendrites—pick up an impulse and carry it toward the cell body; (5) endoplasmic reticulum (rough in this case—ribosomes are attached), the synthetic machinery of the cell (proteins, etc.); (6) cell membrane, semipermeable and the protector of the cell from its environment; (7) cytoplasm (specifically the area here is called axon hillock); (8) myelin sheath (formed by Schwann cells in the PNS and oligodendrocytes in the CNS), the insulator material of the axon; (9) direction of impulse conduction; (10 a, b) axon conducts impulses away from the cell body to contact other neurons, muscle cells, glands, or receptors of many types; (11) terminal branches of the axon.

The Dendrites:
1. are direct extensions of the cytoplasm.
2. are generally multiple.
3. provide an increased surface area, the dendritic zone, to allow for synaptic interaction.

The Axon:
1. There is only one per neuron.
2. This process arises from a conical elevation of cytoplasm which is devoid of rough-surfaced endoplasmic reticulum (Nissl) and this area is called the *axon hillock*.
3. It is usually thinner and longer than the dendrites of the same neuron.
4. It may be surrounded by a *myelin sheath* which is produced by the *oligodendrocytes* in the CNS and by the *Schwann cells* in the PNS. Discontinuities in this myelin sheath occur at intervals known as the *nodes of Ranvier*. Though many axons are myelinated and are referred to as myelinated nerve fibers, numerous others possess no myelin ensheathment and thus are referred to as unmyelinated nerve fibers.
5. At its ending, the axon transmits impulses: (a) to other neurons—the site of this impulse transmission being called a *synapse;* and (b) to effector cells such as muscle fibers or gland cells. The junction with skeletal muscle fibers constitutes a *motor end plate*.

The Action Potential: An impulse traveling along a neuron is an electrical phenomenon initiated by a temporary change in the permeability of the neuron's cell membrane. To understand this change, one must first examine the condition of a resting, or unstimulated, neuron. The membrane possesses specific sites for the active transport of sodium ions (Na^+) and potassium ions (K^+). At these sites, sodium is transported out of the cell, and potassium is transported inward. Both ions tend to return to their original positions through pores, but Na^+ ions are less successful than are K^+ ions. Thus, the unstimulated neuron accumulates a larger concentration of positive ions (both Na^+ and K^+) outside its membrane than in its cytoplasm. A voltmeter would measure this difference as about 70 mV, with the inside of the neuron being negative; this is called the *resting potential* or *membrane potential*.

A sufficient stimulus—whether it be mechanical, chemical, or electrical—causes a radical but temporary change in the permeability of the affected membrane region. The membrane possesses specific channels that can allow sodium to pass, and others for potassium; in a resting membrane both are closed. A stimulus causes the sodium channel to open, and accumulated sodium ions outside the membrane rush into the interior by diffusion. Their number is sufficient to reverse the interior charge, making it about 40 mV positive. This change, in turn, causes the potassium channels to open, allowing a loss of potassium ions from the cytoplasm. Thus, the initial gain of interior positive ions (Na^+) is countered by a loss of positive ions (K^+), and the cytoplasm once again is negatively charged. The charge reversal, from negative to positive to negative, occurs within only a few milliseconds. The phenomenon is termed an *action potential*.

Immediately after an action potential, the sodium and potassium channels close again, and the two types of ions are pumped back to their original sites. During this refractory period of several milliseconds, an additional stimulus will not lead to another action potential.

Initiation of the action potential at any point of a neuron's membrane acts as a stimulus to the adjacent membrane material; therefore, the effect is an action potential flowing along the membrane. The result is that the "message" moves quickly over the length of a motor neuron's axon. It is also the message that flows along and into a muscle fiber that has been stimulated by events at a motor end plate, because the membrane of a muscle fiber can act like that of a neuron.

The Synapse: The synapse is the site of contact between two neurons; it may be, and most commonly is, between an axon and a dendrite; however, contacts between an axon and the cell body and between axons and axons have also been observed. A typical synapse seen between an axon and dendrite (axodendritic synapse) has the following properties:

1. As the axon terminal reaches the synaptic site, it forms a bulbous head called a *bouton*. This bouton, which constitutes the presynaptic element of the synapse, contains numerous mitochondria and specialized vesicles, the synaptic vesicles, which contain the various neurotransmitters (acetylcholine is the primary one).

2. The dendrite, which constitutes the postsynaptic element of the synapse, is separated from the bouton by a cleft which varies in width from 150 to 200 Å.

3. This axo-dendritic synapse is *not* a site where cytoplasmic continuity is established between the axon and the dendrite, as both the pre- and postsynaptic elements are separated by a cleft. However, via the process of synaptic vesicle release, this axodendritic synapse establishes a functional (chemical) continuity across the expanse of the cleft. Numerous chemical transmitters have been identified.

Properties of Several Neurotransmitters

Neurotransmitter	Location	Actions
Acetylcholine	Neuromuscular junctions, autonomic nervous system, and brain	Excites muscles, decreases heart rate, and relays various signals in the autonomic nervous system and the brain
Norepinephrine	Sympathetic nervous system and brain	Regulates activity of visceral organs and some brain functions
Dopamine	Brain	Involved in control of certain motor functions
Serotonin	Brain and spinal cord	May be involved in mental functions, circadian rhythms, and sleep and wakefulness
Gamma-aminobutyric acid	Brain and spinal cord	Inhibits various neurons
Glycine	Spinal cord	Inhibits various neurons

Classification of Neurons

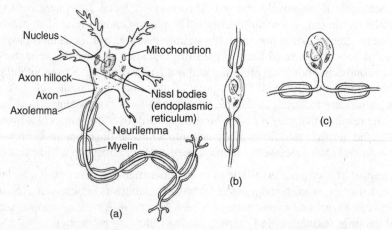

An illustration of the three types of neurons found in the nervous sytem. Multipolar neurons (a) have numerous extensions, whereas (b) bipolar neurons have two extensions and (c) unipolar neurons have one. The details of a neuron are shown in the multipolar neuron.

Multipolar Neurons: Most abundant; somatic and visceral motor, and associational.

Pseudounipolar Neurons (occasionally referred to as **Unipolar Neurons**): Somatic and visceral *sensory* neurons; cell bodies are located in cranial sensory and dorsal root ganglia; peripheral process goes out to receptor and central process travels into the central nervous system.

Bipolar Neurons: Special *sensory* neurons; cell bodies are located in special sense organs; i.e., eye (retina), ear (spiral and vestibular ganglia), and nose (olfactory epithelium).

Groups of Neurons

Nucleus: cluster of neuron cell bodies *within* the central nervous system.

Ganglion: cluster of neuron cell bodies *outside* the central nervous system.

Cortex: layered arrangement of neuron cell bodies on the surface of the cerebrum and cerebellum (gray matter).

Supportive Elements

Neuroglia—Supportive Elements of the Central Nervous System: Neuroglia, the supportive elements of the central nervous system, are of several types:

1. Astrocytes. Astrocytes are fibrous and protoplasmic; their perivascular feet end on capillaries. They are located between capillary (or pia matter) and neurons and are implicated in the blood-brain barrier. Eighty percent of brain capillary surfaces are covered by perivascular end feet of astrocytes.
2. Oligodendrocytes. Oligodendrocytes function in the myelinization of central nervous system axons.
3. Microglia. Microglia are the phagocytic macrophage-like cells of the central nervous system.

Supportive Elements of the Peripheral Nervous System

1. Schwann Cells. Schwann cells surround the axons and form the myelin sheath of peripheral nervous system axons (e.g., axons located in spinal nerves).
2. Satellite Cells. These cells surround nerve cell bodies in the ganglia (e.g., dorsal root ganglia) of the peripheral nervous system.

The Central Nervous System

The central nervous system is made up of the brain and the spinal cord.

Spinal Cord: Before one can appreciate the organization of the cerebral mass and brain stem, it is necessary to understand the basic structural organization found throughout the extent of the spinal cord.

Cross Section View. If one were to examine a cross section through any level of the spinal cord, the following would be seen:

1. A centrally located H-shaped region that contains the cell bodies of multipolar neurons. This H-shaped region is divided into dorsal and ventral columns, or *horns*. Cell bodies responsible for sensory phenomena are located in the dorsal horns, cell bodies for motor phenomena in the ventral horns. This H-shaped region is collectively referred to as the *gray matter*.
2. Peripheral to this H-shaped region, *white matter*, made up primarily of myelinated nerve fibers.

3. Attached to the spinal cord at the apex of the dorsal horn, or column, is the dorsal root of a spinal nerve. The central processes (axons) from the pseudounipolar neurons located in the dorsal root ganglion enter the spinal cord via the dorsal root of the spinal nerve. Attached to the spinal cord at the apex of the ventral horn, or column, is the ventral root of a spinal nerve. The axons from the multipolar neurons located in the ventral horn exit the spinal cord via the ventral root of the spinal nerve.

4. White matter is divided into three masses of fibers known as *funiculi*. These three funiculi are:
    (a) the dorsal funiculus, located between the dorsal midline and the dorsal root,
    (b) the lateral funiculus, located between the dorsal and ventral roots, and
    (c) the ventral funiculus, located between the ventral root and the ventral midline.

Within each funiculus are found bundles of fibers (axons) called *tracts*. The fibers within a specific tract have a common origin, termination, and function and either descend or ascend in the cord.

5. An orderly arrangement of gray and white matter that remains constant throughout the spinal cord, varying only in relative mass.

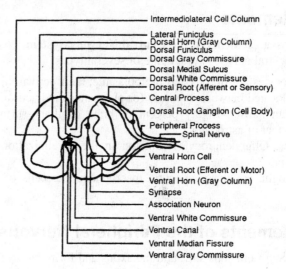

Intermediolateral Cell Column
Lateral Funiculus
Dorsal Horn (Gray Column)
Dorsal Funiculus
Dorsal Gray Commissure
Dorsal Medial Sulcus
Dorsal White Commissure
Dorsal Root (Afferent or Sensory)
Central Process
Dorsal Root Ganglion (Cell Body)
Peripheral Process
Spinal Nerve
Ventral Horn Cell
Ventral Root (Efferent or Motor)
Ventral Horn (Gray Column)
Synapse
Association Neuron
Ventral White Commissure
Ventral Canal
Ventral Median Fissure
Ventral Gray Commissure

Transverse section of spinal cord

Gross Anatomy and Relationships. The spinal cord viewed as a whole also has the following characteristics:

1. It is cylindrical, about ½ inch in diameter and 18 inches in length, and has *cervical* and *lumbar enlargements* due to the involvement of these cord levels with the innervation of the upper and lower limbs, respectively.

2. It runs within the bony *vertebral canal* but is shorter than the canal since vertebral column length exceeds cord length. The spinal cord ends at vertebral level L_1–L_2 (Lumbar 1–2).

3. It is protected not only by the bony vertebral column but also by three connective tissue sheaths known collectively as the *meninges* (dura mater, arachnoid membrane, and pia mater). *Cerebrospinal fluid* is in the subarachnoid space (between arachnoid and pia) and bathes the cord and cushions it from shock.

4. There are 31 pairs of *spinal nerves* that are connected to the cord by *dorsal* and *ventral roots*: 8 *cervical*, 12 *thoracic*, 5 *lumbar*, 5 *sacral*, and 1 *coccygeal*.

5. The spinal nerves exit from the vertebral canal through *intervertebral foramina*.

6. It is because the cord ends at vertebral level L_2 that *lumbar punctures* (spinal taps) can be done safely below that level. (Nerve roots arise from the cord and extend below this level to exit at the specific vertebral level. These roots are collectively called *cauda equina* and are deflected away from the needle and therefore are not damaged.)

The Brain: The brain is divided into three parts: the cerebrum (two cerebral hemispheres), the brain stem, and the cerebellum. The brain stem is, in turn, divided into the medulla, pons, midbrain, and diencephalon. Important facts about the structure and functions of each of the parts follows.

Cerebrum. The cerebrum consists of two hemispheres that are joined by a broad band of commissural fibers, the *corpus callosum*. Eminences on the surface are known as *gyri* and the furrows as *sulci* or *fissures*.

Each cerebral hemisphere is divided into five lobes:

1. **frontal**—contains the major motor areas (motor speech area).
2. **parietal**—is concerned with sensory impressions such as touch, pressure, and pain.
3. **occipital**—is concerned with vision.
4. **temporal**—is concerned with hearing.
5. **insula**—is found deep within the Sylvian fissure.

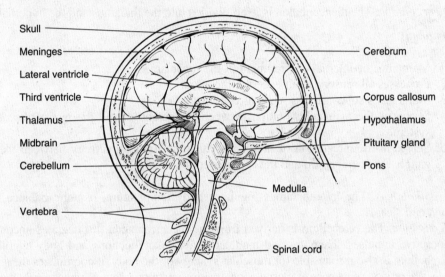

The human brain as seen from the medial aspect. The spinal cord and vertebra are shown in relation to the brain.

The cerebrum is the seat of intelligence, consciousness, and rational behavior, and possesses areas for speech and writing.

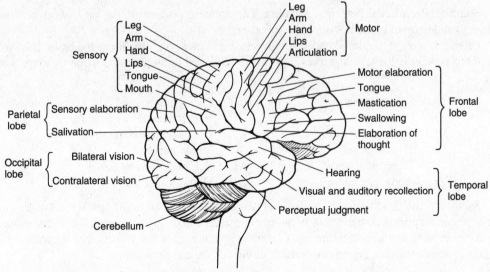

A right lateral view of the cerebrum. Major areas and lobes, and the function they regulate are shown.

Medulla Oblongata. The medulla oblongata is structurally derived from the myelencephalon and is continuous with the spinal cord at the *foramen magnum* and extends to the caudal portion of the pons. The medulla controls movement of eyelids (in blinking), sneezing, coughing, chewing, swallowing, and vomiting, and contains centers for the autonomic control of respiration (breathing), heartbeat (rate and force), contracility of blood vessels, visceral movement (gastric juice production and peristalsis), and glandular secretion (salivation).

Pons. The pons is essentially a crossing and relay station for nerve tracts. It is a conduit through which the cerebral cortex communicates with the cerebellum. It contains the motor nuclei that exert control over facial expression and mastication, and it possesses cell bodies that control lacrimation and salivation, and it serves as a relay station of tactile sensation for the facial system.

Midbrain. The midbrain serves as a relay center for auditory and optic phenomena. It houses the oculomotor nucleus, which controls extraocular movements, and exerts autonomic control over pupillary constriction and the process of accommodation.

Diencephalon. The diencephalon is itself divided into the thalamus and the hypothalamus.

Thalamus.

1. Maintains the internal environment of the organism.
2. Processes all sensory input except olfactation.
3. Maintains a subconscious sense of comfort.
4. Serves as the main relay station between the cerebrum and the rest of the nervous system.
5. Serves in the integration of motor activities via its relay activity between the basal ganglia, the cerebellum and the cerebral cortex.

Hypothalamus. The hypothalamus regulates body temperature, osmotic balance, blood pressure, and sleep.

Cerebellum. The cerebellum is derived from the metencephalon. It integrates unconscious proprioceptive impulses, integrates and modulates vestibular functions and body equilibrium. The cerebellum is also responsible for muscular synergy of the body; it coordinates the smooth, accurate, and orderly sequences of muscular contraction and movement. Without cerebellar influence, muscle activity is disorganized and crude. There is, however, no conscious perception.

The Peripheral Nervous System

The peripheral nervous system is made up of a somatic portion and an autonomic portion.

Somatic Peripheral Nervous System: The somatic portion of the peripheral nervous system is made up of cranial nerves and spinal nerves.

Cranial Nerves. The cranial nerves are those peripheral nerves that leave the brain. It is customary to subdivide the cranial nerves into twelve pairs and to number and name these pairs as follows:

I.	Olfactory nerve	VII.	Facial nerve
II.	Optic nerve	VIII.	Vestibulocochlear (auditory) nerve
III.	Oculomotor nerve	IX.	Glossopharyngeal nerve
IV.	Trochlear nerve	X.	Vagus nerve
V.	Trigeminal nerve	XI.	Spinal accessory nerve
VI.	Abducens nerve	XII.	Hypoglossal nerve

Spinal Nerves. Thirty-one pairs of spinal nerves are connected to the spinal cord. Like any nerve, a spinal nerve is composed of nerve fibers (axons and their Schwann cell sheaths) coursing together outside the central nervous system. Spinal nerves are surrounded by well-organized protective sheaths, i.e., endoneurium, perineurium, and epineurium.

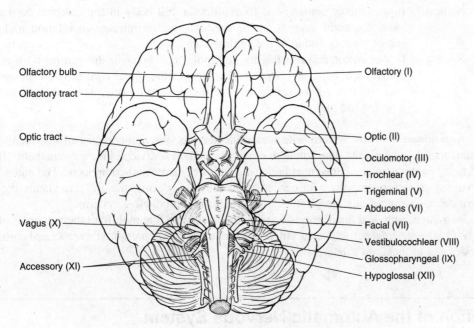

Olfactory bulb — Olfactory (I)
Olfactory tract
Optic tract — Optic (II)
— Oculomotor (III)
— Trochlear (IV)
— Trigeminal (V)
— Abducens (VI)
Vagus (X) — Facial (VII)
— Vestibulocochlear (VIII)
— Glossopharyngeal (IX)
Accessory (XI) — Hypoglossal (XII)

The twelve pairs of cranial nerves as they emerge from the brain.

Spinal nerves contain both sensory and motor fibers.

- Sensory:
  1) from receptors in skin and skeletal muscle (GSA—general somatic afferent),
  2) from receptors in smooth muscle in walls of organs and blood vessels (GVA—general visceral afferent).
- Motor:
  1) to skeletal muscle (GSE—general somatic efferent),
  2) autonomic fibers to smooth muscle, cardiac muscle, and glands (GVE—general visceral efferent).

Sensory Pathway. A typical sensory pathway contains three neurons in a chain from the receptor on the surface of the body to consciousness in the cerebral cortex (Primary: 1°, Secondary: 2°, and Tertiary: 3° neurons).

1° neuron: has its pseudounipolar cell body in the dorsal root ganglion; its peripheral process goes out to the receptor through the spinal nerve; its central process follows the dorsal root and synapses in the CNS with a second-order (2°) neuron.

2° neuron: has its multipolar cell body in the central nervous system; those cell bodies concerned with pain and temperature are found within the spinal cord; those concerned with touch and pressure are localized in the medulla of the brain. The axon of this 2° neuron then crosses the midline and ascends to the thalamus, where it synapses with a third order (3°) neuron.

3° neuron: has its multipolar cell body in the thalamus; its axon ascends to the cerebral cortex.

Voluntary Motor Pathway. A typical voluntary motor pathway contains two neurons from the cerebral cortex to the effector organ in skeletal muscle.

Neuron 1: (upper motor neuron) has its multipolar cell body in the cerebral cortex; its axon descends, crosses in the medulla, and terminates in relation to lower motor neurons found in the ventral horn.

Neuron 2: (lower motor neuron) has its multipolar cell body in the ventral horn of the spinal cord; its axon (efferent fiber) leaves the spinal cord through the ventral root and follows the spinal nerve to the skeletal muscle, where it terminates as a motor end plate.

Autonomic Nervous System: The autonomic nervous system innervates all smooth muscle, cardiac muscle, and glands. The autonomic nervous system is divided into a sympathetic (flight and fight) component and parasympathetic (maintains homeostasis) component. The autonomic nervous system exerts important influences on the intrinsic eye musculature, skin glands, the cardiovascular, gastrointestinal, respiratory, endocrine, and reproductive systems.

Fear, rage, pain, and the like evoke sympathetic activity that mobilizes the resources of the body. Gastrointestinal activity is curtailed; heart rate and blood pressure increase, and coronary arteries and bronchioles dilate.

Summary Action of the Automatic Nervous System

Organ	Sympathetic	Parasympathetic
Heart	Increases rate	Decreases rate
Vasculature	Constricts vessels	Dilates vessels
Blood	Increases pressure	Decreases pressure
Digestive (peristalsis)	Decreases rate	Increases rate
Bladder	Relaxes muscle	Contracts muscle
Bronchial Tree	Dilates	Constricts
Glands	Increases activity	Decreases activity

Reflex Arc

The typical pathway of a reflex may be outlined as follows: sensory receptor on dendrite of dorsal root ganglion cell → ganglion cell → axon of cell → dorsal root → dorsal horn of spinal cord → either directly to motor cell in ventral horn or via internuncial (association) neuron to ventral horn motor cell → axon via ventral root → spinal nerve → effector organ (e.g., muscle).

QUICK RECALL TEST QUESTIONS AND ANSWERS

Choose the Best Answer

1. Among the components of a reflex arc may be cited:

   (A) sensory receptor on dendrite.
   (B) axon of dorsal root ganglion cell.
   (C) dorsal horn of spinal cord.
   (D) all of the above.

2. Which is not a correct statement?

   (A) The end of the spinal cord may be found opposite the disk between the L_1 and L_2 vertebrae.
   (B) The spinal cord has a cervical enlargement which facilitates the innervation of the lower limb.
   (C) Cerebrospinal fluid is produced by the choroid plexus and is found in the subarachnoid space.
   (D) The three membranes known as meninges are the dura, arachnoid, and pia.

3. Of the three types of neurons (classified according to the number of their processes) the cell bodies of _____ are found within the central nervous system (CNS).

   (A) only unipolar (pseudounipolar)
   (B) only bipolar
   (C) only multipolar
   (D) both unipolar and bipolar

4. Supportive elements of the nervous system include:

   (A) astrocytes.
   (B) oligodendrocytes.
   (C) Schwann cells.
   (D) all of the above.

5. An aggregation of nerve cell bodies inside the CNS is typically called a:

   (A) clone.
   (B) colony.
   (C) tract.
   (D) nucleus.

6. The reflex arc is of utmost importance to human beings. Which of the following is NOT a component of the reflex arc?

   (A) medulla
   (B) dendrite (receptor)
   (C) synapse
   (D) ventral horn cell (effector)

7. In an auto accident the driver suffers complete sectioning of several anterior (ventral) roots of spinal nerves. What is the result of such a lesion to the regions supplied by those spinal nerves?

   (A) no neural deficit
   (B) loss of motor activity
   (C) loss of sensation
   (D) loss of sensation and motor activity

8. A patient awaiting selective surgery presents the following symptoms. Which of the following indicate(s) a heightened activity of the sympathetic portion of the autonomic nervous system?

   (A) a yearning for water due to a dry mouth
   (B) sweaty palms
   (C) pale skin
   (D) all of the above

9. Body temperature is regulated by the:

   (A) thalamus.
   (B) medulla.
   (C) cerebellum.
   (D) hypothalamus.

10. The cell bodies of the motor neurons are located in the spinal cord in the:

    (A) intermediolateral cell column.
    (B) dorsal root ganglia.
    (C) dorsal horn (gray matter).
    (D) ventral horn (gray matter).

11. After running to catch the bus for work, an individual experiences a rapid heart rate, an increase in respiratory rate, and an increase in blood pressure. We can attribute these changes to:

    (A) the peripheral nervous system.
    (B) the central nervous system.
    (C) the parasympathetic component of the autonomic nervous system.
    (D) the sympathetic component of the autonomic nervous system.

12. The part of the neuron that conducts impulses away from its cell body is called the:

    (A) axon.
    (B) dendrite.
    (C) node of Ranvier.
    (D) Schwann sheath.

13. The neurotransmitter acetylcholine is released by:

    (A) axon terminals.
    (B) dendrite terminals.
    (C) Golgi apparatus of neuron cell bodies.
    (D) Schwann cells.

14. A patient has suffered a cerebral hemorrhage that has caused injury and nonfunctioning of the primary motor area of his left cerebral cortex. As a result:

    (A) he cannot voluntarily move his right arm or hand or his right leg or foot.
    (B) he feels no sensation on the left side of his body.
    (C) reflexes cannot be elicited on the left side of his body.
    (D) he cannot voluntarily move his right arm or his left leg.

15. _____ give(s) origin to the nervous system.

    (A) Ectoderm
    (B) Mesoderm
    (C) Endoderm
    (D) Ectoderm and endoderm

16. The two cerebral hemispheres of the mammalian brain are connected via the:

    (A) corpus callosum.
    (B) posterior commissure.
    (C) anterior commissure.
    (D) anterior peduncle.

17. We speak of an aggregation of nerve cell bodies in the central nervous system as the site of a (an):

    (A) ganglion.
    (B) nucleus.
    (C) cranial nerve.
    (D) association area.

Answers

1. **(D)** The typical pathway of a reflex may be outlined as follows: sensory receptor on dendrite of dorsal root ganglion cell → ganglion cell → axon of cell → dorsal root → dorsal horn of spinal cord → either directly to motor cell in ventral horn or via internuncial (association) neuron to ventral horn motor cell → axon via ventral root → spinal nerve → effector organ (e.g., muscle).

2. **(B)** The spinal cord viewed as a whole is cylindrical, about ½ inch in diameter and 18 in length, and has cervical and lumbar enlargements due to the involvement of these cord levels with the innervation of the upper and lower limbs, respectively.

3. **(C)** Multipolar neurons are the most abundant; they are somatic and visceral motor, and associational in nature. They are found in the spinal cord and brain (central nervous system). Unipolar (pseudounipolar) neurons are somatic and visceral sensory neurons; their cell bodies are located in cranial sensory and dorsal root ganglia. Peripheral processes go out to receptors and central processes travel into the central nervous system. Bipolar neurons are special sensory neurons; their cell bodies are found in special sense organs, i.e., eye, ear, and nose.

4. **(D)** Neuroglia, the supportive elements of the central nervous system, are of several types: astroytes, oligodendrocytes, and microglia. Supportive elements of the peripheral nervous system include Schwann cells and satellite cells.

5. **(D)** This is a definition and should be memorized.

6. **(A)** Reception via afferent (sensory) receptors, conduction via sensory fibers to the central nervous system (spinal cord), and propagation of the impulses to the efferent (motor) system will then result in appropriate action. Usually most reflex arcs include one association neuron in the spinal cord between their afferent and efferent fibers. The medulla is not a part of the spinal cord; it is a part of the brain, and usually reflex arcs do not utilize higher centers.

7. **(B)** The cell bodies of the motor (efferent) system are located in the ventral horns (gray matter) of the spinal cord and their fibers leave the cord via ventral (anterior) roots which join with the dorsal (sensory) roots to form a spinal nerve. If a spinal nerve were sectioned, loss of both sensation and motor activity would be experienced. In this case only motor functions were interrupted.

8. **(D)** The autonomic nervous system innervates all smooth muscle and glands. The autonomic nervous system is divided into a sympathetic (flight and fight) component and parasympathetic (maintains homeostasis) component. It exerts important influences on the intrinsic eye musculature; skin glands; and the cardiovascular, respiratory, endocrine, and reproductive systems. Fear, rage, pain, etc., evoke sympathetic activity which mobilizes the resources of the body. Gastrointestinal activity is curtailed; heart rate and blood pressure increase; and coronary arteries and bronchioles dilate.

9. **(D)** Many activities are attributed to the hypothalamus. Lesions of this area may produce diabetes insipidus, obesity, sexual dystrophy, and loss of temperature control.

10. **(D)** The gray matter of the spinal cord is divided into two components: motor and receptor. The motor part is comprised of the ventral and intermediolateral columns and gives rise to the ventral roots. Ventral horn cells supply voluntary muscles; intermediolateral cells give rise to preganglionic sympathetic fibers of the thoraco-lumbar system. The receptor portion is located in the dorsal horn. The white matter of the spinal cord is composed of nerve fibers in a network of connective tissue.

11. **(D)** The sympathetic component of the autonomic nervous system mobilizes the body's reserve in case of emergencies.

12. **(A)** Dendrites function in receiving information and conducting it toward the cell body. Axons carry that information away from the cell body and will synapse on dendrites of another neuron.

13. **(A)** The chemical mediator of cholinergic nerve impulses is acetylcholine and is released by the axon terminals.

14. **(A)** Control of these functions is due to crossing of the fibers, and control of the right side is by the left cerebral hemispheres.

15. **(A)** Ectoderm is the germ layer of origin of the nervous system.

16. **(A)** The corpus callosum connects the two cerebral hemispheres in the mammal; association fibers cross in this bundle.

17. **(B)** A group of nerve cell bodies is commonly considered to be the site of a nucleus.

ORGANS OF SPECIAL SENSE

The Eye

The visual system is made up of the eye and complex nerve pathways for interpretation by the cerebral cortex and subcortical centers for the purpose of:

1. Refraction of light rays and the focusing thereof on the retina for the production of an image;
2. Conversion of light rays into a nervous impulse;
3. Transmission to visual centers of the brain for interpretation.

The visual system is composed of the following structures: eyelids, tearing apparatus (lacrimal gland), extrinsic muscles, eyeball, and optic nerve. We will concentrate on the eyeball and optic nerve.

Eyeball and Optic Nerve: The eye is nearly spherical and about 2.5 cm in diameter. The eyeball is composed of three coats—namely, an outer fibrous layer, a middle vascular and pigmented layer, and an inner or retinal layer—and the refractive elements—the cornea, the aqueous humor, the lens, and the vitreous humor.

Two clinical problems concerned with the size of the eyeball must be identified:

1. *myopia* (near-sightedness)—In this condition the eyeball is longer than normal and light rays come to focus in front of the retina.
2. *hyperopia* (far-sightedness)—In this condition the eyeball is shorter than normal and light rays come to focus in back of the retina.

Outer Layer. The outer fibrous tunic is the opaque *sclera* (white of the eye), which anteriorly becomes the transparent, nonvascular *cornea*. The sclera maintains the shape of the eye and gives attachment to the external ("extrinsic") ocular muscles. The cornea is composed of five layers and is one of the refractive elements.

Middle Layer. The middle vascular and pigmented tunic is the *choroid,* which anteriorly becomes the *ciliary body* and the *contractile iris.* The ciliary body, attached to the *lens* via the suspensory ligaments, aids in focusing light rays on the retina. Contraction of the ciliary muscles mediated by the parasympathetic portion (Edinger-Westphal nucleus) of the oculomotor nerve decreases the tension on the suspensory ligaments, allowing the lens to increase in thickness. The *pupil* is the central opening of the iris; its size is regulated by the amount of light present. Two smooth muscles regulate the opening; the constrictor, or sphincter pupillae, is innervated by the parasympathetic system (oculomotor nerve) and reduces the size of the pupil, while the dilator, or dilator pupillae, receives its innervation from the sympathetic system and enlarges the diameter of the pupil.

Inner Layer. The innermost tunic, the retinal layer, consists of ten layers of cells and fibers. Three layers are of neuronal importance:

a. rod and cone layer; here light energy is transformed into chemical and electrical energy;
b. bipolar cells, which allow for internal nerve impulse transmission;
c. ganglion cells which give rise to the *optic nerve.*

There are about 120 million rods and 6 million cones present per eye. The rods contain rhodopsin, or visual purple, which converts photons (basic unit of light) into chemical and then into electrical energy. Rhodopsin is formed from vitamin A; a deficiency of vitamin A may result in night blindness. Rods are very sensitive and function in dim light but yield no color discrimination. Cones contain iodopsin: they are concerned with bright light vision, visual acuity (scotopic vision), and color perception.

Bipolar cells make contact with many rods and cones to receive their impulses which they in turn transmit to the ganglion cells whose axons give rise to the optic nerve. It is estimated that the one million ganglion cells receive information from approximately 130 million rod and cone receptors.

The area at which optic nerve fibers exit is called the *optic disc* or *blind spot.* No photoreception takes place there but the central artery and vein of the retina may be observed there.

Directly in line (visual axis) with the center of the cornea is the *macula lutea.* This area exhibits a high concentration of cones, the center, known as the *fovea centralis,* is the area of most acute vision. The image formed on the retina is inverted; this is inverted again—corrected—by the brain.

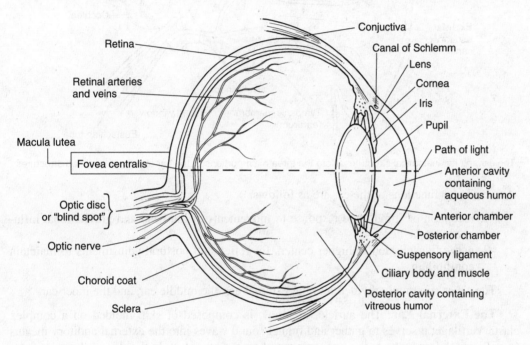

Longitudinal section of the eye.

PATHWAY FOR SEEING

Ganglion cells of the retina → optic nerve → optic chiasm (nasal retinal field fibers cross) → optic tract → lateral geniculate body → optic radiations → visual cortex (area 17 of occipital lobe of cerebrum).

The Ear

The ear, which is located in the temporal bone, essentially serves in a dual capacity. It is an auditory organ for the sense of hearing (40–20,000 cycles/sec) and a vestibular organ monitoring the effects of gravity and position of the head. Hearing utilizes the cochlear mechanism; vestibular functions are modulated by the utricle, saccule, and the three semicircular canals.

Irritative lesions to the vestibular system may result in nystagmus, vertigo, nausea, incoordination, or any other disorders of equilibrium or posture.

The auditory functions of the ear are as follows:

1. reception and conduction of sound waves,
2. amplification of the waves,
3. transduction of the waves into nerve impulses,
4. transmission of the impulse to conscious centers.

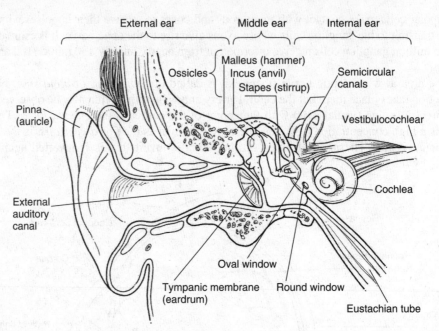

The ear and its anatomical structures. Note the three main portions of the ear and the associated structures.

The vestibular functions of the ear are as follows:

1. reception of stimuli and response to movements of the head and gravitational influences on the head.
2. nerve transmission to higher centers for reflex and postural adjustments to maintain equilibrium.

The ear is commonly divided into the external ear, the middle ear, and the inner ear.

The External Ear: The auricle, or pinna, is composed of skin molded on a complex elastic cartilage; it serves to gather and funnel sound waves into the external auditory meatus (canal), which terminates at the tympanic membrane, or eardrum. In the skin of the meatus are located fine hairs and large sebaceous glands. Coiled, tubular ceruminous glands are also present; they discharge a brownish secretion which, in conjunction with the sebaceous products and desquamated cells, produce a waxy product known as cerumen.

The Middle Ear: The middle ear is a cavity continuous superiorly with the mastoid air cells and inferiorly, via the auditory (Eustachian) tube, with the nasopharynx. The auditory tube is ordinarily closed and serves to equalize the internal and external pressures on the eardrum. Within the cavity are located three ossicles. From external (eardrum) to internal (oval window), they are respectively the malleus (hammer), the incus (anvil), and the stapes (stirrup). These small bones function in transduction: they translate the displacement of the tympanic membrane, produced by sound waves, into mechanical energy.

On the medial wall of the middle ear are the vestibular window (oval) and the cochlear window (round). The vestibular window houses the base of the stapes; the cochlear window is closed by a membrane. Movement of the eardrum sets up vibrations of the stapes in the oval window; these are transmitted to perilymph in the scala vestibuli (bony labyrinth). The movement is transferred to the endolymph in the cochlear duct (membranous labyrinth) and from there to perilymph in the scala tympani and then is dissipated through the movement of the membrane in the round window. Sound vibrations may be transmitted by surrounding bone in case of middle ear disease (deafness); therefore, the outer and middle ear are not absolutely essential for hearing.

The Inner Ear: The internal ear, located in the petrous portion of the temporal bone, consists of a complex series of fluid (endolymph)-filled sacs, the membranous labyrinth, housed within bony cavities (bony labyrinth), which are filled by perilymph. The interconnecting membranous channels serve static and kinetic senses (vestibular) as well as hearing (auditory).

The vestibular apparatus comprises three semicircular canals, utricle, and saccule.

The auditory mechanism is housed in the cochlear duct. Both senses are transmitted by the stato-acoustic nerve (cranial nerve VIII) to the brain. This nerve is also named "vestibulo-cochlear nerve"; in the past it had been called the "auditory nerve."

The Cochlea. The cochlear duct is a helical tube of about 2½ turns housed in its bony labyrinth. The duct separates the bony tube into two channels: the scala tympani and scala vestibuli. At the apex the scala tympani and scala vestibuli communicate at a point termed the helicotrema. The scala vestibuli begins at the oval window and the scala tympani terminates at the round window.

Pulsations are set up in the perilymph of the scala vestibuli by movements of the stapes at the oval window. They are propagated either via the helicotrema directly to the scala tympani or may pass through the vestibular membrane, activate movement in the endolymph of the cochlear duct, and then pass via the basilar membrane into the perilymph of the scala tympani. The pulsations stimulate the receptor (hair) cells located on the basilar membrane and elicit the phenomenon of hearing. Movements of the endolymph, varing with the volume and pitch of the sound waves are registered in specific regions of the organ of Corti. The cochlear division of the stato-acoustic nerve transmits the information to the medulla, then to the midbrain, the thalamus, and, finally, interpretation occurs in the cerebrum.

The Vestibular Apparatus. Head movements are perceived by the three semicircular canals, attached at right angles to the utricle. Displacement of the head causes endolymph to elicit a response in the sensory hair cells of the crista. Position with respect to gravity is monitored by movement of otoliths (calcium carbonate crystals) on the sensory hair cells, in the macula of the utricle and sacculus. The vestibular division of the stato-acoustic nerve (CN VIII) relays the informatin to the medulla, then to the cerebellum, where muscle coordination is elicited.

Semicircular Canals. There are three canals. Each possesses an ampulla with a modified, sensory epithelium (crista ampullaris) which is associated with neuronal reception. Each crista is stimulated by movements occurring in the plane of its specific canal. Rotational movement leads to a compensatory response of the eyes, head and limbs.

Utricle. The sensory epithelium is located in a region known as the macula. Gelatinous material in which are embedded crystals (otoliths) cover the hair cells. Any change in position of the head in space and any linear acceleration will result in pressure from the crystals on the hair cells and a compensatory reaction such as righting of the body and eye coordination.

Saccule. The morphology of the saccule is similar to that of the utricle. The saccule responds to vibrational stimuli.

The Olfactory System

The olfactory system may be visualized as a highly specialized mucous membrane located in the roof of each nasal cavity. Four primary odors—fragrant, acid, burnt, and rancid—are perceived. Olfactory stimulation is caused by gaseous and odiferous substances in solution. Olfactory sero-mucous glands secrete a watery fluid continuously. This allows for reception of dissolved substances and also lessens retention and lingering of stimulation. The receptive cells, bipolar ganglion cells, end in bulbous knobs that possess about ten olfactory hairs; these serve as the sensory receptors. The sense of smell is subject to fatigue; no structural differences are correlated with discrimination of different kinds of odors. Reception follows this route:

Bipolar cells of olfactory epithelium → olfactory bulb → olfactory tract (cranial nerve I) → olfactory stria → olfactory cortex.

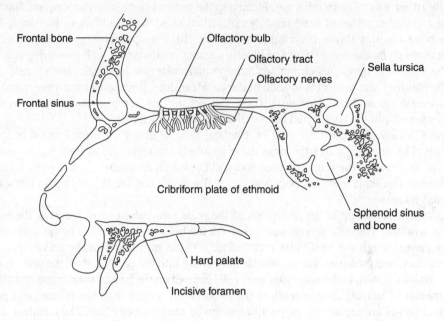

Olfactory System

The Gustatory System

In higher vertebrates the sense of taste is generally restricted to the oral cavity (tongue and epiglottic region). Taste buds are located in vallate (circumvallate), foliate, and fungiform papillae. The receptors in the taste bud are neuroepithelial cells. Substances must be in solution and the four modalities of taste—sweet, sour, salt, and bitter—are specific and regionalized. Sweetness is localized mainly on the tip of the tongue, sour and salt mainly on the central areas, and bitter on the back of the tongue.

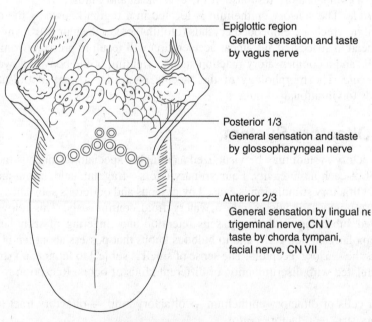

The Tongue: Innervation

Nerves of the Tongue

	General Sensation	Taste	Motor
Anterior 2/3	Lingual, trigeminal, CN V	Chorda tympani, CN VII	Hypoglossal, CN XII
Posterior 1/3	Glossopharyngeal, CN IX	Glossopharyngeal, CN IX	Hypoglossal, CN XII
Epiglottic region of tongue	Superior laryngeal (internal brance), vagus, CN X	Superior laryngeal, CN X	

Organs of Special Sense in Brief

Organ	Receptor	Stimulus	Location
Olfactory mucus membrane	Bipolar cells, olfactory epithelium	Gaseous or odiferous substances in solution	Nasal cavity, cribriform plate
Taste buds	Gustatory cells (neuroepithelial cells), vallate, foliate, fungiform papillae	Sweet, sour, salt, and bitter substances in solution	Tongue and epiglottic region
Eye	Rods and cones	Light waves	Eye
Ear: External membrane	Pinna, tympanic	Sound waves	Ear
Middle	Ossicular chain to oval window	Sound waves	Ear
Internal cochlea scala vestibula scala tympani basilar membrane	Organ of Corti	Pulsations (vibrations) converted to electrical stimulus	Ear
Vestibular apparatus semicircular canals (crista ampularis) utricle (macula) saccule	Hair cells	Movement (position of head), vibration	Ear

QUICK RECALL TEST QUESTIONS AND ANSWERS

Choose the Best Answer

1. Which of the following sequences is correct for sound transmission?

    (A) tympanic membrane, malleus, stapes, incus, and cochlea
    (B) tympanic membrane, malleus, incus, stapes, and cochlea
    (C) tympanic membrane, auditory tube, middle ear, and inner ear
    (D) tympanic membrane, incus, malleus, stapes, and cochlea

2. Hearing utilizes the _____ mechanism.

    (A) cochlear
    (B) utricle
    (C) saccule
    (D) semicircular canal

3. All of the following structures are located in the middle ear except:

    (A) opening of Eustachian tube.
    (B) passage to mastoid air cells.
    (C) oval window.
    (D) cochlear duct.

4. The hair cells of the inner ear are located in the:

    (A) organ of Corti.
    (B) macula of the utricle.
    (C) crista ampullaris.
    (D) A, B and C.

5. The receptors (specialized neuroepithelium) for the perception of sound are the:

    (A) spiral ganglion cells.
    (B) hair cells of the macula.
    (C) hair cells of the organ of Corti.
    (D) cells of the crista ampularis.

6. The Eustachian tube provides a communication between the:

    (A) inner ear and the cranial cavity.
    (B) outer ear and middle ear.
    (C) middle ear and mastoid air cells.
    (D) middle ear and nasopharynx.

7. Which of the following is the structure of the eye that is responsible for holding the lens in its normal position?

    (A) iris
    (B) cornea
    (C) anterior chamber
    (D) ciliary body

8. Three layers of neuronal elements are intimately involved in the transmission of light. The first components of that chain are the:

    (A) ganglion cells.
    (B) bipolar cells.
    (C) rods and cones.
    (D) connective tissue cells.

9. The vision of a near-sighted individual may be corrected by:

    (A) a convex lens.
    (B) a biconvex lens.
    (C) a biconcave lens.
    (D) none of the above.

10. The region of the retina where vision is most acute is known as the:

    (A) ciliary body.
    (B) vitreous humor.
    (C) conjunctiva.
    (D) fovea centralis.

11. Which of the following components of the eye is/are considered to refract light?

    (A) cornea
    (B) aqueous humor
    (C) lens
    (D) all of the above

12. Sound vibrations received by the tympanic membrane are transmitted to the ossicular chain. The foot plate of the stapes is located in the:

    (A) oval window (vestibular).
    (B) round window (cochlear).
    (C) helicotrema.
    (D) organ of Corti.

13. There are about 120 million rods and 6 million cones present per eye. The rods are very sensitive and function:

    (A) in colorful situations.
    (B) in bright light.
    (C) in dim light.
    (D) where the intensity of light is no consideration.

14. The eyeball is composed of three coats—namely an outer fibrous layer, a middle vascular and pigmented layer, and an inner or retinal layer. The outer layer comprises the:

    (A) extraocular muscles and sclera.
    (B) sclera and cornea.
    (C) iris and ciliary body.
    (D) conjunctiva and choroid.

Answers

1. **(B)** The auditory ossicles, malleus, incus and stapes, form a lever system that converts the vibrations of the air impinging on the tympanic membrane into mechanical energy to oscillate the foot plate of the stapes in the vestibular (oval) window.

2. **(A)** The ear, which is located in the temporal bone, essentially serves in a dual capacity. It is an auditory organ for the sense of hearing (40–20,000 cycles/sec) and a vestibular organ monitoring the effects of gravity and position of the head. Hearing utilizes the cochlear mechanism; vestibular functions are modulated by the utricle, saccule, and the three semicircular canals.

3. **(D)** The middle ear is a cavity continuous superiorly with the mastoid air cells and inferiorly, via the auditory (Eustachian) tube, with the nasopharynx. Within the cavity are located the three ossicles. On the medial wall of the middle ear are the vestibular window (oval) and the cochlear window (round). The vestibular window houses the base of the stapes; the cochlear window is closed by a membrane.

4. **(D)** Movements of the endolymph, varying with the volume and pitch of the sound waves are registered in specific regions of the organ of Corti. Head movements are perceived by the three semicircular canals, attached at right angles to the utricle. Displacement of the head causes endolymph to elicit a response in the sensory hair cells of the crista.

5. **(C)** Pulsations are set up in the perilymph of the scala vestibuli by movements of the stapes at the oval window. Movements of the endolymph, varying with the volume and pitch of the sound waves, are registered in specific regions of the organ of Corti.

6. **(D)** The middle ear is a cavity continuous superiorly with the mastoid air cells and inferiorly, via the auditory (Eustachian) tube, with the nasopharynx. The auditory tube is ordinarily closed and serves to equalize the internal and external pressures on the eardrum.

7. **(D)** The middle vascular pigmented tunic is the choroid, which anteriorly becomes the ciliary body and the contractile iris. The ciliary body, attached to the lens via the suspensory ligaments, aids in focusing light rays on the retina. Contraction of the ciliary muscles mediated by the parasympathetic portion (Edinger–Westphal nucleus) of the oculomotor nerve decreases the tension on the suspensory ligaments, allowing the lens to increase in thickness.

8. **(C)** The innermost tunic, the retinal layer, consists of ten layers of cells and fibers. Three layers are of neuronal importance:

    (a) rod and cone layer; here light energy is transformed into chemical and electrical energy;

    (b) bipolar cells, which allow for internal nerve impulse transmission;

    (c) ganglion cells which give rise to the optic nerve.

9. **(C)** Anterior-posterior diameters of eyeballs vary. A long eye is considered near-sighted or myopic; light rays come to focus before they reach the retina; therefore, a concave lens is needed for correction. A short eye results in far-sightedness or hypermetropia; light rays would come to focus in back of the retina and, therefore, a convex lens is needed for correction.

10. **(D)** Light must penetrate the retina to reach the rods and cones. The fovea centralis is the central portion of the macula lutea; it is the region of sharpest vision. It is thinner than the rest of the retina and only cones are present. Rods are absent from this area. Cones are regarded as color receptors, whereas rods are achromatic receptors of low-intensity light.

11. **(D)** The path of light starts at the cornea; it then enters the anterior chamber which contains the aqueous humor. Next it encounters the lens and then enters the posterior chamber filled with vitreous humor.

12. **(A)** Pulsations are set up in the perilymph of the scala vestibuli by movements of the stapes at the oval window. The pulsations stimulate the receptor (hair) cells located on the basilar membrane and elicit the phenomenon of hearing.

13. **(C)** Rods are very sensitive and function in dim light but yield no color discrimination. Cones contain iodopsin: They are concerned with bright light vision, visual acuity (scotopic vision), and color perception. Directly in line (visual axis) with the center of the cornea is the macula lutea. This area exhibits a high concentration of cones, the center, known as the fovea centralis, is the area of most acute vision.

14. **(B)** The outer fibrous tunic is the opaque sclera (white of the eye), which anteriorly becomes the transparent, nonvascular cornea. The sclera maintains the shape of the eye and gives attachment of the external ("extrinsic") ocular muscles. The cornea is composed of five layers and is one of the refractive elements.

ENDOCRINE SYSTEM

Two systems modulate, integrate, and control the activities of the body: the nervous and endocrine systems. The response in nervous control is rapid whereas control via the endocrine system is fairly slow and longer lasting. The organs of the endocrine system are ductless glands composed of secretory epithelial tissue. Endocrine glands secrete their products, called hormones, into the surrounding tissue fluid. The secretory products then diffuse into connective tissue surrounding the secretory epithelium. In most cases, the secretory products then enter capillaries in the connective tissue and are subsequently carried to their target organ as a component of the blood. Hormones may be proteins, peptides, amino acids (or amino acid derivatives), steroids, or prostaglandins (derivatives of essential fatty acids). The product of the target organ may also feed back on the organ that stimulated its activity and production and thus manipulate its cycle of function. It may shut off the supply of stimulating hormone; this activity is called a negative feedback. The controlling mechanism can be thought of as a neuro-endocrine-somatic tissue relationship, or the brain affecting the pituitary gland, which in turn affects the target organs, which then elicit their effect upon the body tissues and cells.

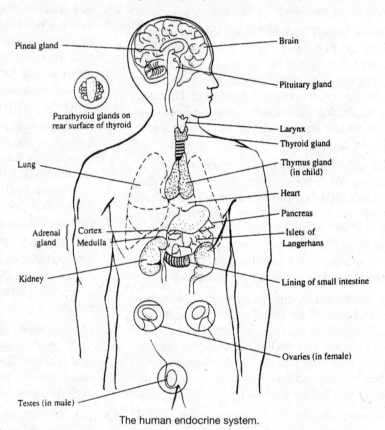

The human endocrine system.

The Pituitary Gland (Hypophysis)

The pituitary gland is divided into an anterior and a posterior lobe according to embryonic origin. The anterior lobe (adenohypophysis) originates from the oral epithelium of the roof of the mouth in the embryo (Rathke's pouch). The posterior lobe (neurohypophysis) originates from the ventral region of the diencephalon region of the embryonic brain (infundibulum).

Three cell types are found in the anterior lobe: chromophobes 50%; acidophils 40%; basophils 10%. Chromophobes are considered to be resting cells.

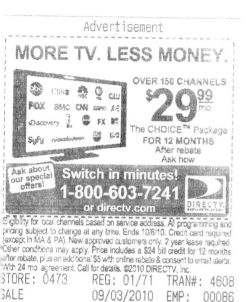

... th; acts on liver to produce somatomedins that act

... cation is complete, giantism
... tion is complete, acromegaly

... hormone production

... hic hormone (LTH) or prolactin

... at was already stimulated by estrogen and proges-
... ast trimester of pregnancy
... ion
... e corpus luteum

... lt in hypogonadism

... eta and Delta Cells):

... (TSH)

(1) ... gland to produce its hormones T_3 (triiodothyronine) and T_4 (tetraiodothyronine or thyroxin)
(2) Modulates the iodide trapping mechanisms
(3) Hypersecretion—goiter, exophthalmos
(4) Hyposecretion—diminished thyroid function and lethargy

b. Adrenocorticotropic hormone (ACTH)

(1) Stimulates the adrenal cortex to produce glucocorticoids (cortisol, etc.)
(2) Does *not* stimulate mineralocorticoid activity (aldosterone production)
(3) Affects production of adrenal androgens

c. Melanocyte stimulating hormone (MSH) or intermedin

This hormone causes the dispersion of pigment in the chromatophores of the skin of cold-blooded vertebrates and a darkening of the skin results; the action of MSH allows for quick changes in the skin color in response to changes in the external environment.

2. **Delta cells**

a. Luteinizing hormone (LH) in female; Interstitial cell stimulating hormone (ICSH) in male

(1) In the female this hormone is necessary for preovulatory development of the ovarian follicle, ovulation, and formation of the corpus luteum.
(2) In the female it modulates the production of estrogen and progesterone.
(3) In the male this hormone stimulates the interstitial cells of the testes, which results in a secretion of testicular androgens.

b. Follicle stimulating hormone (FSH)

(1) In the female this hormone stimulates the growth of the ovarian follicle.
(2) In the male FSH stimulates the testes to produce sperm (spermatogenesis).

Hormones of the Neurohypophysis: The function of this portion of the pituitary gland is to store and release the hormones oxytocin (produced by the paraventricular nucleus of the hypothalamus) and vasopressin or antidiuretic hormone (ADH, produced by the supraoptic nucleus of the hypothalamus).

1. *Oxytocin*

    a. Stimulates the contraction of the smooth muscle of the uterus and may play some role in the initiation of labor.

    b. Stimulates the ejection of milk by affecting the myoepithelial cells of the breast tissue (mammary gland).

2. *Vasopressin; antidiuretic hormone (ADH)*

    a. Acts upon the renal tubules to aid water resorption and thereby restricts diuresis; a lack of hormone results in the condition known as diabetes insipidus (the production of large volumes of dilute urine, polyuria).

The Pituitary Portal System: In humans the pituitary gland receives its blood supply via the right and left superior and the right and left inferior pituitary arteries from the internal carotid artery system. These vessels supply the hypothalamic areas, the pituitary stalk, and the posterior lobe. The anterior lobe, however, receives no arterial blood supply. The entire blood supply to the anterior lobe is derived from the pituitary portal veins. These veins arise from the capillary network of the median eminence and the infundibular stem. The vascular tufts of the primary capillary system are in close relationship with the nerve endings of the hypothalamo-hypophyseal tract. It is hypothesized that upon excitation these nerve fibers liberate their secretory products into this system, which then, via the portal veins, transports these neurosecretory products to the sinusoids of the anterior lobe. It is in this manner that the activity of the anterior lobe is governed by the hypothalamic areas.

Negative Feedback: The control of secretion of TRH, GnRH, and CRH is exerted by the concentration of the products of the target glands in the bloodstream. Therefore, hypothalamic and pituitary secretion is modulated (controlled) via a "Negative Feedback."

The Thyroid Gland

The thyroid gland is derived from a diverticulum of the pharynx. Its structural unit is the follicle; the follicle is composed of a unit of epithelial cells that surround a colloid space. Colloid is located extracellularly and contains thyroglobulin. The function of the thyroid gland is to produce the thyroid hormones (T_3 [triiodothyronine] and T_4 [thyroxin]), which affect the rate of metabolism of all the tissues of the body.

The iodides consumed in our food and water are absorbed and carried to the iodide pool in the extracellular fluid via the circulatory system. Five basic events can be identified in thyroid hormone production: (a) trapping iodide; (b) oxidation of iodide to organic iodine; (c) synthesis of hormone; (d) storage of hormone as the thyroglobulin moiety in the follicle; and (e) release of the hormone into the circulation. TSH from the anterior pituitary influences greatly the trapping mechanism; thiocyanates block this mechanism, and thiouracil blocks the oxidation and synthetic steps. These compounds are classified as antithyroid agents.

The hormone thyrocalcitonin is produced by the parafollicular cells or C cells of the thyroid gland. This hormone is an antagonist of parathyroid hormone and it functions to lower the serum calcium level and to enhance the deposition of calcium in bone. It lowers blood calcium levels by inhibiting bone resorption.

Action of Thyroid Hormones (T3 and T4):

1. Control the rate of metabolism.
2. Control the growth, maturation, and differentiation of the organism.
3. Influence nervous system activity.

Problems Associated with Thyroid Function:

1. **Cretinism.** Congenital failure of proper development of the thyroid gland. The cretin is a dwarf—physically and mentally.
2. **Myxedema.** Acquired thyroid deficiency in the adult. This deficiency can be of two types:

   a. Thyroid deficiency due to thyroidectomy, neoplasms, thyroiditis, and so forth.
   b. A pituitary deficiency in the secretion of TSH.

   The thyroid in these cases appears atrophic, hard, and fibrous. The clinical picture is the presentation of a patient who is fairly heavy, phlegmatic, and devoid of expression; his skin is rough and dry and sensitive to cold. The patient is sluggish mentally and physically. Laboratory tests would show a low basal metabolic rate, low protein bound iodine, and a high serum cholesterol level.
3. **Goiter.** Any enlargement of the gland not due to neoplasm or inflammatory disease. Endemic goiters are due to lack of intake of iodine (less than 10 mg/day) caused by deficiency in the soil and water. This interferes with hormone production, results in increased TSH production, thyroid compensatory hypertrophy, and eventual exhaustion of the gland.
4. **Hyperthyroidism.** Graves' disease. Increased activity by the organ. The patient exhibits loss of weight, nervousness, irritability, increased metabolic rate, rapid heart rate, sweating, and so forth. Exophthalmos, a protrusion of the eyeballs, is exhibited and thought to be due to an increased production of TSH. Hyperthyroidism may be an adjunct to the development of a goiter or may arise de novo.

The Parathyroid Glands

There are usually four parathyroid glands, which are embedded in the thyroid gland. The parathyroid glands produce parathyroid hormone, which governs the metabolism of calcium and phosphorus. Calcium levels regulate parathyroid production of hormone. The parathyroids are essential to life; their removal results in cramps, convulsions, tremors, and eventually death due to tetany. The condition is due to the increased irritability of the muscular and nervous system caused by the decrease of calcium levels in the blood and body fluids. The activity of the parathyroids depends on the level of ionized calcium and phosphate ions in the serum.

Problems Associated with Parathyroid Function:

1. **Hypoparathyroidism.** This condition results in a decrease in urinary excretion of phosphorus and its concomitant rise in the serum; this results in a shift in the calcium-phosphorus serum levels and a decline in calcium resorption from bone. The fall in serum calcium will produce tetany. Low serum levels of calcium may also be influenced by deficient intake of calcium, deficiency of vitamin D in the diet, problems with intestinal absorption, or increased demand for calcium during pregnancy.
2. **Hyperparathyroidism.** Tumor is the most frequent cause of this condition. In this condition urinary phosphorus excretion is elevated and serum levels are decreased. Calcium resorption from bone is increased and serum levels rise. The glomerular filtrate is saturated and stones may form. Secondary renal disease may occur. Bones become decalcified and fractures result. Calcitonin lowers the blood calcium level.

The Pancreas

The pancreas is both an endocrine and exocrine gland. The endocrine portion consists of the islets of Langerhans. The function of the islets of Langerhans is to produce insulin by the beta cells and glucagon by the alpha cells. A deficiency of insulin production results in the disease known as diabetes mellitus (elevated blood sugar level). The beta cells do not seem to depend on any outside trophic influences and the primary physiologic stimulus for insulin production seems to be the level of the blood sugar.

Insulin promotes the removal of glucose from the blood and also the conversion of glucose to glycogen in muscle and liver. It increases the rate of oxidation of glucose in the tissues, the conversion of carbohydrates into fats, the mobilization of fatty acids from adipose tissue, and the rate of protein synthesis.

Glucagon is the glycogenolytic hormone produced by the alpha cells of the pancreas; its principal action is to stimulate the conversion of glycogen to glucose by the liver. Glucagon also increases the peripheral utilization of glucose; therefore, it should not be referred to as simply the antagonist of insulin. Its secretion is controlled by the concentration of blood glucose and blood insulin levels. If insulin levels rise and blood glucose levels drop, glucagon secretion increases.

Two other cell types commonly associated with the islets are D cells, which produce somatostatin which inhibits glucagon release and decreases pancreatic exocrine functions, and F cells, which produce a polypeptide which inhibits pancreatic exocrine secretion and also decreases bile secretion.

The Adrenal Glands

The adrenal glands are composed of a cortex and a medulla. The cortex is derived from mesoderm, whereas the medulla is derived from neural crest cells. In fetal life the adrenal is composed almost completely of cortex, but after birth the entire fetal cortex rapidly degenerates and is replaced by the adult cortex and medulla. The cortex, which produces the mineralocorticoids and glucocorticoids, is divided into three zones: (a) the most peripheral zona glomerulosa; (b) the intermediate zona fasciculata; and (c) the zona reticularis bordering the medulla.

ADRENAL CORTEX

The zona glomerulosa is rich in lipids, especially cholesterol, from which the mineralocorticoids are formed. Aldosterone is the most powerful mineralocorticoid. Mineralocorticoids function in the retention of water, sodium, and chloride, and increase urinary loss of potassium and phosphorus by action on the renal tubules. This regulation of the electrolytes is essential to life. No pituitary control is present.

The zona fasciculata and reticularis are the sources of the glucocorticoids; i.e., 17-hydroxycorticosteroids. Corticosterone (hydroxycorticosterone), cortisone (compound E), and hydrocortisone (cortisol or compound F) are the most widely known compounds. The levels of these hormones are increased by ACTH; they are gluconeogenic in nature. They convert amino acids into sugar instead of protein and in this way increase blood sugar and liver glycogen levels. Cortisone—in addition to influencing protein, carbohydrate, and fat metabolism—(a) affects the permeability of cell membranes; (b) interferes with the antigen-antibody response by inhibiting antibody formation; and (c) suppresses the inflammatory response. Cortisone, however, relieves only the symptoms of disease without influencing the cause.

The zona reticularis is responsible for the production of the sex hormones or 17-ketosteroids. The action of these hormones is no different from the action of the estrogens, androgens, and progesterone produced by the testes and ovaries; i.e., they masculinize the body and increase the synthesis of amino acids and protein from nitrogen; they favor the retention of nitrogen, phosphorus, potassium, sodium, and chloride. ACTH has some control of these hormones.

Problems Associated with Adrenal Cortex Function:
1. Hypofunction or *chronic adrenal insufficiency.* Addison's disease. This condition is due to inadequate amounts of steroid hormones. Deficiency of glucocorticoids makes the patient easily susceptible to stress; deficiency of mineralocorticoids leads to a fall in serum sodium and rise in serum potassium. These patients lack proper resistance to infection and are easily deyhdrated. Patients exhibit general languor and debility, a

very weak heart, irritability of the stomach, and a peculiar change in skin color due to the deposition of melanin; this feature is highly characteristic.

2. Hyperadrenalism

    a. Overfunction of zona glomerulosa—aldosteronism (Conn's syndrome).
    b. Overfunction of zona fasciculata—(Cushing's syndrome).
    c. Overfunction of zona reticularis—adrenal virilism (Adrenogenital syndrome).

Primary Aldosteronism—Conn's Syndrome:
Characterized by:

1. Periodic severe muscular weakness or paralysis.
2. Intermittent tetany and paresthesia.
3. Hypertension.
4. Renal disfunction.

Cushing's Syndrome:
Characterized by:

1. Painful adiposity of face, neck, and trunk (full moon face)
2. Excess hair growth in the female and preadolescent males.
3. Peculiar body striations.
4. Sexual dystrophy.
5. Muscular weakness and atrophy.
6. Hypertension.

Adrenal Virilism—Adrenogenital Syndrome:
Characterized by:

1. Excess hair growth.
2. Virilism.
3. Excessive muscularity.

ADRENAL MEDULLA

The adrenal medulla develops from the neural crest. The cells of the adrenal medulla are modified ganglion cells and receive stimulation from the preganglionic fibers whose cell bodies are located in the intermediolateral cell columns of the spinal cord in the thoracolumbar segments dealing with the sympathetic outflow of the autonomic nervous system. Sectioning of the splanchnic nerves to the adrenal medulla will result in cessation of secretion, while stimulation of these nerves enhances secretion markedly. The function of the adrenal medulla is to secrete the catecholamines adrenalin (epinephrine) and noradrenalin (norepinephrine).

In general these hormones help the body in frightful and stressful situations. They affect the vascular system (vasoconstriction), the heart (increased rate), respiration, carbohydrate metabolism (increased blood glucose levels), the pupillary dilators, the intestines, and uterine musculature.

A clinical picture of noradrenalism during which these pressor amines are produced in excess will show: (a) hypertension; (b) headache; (c) palpitation; (d) dyspnea; (e) weakness; and (f) chest and/or abdominal pain, etc.

The Testes

The testes function in the production of sperm and in the production of the male sex hormone testosterone. Testosterone promotes and maintains the development of the male accessory genital organs (prostate and seminal vesicles) and secondary sex characteristics, i.e., beard growth, hair growth (pubic, axilla, trunk, and limbs), and scrotal growth. It maintains spermatogenesis, is responsible for the deepening of the voice, the greater muscular development of men, sex urge, and acne at puberty. It also exerts an influence on nitrogen, electrolyte, and water balance within the system. Both males and females produce estrogens and androgens; it is the ratio of the two which determines male and female characteristics.

Steroidogenesis is similar in the ovary and the testis; the difference is in the predominance and quantity of the secretions. The androgen testosterone is the predominant secretion of the testis, while in the ovary the estrogen estradiol and the progestin progesterone predominate.

Actions of LH and FSH in the Male: These hormones act on the testis to promote:
1. androgen secretion by the interstitial cells of Leydig.
2. spermatogenesis.

Hormonal Control of Spermatogenesis:
1. Pituitary secretions regulate spermatogenic activities.
2. Interstitial-cell-stimulating hormone (ICSH) affects seminiferous tubules via androgen secretion.
3. FSH affects maturation of spermatids.
4. FSH and GH maintain spermatogenesis.

Androgenic and Anabolic Actions of Testosterone:
1. Maintenance of spermatogenesis.
2. Maintenance of structure and function of the accessory sex organs.
3. Promotion of secondary sex characteristics (size of genitalia, voice, glandular secretions, muscle development, and hair distribution).
4. Normal development and body growth.
5. Psychological balance.
6. Suppression of LH via feedback mechanism.

The Ovaries

Like the testes, the ovaries are endocrine glands. They have two functions. Ovaries are the site of gamete production. They are also a major site of steroidogenesis, specifically the production of estrogens and progesterones. These steroid hormones are responsible for the development of secondary female sex characteristics, mammary gland development, and preparing the uterus for implantation of the fertilized egg.

Ovarian Cycle: It occurs from menarche to menopause, is typically 28 days long, and can be divided into two phases:

1. follicular or estrogenic
2. luteal or progestational

Menstrual Cycle

The ovarian cycle and the menstrual cycle of the uterus are integrated. The menstrual cycle can be divided into four phases:

1. menstrual phase (days 1–5);
2. proliferative or follicular phase (days 6–13), followed by ovulation (day 14);
3. secretory or luteal phase (days 15–25);
4. ischemic phase (days 26–28).

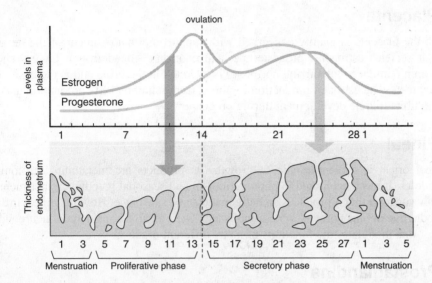

The menstrual cycle. Menstruation proceeds for several days, then the proliferative stage extends from day 6 to day 14, when ovulation occurs. The secretory stage extends from day 15 to 28 to complete the cycle. Note the levels of estrogen and progesterone during the various stages. The thickness of the endometrial lining is also shown, and the effects of the hormones on its development is illustrated by the vertical arrows.

Uterine Changes during the Menstrual Cycle: Menses (days 1–5) involves the sloughing off of necrotic endometrium, blood, and uterine fluid, which is discharged as menstrual flow. During the proliferative phase (days 6–13), the primary hormonal stimulus is estrogen from the follicle, which promotes proliferation of uterine epithelium and glandular tissue. Ovulation generally occurs on day 14 of the cycle. During the postovulatory phase (days 15–25), the uterus is under the combined effects of estrogen and progesterone from the corpus luteum. This hormonal milieu promotes increased vascularity, further development of glands, their increased secretory activity (including glycogen accumulation), hypertrophy, and fluid accumulation. These changes prepare the uterus for implantation of a fertilized ovum, should fertilization occur. If fertilization does not occur, the corpus luteum begins to regress after day 25, leading ultimately to the onset of menses.

Hormonal Control of the Menstrual Cycle: The suppressed (and even declining) plasma gonadotropin (FSH and LH) levels during the follicular phase are due to the negative feedback inhibitory effects of estrogen being secreted from developing follicles. The small, abrupt rise in plasma estrogen is believed to trigger the ovulatory LH surge (by suspension of negative feedback or by positive feedback). During the luteal phase negative-feedback suppression is reestablished, but in this period feedback is due to the combined effects of estrogen and progesterone. Luteal failure occurs at about 26 days. It results in an abrupt withdrawal of estrogen and progesterone and hence in a release of feedback inhibition, which accounts for the rise in FSH and LH at the beginning of a new cycle.

Female Contraception

Female oral contraceptives represent combinations of synthetic progestational compounds (19-nortestosterone derivatives such as norgestrol and neorethindrone) with synthetic estrogen. The original rationale behind the pill was that the synthetic progestin in the presence of estrogen would block the ovulatory LH surge. The progestins are effective because they also cause the cervical mucus to produce an environment (like that in the luteal phase) hostile to sperm.

The Placenta

Although the placenta is mainly concerned with support and nourishment of the developing embryo, it secretes estrogens, progesterone, and chorionic gonadotropin. Excess chorionic gonadotropin (similar to luteinizing hormone) is excreted in the urine and is the basis of most pregnancy tests. The estrogen production by the placenta inhibits FSH production and in this manner inhibits follicle development during pregnancy.

The Pineal

The pineal organ is a diencephalic outgrowth. Its products are melatonin, serotonin, and methylindoles. It has been linked to photoperiodism and seasonal breeding; experimental evidence now suggests that it produces an antigonadotropic substance. How the pineal influences the reproductive organs remains to be established. The pineal is considered a neuroendocrine transducer that modulates the functions of many different organs.

The Prostaglandins

Prostaglandins (PGs) are hormonelike substances that play a role in cellular metabolism. Their function, unlike that of hormones, is limited to immediate areas; in this respect they may be labeled as tissue hormones. These substances, which are derivatives of prostanoic acid, are C_{20} fatty acids containing a five-membered ring; they are found in almost every type of human and animal tissue and elicit a multitude of effects. Prostaglandins exert control over processes such as reproduction, inflammation, nerve impulse transmission, blood pressure and blood clotting, smooth muscle activity, and hormone secretion.

The Small Intestine

Food materials stimulate the secretion of certain hormones by the neuroendocrine cells of the gastrointestinal mucosa. These hormones may be summarized as follows:

1. **Secretin:** from duodenal mucosa—stimulates pancreatic juice secretion, which is low in enzymatic content.
2. **Pancreozymin:** from duodenal mucosa—stimulates pancreatic juice secretion rich in enzymes.
3. **Cholecystokinin:** from duodenal mucosa—stimulates the contraction and emptying of the gallbladder.
4. **Enterogastrone:** from duodenal mucosa—inhibits motility and depresses the acid secretion by the stomach.
5. **Gastrin:** from pyloric region of stomach—enhances acid secretion by the stomach.

QUICK RECALL TEST QUESTIONS AND ANSWERS

Choose the Best Answer

1. Follicle-stimulating hormone is to estrogen as luteinizing hormone is to:

   (A) progesterone.
   (B) testosterone.
   (C) vasopressin.
   (D) luteotrophic hormone.

2. Which of the following patterns would you expect to find in the blood one hour after a rich meal?

	Blood Sugar	Insulin
(A)	high	low
(B)	low	low
(C)	high	high
(D)	low	high

3. During the follicular phase of a normal menstrual cycle, ovarian changes occur that are due to pituitary secretions of:

   (A) FSH only.
   (B) LH only.
   (C) oxytocin.
   (D) FSH and LH.

4. Growth hormone releasing factor is:

   (A) a precursor of growth hormone.
   (B) the same as growth hormone (somatotropin).
   (C) a hypothalamic releasing factor.
   (D) a dietary stimulant regulating positive nitrogen balance.

5. Glucagon, which is produced by the pancreas, and epinephrine, which is produced by the adrenal glands, are hormones that:

   (A) raise blood sugar level.
   (B) lower blood sugar level.
   (C) do not affect blood sugar markedly.
   (D) markedly increase liver glycogen.

6. Testosterone is produced by:

   (A) spermatogonia of the testes.
   (B) interstitial cells of the testes (Leydig cells).
   (C) the glans penis.
   (D) the prostate gland.

7. Hypersecretion of the hormone _____ will result in acromegaly (giantism).

   (A) TSH—thyroid stimulating hormone
   (B) STH—somatotropin (growth hormone)
   (C) ACTH—adrenocorticotropic hormone
   (D) thyroxin

8. A lack of iodine in the diet usually is associated with which disorder?

   (A) acromegaly
   (B) goiter
   (C) rickets
   (D) skin rash

9. Each of the following is under control of the adenohypophysis EXCEPT the:

   (A) thyroid.
   (B) adrenal medulla.
   (C) testis.
   (D) adrenal cortex.

10. The structure(s) responsible for the production of progesterone is/are:

    (A) ovarian follicle.
    (B) corpus albicans.
    (C) corpus luteum.
    (D) corpus spongiosum.

11. The pituitary (master) gland releases a gonadotrophic hormone that stimulates the production of testosterone by:

    (A) spermatogonia.
    (B) interstitial cells of Leydig.
    (C) Sertoli cells.
    (D) epididymis.

Directions: For questions 12–17, choose the letter word or phrase that is most closely associated with the given item. You may use a letter choice more than once, or not at all.

    (A)   Placenta
    (B)   Hypothalamus
    (C)   Adrenal cortex
    (D)   Saliva

12. Chorionic gonadotropin

13. Relaxin

14. Cortisol

15. Ptyalin

16. Vasopressin

17. Maltase

Directions: For questions 18–26, choose the letter word or phrase that most closely matches the description. You may use a letter choice more than once, or not at all.

    (A)   Thyroid
    (B)   Parathyroid
    (C)   Thymus
    (D)   Adrenal

18. Regulates the resorption of calcium from bone

19. Produces mineralocorticoids and glucocorticoids

20. Removal results in muscle spasms, tetany, and death

21. Oversecretion can cause an individual to have bulging eyeballs

22. Insufficiency can lead to mental and physical sluggishness

23. Plays a dominant role in the development of a competent immune system

24. Chromaffin cells of the adrenal medulla are derived from:

    (A) the thyroglossal duct.
    (B) mesothelium of the Wolffian ridge.
    (C) endoderm.
    (D) neural crest ectoderm.

25. Which of the following hormones is the product of a pituitary acidophil (alpha cell)?

    (A) lutinizing hormone (LH)
    (B) follicle stimulating hormone (FSH)
    (C) thyroid stimulating hormone (TSH)
    (D) lactogenic hormone (LTH) or prolactin

26. All of the following may be considered as secondary sex characteristics of the male EXCEPT:

    (A) increase in sex drive.
    (B) external genitalia.
    (C) pattern of hair and beard growth.
    (D) development of a deeper voice.

Answers

1. **(A)** FSH stimulates the production of estrogen by the developing follicle. LH stimulates the production of progesterone by the corpus luteum.

2. **(C)** Langerhans described the beta cells (within the islets of Langerhans) of the pancreas, which produce insulin that affects the metabolism of glucose directly. Fat and protein are indirectly affected. After a meal the level of blood sugar rises, eliciting the production of insulin, which stimulates the absorption of glucose by the cells and helps in its conversion to glycogen. Insulin deficiency leads to high blood sugar levels and the disease called diabetes mellitus.

3. **(D)** The pituitary and ovaries have a reciprocal effect upon each other. FSH (follicle stimulating hormone) from the pituitary elicits estrogen production from the developing follicle. When estrogen concentrations reach a certain blood level, it inhibits FSH production. At that time, the egg is discharged and the cells lining the follicle come under the influence of another gonadotrophin LH (luteinizing hormone), which influences the development of the corpus luteum.

4. **(C)** The releasing factors that have been isolated and identified to date are produced in hypothalamic areas.

5 **(A)** Glucagon is released into the bloodstream in response to diminishing blood sugar levels. The main action of glucagon is to promote liver glycogenolysis; as a consequence glycogen stores of the liver diminish. Epinephrine secreted by the adrenal medulla has the same general effect. Epinephrine is an important factor in the normal organism for counteracting the hypoglycemic action of insulin.

6 **(B)** Most researchers feel that the interstitial cells of Leydig of the testis are the source of androgen and

possibly testicular estrogen. The most potent androgen is testosterone.

7. **(B)** Acromegaly and (or) giantism is due to overactivity of the alpha cells of the pituitary which secrete growth hormone. If a person is affected before puberty, he or she will develop into a fairly well-proportioned giant. After maturity, an increase in the size of the hands and feet and massive development of the bones that make up the face are consequences. In the adult, strictly speaking, the term *acromegaly* must be applied to this condition.

8. **(B)** Acromegaly is a result of pituitary oversecretion of growth hormone. Lack of iodine will result in goiter development of the thyroid gland. Rickets is due to a vitamin D deficiency. A skin rash is not a specific lesion that can be associated with only one specified cause, as can the others listed.

9. **(B)** The adrenal medulla can be considered to house the post ganglionic neurons for part of the sympathetic portion of the autonomic nervous system and is responsible for epinephrine and norepinephrine production.

10. **(C)** Progesterone is produced by the corpus luteum.

11. **(B)** The interstitial cells are stimulated by ICSH (interstitial cell stimulating hormone), a gondadotrophin of the pituitary, to produce androgens. Testosterone is an androgen.

12. **(A)** Chorionic gonadotropin is produced by the placenta and acts with other reproductive hormones to maintain pregnancy.

13. **(A)** Relaxin is a product of the ovaries and placenta and functions in relaxing the pelvic ligaments during parturition.

14. **(C)** Cortisol is produced by the adrenal and is active in the conversion of proteins to carbohydrates.

15. **(D)** Ptyalin (salivary amylase) is found in saliva and initiates starch digestion.

16. **(B)** Vasopressin (ADH) elaborated by the hypothalamus and secreted from the posterior pituitary has an antidiuretic action on the kidney tubules.

17. **(D)** Maltase, a component of saliva, participates in starch digestion.

18. **(B)** It is believed by some that parathyroid hormone acts upon bone, eliciting changes in calcium and phosphrous. Osteoclasts are the cells stimulated by parathyroid hormone to facilitate the resorption of calcium and phosphorus from bone. Administration of parathyroid hormone to animals without parathyroids results in an increase of phosphorus excretion in the urine, a fall in serum inorganic phosphorus levels, an increase in serum calcium, and an increase of calcium excretion in the urine.

19. **(D)** The function of the adrenal cortex is to secrete sex hormone—androgens, estrogens, and progesterone; corticosteriods—glucocorticoids; and mineralocorticoids. These are all steriod hormones. The functional aspects of mineral and carbohydrate control by the adrenal are far more important than the influence it has on the reproductive organs (reproduction).

20. **(B)** Tetany is a state of increased neuromuscular excitability caused by a decrease in serum calcium. This can exhibit itself by numbness, cramps, spasms, loss of consciousness, convulsions, and possible death.

21. **(A)** Symptoms of hyperthyroidism can be listed as loss of weight, nervousness, irritability, rapid pulse, sweating, protrusion of the eyeballs (exophthalamus), and goiter.

22. **(A)** Hypothyroidism results in sluggish mental and physical behavior. Pulse rate is down and skin appears dry.

23. **(C)** Lymphocytes, which participate in such immunologic activities as delayed hypersensitivity reactions and graft rejection, are able to do so because of the influence of the thymus. Stem cells for this population are thought to pass through the thymus, and having come under its influence seed more peripheral lymphoid organs with their progeny. Removal of the thymus from newborn animals seriously impairs their immunologic system because of the lack of thymic influences.

24. **(D)** The thyroglossal duct is the path that the thyroid gland takes in its descent from the base of the tongue to its final position in the neck. As far as the adrenal gland is concerned, the cortex has its origin from mesodeum while the medulla is derived from ectoderm, neural crest origin in conjunction with the anlage of the sympathetic nerve cells.

25. **(D)** Luteinizing hormone and follicle stimulating hormone are products of delta cells. Thyroid stimulating hormone and melanocyte stimulating hormone are produced by beta cells. Lactogenic hormone is secreted by alpha cells.

26. **(B)** At the time of puberty usually an increase in sex drive, beard growth, and development of a deeper voice are experienced. The external genitalia are part of the organism and will develop and grow as the organism does. They are genetically determined and are a primary characteristic of the male.

REPRODUCTIVE SYSTEM

Reproductive Organs

Male: Seminiferous tubules of the testis, epididymis, vas deferens, seminal vesicles, prostate, prostatic urethra, membranous uretha, penile urethra, glans penis.

Female: Ovaries, oviduct, uterus, vagina, the breasts (accessory organs containing mammary glands).

Hormonal Control

For a detailed discussion of the hormonal interactions concerning the reproductive system, the reader is referred to the section dealing with the endocrine system. However, the cyclic activity of the female organism is briefly summarized because of its importance.

The reproductive cycle in mammals is regulated by the gonadotrophic hormones secreted by the anterior pituitary gland. In females, FSH (follicle-stimulating hormone) stimulates growth of the ovarian follicles and the ultimate development of Graafian follicles. LH (luteinizing hormone), a *steroidogenic* hormone, stimulates the synthesis and secretion of the steroid hormones estrogen and progesterone by the cells of the ovarian follicles. When the blood LH reaches a peak, ovulation occurs and the eggs are released from the Graafian follicles. Under the influence of LH, the cells of the collapsed ovarian follicles develop into corpus lutea and continue to synthesize and secrete estrogen and progesterone. Both estrogen and progesterone cause the inner lining of the uterus to prepare for implantation of the embryos. The anterior pituitary gland and the ovaries have a reciprocal effect on each other. As the concentration of estrogen and progesterone in the blood increases, FSH and LH production are respectively inhibited and, ultimately, the corpus lutea cease to function. If fertilization and subsequent pregnancy occur, the corpus lutea continue to function in steroidogenesis until the developing placenta takes over this function. However, if fertilization does not occur, the reproductive cycle begins anew.

Gametogenesis

The production of gametes (egg and sperm) within the gonads (ovary and testis) is referred to as gametogenesis. Most of the cells of the body (i.e., the somatic cells) are diploid. In humans, the total chromosome number is 46 (22 pairs plus an X and a Y in males, 22 pairs plus X and another X in females). In contrast, gametes have a haploid number of chromosomes. Therefore, a reduction in chromosome number from the diploid to the haploid condition must occur during gametogenesis. This reduction in chromosome number occurs when the primary oocytes and spermatocytes undergo the meiotic divisions associated with gametogenesis.

During gametogenesis in males, four functional sperm are produced from each primary spermatocyte that undergoes meiosis. In contrast, during gametogenesis in females, one functional ovum and three polar bodies are produced from each primary oocyte that undergoes meiosis.

Mature Gametes

Types of Eggs: Alecithal eggs have no yolk; examples are human and most other mammalian eggs. Microlecithal eggs have a small amount of yolk that is distributed equally; examples are sea urchin eggs. Telolecithal eggs have a very large amount of yolk. The small amount of nonyolky cytoplasm is concentrated at the animal (or upper) pole of the egg; examples are fish, reptile, and bird eggs. Centrolecithal eggs show a concentration of yolk in their center; insect eggs are the prime example.

Semen: In mammals semen is a fluid secreted by the male accessory sex glands, namely the prostate, seminal vesicles, and bulbourethral glands. Fructose is added by the prostate, as are acid phosphatase, citric acid, calcium, and fibrinolysin. The seminal vesicles add phosphorylcholine. The vas deferens is just a tube through which sperm are transported from the testes to the urethra. Between 3 and 4 ml of semen comprise one ejaculation, which contains between 300 and 400 million sperm cells.

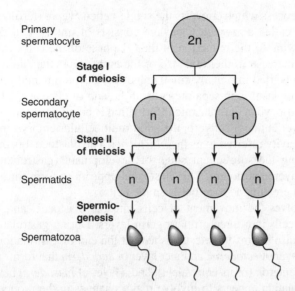

The formation of sperm cells by the process of meiosis and spermiogenesis.

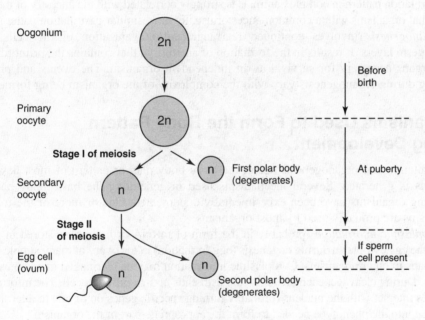

Egg cell production.

OVERVIEW OF DEVELOPMENT
Stages in Development

Conversion of the male and female gametes of an animal into a functional multicellular organism normally involves a predictable series of stages: fertilization, cleavage, blastulation, gastrulation, and organogenesis.

Fertilization involves two fusion events—gamete fusion (fusion of the outer membranes of the gametes) and pronuclear fusion (fusion of the haploid nuclei of the gametes). Fertilization results in the formation of the zygote (fertilized egg). The two fusion events of fertilization serve two functions in development. As a result of gamete fusion, the egg is activated to begin development. As a result of pronuclear fusion, the chromosome number of the zygote nucleus is restored to the diploid number characteristic of the species.

Cleavage is the process which converts the single-celled *zygote* (fertilized egg) into a solid multicellular embryo called a *morula*. Cleavage consists of mitotic cell divisions which are usually quite rapid owing to the reduction in the G1 phase of the cell cycle. These divisions therefore cause little increase in the total size of the embryo. At the end of cleavage a single large cell has been converted into many small cells. Any developmental information stored in regions of the egg cytoplasm is in separate cells at the end of cleavage. The cleavage pattern is frequently asymmetric when cytoplasmic information is being partitioned into specific cells.

Blastulation (in vertebrates) converts the solid multicellular embryo into an embryo containing a fluid-filled cavity referred to as the *blastocoel*. The blastocoel is the space into which cells will move during the subsequent stage of development (gastrulation) to convert the embryo into a multilayered structure. The blastocoel appears to form through loss of cell-to-cell attachments, thus creating a space between the cells.

Gastrulation involves the movement of cells into the blastocoel and the rearrangement/reorganization of the cells into three primary germ layers. During gastrulation, the basic body plan of the organism also begins to be established. At the end of gastrulation, the embryo typically has an external layer of *ectoderm*, an inner layer of *endoderm* that forms a primitive gut tube referred to as the archenteron (or its equivalent), and a layer of *mesoderm* between the ectoderm and endoderm. Gastrulation appears to involve major changes in the properties of the affected cells, since they have to alter their attachments to neighboring cells and become actively motile. The gastrulation pattern in complex animals is strongly correlated with the ancestry of the organisms in that organisms with a common ancestor usually have similar gastrulation patterns.

Organogenesis involves continued rearrangement/reorganization of the cells of the primary germ layers. It results in the formation of an embryo that contains the primordia of all of the organs necessary for survival as an independent organism. The events and processes occurring during organogenesis vary with the complexity of the organism being formed.

Mechanisms Used to Form the Body Pattern During Development

As gastrulation and organogenesis occur, the basic body plan or pattern of most developing organisms is generated. Several mechanisms used in generating the basic body pattern in developing organisms have been experimentally documented. One or more of the following mechanisms are probably used by most organisms.

Cytoplasmic information (probably in the form of mRNA or protein) is stored in specific areas of the egg cytoplasm during oogenesis (egg formation) in the ovary of many simple animals and perhaps in other organisms. Cytoplasmic information may be rearranged in response to fertilization. During cleavage, each area of cytoplasm ends up in a different cell. The informational molecules interact with the nucleus (probably turning specific genes on or off) to alter the cell's phenotype into the phenotype needed to form the appropriate part of the organism.

Use of cytoplasmic information as a pattern-generating mechanism can be easily demonstrated by removing individual cells from early embryos and noting which structures are missing later in development. If cytoplasmic information is the major mechanism involved, the parts normally formed by the missing cells will not form in the embryos from which the cells have been removed, but all other structures in the embryos will form normally.

This mechanism appears to be used most often in animals with relatively simple body patterns. Cytoplasmic information does not appear to be a major mechanism in birds or mammals. Most organisms that use cytoplasmic information also use cell-cell interactions to "fine-tune" formation of most complex organs.

Cell-cell interactions occur in all animal embryos that have been investigated so far. Cells in the developing embryo interact (through surface-surface interactions or by transferring chemical signals) to alter each other's phenotypes. This process is also called *induction*. Cell-cell interaction is frequently used to cause the parts of an organ to form in the correct relationship to each other but is not capable of generating an initial asymmetry in an embryo.

Cell-cell interaction can be experimentally detected by separating the cells between which interactions are suspected. If all cells involved still form their normal phenotypes after separation, cell-cell interaction (at least during the period following the separation) is clearly not essential in generating those phenotypes. Cell-cell interaction is also indicated if removal of one or more cells during cleavage results in failure to form structures normally created by neighbors of the cells that were removed. Cell-cell interaction appears to be the predominant identifiable developmental mechanism in vertebrates, especially in birds and mammals.

Cell-environment interactions have not been as thoroughly studied as cytoplasmic localization and cell-cell interactions, but have been demonstrated experimentally in several species. Embryos of birds and frogs appear to use gravity to produce initial differences between cells at the top (animal pole) and the bottom (vegetal pole) of the embryo.

Cell-environment interactions may be detected either by altering the environmental factors involved or by altering the orientation of the embryo relative to the factors and then observing the resulting developmental pattern. If cell-environmental interactions are involved, the orientation of the structure in the embryo will consistently follow the orientation of the environmental factor.

DEVELOPMENT IN HUMANS

Fertilization

During fertilization, the male and female gametes unite in the ampulla of the oviduct (Fallopian tube). At the time of ovulation, the egg is a secondary oocyte (arrested at metaphase II of meiosis) and is surrounded by a zona pellucida, an extracellular coat, and a cumulus oöphorus (an outer cellular coat composed of ovarian follicle cells). Following ovulation, the egg enters the ostium of the oviduct and is transported into the ampulla by ciliary movement and contractions of the musculature of the oviduct.

Sperm, deposited in the vagina during intercourse, pass into and through the uterus and then into and through the oviduct. Passage of the sperm through the female reproductive tract occurs as a result of the contractions of the musculature of the uterus and oviduct. During transport through the uterus and oviduct, sperm are exposed to secretions of these organs and undergo capacitation. During capacitation, sperm motility is increased and important alterations occur in the sperm plasmalemma. Following capacitation, the sperm are capable of interacting with the egg in order to undergo the acrosome reaction and the subsequent events of fertilization.

When the sperm reach the egg in the ampulla of the oviduct, the acrosome reaction occurs and hyaluronidase associated with the sperm causes dispersal of the cumulus oöphorous. Subsequently, the sperm bind to and then penetrate the zona pellucida. At this point, the sperm contacts the oolema and gamete fusion occurs. Of the approximately 350 million sperm deposited in a single ejaculation, only about 350 reach the egg in the ampulla of the oviduct. Although only one sperm will participate in gamete fusion, the other sperm are essential for dispersal of the cumulus oöphorous.

Following gamete fusion, the sperm pronucleus is taken into the egg cytoplasm, the secondary oocyte completes the second meiotic division, and the haploid female pronucleus is formed. When the male and female pronuclei come into close proximity, their nuclear envelopes break down. The maternal and paternal chromosomes intermingle and return the chromosome number to the diploid condition. Fertilization is now complete, and the fertilized egg is referred to as a *zygote*.

Cleavage

About 24 hours after pronuclear fusion, the zygote begins to undergo cleavage. As cleavage occurs, the multicellular embryo is transported through the oviduct. The embryo usually enters the uterus at the 12- to 16-cell stage. At the 16-cell stage, the embryo consists of several internally located blastomeres surrounded by a larger number of externally located blastomeres and is referred to as a *morula*.

Blastocyst Formation

After the morula stage, when the embryo enters the uterus, the outer blastomeres begin to absorb fluid. As the number of blastomeres in the embryo increases, fluid begins to accumulate in the extracellular space surrounding the internally located blastomeres. As a result, the innermost blastomeres and outer blastomeres of the embryo become separated by an enlarging fluid-filled space. The embryo is converted into a blastocyst. The blastomeres located on the exterior of the blastocyst are referred to as the *trophoblast/trophectoderm*, while the blastomeres located internally are referred to as the *inner cell mass/ICM/embryoblast*. The fluid-filled space that forms between the ICM and trophoblast is referred to as *blastocyst cavity*.

The blastocyst stage in mammals is sometimes equated with the blastula stage of embryonic development. However, the blastocyst stage should be considered a preblastula stage. Subsequent to the formation of the blastocyst, the cells of the inner cell mass become reorganized into a two-layered disclike structure that is similar to the blastula stage of a bird embryo.

Implantation in the Uterus

During the sixth day of development, the blastocyst begins the implantation process by which it invades the uterine tissue to establish contact with the maternal circulation. The wall of the uterus consists of the inner endometrium, the myometrium, and the outer perimetrium. *Endometrium* (uterine mucosa, an epithelium and underlying connective tissue) lines the uterus; *myometrium* forms the thick, middle muscular layer; and *perimetrium* covers the outside of the organ. When the blastocyst arrives the *uterine mucosa* is in the *secretory* or *progestational* phase. Uterine arteries are dilated, glands are enlarged, mucin and glycogen are being produced, and the tissue resembles a sponge. Implantation usually occurs either along the anterior or posterior wall of the uterus.

Second Week (Bilaminar Germ Disc Formation)

As the blastocyst embeds, the trophoblast differentiates into an inner *cytotrophoblast* and an outer *syncytiotrophoblast* layer. Syncytiotrophoblastic processes invade the endometrial epithelium and stroma. *Lacunae* (spaces) soon appear in the syncytiotrophoblast and fill with maternal blood and secretions; this nutritive material, called *embryotroph,* reaches the embryoblast by diffusion (a primitive uteroplacental circulation). The embryoblast differentiates into *endoderm* and *ectoderm* (two of the three primary germ layers), which form a flat disc known as the *bilaminar germ disc*. Between the cytotrophoblast and ectoderm layer the *amniotic cavity* develops, while beneath the ectoderm, the single layer of endoderm proliferates to form the definitive *yolk* sac. As development proceeds, the extraembryonic coelom, the cavity between the embryoblast and the trophoblast, expands and the large *chorionic cavity* is formed. Within the chorionic sac, the embryo and its amnion and yolk sac are suspended. Extraembryonic mesoderm lines this cavity and covers the embryoblast, thus connecting it to the trophoblast. As soon as blood vessels develop this connecting stalk will become the *umbilical cord.*

Highlighting this period is the development of the *primitive streak* on the surface of the ectoderm facing the amniotic cavity. The primitive streak functions as the *blastopore* during gastrulation. The cephalic end of this streak is known as the *primitive node*. During gastrulation, mesoderm cells segregate from the ectoderm layer and migrate between the ectoderm and endoderm by way of the primitive streak. In this manner the third primary germ layer, the *mesoderm* is formed between the ectoderm and endoderm except at the prechordal plate (buccopharyngeal membrane) and cloacal membrane.

The *allantois* appears as an outpocketing in the caudal end of the primitive gut around day 16. It stores excretory products in lower forms; it remains rudimentary in humans but plays a vital role as a source of vascular stem cells. During this period, formation of the *somites* from *mesoderm* and the initiation of the formation of the *central nervous system* from *ectoderm* begins. Mesoderm also gives rise to the blood vessels which eventually connect the placenta and the embryo.

Derivatives of the Germ Layers

Ectoderm	Mesoderm	Endoderm

1. Epidermis of the skin
  • Hair and nails
2. Epithelium of the organs
  • Eye: retina, lens, cornea, and conjunctiva; lacrimal gland
  • Ear: external auditory meatus and membranous labyrinth
  • Nose: olfactory epithelium and glands of the nasal cavity and paranasal sinuses
3. Nervous system (central and peripheral)
  • Pia and arachnoid
  • Pineal gland and posterior lobe of pituitary
  • Adrenal medulla
4. Epithelium and glands of the lips, cheeks, gums, hard palate, and the parotid, submandibular, sublingual, and all minor salivary glands
5. Anterior lobe of pituitary gland
6. Enamel of the teeth
7. Muscles of the iris and the sweat glands
8. Epithelium of anal canal and vestibule of vagina
	1. Connective tissue
	  • Bone and cartilage
	2. Synovial membranes
	3. Lymphoid tissue
	  • Tonsils and lymph nodes
	4. Contents of the eye not developed from ectoderm
	5. Middle and internal ear
	  • Not membranous labyrinth or tympanic aspects
	6. Dura and microglia
	7. Teeth (except for enamel)
	8. Cortex of adrenal gland
	9. Serous membranes
	  • Pleura, pericardium, peritoneum, and tunica vaginalis testis
	10. Muscle
	  • Striated, smooth, and cardiac
	11. Endothelium of the cardiovascular and lymphatic system
	12. Bone marrow, blood, and spleen
	13. Urogenital organs
		1. Epithelium of the digestive tract, tongue and taste buds, liver, biliary system, and pancreas
		2. Epithelium of the thyroid, parathyroid, and thymus
		3. Epithelium of the respiratory tract, larynx, trachea, bronchi, and alveoli
		4. Epithelium of the genito-urinary system

Third–Eighth Week (Germ Layer Derivatives)

During this period the main organ systems become established and external body features such as limb buds, face, ear, nose, and eyes become apparent.

At 8 weeks the fetus stage has been reached and the dramatic changes leading to organ formation have occurred. The embryonic period now enters a phase of remarkable growth until the *conceptus* is ready for delivery.

Fetal Membranes and Placenta

The fetal membranes are the: amnion, yolk sac, allantois, and chorion. Although these membranes originate from the zygote, only the *yolk sac* and *allantois* contribute cells to embryonic structures.

The Amnion: The amniotic cavity is filled with fluid derived from the maternal circulation and from excretory products of the fetus. Amniotic fluid is swallowed by the fetus and taken up by the gastrointestinal system. The embryo, suspended by the umbilical cord, floats in the amniotic fluid. Amniotic fluid:

1. serves as a cushion and absorbs jolts,
2. allows the fetus to move,
3. helps in temperature regulation,
4. separates the amnion from the embryo,
5. provides a hydrostatic wedge during birth.

The Yolk Sac: The yolk sac is formed in the chorionic cavity and is connected to the umbilical cord. No yolk storage takes place in the human. However, the yolk sac plays a role in:

1. nutrient transfer before placental circulation is established,
2. blood cell development,
3. formation of the primordial germ cells.

The Allantois: This structure serves in the following manner:

1. It contributes to blood cell formation.
2. The allantoic blood vessels become the umbilical arteries and vein.
3. Via the urachus the bladder is connected to the umbilicus.

The Placenta:
Structure. The placenta is composed of two parts:

1. The maternal part, derived from the endometrial decidua basalis
2. The fetal part, derived from the chorionic villi

Decidua. The decidua is the functional layer of the endometrium during pregnancy. Three zones are differentiated:

1. Decidua basalis—this is the part deep to the conceptus, which forms the maternal placenta.
2. Decidua capsularis—this is the part superficial to the conceptus and closest to the uterine cavity.
3. Decidua parietalis—this is the term applied to the remaining portion of the uterine mucosa.

Chorionic Component. Originally the entire chorionic sac is covered by villi; however, around week 8, the villi not associated with the decidua basalis start to degenerate. The villi in relation to the decidua basalis increase in number and size and become the functional fetal portion of the placenta. The maternal and fetal components form an intimate anatomical and functional unit.

Function. Deoxygenated blood is carried from the fetus via the umbilical arteries to the placenta (villi). No mixing of maternal and fetal blood occurs. Exchange takes place over the endothelial barrier of the fetal vessels. Oxygenated blood passes into fetal placental veins, which form the umbilical vein, which supplies the fetus.

The main functions of the placenta are:

1. exchange of metabolic and gaseous products,
2. synthesis of glycogen, cholesterol and fatty acids,
3. synthesis of hormones,
4. transmission of antibodies.

Fetal and Neonatal Circulation

The cardiovascular system is designed to meet the needs of the fetus and at birth to adapt quickly to the demands of a new circuit and environment.

Fetal Circulation: Placenta → umbilical vein → ductus venosus of liver (half of the blood bypasses in this manner the hepatic circulation) → inferior vena cava → right atrium → foramen ovale, between right and left atria (blood bypasses the pulmonary circuit) → left atrium → left ventricle → ascending aorta → descending aorta → two umbilical arteries → placenta.

Blood that enters the right ventricle from the right atrium leaves via the pulmonary artery but bypasses the pulmonary circuit by passing through the ductus arteriosus, which connects the pulmonary artery to the aortic arch. In this manner blood reaches the aorta.

Changes at Birth: Due to a cessation of placental blood flow and the activation of the respiratory system because of pressure on the thoracic cavity and the replacement of amniotic fluid by air in the bronchial tree, certain changes are necessary:

1. Ductus arteriosus closes due to muscular constriction of its wall.
2. Blood flow through the lungs increases and results in a rise of pressure in the left atrium.
3. Right atrial pressure drops due to cessation of placental circulation.
4. The above pressure differentials result in the closing of the foramen ovale and complete pulmonary circulation is established.
5. The umbilical arteries close.
6. The umbilical vein and ductus venosus close.

Adult Derivatives

Fetal structure		Adult structure
(1) umbilical vein	→	ligamentum teres
(2) ductus venosus	→	ligamentum venosuum
(3) umbilical arteries	→	(a) superior vesicle arteries
		(b) medial umbilical ligaments
(4) foramen ovale	→	fossa ovalis
(5) ductus arteriosus	→	ligamentum arteriosum

Multiple Pregnancy

Twinning: Twinning occurs in about 1% of normal births; about two-thirds are of the *dizygotic* (fraternal) twin type. The frequency of dizygotic twins increases with the age of the mother and is influenced by heredity. (No age correlation exists as far as *monozygotic* [identical] twins are concerned.) If a first pregnancy results in twins, subsequent twinning is about three to five times greater than in the normal population. The *genotype* of the mother seems to be the key determining factor in the frequency of twin births.

Monozygotic Twins (Identical Twins). A single oocyte and sperm are involved. Two inner cell masses form within a single trophoblast at the blastocyst stage. Each inner cell mass subsequently develops into an embryo. These embryos have a common placenta and chorionic cavity but possess separate amniotic cavities. These individuals have the same sex and blood groups, and a strong resemblance in external features. (Their phenotypes and genotypes are identical.)

Dizygotic Twins (Fraternal Twins). Two separate oocytes and two separate sperm are involved. Both zygotes are totally different genetically. They may or may not be of the same sex. These zygotes implant independently and develop their own placenta and membranes. (Fraternal twins are not identical in phenotype and genotype. They are no more similar than any other non-twin siblings.)

Triplets: Triplets occur once in about 8,000 pregnancies. They may result from:

1. one zygote and therefore be identical,
2. two zygotes, and therefore give rise to one set of identical twins and one independent infant,
3. three zygotes and result in three independent individuals.

Types of multiple births higher than triplets are rare but similar combinations do occur.

QUICK RECALL TEST QUESTIONS AND ANSWERS

Choose the Best Answer

1. Which of the following does not contribute to the formation of semen?

    (A) prostate
    (B) seminal vesicles
    (C) bulbo-urethral glands
    (D) vas deferens

2. The human female has a karyotype of:

    (A) 23 pairs of autosomes and an X and a Y.
    (B) 23 pairs of autosomes and two X's.
    (C) 22 pairs of autosomes and an X and a Y.
    (D) 22 pairs of autosomes and two X's.

3. During gametogenesis (spermatogenesis) in the male, the second meiotic division takes place between:

    (A) the zygote and spermatid.
    (B) the primary germ cells and haploid gametes.
    (C) the secondary spermatocyte and spermatid.
    (D) the spermatid and spermatozoan.

4. Human sperm and ova are similar in the respect that they:

    (A) are haploid.
    (B) both possess flagella, which give them good mobility.
    (C) are approximately the same size.
    (D) both carry the identical genetic information.

5. Vasectomy is becoming a fashionable form of birth control in our society. In a vasectomy the _____ is/are cut, a portion is removed, and the stumps are sutured.

    (A) epididymis
    (B) vas deferens
    (C) oviducts
    (D) urethra

6. The basic scientific finding that finally led to the development of the oral contraceptive (pill) used by many females in our society was that the pre-ovulatory surge of LH can be prevented by the administration of:

    (A) FSH.
    (B) estrogen.
    (C) progesterone.
    (D) ICSH.

7. During gamete production in the human female, the cell that undergoes the reduction divisions (meiosis) eventually produces _____ functional egg(s).

    (A) 4
    (B) around 300
    (C) 8
    (D) 1

8. The sperm count of a normal 25-year-old male is:

    (A) 1 million/ml.
    (B) 100 million/ml.
    (C) 100,000/ml.
    (D) 4 million/ml.

9. Sperm utilize the substance _____ to penetrate the cumulus oöphorus of the egg in fertilization.

    (A) spermatase
    (B) chondroitin sulfatase
    (C) hyaluronidase
    (D) deoxyribonuclease

10. During the process of meiosis in the human male four functional sperms are produced, whereas in the female one functional egg and three _____ are the result.

    (A) zygotes
    (B) follicles
    (C) polar bodies (polocytes)
    (D) blastocysts

11. Conversion of a haploid cell into a diploid cell occurs during _____ in most animals.

    (A) fertilization
    (B) organogenesis
    (C) cleavage
    (D) blastulation

12. Ectoderm, mesoderm, and endoderm form as distinct layers during _____ in most animal embryos.

    (A) fertilization
    (B) organogenesis
    (C) cleavage
    (D) gastrulation

13. The process of _____ converts the single-celled zygote into a multicellular structure in most animal embryos.

    (A) fertilization
    (B) organogenesis
    (C) cleavage
    (D) gastrulation

14. Different cell types (muscle, brain, liver, etc.) within a single human body:

    (A) have genetically identical nuclei (contain the same genes) and express (transcribe) the same genes.
    (B) have genetically different nuclei (do not contain the same genes) but express (transcribe) the same genes.
    (C) have genetically identical nuclei (contain the same genes) but express (transcribe) different genes.
    (D) have genetically different nuclei (do not contain the same genes) and express (transcribe) different genes.

15. Gastrulation involves:

    (A) rapid cell division forming a multicellular embryo.
    (B) formation of ectoderm, mesoderm, and endoderm.
    (C) conversion of a larva into an adult.
    (D) formation of sperm and eggs.

16. The process of embryonic development which most closely follows after fertilization is:

    (A) metamorphosis.
    (B) organogenesis.
    (C) cleavage.
    (D) blastulation.

17. Gametogenesis involves:

    (A) rapid cell division forming a multicellular embryo.
    (B) formation of ectoderm, mesoderm, and endoderm.
    (C) conversion of a larva into an adult.
    (D) formation of sperm and eggs.

18. Fertilization involves:

    (A) rapid cell division forming a multicellular embryo.
    (B) formation of ectoderm, mesoderm, and endoderm.
    (C) conversion of a larva into an adult.
    (D) fusion of haploid cells to form a zygote.

19. Cleavage involves:

    (A) rapid cell division forming a multicellular embryo.
    (B) formation of ectoderm, mesoderm, and endoderm.
    (C) conversion of a larva into an adult.
    (D) formation of sperm and eggs.

20. The food reserves which will support the development of a human embryo are:

    (A) stored in the unfertilized egg or ovum.
    (B) stored in both the unfertilized egg and the sperm.
    (C) transferred to the embryo by the epithelium of the female reproductive tract.
    (D) transferred to the embryo from maternal blood in the endometrium of the uterus.

Answers

1. **(D)** Semen is a fluid secreted by the male accessory sex glands—namely, the prostate, seminal vesicles, and bulbo-urethral glands. Fructose is added by the prostate, as are acid phosphatase, citric acid, calcium, and fibrinolysin. The seminal vesicles add phosphorylcholine. The vas deferens is just a tube through which sperm are transported from the testes to the urethra.

2. **(D)** Forty-four autosomal chromosomes are present in every diploid cell of the human body. Mature gametes, however, are haploid. The total chromosome number of the human being is 46 (male 44 plus X and Y; female 44 plus X and X).

3. **(C)** The production of gametes, or sex cells—egg and sperm—is known as gametogenesis. Because an individual possesses an equal amount of genetic material from both parents and the same number of chromosomes as either parent, a reduction to one half that number must be accomplished in the development of the egg and sperm. The second meiotic division takes place between the secondary spermatocyte and spermatid.

4. **(A)** Human sperm and ova are similar in the respect that they both carry a haploid chromosomal complement. After fertilization the diploid composition is again found.

5. **(B)** Vasectomy involves an interruption of the vas deferens in the male.

6. **(C)** While on the pill the female produces no new eggs and is kept in the progestational phase (second half) of the menstrual cycle.

7. **(D)** During meiosis in the female one functional gamete (egg) and three polar bodies are produced.

8. **(B)** Between 3 to 4 ml of semen make up one ejaculate, which contains 300–400 million sperm cells.

9. **(C)** Hyaluronidase, an enzyme carried by sperm, is capable of hydrolysis of hyaluronic acid, promoting fertilization (penetration of sperm). Hyaluronidase is medically used to promote the diffusion and absorption of many injected medications.

10. **(C)** In the human male four functional cells (sperms) are produced, whereas in the human female one functional cell (egg) and three polar bodies (polocytes) are produced during meiosis.

11. **(A)** Fusion of the haploid sperm with the egg (which eventually becomes haploid) produces a diploid zygote.

12. **(D)** Gastrulation completes formation of a three-layered embryo with ectoderm, endoderm, and mesoderm. In some animals, both endoderm and mesoderm form during gastrulation. In other animals, part of the endoderm may be in place at the beginning of gastrulation, so gastrulation completes endoderm formation and forms the mesoderm.

13. **(C)** Cleavage converts the single-celled zygote into a multicellular embryo. Cleavage consists of rapid mitotic cell division.

14. **(C)** Different cell types form by activation of different sets of genes. In most cases studied so far, no permanent changes occur in the genetic makeup of the different cells. The exceptions include lymphocytes, in which genetic rearrangements occur in the process of forming antibodies and T-cell receptors.

15. **(B)** Gastrulation completes formation of a three-layered embryo with ectoderm, endoderm, and mesoderm. In some animals, both endoderm and mesoderm form during gastrulation. In other animals, part of the endoderm may be in place at the beginning of gastrulation, so gastrulation completes endoderm formation and forms the mesoderm.

16. **(C)** Mitotic cell division (called cleavage) must occur after fertilization to produce a sufficient number of cells to form the parts of the embryo.

17. **(D)** Gametogenesis is the process of converting body cells into sperm or eggs. In most animals, this process involves meiosis to convert diploid body cells into haploid cells and differentiation of body cells into the highly specialized cells called sperm and eggs.

18. **(D)** Fertilization involves fusion of a sperm with an egg. The initial fusion typically activates the egg to begin development; the fusion of the haploid nucleus from the sperm with a haploid nucleus in the egg forms the diploid nucleus of the embryo.

19. **(A)** Cleavage converts the single-celled zygote into a multicellular embryo. Cleavage consists of rapid mitotic cell division. Mitotic cell division must occur after fertilization to produce a sufficient number of cells to form the parts of the embryo.

20. **(D)** In humans and other mammals with deep implantation, some nutrients may be taken up from the lumen of the female reproductive tract prior to implantation, but most of the food reserves which support development are transferred from maternal blood (which forms a pool around the implanted embryo in the endometrium of the uterus) into the embryo. In the fully implanted embryo, this occurs in the placenta.

DEFENSE AGAINST FOREIGN ORGANISMS AND ABNORMAL CELLS

Routine defense against foreign organisms which are not adapted to function as parasites is primarily due to *barrier layers* at body surfaces. *Clot formation* reduces foreign organism entry following mechanical damage to a barrier layer. *Innate defense mechanisms* destroy most nonpathogenic organisms which have passed barrier layers, destroy many types of abnormal host cells, and reduce the numbers of newly encountered pathogenic organisms until a specific immune defense can be established. *Specific immune responses* require time to develop following the initial exposure to a particular organism, but are capable of completely wiping out most infections under optimal conditions. The specific components of a foreign organism that are responded to by a specific immune response are called antigens.

Barrier Layers

Barrier layers protect all body surfaces that may be exposed to foreign organisms. These barrier layers include the skin and the inner luminal surface of the tubular organs of the respiratory, digestive, urinary, and reproductive systems. A typical barrier layer consists of a surface epithelium and an underlying connective tissue layer. The tight junctions between the cells in the epithelium prevent movement of organisms across the barrier through extracellular spaces. The connective tissue layers underlying the epithelium provide mechanical strength to the barrier.

Organs in which the barrier function is reduced as an adaptation to the requirements of the physiological processes occurring across the barrier are protected by mechanisms which reduce the chance of living foreign organisms reaching the organ. The lungs have a very thin lining to allow efficient gas exchange and are protected by the mucus layer in the nose, trachea, and bronchi; the small intestine has a simple columnar epithelium to allow effective food absorption and is protected by the acidic environment in the stomach; and the uterus has a thin lining, which allows embryos to penetrate into the endometrium, and is protected by the mucus plug in the cervix. The cavities communicating with these organs are also populated with nonpathogenic microorganisms which compete with pathogens and reduce the chance of their successful entry.

As a result of the effectiveness of barrier layers, infections usually result from either mechanical damage to a barrier layer or penetration of a barrier layer through specific pathogenic mechanisms which evolved in the pathogens as ways to enter the host.

Clot Formation

A clot provides a temporary barrier when an epithelium (normal barrier) is damaged. Clot formation can be initiated by either blood vessel damage or tissue damage and involves a cascade of sequential clotting factor reactions which culminate in deposition of a fibrin clot blocking access to the damaged area.

Innate Defense Mechanisms

Purely innate or paraimmune mechanisms require no prior exposure to a particular foreign organism before the mechanisms can function at full efficiency. This is partly because innate mechanisms are directed at features shared by groups of foreign organisms and typically have less specificity than specific immune mechanisms.

Unfortunately, innate mechanisms are less capable of completely destroying an invading population of foreign organisms than are specific immune mechanisms. Therefore, innate mechanisms may destroy small invasions if the organisms lack effective mechanisms of avoiding destruction, but usually serve to hold larger, more pathogenic invasions in check until a specific immune response can develop. In other words, your innate mechanisms usually keep you alive long enough to generate a specific immune response to finish off the infection.

In addition, some innate mechanisms also serve as effectors for specific immune responses and may chemically enhance specific immune responses. In general, defense mechanisms are closely integrated.

Numerous innate mechanisms have been identified. A few typical examples are listed below.

1. *Neutrophils* are granular leukocytes which are intrinsically capable of phagocytosis of some types of bacteria. This response is vastly increased by innate complement activation or by specific immune responses which deposit antibodies and complement on the bacteria.

2. *Macrophages* are monocyte-derived connective tissue cells which are intrinsically capable of phagocytosis of some types of bacteria. This response is vastly increased by innate complement activation or by specific immune responses which deposit antibodies and complement on the bacteria.

3. *Natural killer (NK)* cells are lymphocytes which are intrinsically capable of killing some types of cancer cells and some types of virus-infected cells. Additional types of abnormal or foreign cells are killed if the NK cells are activated by cytokines secreted by helper T lymphocytes or if the target cells are coated with antibodies produced by a specific immune reaction.

4. Some types of bacteria spontaneously activate *complement* proteins by the alternate pathway, resulting in killing the bacteria. Complement proteins are innate components of blood plasma and tissue fluid. Interaction between some innate inflammatory response proteins and some bacteria increases complement activation. Complement is also activated very efficiently by many of the classes of antibodies produced in specific immune responses.

5. Release of *interferon* by virus-infected cells is an innate response which makes surrounding cells more resistant to virus infection.

Specific Immune Mechanisms

Specific immune responses require prior exposure to the same or a very similar foreign organism to be fully effective because initial exposure to a foreign organism causes a primary immune response, which is much slower and less efficient than the secondary immune response which is triggered by subsequent exposure to the same organism. As a result, natural immunization against a pathogenic foreign organism will only occur if the infection is successfully held in check by innate mechanisms while the specific immune response develops.

This problem may be overcome by immunizing the host prior to the initial exposure to the pathogenic organism. Immunity may be clinically produced through two processes.

Passive immunization is achieved by transfer of antibodies directed against a foreign organism from one organism to another. This causes the recipient to immediately but temporarily become immune to the foreign material.

Passive immunization occurs naturally in mammals as a result of antibodies transferred from the mother to the fetus across the placenta and to the newborn in milk. Passive immunization is used clinically in cases in which a functional immune response is needed more quickly than it can be generated by active immunization; for example, in a patient who was bitten by a rabid animal and who did not begin active immunization soon enough to be sure that rabies shots would generate active immunity in time to prevent rabies.

Passive immunization can be used only with antibodies because transferred cell-mediated immune components could reject the body of the recipient. In addition, passive immunization is undesirable when it is not essential because the injected antibodies reduce the effectiveness of simultaneous active immunization.

Active immunization is achieved by exposure of the patient to a nonpathogenic form of a foreign organism or to isolated components of a foreign organism. This results in a primary immune response which produces immunity against the foreign organism after a delay of days or weeks. Subsequent exposure to the same foreign organism results in a secondary immune response which produces a rapid and effective response.

Patterns of Specific Immune Responses

The principal response mechanisms of the immune system are traditionally divided into cell-mediated responses and humoral or antibody-mediated responses. With the exception of a few situations, both of these responses require interactions with helper T lymphocytes.

Type of Specific Immune Response

	Cell-mediated Immunity	Antibody-mediated Immunity
Targets of response	Virus infected cells, cancer cells, transplanted cells	Bacteria, viruses, foreign molecules
Lymphocytes involved	Activated cytotoxic T (T_c) lymphocytes	Activated B lymphocytes which differentiate into plasma cells
Effector mechanisms	Cell-mediated killing of target cells and organisms	Antibody-mediated killing of target cells and organisms

Both types of responses involve receptors (T cell receptors on T_c and antibodies on B lymphocytes) that are generated by random recombination of gene segments which code for the variable regions of the receptors. This generates an enormous number of receptor specificities. After the initial recombination during the development of the lymphocytes, the cells undergo positive selection for cells bearing functional receptors and negative selection against cells bearing receptors reactive against components of the organism's own body. Cells which fail either test die in the formative organ. The cells that pass both tests leave the formative organ as potentially functional lymphocytes which require activation to become fully functional. At this point, only a few lymphocytes will react effectively with any particular foreign component. Successful activation triggers proliferation of the cells whose receptors interact effectively with abnormal or foreign components, and some of the resulting cells remain as memory cells. As a result, a second exposure to the same components results in a much faster response because the process is beginning with many more cells.

Cytotoxic T Lymphocyte Responses

In a cell-mediated response, T_c lymphocytes recognize viral or abnormal peptides displayed on major histocompatibility complex class I (MHC I) molecules on the surface of body cells. T cell receptor molecules on the T_c cells specifically recognize the peptides and closely associated CD8 molecules on the T_c cells recognize the MHC I molecules. If a peptide is recognized by a T cell receptor on an activated T_c, the cell displaying the peptide on its MHC I is killed. Cell-mediated killing of target cells and organisms may involve secretion of perforins (pore-forming proteins) onto the target cells or may involve secretion of cytokines which stimulate receptors on the target cells and trigger programmed cell death through apoptosis.

Antibody Structure

A functional antibody contains a Y-shaped unit structure consisting of two heavy-chain–light-chain pairs joined by disulfide bonds and containing two antigen-binding sites. Each arm of the Y is formed by one of the light-heavy chain pairs. The base of the Y is formed by the parts of the two heavy chains which extend past the light chains.

Antibodies are subdivided into classes or isotypes based on the type of heavy chain found in the molecule as shown in the following table.

Each light and heavy chain has a variable region formed by rearrangement of DNA segments in the corresponding gene during the development of the B lymphocyte and a constant region characteristic of the category of polypeptide. An antigen binding pocket in an antibody is formed by the association of variable regions of a light plus a heavy chain. The large number of variable segments and the process of recombining them during B lymphocyte development results in an enormous number of antibody specificities in each individual.

Immunoglobulin class	Subclass	Heavy chains	Light chains
IgA			
	IgA1	alpha1	kappa or lambda
	IgA2	alpha2	kappa or lambda
IgD		delta	kappa or lambda
IgE		epsilon	kappa or lambda
IgG			
	IgG1	gamma1	kappa or lambda
	IgG2	gamma2	kappa or lambda
	IgG3	gamma3	kappa or lambda
	IgG4	gamma4	kappa or lambda
IgM		mu	kappa or lambda

Cell surface receptor forms of IgM and IgD and circulating forms of IgE and IgG consist of single fundamental units (two heavy chains plus two light chains). IgA occurs as single fundamental units and also occurs in a complex containing two of the fundamental units joined by a J polypeptide. IgA which has been transported across an epithelium contains an additional secretory polypeptide. Circulating IgM consists of an assembly of five antibody fundamental units plus a J polypeptide.

IgD exists only as a cell surface receptor in unstimulated B lymphocytes. IgM functions primarily within blood vessels. Because IgG can function within blood vessels and is easily moved across blood vessel walls in tissue fluid, it is the primary antibody in connective tissues. IgG is also moved across the placenta from the mother to the fetus during late pregnancy. IgA is transported across lining epithelia in the digestive and respiratory systems and functions on the mucosal surfaces. IgE also occurs on and below the same surfaces, and apparently evolved as a defense against parasitic worms. Its ability to trigger mast cell secretions unfortunately also results in allergies.

In an antibody-mediated response, foreign components bind to antibodies on the surfaces of B lymphocytes and stimulate the B lymphocytes to proliferate and differentiate into plasma cells which secrete antibodies of the same specificity as the antibody receptors which were triggered. The antibodies then bind specifically to proteins or carbohydrates on the surface of the target cells.

Antibody-mediated killing of target cells and organisms may involve activation of complement, resulting in pore formation in the plasma membranes of the target cells. Antibodies bound to target cells can also trigger killing of eukaryotic target cells by NK cells or macrophages through the process of antibody-dependent cellular cytotoxicity (ADCC) or can act alone or with activated complement to trigger phagocytosis followed by intracellular killing of bacteria by neutrophils and macrophages.

Helper T Lymphocytes

Helper T lymphocytes (T_h, CD4$^+$) are essential to provide chemical stimuli to the responding cells in almost all cell-mediated and antibody-mediated responses. T_h lymphocytes function by secreting cytokines which stimulate T_c or B lymphocyte activation and function and which may also activate macrophages and NK cells.

T_h lymphocytes are activated by interaction with an antigen-presenting cell presenting a fragment of a molecule (an antigen) recognized by the receptors on the T_h lymphocyte. The antigen must be presented on a major histocompatibility class II (MHC II) molecule and the antigen-presenting cell must provide appropriate costimulation. Antigen presentation without costimulation appears to inactivate T_h lymphocytes.

Antigen-Presenting Cells

Antigen-presenting cells are essential in activation of T_h lymphocytes. Macrophages and B lymphocytes can act as antigen-presenting cells under some circumstances, but interdigitating dendritic cells appear to be the most important antigen-presenting cells for T_h activation in intact organisms. These cells take in foreign material by phagocytosis or pinocytosis and partially degrade the molecules, then bind fragments to MHC II molecules and present them on the cell surface. Antigen-presenting cells must also provide T_h lymphocytes with costimulation signals on the antigen-presenting cell surfaces, usually in the form of B7 molecules. Antigen-presenting cells are also involved in activation of T_c lymphocytes, but the process is not well understood.

A separate population of follicular dendritic cells appear to be critical in developing and maintaining B cell populations for antibody-mediated responses. Follicular dendritic cells apparently accumulate antigen complexed with antibody on their cell surfaces by binding to receptors for antibody and complement. This bound antigen is available for interaction with B cells, both during their development and during memory cell maintenance.

Development of T Lymphocytes

Bone marrow is where most unspecialized lymphocytes appear to be produced. Most T lymphocytes leave the bone marrow and differentiate in the thymus. While in the thymus, developing T lymphocytes rearrange DNA segments within their T cell receptor (TCR) genes to form a functional TCR. A functional TCR usually contains one alpha and one beta polypeptide complexed with a CD3 complex of additional polypeptides. A smaller number of T lymphocytes have TCR with gamma and delta polypeptides in place of the alpha and beta polypeptides. Each alpha, beta, gamma, and delta polypeptide has a variable region formed by rearrangement of DNA segments in the corresponding gene and a constant region characteristic of the category of polypeptide. An antigen-binding pocket in a TCR is formed by the association of variable regions of an alpha plus a beta polypeptide or by association of variable regions of a gamma plus a delta polypeptide.

Positive and Negative Selection of T Lymphocytes in the Thymus

As they begin to express TCR on their surfaces, developing T lymphocytes initially express both CD4 and CD8 on their surfaces as well. Developing T lymphocytes whose TCR fails to interact with either MHC I or MHC II die as a result of the initial positive selection for cells with minimally functional TCR. If the TCR interacts more effectively with MHC I, the T lymphocyte loses CD4, retains CD8, and becomes a T_c. If the TCR interacts more effectively with MHC II, the T lymphocyte loses CD8, retains CD4, and becomes a T_h. Subsequently, both T_c and T_h lymphocytes which interact too strongly with antigens presented on MHC I and MHC II in the thymus die in the process of negative selection. The components used in negative selection appear to include most of the normal body components which could easily be presented by MHC I or MHC II. As a result, the T_c and T_h lymphocytes leaving the thymus have functional TCR which do not react excessively with normal components from the organisms' own cells. The tendency of presentation of an antigen without appropriate costimulation to inactivate a T_c or T_h lymphocyte appears to protect most individuals adequately against any remaining T lymphocytes carrying TCR reactive with normal body components, but these selection processes clearly fail in cases of autoimmune responses.

Development of B Lymphocytes

B lymphocytes appear to complete their differentiation in the bone marrow where they are initially produced and emerge into the circulation as mature B lymphocytes with antigen specificity.

Development of a functional B lymphocyte requires genetic recombination in the genes which code for the amino acid sequence of the immunoglobulin light and heavy chains. Light chains are coded for by a kappa gene or a lambda gene, only one of which will be used in a particular B lymphocyte. Heavy chains are coded for by a single set of heavy chain genes, each of which contains a constant region segment for each of the classes or isotypes of antibodies.

Heavy chain recombination occurs initially, followed by light chain recombination. Failure to generate a functional antibody apparently results in cell death in a process similar to positive selection in the thymus, but the detailed interactions are not understood. In addition, developing B lymphocytes producing antibodies which are excessively reactive toward normal body components present in bone marrow are also eliminated in a process which is apparently similar to negative selection in the thymus. The antibodies at this point are present on the B lymphocyte cell surface as IgM and IgD molecules which serve as cell surface receptors.

Exposure to an antigen which reacts with cell surface IgM or IgD begins the process of activation of the B lymphocyte. With the exception of a few polymeric antigens, material which binds to the immunoglobulin receptors on a B lymphocyte is internalized, processed, and returned to the surface of the B lymphocyte on MHC II molecules. The B lymphocyte must then present the antigen on its MHC II molecules to a T_h lymphocyte and be stimulated by the cytokines secreted by the T_c before the B lymphocyte is activated.

Activation triggers proliferation of the B lymphocyte. Some of the progeny remain as memory B lymphocytes, but most of the progeny differentiate into plasma cells which secrete antibodies. During differentiation into plasma cells, the functional heavy chain gene is altered by deletion of at least the delta and mu segments, resulting in secretion of antibodies of IgA, IgE, or IgG classes. This process is called class or isotype switching. During the activation process, mutations also occur which result in small changes in amino acid composition of the antigen-binding site and the resulting cells compete for antigen, with cells carrying more effective receptors becoming more frequent and the secreted antibodies becoming more specific.

Reactive Lymphoid Organs

Reactive organs or secondary lymphoid organs are locations in which lymphocytes provide surveillance of body cavities connected to microbe-containing environments or surveillance of body fluids. All of these organs contain B lymphocyte-rich follicles or nodules and associated T lymphocyte-rich areas. Secondary lymphoid organs can be classified into two functional and organizational patterns.

1. *External cavity screening organs* are located in the walls of tubular organs which routinely contain microorganisms. *Diffuse lymphoid tissue* (populations of lymphocytes and innate response cells) in the subepithelial connective tissue in the walls of the digestive, respiratory, urinary, and reproductive systems is involved in surveillance of the contents of those organ lumens and walls. The *tonsils* in the wall of the posterior part of the pharynx are involved in surveillance of organisms in the oral cavity. *Peyer's patches* in the wall of the ileum are involved in surveillance of organisms in the lower small intestine. The *appendix* extending from the blind end of the large intestine is involved in surveillance of organisms in the large intestine.

2. *Fluid screening organs* are interposed in the circulatory system. *Lymph nodes* are expanded areas in lymphatic vessels which contain aggregates of lymphoid tissue. They are involved in surveillance of organisms in lymph. Because lymph is tissue fluid which has just left organs, its contents represent a sample of any organisms which have invaded the organs of the host organism. The *spleen* (along with some areas in bone marrow) is involved in surveillance of organisms in blood. The spleen receives blood from the systemic circulation. The blood is intimately exposed to lymphocytes and macrophages while in the spleen.

QUICK RECALL TEST QUESTIONS AND ANSWERS

Choose the Best Answer

1. Antibodies are synthesized by:

   (A) the liver.
   (B) granulocytes.
   (C) platelets.
   (D) B lymphocytes and plasma cells.

2. B lymphocytes initially develop in:

   (A) bone marrow.
   (B) the thymus.
   (C) the wall of the digestive tract.
   (D) the wall of the reproductive tract.

3. Most T lymphocytes develop their antigenic specificity in:

   (A) bone marrow.
   (B) the thymus.
   (C) the wall of the digestive tract.
   (D) the wall of the reproductive tract.

4. Helper T lymphocytes may contribute to an immune response by:

   (A) producing antibodies.
   (B) stimulating the production or activity of cytotoxic T lymphocytes.
   (C) killing virus-infected cells.
   (D) releasing clotting factors to restore a barrier layer.

5. Cytotoxic T lymphocytes respond effectively to:

   (A) bacteria.
   (B) virus-infected cells.
   (C) toxic food molecules.
   (D) plant pollens

6. The "non-specific immune" or paraimmune (early phase inflammatory) system in humans does not require prior exposure to most foreign organisms in order to mount a rapid response; the specific immune system responds only to an initial exposure to a foreign organism after a delay of approximately a week.

   (A) TRUE
   (B) FALSE

7. The "non-specific immune" (early phase inflammatory) system in humans does not involve cell-mediated responses; the specific immune system does use cell-mediated responses to some targets.

   (A) TRUE
   (B) FALSE

8. The initial mechanism that acts to prevent infection of a normal human body by most types of bacteria is:

   (A) skin.
   (B) blood clotting.
   (C) inflammatory or paraimmune reactions.
   (D) specific immune reactions.

9. For maximum effectiveness, _____ require previous exposure to the same (or a very closely related) foreign organism.

   (A) skin barrier functions
   (B) blood clotting reactions
   (C) inflammatory or paraimmune reactions
   (D) specific immune reactions

10. Lymph nodes respond to foreign organisms present in:

    (A) the lumen of the digestive tract.
    (B) the lumen of the respiratory tract.
    (C) the lumen of the reproductive tract.
    (D) tissue fluid draining from many organs and body regions.

11. The spleen responds to foreign organisms present in:

    (A) the lumen of the digestive tract.
    (B) the lumen of the reproductive tract.
    (C) tissue fluid draining from many organs and body regions.
    (D) blood.

12. Peyer's patches respond to foreign organisms present in:

    (A) the lumen of the digestive tract.
    (B) the lumen of the respiratory tract.
    (C) the lumen of the reproductive tract.
    (D) tissue fluid draining from many organs and body regions.

13. A foreign protein, when introduced into the body, is recognized and elicits an immunologic response; this substance is known as a(an):

    (A) antigen.
    (B) antibody.
    (C) complement.
    (D) vitamin.

Answers

1. **(D)** Membrane-bound antibodies (IgM and IgD) are synthesized by B lymphocytes. After antigen stimulation, B lymphocytes proliferate and most of their progeny become plasma cells, which secrete IgM, IgG, IgA, or IgE.

2. **(A)** B lymphocytes primarily develop in bone marrow, then migrate to secondary lymphoid organs as naive B lymphocytes. Some B lymphocytes may develop in other locations.

3. **(B)** Most developing T lymphocytes initially form their T cell receptors (TCR) while in the thymus. Some T lymphocytes may develop in the gut wall or in other locations.

4. **(B)** Most helper T lymphocytes primarily either stimulate macrophage activity and stimulate proliferation and function of cytotoxic T lymphocytes or stimulate development of B lymphocytes. Some T lymphocytes with helper T lymphocyte surface markers may kill virus-infected cells.

5. **(B)** Cytotoxic T lymphocytes respond most effectively to virus-infected cells.

6. **(A)** Inflammatory or paraimmune responses use cells and molecular components which are produced routinely in the body, so the first exposure triggers an effective response. Specific immune components are present in very small numbers until they are stimulated to proliferate by exposure to a particular foreign organism. The requirement for proliferation before an effective response can occur results in a delay.

7. **(B)** Both systems use cell-mediated responses. Inflammatory responses usually use macro-phages and commonly use neutrophils against bacteria and natural killer cells against virus-infected cells. Specific immune responses almost always use helper T lymphocytes and use cytotoxic T lymphocytes against virus-infected cells.

8. **(A)** Skin is the initial barrier against most bacteria. The other mechanisms come into play if the skin (or respiratory of gut lining) is penetrated.

9. **(D)** Specific immune components are present in very small numbers until they are stimulated to proliferate by exposure to a particular foreign organism. The requirement for proliferation before an effective response can occur results in a delay. Prior exposure results in generation of memory T and B lymphocytes which allow a rapid, effective response.

10. **(D)** Lymphatic fluid entering the lymph nodes originates from tissue fluid in the organs being drained by the lymphatic vessels. Any foreign organisms present in the tissue fluid are exposed to T and B lymphocytes in the lymph nodes.

11. **(D)** Blood circulating through the spleen passes through sinuses, which allow exposure of any foreign materials in the blood to T and B lymphocytes in the spleen.

12. **(A)** Peyer's patches contain specialized intestinal lining cells (M cells) which pass foreign materials from the intestinal lumen of the digestive tract to the T and B lymphocytes in the Peyer's patch.

13. **(A)** Any substance that has the ability to elicit an immunological response, such as the production of antibody that is specific to that substance, is considered an antigen.

GENETICS

Chromosomes within the nucleus of the cells are the source of DNA (deoxyribonucleic acid), the inheritable material; chromosomes contain specific units called genes, which are arranged in linear order on the chromosomes. Genes are paired elements, held together in a specific linkage arrangement. One member of each pair of genes separates during germ cell production; therefore, each germ cell contains only one set. An allele is one of a pair of genes that occupies the same locus on homologous chromosomes. Genotype refers to the genetic make-up of the organism. The genotype is expressed via phenotypic characteristics that are visible and observable under normal circumstances.

Mendel is responsible for the discovery of several intriguing phenomena:

1. He showed that each member of a pair of genes will be found in a different gamete; they were contributed to that individual by his parents and underwent no change such as blending while they were associated. This is Mendel's first law (law of segregation), which affirms that *allelomorphs segregate*.
2. Mendel also documented that the distribution of members of one pair has absolutely no bearing on the distribution of another pair. For example, if an individual possesses one pair of alleles Y and y, and another pair Z and z, the individual will produce approximately equal numbers of gametes of the four possible chance combinations of one member from each pair (YZ; Yz; yZ; yz). This law is known as independent assortment; the law does not apply to linked genes but only to genes located on different chromosomes. Independent behavior of chromosomes during meiosis is essential.

Mendel also showed that certain characteristics mask other traits; this phenomenon is known as dominance.

Genetic phenomena are best explained and demonstrated by problem solving, and it will be attempted in this manner.

Mendelian Characteristics

Dominance: Dominance is expressed in terms of a pair of alleles. A gene which produces and expresses the same characteristic whether it is present alone (in the heterozygous state matched to a gene not possessing the same trait) or with a gene possessing the same trait (in the homozygous state) is said to be dominant to the allele with which it is paired. The allele which is ineffective in the expression of its trait in the heterozygote is said to be recessive to the dominant. Let us illustrate with the following example.

The trait of green eyes did not occur in the F_1 (offspring from parents) but made its appearance in the F_2 (offspring of F_1 or offspring of offspring from the parents) generation. We are dealing with a recessive trait that is being masked by a dominant one. AA (brown eyes) bred with aa (green eyes) results in all F_1, Aa (genotypically heterozygous but phenotypically A; all brown eyes). Breeding of the offspring Aa with Aa results in 1 AA 2 Aa 1 aa genotype and 3:1 phenotype. The above demonstrates a one factor cross.

Let us now demonstrate several typical two-factor crosses:

1. Crossing of two types of organisms yields the classical 9:3:3:1 ratio. The cross would be considered an expression of phenotypic ratio.

   The example calls for a cross between individuals possessing a genetic makeup of RrSs × RrSs. Construct the Punnett square below and see the results in a 9:3:3:1 phenotypic ratio.

	RS	Rs	rS	rs
RS	RRSS	RRSs	RrSS	RrSs
Rs	RRSs	RRss	RrSs	Rrss
rS	RrSS	RrSs	rrSS	rrSs
rs	RrSs	Rrss	rrSs	rrss

R__S__ or RS = 9
R__ss or Rss = 3
rrS__ or rrS = 3
rrSS or rrss = 1

2. In rabbits, rough coat is dominant over smooth coat. Brown is dominant over gray fur color. A rough, brown male is mated to a couple of smooth, gray females. The offspring are counted as: 18 rough, brown; 21 rough, gray; 16 smooth, brown; 24 smooth; gray. If this male had been mated to a female of his own genotype, what proportion of the offspring would have exhibited rough, gray coats? The answer is 3 out of 16 and is obtained in the following manner.

Basic genetic knowledge is applied.

rough   = (dominant)
smooth = (recessive)
brown   = (dominant)
gray   = (recessive)

The male is crossed to several smooth gray females; they had to be homozygous recessive genotype. Because all four combinations appeared, we can assume that the male was genotypically heterozygous even though he appeared phenotypically dominant. If first we crossed this heterozygous male RrBb × rrbb, the result would be RrBb; Rrbb; rrBb; in other words, the four combinations given. Now let us cross the RrBb male × RrBb female; the following combinations would have to be considered in both male and female: RB; Rb; rB; rb. If these are crossed, we find 3 out of 16 possess rough gray coats (namely, RRbb; Rrbb and Rrbb).

Incomplete Dominance: Seeds from a self-pollinated gold flowering plant produce 56 charcoal, 130 gold and 61 beige flowering plants. The plant is heterozygous with incomplete dominance of its traits.

The phenomenon illustrated here is incomplete dominance (blending of two traits). Let us assume:

charcoal C
beige   B
gold   BC

Cross: → BC × BC
Result: 1 BB (beige)
           2 BC (gold)
           1 CC (charcoal)

Backcross: A backcross consists of crossing a dominant phenotype with a pure homozygous recessive. In this manner a breeder can determine if the phenotype is heterozygous or homozygous. The backcross is used, therefore, to determine if a line is genotypically pure.

Probability Ratios: Genetic ratios are probability ratios. If, for example, we mate (B = black dominant; b = gray recessive) two heterozygous black squirrels (Bb) and 4 offspring are produced, the ratio of 3 black and 1 gray should be probable. However, what are the chances of all black and all gray litters?

Many crosses of heterozygous (Bb) animals will result in a fairly close 3:1 ratio. We, therefore, can see that we have 3 chances out of 4 to produce an individual exhibiting the dominant trait, and 1 chance out of 4 to show the recessive trait.

Therefore, to produce black squirrels (BB or Bb, 3 out of 4) we multiply ¾ × ¾ × ¾ × ¾ = $^{81}/_{256}$; to produce gray squirrels (bb, 1 out of 4) we multiply ¼ × ¼ × ¼ × ¼ = $^{1}/_{256}$.

Polygenic Traits

In morning glories, genes C and P are necessary for pink flowers. In the absence of either (ccP__ or C__pp) or both (ccpp) of these genes, the flowers are blue. What will be the result of the following crosses as far as flower color of the offspring and proportion of the offspring are concerned? Cross a. Ccpp × ccPp = 1 pink: 3 blue; b. ccpp × CcPp = 1 pink: 3 blue.

In essence, the expression of pink requires C__P__, and all others will be blue. The offspring may be Cc or cc with equal probability (i.e., 50%); the same is true for Pp and pp (50%). If the chance of C__ is 0.5 and the chance of P__ is 0.5, then the chance of C__P__ is 0.5 × 0.5 = 0.25. Thus, ¼ will be pink and ¾ will be blue.

Sex Determination: A male carries an XY and a female an XX complement of chromosomes. If a male embryo were to result, the sperm that fertilizes an egg would have to possess a Y chromosome.

Sex-Linked Traits: Both sexes carry a complete complement of sex-linked genes. A female, however, with the XX arrangement will exhibit a recessive gene only if it has received it from both parents (a rare event if we are dealing with an uncommon gene of the population), whereas in the male with the XY arrangement the recessive gene cannot be masked since there is no partner X chromosome and, therefore, a larger number of recessive genes are expressed (examples are hemophilia and color blindness). A man receives his X chromosome from his mother and passes it on to his daughters, not his sons. His daughters in this respect are the carriers of his sex-linked traits and their sons will be the affected ones. Let us illustrate with an example. The normal czarinas of Russia produced sons suffering from hemophilia, a disease that is caused by a sex-linked recessive gene, h. The more dominant gene, H, produces normal blood clotting. Genotypically, these women must have carried Hh (X_H and X_h). A daughter, depending on the father (X_HY or X_hY), could have carried X_HX_h or X_HX_H whereas a son could have been born with either an X_HY or an X_hY (hemophilic) chromosal complement.

Another way of expressing a sex-linked or, strictly speaking, sex-limited phenomenon is shown in the example below.

A cattle breeder has in his herd a y-linked trait that produces white stockings. A calf sired by a white-stockinged bull is born. The breeder determines that the chances of white stockings by this inheritance are 50%. If the calf born had been a female, the chances of exhibiting the trait (or serving as a carrier) were zero. The explanation is that the male may contribute gametes containing either X or Y chromosomes, but the female can contribute only gametes containing X chromosomes. If the X chromosome is contributed by the male, an unaffected female offspring will result; if the Y chromosome is contributed by the male, an affected male offspring will result. These two possibilities are of equal probability (i.e., 50%). If the sex of the offspring is known, there is no doubt about whether it has the trait. All males (100%) and no females (0%) would have the trait. Females could not even be carriers for a Y-linked trait.

Mutation: A mutation may be thought of as a sudden change in the genetic makeup of the organism. It may be beneficial or harmful. It may occur spontaneously or may be experimentally produced with chemicals, X-rays, cosmic rays, and so forth. It may or may not be passed on to the next generation because, for example, it may be lethal or otherwise preclude reproduction.

Blood Types: The ABO blood grouping system is explained on the basis of a single trial-lelic system with genes A, B, and O operating at a single genetic locus. Phenotypic and genotypic characteristics may be expressed as follows:

Phenotype	Genotype
A	A/A; A/O
B	B/B; B/O
O	O/O
AB	A/B

The A and B genes appear to be codominant; they are dominant over O, which is recessive.

As can be seen from the above table, there are four major blood types and the explanation as to universal donor and recipient is based on the following:

Type	Agglutinogens on Cells	Agglutinins in Serum and Plasma
AB—can receive A, B, AB, or O (universal recipient)	A,B	none
A—can receive A, O	A	anti b
B—can receive B, O	B	anti a
O—can receive only O, but can give to all; therefore, O is the universal donor	O	anti ab

Rh Factor: Rhesus (Rh) agglutinogen is present in humans and is represented by a dominant gene R. The agglutinogen of an Rh positive fetus passes across the placenta, enters the maternal bloodstream, and elicits the production of an agglutinin (antibody) by the mother. The agglutinin passes into the circulation of the fetus and if present in sufficient concentration can produce agglutination, at times fatal to the developing fetus.

Mode of Inheritance of Some Common Human Traits: Among the human traits inherited as single-gene dominants are:

a) brachydactyly (short digits),
b) white forelock in the hair,
c) blue sclera (white of the eye),
d) Rh-positive blood.

Among the traits inherited as recessives:

a) albinism (lack of skin pigment),
b) alkaptonuria (urine turns black).

Sex-linked traits:

a) hemophilia,
b) color blindness.

Crossing-Over: During the process of meiosis a recombination of genetic material is possible. One way this is effected is through crossing-over. In crossing-over, comparable portions of chromatids are exchanged. Because crossing-over is more the rule than the exception, we shall illustrate it with two diagrams. These portions may differ in alleles but they do carry the same gene sites (loci) and control the same specific trait, as, for example, eye color.

Let us start with one pair of homologous chromosomes:

As illustrated, replication results during the first part of meiosis in four chromatids:

Of the four chromatids, two may exchange materials in a process known as crossing-over:

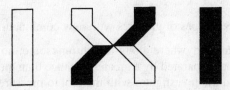

The configuration shown by the central two chromosomes is termed a chiasma, the region where crossing-over occurs. After separation in the second reduction division of meiosis, the resulting chromatids include two recombinants, having new combinations of genetic material.

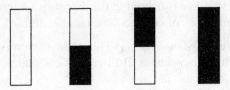

We shall next illustrate crossover using two specific genes.

Parents
```
|     |
A     a
|  +  |
B     b
|     |
```

Two gametes unite and form a new hybrid individual (F₁).

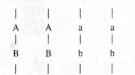

Without crossover these four gametes are produced:

With crossing-over these four gametes are produced:

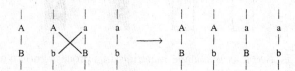

and the result is two new types of gametes with new combination of genes.

Crossing-over may occur anywhere along the chromosome; however, the recombination frequency is higher for genes separated by a greater distance than those that are close together. Crossing-over has provided the investigator with the tool to measure distances between genes and make chromosome maps.

Abnormalities in Chromosome Number: Chromosomes can be identified in somatic cells and a *karyotype,* a standardized display of an individual's chromosomes, can be constructed. Chromosomes vary in size and shape but the number is species specific. In humans the chromosome number is 46. A karyotype is helpful in the diagnosis of genetic abnormalities.

In humans some abnormalities of chromosome number are:

Down's syndrome (formerly called mongolism) This phenomenon is most often characterized by three, instead of two, chromosomes 21 in group G; a total number of 47 chromosomes are present in these individuals.

Turner's syndrome Females possess only one X chromosome (not the normal female XX). Total number of chromosomes present is 45.

Klinefelter's syndrome This syndrome is characterized by the presence of two X chromosomes and a Y, which results in 47 chromosomes being present.

Epistasis (or Gene Interaction): In morning glories, genes *C* and *P* are necessary for pink flowers. In the absence of either (*ccP__* or *C__ pp*) or both (*ccpp*) of these genes, the flowers are blue. What will be the result of the following crosses as far as flower color of the offspring and proportion of the offspring are concerned?

$$Ccpp \times ccPp = 1 \text{ pink} : 3 \text{ blue};$$
$$ccpp \times CcPp = 1 \text{ pink} : 3 \text{ blue}$$

In essence, the expression of pink requires $C\_P\_$, and all others will be blue. In this example, the epistasis is of the complementary interaction type. The offspring may be Cc or cc with equal probability (i.e., 50%); the same is true for Pp and pp (50%). If the chance of $C\_$ is 0.5 and the chance of $P\_$ is 0.5, then the chance of $C\_P\_$ is $0.5 \times 0.5 = 0.25$. Thus, ¼ will be pink and ¾ will be blue.

Polygenic Traits: Certain conditions are determined by genes at several loci. Each of the genes involved has a small effect that may be additive. Expression of this kind of trait is usually very sensitive to environmental influences.

Lethal Genes: Certain genes are lethal in the homozygous condition and cause the demise of the organism. An example is yellow coat in mice. If two hybrid yellow mice are mated, the typical 1:2:1 genotypic ratio results—namely, ¼ homozygous dominant (yellow dead embryos), ½ hybrid (yellow mice), and ¼ homozygous recessive (wild type or agouti mice), but the phenotypic ratio among the live born mice is 2 yellow : 1 gray.

Modifying Genes: These genes affect the performance of other genes but apparently exhibit no trait of their own. If, for instance, in mice the gene for black hair is present, the gene for agouti color will elicit a yellow banding. When it is absent there is no effect.

Paternity Exclusion and Reassignment of Misassigned Infants

1. Paternity will be excluded if the child

    a. has an antigen that is present in neither the mother nor the putative father;
    b. does not have an antigen that the putative father has and would have had to give to his progeny (for example, a type O child and a type AB putative father).

2. Correct reassignment of infants misassigned to parents in a hospital is often achieved by looking for any of the following kinds of incompatibilities between the infants and the couples and then assigning each infant to the couple with which only compatibilities exist:

    a. The child has an antigen present in neither spouse;
    b. The child lacks one or more antigens that either or both spouses would have had to give him/her.

3. Increased probability of exclusion of a falsely accused male or of correct parental reassignment of misassigned infants results if several kinds of blood groups, HLA, and some of the following kinds of other genetically determined proteins are also included in the studies: hemoglobins, serum proteins, red cell enzymes, and several other enzymes.

QUICK RECALL TEST QUESTIONS AND ANSWERS

Choose the Best Answer

1. Alleles are genes that:

   (A) arise during the cross-over process.
   (B) are linked to one chromosome only.
   (C) are always sex-linked and are transmitted from mothers to their sons.
   (D) occupy corresponding positions on homologous chromosomes.

2. The ABO blood group is transmitted in humans as alleles A and B that are codominant, occurring at the same genetic locus as a recessive allele O. In some cases it may be utilized to assist in determining paternity or in reuniting a lost child with his or her biological parents.

   A woman of blood type O claims a child of blood type AB, and alleges that the father is a man of blood type B. The most likely explanation is that:

   (A) these are the biological parents.
   (B) she is the mother but the man is not the father.
   (C) neither is a possible parent of the child.
   (D) she is not the mother but the man's blood type does not rule him out as the father.

3. Seeds from a self-pollinated gold flowering plant produce 56 charcoal, 130 gold, and 61 beige flowering plants. The plant is:

   (A) unhealthy.
   (B) heterozygous recessive.
   (C) heterozygous with incomplete dominance.
   (D) heterozygous with complete dominance.

4. In ant lions the gene for dull teeth is dominant D. The recessive gene d produces sharp teeth. Another gene T, when homozygous, produces dark-brown coats. Its allele t, when homozygous, produces albino coats. The heterozygote Tt is chocolate colored.

   If a chocolate-colored, dull-tooth male whose father was sharp toothed is mated to a chocolate, sharp-toothed female, what is the probability that an albino, sharp-tooth offspring will be produced?

   (A) $\frac{1}{16}$
   (B) $\frac{2}{16}$
   (C) $\frac{4}{16}$
   (D) $\frac{12}{16}$

5. A mink breeder finds that 50% of the offspring are aa. What genotype were their parents?

   (A) aa × aa
   (B) Aa × Aa
   (C) AA × aa
   (D) Aa × aa

6. During metaphase of mitosis:

   (A) there is a dissolution of the chromosomal material.
   (B) the centrioles with asters are at the opposite poles.
   (C) the cell membrane starts to reappear.
   (D) the nuclear membrane disappears.

7. A hog breeder would use a backcross to:

   (A) produce a bigger and healthier strain.
   (B) produce a larger number of offspring.
   (C) maintain a pure line of desirable traits.
   (D) determine if a particular hog is genotypically pure.

8. Rh-related hemolytic anemia of the newborn (erythroblastosis foetalis) may result when the:

   (A) father, mother, and fetus are all Rh negative.
   (B) father and mother are Rh positive, but the fetus is Rh negative.
   (C) mother is Rh negative and the fetus is Rh positive.
   (D) mother is Rh positive and the fetus is Rh negative.

9. In rabbits, rough coat is dominant over smooth coat. Brown is dominant over gray fur color. A rough, brown male is mated to a couple of smooth, gray females. The offspring present the following ratios: 18 rough, brown, 21 rough, gray; 16 smooth, brown; 24 smooth, gray. If this male had been mated to a female of his own genotype, what proportion of the offspring would have exhibited rough, gray coats?

   (A) 4 out of 16
   (B) 3 out of 32
   (C) 3 out of 16
   (D) 12 out of 16

10. Twinning is an interesting biological phenomenon. Identical twins usually result from fertilization of:

    (A) two eggs by one sperm.
    (B) one egg by two sperm.
    (C) one egg by one sperm and separation of cells during early development.
    (D) one egg and one polar body.

11. A man with blood cell genotype B/O marries a woman with type A/B. Their offspring could have:

    (A) A/B, B/B, A/O, B/O.
    (B) A/B and B/O only.
    (C) A/O and B/B only.
    (D) none of the combinations above.

12. Two people are planning to have a family. The woman has blood type A/A and the man B/B. Their children might have the following:

    (A) A and B.
    (B) B only.
    (C) A/B only.
    (D) A and B and A/B.

13. Alleles are genes that:

    (A) arise during the cross-over process.
    (B) are linked to one chromosome only.
    (C) are always sex-linked and are transmitted from mothers to their sons.
    (D) occupy corresponding positions on homologous chromosomes.

14. Phenotype may be defined as:

    (A) genetic makeup of an individual.
    (B) hidden traits of an individual.
    (C) unrelated characteristics.
    (D) visible expression of genotype.

15. The czarinas of Russia and the queens of England produced sons suffering from hemophilia, a disease that is caused by a sex-linked recessive gene, h. The more common dominant gene, H, produces normal blood clotting. Genotypically, these women must have carried:

    (A) HH.
    (B) Hh.
    (C) hh.
    (D) none of the above.

16. The hematology laboratory reports to the surgeon that his patient's blood clumped with both anti A and anti B serum. The patient's blood type is:

    (A) AB.
    (B) A.
    (C) B.
    (D) O.

17. The hematology laboratory reports to the surgeon that his patient's blood clumped with both anti A and anti B serum. In this case, what percentage of the population would the surgeon expect to have the blood type of the patient?

    (A) 47
    (B) 41
    (C) 15
    (D) 3

18. The ABO blood grouping system is explained on the basis of a single triallelic system with genes A, B, and O operating at a single genetic locus. Phenotypic and genotypic characteristics may be expressed as follows:

Phenotype	Genotype
A	A/A; A/O
B	B/B; B/O
O	O/O
AB	A/B

    The A and B genes appear to be codominant; they are dominant over O, which is recessive. Transfusions have become relatively safe under this system. The universal recipient is considered to be type:

    (A) A.
    (B) B.
    (C) O.
    (D) AB.

19. The ABO blood grouping system is explained on the basis of a single triallelic system with genes A, B, and O operating at a single genetic locus. Phenotypic and genotypic characteristics may be expressed as follows:

Phenotype	Genotype
A	A/A; A/O
B	B/B; B/O
O	O/O
AB	A/B

The A and B genes appear to be codominant; they are dominant over O, which is recessive. Which of the following agglutinogens do these individuals carry on their red blood cells?

(A) A
(B) B
(C) O
(D) A,B

20. The ABO blood grouping system is explained on the basis of a single triallelic system with genes A, B, and O operating at a single genetic locus. Phenotypic and genotypic characteristics may be expressed as follows:

Phenotype	Genotype
A	A/A; A/O
B	B/B; B/O
O	O/O
AB	A/B

The A and B genes appear to be codominant; they are dominant over O, which is recessive. A person of blood type A can receive blood of type(s):

(A) A.
(B) B; A.
(C) O.
(D) A; O.

Answers

1. **(D)** An allele is one of a pair of genes that occupies the same locus on homologous chromosomes.

2. **(D)** This woman is not the mother. She can contribute only the O gene, and this child must receive an A gene from one parent and a B gene from the other parent. The man cannot be ruled out as the father with the limited information given, since he can contribute a B gene to a child.

3. **(C)** The phenomenon illustrated here is incomplete dominance (blending of two traits). Let us assume:

charcoal C
beige B
gold BC
Cross: BC × BC
Result: 1 BB (beige)
2 BC (gold)
1 CC (charcoal)

4. **(B)** Basic genetic knowledge applies:

dull teeth—D
sharp teeth—d
dark-brown—T
albino—t
chocolate—Tt

The male is TtDd; the female Ttdd; want ttdd offspring; what proportion? The male provides us with the following TD, Td, tD, td. The female provides us with the following Td, Td, td, td. $\frac{2}{16}$ of the offspring will be ttdd.

5. **(D)** Use your basic genetic knowledge.

(1) 100% aa
(2) 25% AA, 50% Aa, 25% aa
(3) 100 Aa
(4) 50% Aa, 50% aa

6. **(B)** During metaphase of mitosis the centrioles with asters are at the opposite poles; the chromosomes are at the equator of the cell.

7. **(D)** A backcross consists of crossing a dominant phenotype with a pure homozygous recessive. In this manner the breeder determines if the phenotype is heterozygous or homozygous.

8. **(C)** Multiple alleles determine the human blood types. The common blood types are A, B, AB, and O. Red blood cells of a person classified as Type A contain Agglutinogen A and their serum contains Agglutinin b. Type AB contains agglutinogens A and B but no agglutinins. Type O possesses no agglutinogens but the serum carries a + b agglutinins. Rhesus (Rh) agglutinogen is present in humans and is represented by a dominant gene R. The agglutinogen of an Rh positive fetus passes across the placenta, enters the maternal bloodstream, and elicits the production of an agglutinin (antibody) by the mother. The agglutinin passes into the circulation of the fetus, and if present in sufficient concentration can produce agglutination, at times fatal to the developing fetus.

9. **(C)** Basic genetic knowledge applies:

rough—R (dominant)
smooth—r (recessive)
brown—B (dominant)
gray—b (recessive)

The male is crossed to several smooth gray females; the females had to be homozygous recessive genotype. Since all four combinations appeared, we can assume that the male was genotypically heterozytous even though he appeared phenotypically dominant. If first we crossed this heterozygous male RrBb × rrbb, the result would be RrBb, rrBb; rrbb; Rrbb—in other words, the four combinations given. Now let us cross the RrBb male × RrBb female; the following combinations would have to be considered in both male and female: RB, Rb; rB; rb. If these are crossed, we find that 3 out of 16 possess rough gray coats (namely, RRbb; Rrbb and Rrbb).

10. **(C)** Identical twins arise from the same egg. One egg is fertilized by one sperm and a splitting (separation) occurs during early development. Fraternal twins arise from the fertilization of two eggs, each by one sperm. Identical twins always are the same sex. Fraternal twins may be of either sex (50–50 proposition).

11. **(A)** The ABO blood grouping system is explained on the basis of a single triallelic system with genes A, B, and O operating at a single genetic locus. Phenotypic and genotypic characteristics may be expressed as follows:

Phenotype	Genotype
A	A/A; A/O
B	B/B; B/O
O	O/O
AB	A/B

The A and B genes appear to be codominant; they are dominant over O, which is recessive.

12. **(C)** The ABO blood grouping system is explained on the basis of a single triallelic system with genes A, B, and O operating at a single genetic locus. Phenotypic and genotypic characteristics may be expressed as follows:

Phenotype	Genotype
A	A/A; A/O
B	B/B; B/O
O	O/O
AB	A/B

The A and B genes appear to be codominant; they are dominant over O, which is recessive.

13. **(D)** An allele is one of a pair of genes that occupies the same locus on homologous chromosomes.

14. **(D)** Genotype refers to the genetic makeup of the organism. The genotype is expressed via phenotypic characteristics that are visible and observable under normal circumstances.

15. **(B)** Hemophilia, a frequent disease of the royal houses of Europe, is a bleeding disorder transmitted through a sex-linked recessive gene. It results in abnormal coagulation; hemophilia A is the classical true hemophilia, resulting from a deficiency of factor VIII.

16. **(A)** Four primary blood groups are found in humans: O (47%), A (41%), B (9%), and AB (3%). These blood groups are based on the presence or absence of antigens (agglutinogens) on red blood cells and antibodies (agglutinins) in the serum.

17. **(D)** Four primary blood groups are found in humans: O (47%), A (41%), B (9%), and AB (3%). These blood groups are based on the presence or absence of antigens (agglutinogens) on red blood cells and antibodies (agglutinins) in the serum.

18, 19, and 20.

(D) As can be seen from the table, there are four major blood types, and the explanation as to universal donor and recipient is based on the following:

Type	Agglutinogens on Cells	Agglutins in Serum and Plasma
AB—can receive A, B, AB, or O (universal recipient)	A, B	none
A—can receive A, O	A	anti b
B—can receive B, O	B	anti a
O—can receive only O, but can give to all; therefore, O is the universal donor	O	anti ab

THE ANIMAL KINGDOM
Distribution of Living Organisms

Every living organism has a distinct yet interactive role, a place, and a mode of life, which are determined by that individual's structure and physiological makeup. The earth represents diverse *habitats* (places where one lives), which are characterized by conditions such as temperature, moisture, soil conditions, terrain, pressure, chemical cycles (gases and minerals), sunlight, seasonal variations, and others; organisms (species) must adapt and adjust their *life cycles* to the *climate* they live in. No species lives in a vacuum and is entirely independent; all are part of an integrated, systematically functioning, living (dynamic) *community* that includes many varieties of plants, animals, viruses, etc.

Although many populations of different species live together as a *community,* and although *turnover* is continuous, automatic, and self-adjusting, the result is an internally balanced community; there is a remarkable numerically steady state that is determined essentially by food supply, reproduction, and protection of the bonds of interdependency of community members.

Six factors are important to any habitat.

1. *Temperature* controls the speed of every reaction; raising the temperature by 10°C doubles the speed. Although there exists a large range of temperature, most life exists in a narrow range; species have limits, and most are destroyed by excess at either end of the scale. Warm-blooded organisms (mammals and birds) possess internal regulation of body temperature, whereas cold-blooded animals (fishes, reptiles, amphibians, and invertebrates) do not and their function is directly related to their external environment. The oceans represent a fairly stable environment, and marine organisms are less prone to seasonal variations. Many land animals have adapted to seasonal changes by migration or hibernation.

2. *Moisture* (water) is critical to the existence of life since it is a solvent (minerals used by plants), a constituent of tissues, and the medium in which many species live and breed. The water cycle (evaporation, cloud formation, precipitation, drainage, and soil percolation) is dynamic and continuous (between sea, land, and air) and affects every particle of the universe. Also, water prevents rapid temperature fluctuations, a critical element in homeostasis.

3. *Soil conditions* are a crucial factor. The chemical makeup of the soil determines the presence or type of plants and, in some cases, the animals of the region. Texture and porosity play a role in moisture content, pH, and the presence or absence of burrowing animals. Slope affects drainage, while exposure to sunlight modulates absorption of heat.

4. *Pressure* varies with elevation (atmospheric pressure reflected in barometric reading) and with depth (water pressure: 15 pounds/10 meters equals one atmosphere of pressure). Availability of oxygen decreases with increasing altitude and depth. People living at high altitudes have higher red blood cell (erythrocyte) counts to compensate.

5. *Chemical interchange* occurs continuously in all habitats. Here are three good examples:

   a. Oxygen derived from air and water serves the oxidative machinery of life; after usage it returns to the life cycle in the form of carbon dioxide or, combined with hydrogen, as water. Carbon dioxide is used in the process of photosynthesis; some of the oxygen released is utilized by plants in respiration, but most is returned to the environment.

   b. Nitrogen is utilized directly by nitrogen-fixing bacteria to produce plant proteins; after utilization by animals these become animal proteins, and their eventual metabolic fate results in nitrogeneous wastes. These wastes are converted by bacteria into nitrites and ammonia with release of nitrogen into the atmosphere; the nitrites are converted into nitrates, which again are utilized to make plant proteins.

   c. Carbon is the backbone of protoplasm; it is derived from carbon dioxide (via photosynthesis) and synthesized into carbohydrates, which, together with proteins and fats, comprise the tissues of all plants and animals. Metabolism returns carbon for recycling as carbon dioxide.

6. *Sunlight* provides all the energy utilized by most living organisms. Energy is transformed from one type to another, but it is neither created nor destroyed. Lavoisier (1743–1794) showed that processes of organisms conform to the First Law of Thermodynamics—namely, the total amount of energy in a system is constant but is capable of transformation. Radiation from the sun includes heat, visible light, and ultraviolet radiation. Solar radiation, especially of the longer wavelengths, controls most climatic variations because of the effects of soil heating, water evaporation, and air expansion. Light controls the photoperiod responsible for the flowering of plants and the migration of animals.

Interrelationships of Animals

Competition for food, shelter, and mates is considerable; some organisms (termites, bees), however, have developed a cooperative society based on distinct roles (workers, protectors, reproducers, nurses, etc.). Plants (producers—autotrophs) commonly compete for sunlight (energy), minerals, and water. The passing of energy from one organism to another constitutes the *food chain* or pyramid; the small (more abundant) are eaten by the large (fewer in number). Plants are eaten by *herbivores* (primary consumers); these in turn are eaten by *carnivores* (secondary consumers); and as larger carnivores eat smaller ones, the energy is passed along the chain. As the energy is transferred through the predator chain, the total declines progressively, and successive members are usually larger in size but fewer in number. Organisms eaten by a predator are called *prey;* an organism that consumes its own species is considered a *cannibal,* and one that devours dead material is a *scavenger.*

Factors such as disease control the number of organisms in the food chain; organisms such as viruses, rickettsias, bacteria, protozoans, parasitic worms, and arthropods which by themselves are populations also control the populations on/in which they live. The *parasite* obtains its food from its host, generally harming the host. *Ectoparasites* (lice) live *on* the host, while *endoparasites* (trichina worm) live *in* the host (gut or tissues). Some parasites such as the tick are intermediate hosts, as demonstrated in the transmission of Rocky Mountain spotted fever. Parasites that may destroy the host are called *pathogenic,* and are a considerable element in the regulation and control of the host population. All viruses are parasitic, and bacteria that lack photosynthetic abilities (are saprotrophic) are also parasitic.

The long-term relationship of two organisms of different species is commonly referred to as *symbiosis.* When one gains without harming the other, we speak of *commensalism* (barnacles on whales and epiphytes—plants—that grow on another host plant); in *mutualism* both parties are benefited (the flagellate in the termite digests the wood the termite eats, and the tick bird on the rhinoceros eats ticks, and cleans and warns the larger animal of danger).

Saprophytism is the obtaining of food from dead or decaying material (bacteria of decay and filamentous fungi are examples); the saprophytes essentially function to release chemicals back to the food chain. Without their role many essential elements would soon be unavailable, and the balance of energy transfer and transformation would be disturbed.

As previously emphasized, no organism can be successful in isolation because every specialized being depends on others for some product or process. The smallest congregation of like organisms is the *family;* a larger number constitutes a *population.* The key element of a population is the fact that its members interbreed with one another; all populations are composed of *species.* Reproductive barriers exist between species. Speciation has many causes, such as separation by differences in climate, mountain ranges, rivers, or just distance. Only inheritable variations (e.g., skin color) controlled by genes are transmitted to new generations; acquired ones (e.g., muscle build) die with the individual. Individual variations of the members of a species are denoted as *polymorphism,* and the differences due only to sex are referred to as dimorphism.

All organisms live together in a dynamic state under the influence of environmental (chemical and physical) factors; not all are friendly since natural enemies exist for every species (they consume one another or compete for the same food source). Protective adaptation helps in survival. Many organisms blend well into their surroundings (polar bears are white), so that they are hard to see; some organisms such as the flounder can adapt readily to several backgrounds, and others (insects are good examples) mimic their surroundings (butterflies look like flowers and leaves).

Another process facilitating survival is *holotropism,* which denotes eating other living cells as a whole.

All the processes discussed so far are self-limiting. Parasitism, saprotrophism, and holotrophism (known collectively as heterotrophic forms of nutrition) merely affect distribution of foodstuff without adding resources.

In order for the evolutionary process to progress, a new way of synthesizing organic material was needed. Organisms evolved that could utilize external energy to produce organic compounds; we now speak of *autotrophs.* Two types evolved. Organisms that could utilize inorganic material, break the chemical bonds, and convert this energy into metabolic products (specifically, carbohydrates) appeared, and the process became known as *chemosynthesis* (carried out by chemosynthesizers).

The sun, however, came to the rescue as an energy source to solve the food problem. Light-trapping mechanisms evolved and the substance chlorophyll saved the day. The process of converting CO_2 and water into food is called *photosynthesis.*

Population Dynamics

According to their mode of mobility, organisms are classifed as *free-living* (the organism gets around by itself) or *sessile* (it is fixed to another structure). Among both groups there are *solitary* (independent) individuals and others that live in colonies (groups).

All organisms of one species that live in a definable area comprise a population that has distinct organizational features.

As part of the group dynamics of a population, certain factors must be considered:

1. **population density**—the number of organisms in a unit of area,
2. **birth rate**—the number of new organisms per unit of time,
3. **mortality rate**—the number of organisms dying per unit of time,
4. **reproductive or biotic potential**—the potential of a population to increase its numbers under optimal conditions.

Populations are usually considered in terms of the number per unit occupying a given area. As mentioned before, the number of larger organisms is considerably smaller. *Biotic potential* (maximum rate of increase) is continuously checked by *environmental resistance* (competition, disease, inclement climate, etc.). When a population settles in a new area, growth at first is slow (lack of mates), then increases rapidly (exponentially), and finally levels off as an equilibrium is reached because of limits of food supply, the settling of suitable habitats, and the increase of parasites and predators. Usually, as a population increases the environmental resistance, which initially was low, also increases as a result of population density.

A dynamic community of different plants and animals (interdependent) evolves to form an *ecosystem* with the physical environment. No situation is permanent; and although some changes occur rapidly, most are due to a sequential *succession* (lake-pond-swamp-grassland). No one species is present in every corner of the world; geography (geographical range) and environment (ecological range) are key elements. Physical (land and water), climatic (temperature and moisture), and biological (food and predators) barriers are limiting factors to the spread of populations.

Each species requires certain minimal elements for growth and reproduction; this fact led Liebig in 1840 to formulate the "law of the minimum," which states that the rate of growth of an organism is limited by the factor present in the scarcest amount. Too much of a certain factor, according to Shelford (1913), can be just as limiting since the well being of a species is determined by its *range of tolerance.* Organisms are usually more sensitive during development and early and late in life. The range varies greatly from factor to factor. *Stenothermic* organisms can tolerate only slight variations in temperature, while *eurythermic* organisms are able to survive a wide range.

Major Environments–Habitats

1. **Water:**

   a. *Salt Water.* Over 70 percent of the earth is covered by salt water, and the environment, although varying widely overall, is quite stable in a specific region in regard to temperature (a range of 35°C), gas composition, and salinity (30–37 parts of salt per thousand). Ocean currents affect movements of marine organisms and the adjacent regional climate. Tidal fluctuations affect organisms in the shore region. Depth varies, pressure increases with depth, and light decreases with depth (about a 600-ft. limit).

   b. *Fresh Water.* Freshwater bodies are scattered in their distribution, have less volume and depth, and exhibit great variability in temperature, gas composition, mineral content, light penetration, and mobility. Organisms living in fresh water, because of its low salinity (low osmotic pressure), have had to develop organs for effectively regulating the osmotic pressure. Unlike oceans, freshwater bodies are subject to periodic drying, changing flow rates, and high turbidity.

2. **Land or Terrestrial Habitat:** The greatest variability is present on land, when one considers minerals, topography, temperature, water content, air movement, and light. Temperature and moisture vary tremendously with the seasons, altitude, latitude, and with topography. Soil and air temperatures vary as much as 120°C.

Learning, Conditioning, Rhythms

1. **Learning:** Many definitions of learning exist, but the process of learning, simply defined, is a change in the behavior of an organism based on some experience or practice. Many organisms have been very successful without much learning; their inborn patterns or instincts allow them to compete for food, find shelter, mate, and live out their life spans. Familiar examples of instinctive behavior are spiders spinning webs (specific patterns), birds building nests and migrating and returning, and fish returning to spawning grounds thousands of miles away. More complex, but still instinctive, are societies of bees and ants where a definite division of labor exists. Humans, on the other hand, although high in the evolutionary scale, must learn from their interaction with the environment and use that knowledge to succeed; for many years a human child is quite dependent, while most animals from day 1 are quite independent. Changes in behavior are often hard to assess but might include:

   a. a new pattern of the organism, and
   b. a change in the response to a stimulus not previously exhibited.

2. **Conditioning:** Many of our actions seem automatic, and in most instances we cannot attribute definite reasons for them. These behaviors (responses) may be learned even though we have no recollection of the learning process. On the other hand, many actions are unlearned reflexes. An example of the latter is the fact that the autonomic nervous sytem (sympathetic and parasympathetic) allows an organism to adapt to certain phenomena. When we walk into bright sunlight the sphincter pupillae contracts, but if we enter a dark area the dilator opens the pupillary opening; the sphincter is under parasympathetic, and the dilater under sympathetic, control. For close vision (reading) convergence and change in the shape of the lens allow the eye to accommodate. Salivary secretion (parotid, submandibular, and sublingual glands) and tearing by the lacrimal gland of the eye are other superb examples of these homeostatic reflexes. Fright produces an increase in heart rate, blood pressure, and metabolic states to prepare an organism to cope; all this takes place at the subconscious level.

Classical Conditioning. Some actions, however, can be learned by a process called *classical conditioning,* that is, learning to associate two previously linked phenomena. First reported by Pavlov in 1927, it is exemplified by the responses of dogs to the introduction of food. When a dog sees or smells food, it is stimulated to begin a reflexive behavior—secretion of saliva. Pavlov restrained dogs in a harness and then simply used an auditory stimulus such as a bell. When the bell was rung, the dog did not secrete saliva. When food alone was provided, the expected salivary secretion occurred. If, thereafter, the two stimuli—bell and food—were presented for some time simultaneously, salivary secretion occurred. After many trials, the bell alone elicited the salivary response; the dog had learned to react to a different stimulus via conditioning. In 1920 Watson showed the same reaction in an 11-month-old baby, who was conditioned by a loud noise and the presentation of a furry object to eventually be frightened by fur alone. Many of the results of conditioning can be reversed through reconditioning the organism to a different association.

Pavlov identified five components of classical conditioning:

1. unconditioned stimulus—the food; it automatically stimulates salivation;
2. conditioned stimulus—the bell; it is neutral at the beginning but eventually effective and undistinguishable;
3. reinforcement—the pairing of two stimuli;
4. unconditioned response—salivation—the automatic response by the parasympathetic division of the autonomic nervous system;
5. conditioned response—the bell—the response as a result of learning by the central nervous system; the unconditioned and conditioned stimuli function as one.

Five other aspects of conditioning should be mentioned.

1. Extinction. The conditioned response can be reversed. Pavlov showed that, after an animal was conditioned, if for some time thereafter only the bell was rung without food being offered, the flow of saliva started to decrease and eventually stopped.
2. Spontaneous Recovery. In this set of experiments, Pavlov let a response achieve extinction and then gave the animal a long rest from the experimental protocol. After this rest the bell was rung and the response reappeared. This spontaneous recovery may explain phenomena we all experience, such as fears or preferences for certain things for which we have no conscious basis.
3. Stimulus Generalization. In these experiments, Pavlov was able to show that somewhat different but basically similar stimuli (e.g., different tones of music) may evoke the same response and effect. The more similar the new stimulus is to the familiar one, the stronger the response usually will be.
4. Stimulus Discrimination. In another set of experiments, food was offered to animals only at the sound of a specific bell, and salivation was elicited only when that particular bell was rung. The animal did not salivate at the ringing of a different bell; it had learned to discriminate between different stimuli.
5. Onset of Neurotic Behavior. In 1927 Pavlov also observed that, after an animal had learned stimulus discrimination and then the difference between the two stimuli was decreased to the point where the animal could not recognize it, the animal's behavior became unpredictable and aberrant.

In general, conditioning is best accomplished when a short interval between stimuli is used and when positive phenomena are elicited or are the end result. Conditioning is also enhanced when the stimulus is truly different (strong and novel) from many of the background stimuli.

Operant Conditioning. The results described above are due chiefly to the influence of the learning process on autonomic reflexes. However, other forms of behavior are also of consequence in reactions to stimuli. When, for instance, a cat is introduced into a new environment, the animal will react by exploring and marking its territory. In this case, the organism itself is acting on the environment, as Skinner demonstrated in the 1930s with the help of a box and a food bar to reward the animal for a certain action.

In 1938 Skinner observed that a rat placed in a box explored actively and even pressed a bar that released a pellet of food. At first the animal did not make an association but soon learned to connect the pressing of the food lever with the dispensing of food and a reward for the action of pressing. The key element in this situation is that reinforced operant behavior is repeated (the lever is pressed frequently), while nonreinforced activities are quickly abandoned. Extinction, spontaneous recovery, and stimulus generalization and discrimination are also part of operant behavior.

Instrumental Conditioning (Operant) and the Law of Effect. In 1898 Thorndike addressed similar issues and found that, when cats were placed in a box and had to learn to open the door in order to obtain food, the reward enhanced their conditioning. The law of effect essentially states that, when a stimulus is followed by a reward, the response is strong, consistent, and likely to be repeated by the experimental subject.

Certain factors called *reinforcers* have been identified by psychological researchers:

1. Primary—in animals, food and water.
2. Secondary—love and affection, shown, for example, by petting.
3. Immediate—a reward given on accomplishing a feat produces the most efficient learning.
4. Constant—repeated (short-interval) stimuli result in very efficient and rapid learning.
5. Partial—extinction is less apt to occur if there is at least partial reinforcement.

Operant Escape—Escape Learning. When an animal is exposed to an unpleasant stimulus (shock), it will quickly learn to leave the environment to avoid the experience.

Operant Avoidance—Active Avoidance Learning. If an animal is conditioned to a warning signal (bell) and knows that a shock will follow it will heed the warning and rapidly leave the hostile environment.

Aversive Conditioning. In this experimental setup the unconditioned stimulus is offensive and is of negative value to the organism. In this case the organism (e.g., after a shock is administered) not only exhibits a specific response such as muscular twitching but also develops a generalized "fear reaction," which results in modification of heart rate, respiratory activity, sweating, etc.

Primary Activities. Many activities occur as the organism goes through life, but some very organized ones are limited to early development. Human beings are fairly helpless, but other animals (e.g., rats) on day 1 can perform highly complex motor patterns independently. Two classical phenomena of rat behavior will serve as examples:

1. Suckling. Suckling involves some very complicated sensory input aspects, helps meet the nutritional needs of the organism, is an effective reinforcing activity leading to other skills, and provides thermal support and transport for the young. In order for suckling to occur, the mother's nipple must be coated by amniotic fluid, saliva, or both; the pup in utero swallows and excretes amniotic fluid during the last trimester and it is that familiarity with the substances that directs the pup's first act of suckling. Also, because the mother licks the pups and the nipples (milk-line), saliva is a behavioral stimulus. The key factor in this primary activity is that it is the animal's previous exposure to the stimulus that leads it to react to it (it has had gustatory and olfactory clues). Thereafter, however, the pup's saliva becomes the stimulus. Ability of the pup to adapt to its new environment is categorized as developmental plasticity.
2. Huddling. This activity is undertaken by neonates and is beneficial in temperature regulation, which results in less energy expenditure by the young (a homeostatic response). Huddling is not a self-serving mechanism; it benefits the whole brood. An animal starting at the periphery will eventually end up in the center, and so on; the shifting of places helps the group to survive and to adapt to and identify with littermates. Young animals that know their littermates will find their nest readily.

Conditioning and Biofeedback. Biofeedback manipulation is an attempt by the physician to let the individual know what his/her spontaenous functions—heart rate, blood pressure, respiratory activity, skin and internal body temperature, brain waves, peristaltic activity, muscular activity—are at a particular time and circumstance. Patients learn, for example, to recognize when their muscles are tense and may with conditioning be able to relax them to avoid spasms or relieve tension; in the same way vascular headaches may perhaps be avoided. In these procedures patients learn to manipulate and control nonconscious processes. Although results have been mixed, this arena has excited the imagination of researchers and is undergoing active analysis.

3.   Rhythms—Biological Clocks: Interest has mainly focused on rhythms that appear in close approximation with natural periodicities such as day-night cycles; tidal rhythms; monthly, seasonal and annual phenomena; circadian rhythms (about 24 hours); and circatidal rhythms (12-hour cycles in marine organisms).

Rhythms are present from the cellular to the tissue-organ-system-organismal level, and from unicellular organisms to humans. Circadian rhythms persist even when the cues for the cycle are deleted. When cues are controlled, cycles are extremely constant and exact, but in the wild they tend to vary slightly. There is considerable evidence that endogenous and autonomic, genetically controlled mechanisms account for the persistence of rhythms.

Most living things, both animals and plants, show a circadian rhythm of activity and rest. It is well documented that humans perform differently on physiological and psychological tests at different periods of the day and night. Local time is not a critical factor, as has been well established by shift workers who work at night and sleep during the day; the shift worker's temperature is falling during the daytime, while in the rest of the population, which is working, temperatures are rising. The shift workers at the same time exhibits low levels of adrenal steroids, while in the rest of the population levels are high. These are relevant examples that the body's biological clock adjusts to the mechanical clock of society.

Characteristics of Rhythms. Rhythms are usually described in terms of four characteristics.

1.   *Period*— the number of times required to complete the cycle; it is the time between peaks.
2.   *Frequency*—the number of times that a peculiar event, such as sleeping occurs.
3.   *Phase*—time location when a specific event occurs in a particular organism; the highs and lows of a substance are phase phenomena. Adrenal corticosteroid levels in day and night workers can be described as 180 degrees out of phase;
4.   *Amplitude*—the extent (amount) of change that takes place (e.g., body temperature varies as much as 2° during one cycle).

Factors that Affect Rhythms. Among the commonly cited factors that influence rhythms are these six:

1.   geomagnetic fields,
2.   cosmic rays,
3.   electric fields,
4.   X-rays,
5.   light and darkness,
6.   atmospheric pressure.

Cycles can be disrupted by many factors; commonly cited ones are shift work, jet travel, and space flight.

Importance of Rhythms. As a consequence of our daily circadian rhythms we have a susceptibility or a resistance to drugs, stress, allergy, pain, infection, and many other factors. The responsiveness to different regimens, doses, and procedures have ramifications in therapeutic plans. The outcome of surgical procedures and the effect of anesthetic agents certainly are influenced by rhythms and the time they were performed and administered, respectively. Pain tolerance, for instance, shifts according to the time of day (more pain is experienced at night). What is just an annoyance at one time in the cycle is fatal at another point. Births and deaths mainly occur at night and in the early morning. Ulcers, allergies, and psychoses are more prevalent in the spring. Arctic hysteria is a winter phenomenon. In humans, deaths from arteriosclerotic disease peak in January and suicides in May.

To illustrate the importance of rhythms in every activity, here is a partial list of the factors they influence:

1. Body and skin temperature
2. Blood pressure
3. Pulse rate
4. Respiration
5. Blood sugar levels and glucose tolerance
6. Hemoglobin levels
7. Protein utilization and amino acid levels
8. Production and breakdown of ATP
9. Adrenal hormone levels
10. Urinary production, volume, and rate and urinary electrolytes
11. Mitosis
12. Enzyme activities
13. EEG rhythms
14. Stamina and physical vigor
15. Emotional state
16. Metabolic rate
17. Pancreatic enzymatic activity and insulin production

QUICK RECALL TEST QUESTIONS AND ANSWERS

Choose the Best Answer

1. The relationship of two organisms living together for their mutual benefit is classified as:

    (A) symbiosis.
    (B) commensalism.
    (C) saprophytism.
    (D) parasitism.

2. The stimulus that induces migration in animals is:

    (A) hydrotrophic.
    (B) photoperiodic.
    (C) geotrophic.
    (D) hydroperiodic.

3. The functional role that an organism plays in a community is referred to as its:

    (A) habitat.
    (B) home range.
    (C) niche.
    (D) environment.

4. Some marine animals have unusual rhythms of behavior because:

    (A) tides function as the external determinant.
    (B) their eyes perceive only ultraviolet light.
    (C) the moon hypnotizes them.
    (D) circadian rhythms do not affect them.

5. If a new species were to develop, which of the following phenomena would have to be considered as having played a predominant determining role?

    (A) geographical isolation
    (B) migration every year
    (C) extensive outbreeding
    (D) extensive inbreeding

6. The ecological niche of an organism denotes:

    (A) where the organism lives.
    (B) on whom the organism feeds.
    (C) the status of an organism within the ecosystem.
    (D) the habits of the organism.

7. An ecosystem is composed of:

    (A) producers.
    (B) consumers.
    (C) decomposers and nonliving components.
    (D) all of the above.

8. Which of the following statements is not correct?

    (A) Most life exists in a narrow range of temperature.
    (B) Cold- and warm-blooded organisms possess internal regulation of body temperature.
    (C) Water is a critical component of life.
    (D) Texture and porosity of the soil play a role in moisture content.

9. Which of the following is not considered under the phenomenon of conditioning?

    (A) stimulus
    (B) response
    (C) reinforcement
    (D) phototropism

Answers

1. **(A)** Symbiosis is defined as association of organisms from which each member derives some advantage. Commensalism is defined as association of organisms which share the same food and so forth (one utilizing the leftovers from the other). Saprophytism is defined as organisms living on dead organisms or products of living ones; they bring about putrefaction or decay. Parasitism is defined as organisms that live in or on their hosts and feed on their tissues or their products.

2. **(B)** Alternating periods of light and darkness and the proportion thereof is extremely important to the functioning (cycles) of plant and animal life observed.

3. **(C)** A niche is defined as the position or status that an organism occupies with respect to the other organisms with which it associates.

4. **(A)** Tides are important determinants for some marine animals.

5. **(A)** Geographical isolation is a most important factor for the development of a new species.

6. **(C)** An ecological niche defines the status of an organism within a particular community. An organism has a habitat which denotes where an organism lives. The niche places it in relation to the other organisms that live in the same surroundings (e.g., it will indicate who the organism feeds on and who feeds on it).

7. **(D)** An ecosystem such as a pond may be divided into a nonliving part that is composed of the water, gases, inorganic salts, and many organic compounds and a living entity that is made up of:

   (1) producers—the green plants
   (2) consumers—insects, crustacea, fish, etc.
   (3) decomposers—bacteria and fungi

8. **(B)** Cold-blooded organisms do not possess internal regulation of body temperature.

9. **(D)** Phototropism is a response to light by a plant.

EVOLUTION

The cornerstone of evolution is the fact that species arise from preexisting species.

Key People and Concepts

Aristotle (384–332 B.C.) philosophized that living organisms represent a succession and progression of more suitable forms, rather than random creations.

Redi (1627–1697) showed by experiment that organisms do not arise spontaneously from nonliving material; he demonstrated that maggots did not appear in meat unless the meat was exposed to flies, which laid their eggs on it.

Spallanzani (1729–1799) repeated Redi's work and showed that no life appeared in solutions first boiled and then protected from air.

Lamarck (1744–1829) believed that simple animals and plants are spontaneously generated but that lineage presents a series of evolutionary forms and that there can be independent branching and development. However, his incorrect ideas of inherited characteristics and of use and disuse of parts overshadowed his correct ideas that individual variations are retained because of adaptive value and that these variations lead to the emergence of different species suited for particular environments.

John Ray (1627–1705) was the first to attempt to define a species and to point out the difference between constant and incidental features of organisms.

Louis Pasteur (1822–1895) showed that life cannot arise in a medium from which all living things are excluded.

Charles Darwin (1809–1882) and *Alfred Russel Wallace* (1823–1913) documented the fact that natural processes can bring about a gradual development of new types.

Alfred Russel Wallace sent a manuscript to Darwin that dealt with the tendency of organisms to depart from the original type. Wallace had observed the same things as Darwin had on his voyage on the *Beagle,* and Darwin, being the scholar and gentleman he was, forwarded Wallace's article for publication and included a short article on his own observations. The failure of the articles to arouse much interest gave Darwin the impetus to proceed with his own work, and in 1859 he published his *Origin of Species by Natural Selection.* He argued two main premises:

1. No two members of a species are exactly alike even if they have the same parents.
2. Some variations are advantages, giving the organism the chance to branch out into new environments and to enlarge its numbers, whereas others are detrimental and diminish its chances of survival.

These premises lead to the conclusion that a population is likely to change in the relative frequency of its various characteristics (i.e., it *evolves*), because of the *natural selection* of some characteristics over others. The environment was cited as a major cause of natural selection, because it weeds out organisms with unfavorable characteristics and strengthens those with favorable variations.

As one can gather, the modern theory of evolution is not the work of a single individual, but it was Darwin, via his careful documentation and voluminous writings, who marshaled the evidence.

Mechanisms of Evolution on a Small Scale (Microevolution)

Two conceptual frameworks have heavily influenced modern thinking about microevolution. These are not competing explanations, but represent two ways of describing the same pattern. Both conceptual frameworks view evolution as occurring in *populations,* which are groups of organisms of one species that occur in the same place at the same time.

Evolution by natural selection (as proposed by Darwin and Wallace) occurs because of the following patterns.

1. Organisms within a population vary in their characteristics.
2. At least some of the variations in a population are inheritable.
3. More organisms are produced in each generation than live to reproduce.
4. Organisms with some variations within a population (the best-adapted variations) are more likely to survive and reproduce than are other organisms.

Evolution may also be viewed as occurring as a result of failure of the genetic equilibrium described by Hardy and Weinberg. The Hardy-Weinberg Law in population genetics states that as long as 5 conditions are reasonably well met, gene frequencies in a population will be constant. In other words, no evolution will occur. Therefore, violations of these conditions could result in evolution. The 5 conditions for the Hardy-Weinberg Law to be valid are as follows:

1. The population must be large enough that random fluctuations in gene frequency are unimportant. This usually requires population sizes of hundreds or thousands of organisms.
2. Mating in the population must be random, or at least no mate selection based on phenotypes must occur.
3. No net gene flow (selective immigration or emigration of organisms or reproductive structures) may occur into or out of the population.
4. No net mutations may occur in the population. This requirement can be met if mutational equilibrium exists (if changes offset each other).
5. No natural selection (differential survival and/or reproduction based on phenotypes) may occur in the population.

Current views of mechanisms of microevolution incorporate multiple possible mechanisms of evolution. Evolution requires production of genetic variations in a population followed by selective removal of some of the variations, resulting in change in the genetic composition and the typical phenotypes in the population.

Genetically based variations in a population are created by three mechanisms:

1. **Mutation** of existing genes to form new alleles is the only process which can create new forms of genes. Most new forms of genes are less functional than the existing forms, but a few mutations do turn out to be beneficial. Although mutation is the only process that can create new forms of genes, the rates at which mutations occur under normal conditions are very low (usually $\frac{1}{100,000}$ to $\frac{1}{1,000,000}$). Therefore, although mutations are essential in advance of most large-scale evolutionary changes, mutations do not usually contribute to the visible rate of evolutionary change.
2. **Gene flow** is movement of genetic information between populations, usually in the form of spores, seeds, or organisms but occasionally in the form of gametes (eggs or sperm) or pollen. Gene flow does not create new forms of genes, but gene flow can move a new form of a gene from a population in which it exists into a population in which it does not exist. The effect on the population into which the new form of the gene was moved is the same as if the new form of the gene was created in the population by mutation. Gene flow is usually slow in stable ecosystems with well-defined boundaries, but may be rapid in unstable ecosystems.
3. **Recombination of existing genes** into all possible combinations is the major mechanism increasing genetic variations in populations. *Crossing-over* exchanges material between homologous chromosomes during prophase I of meiosis. *Independent assortment* of chromosomes at the transition from metaphase I to anaphase I of meiosis shuffles chromosomes so that the entire set of chromosomes from one parent is unlikely to be passed on to one offspring. *Fertilization* combines genetic information from two parents into a new individual. *Chromosomal rearrangements* (translocations, etc.) can

produce new genetic combinations in some cases, but are much less frequent than recombination due to meiosis or fertilization. Recombination does not create new forms of genes, but instead "shuffles" existing genes into new combinations. Recombination therefore creates new combinations of genes, and the combination of genes is what determines the genetically controlled aspects of the phenotype of the organism.

Genetically based variations in a population are decreased by two mechanisms:

1. Selective loss of organisms due to *natural selection* will reduce genetic variation and may or may not result in evolutionary change. *Stabilizing natural selection* removes all extreme phenotypes equally. This decreases the variation in the population without changing the average or "typical" characteristics and therefore causes no apparent evolution. *Directional natural selection* differentially removes some extreme phenotypes but not others. This causes a change in the average characteristics of the population (i.e., evolution), with characteristics selected against becoming less frequent. *Disruptive natural selection* favors extreme phenotypes over the average phenotype(s). This may eventually result in creating two or more distinct sets of characteristics or phenotypes (i.e., evolution). Under extreme conditions these phenotypes may evolve into separate species if they become too different to interbreed.

2. Nonselective changes in gene frequency due to *small population sizes* usually reduce genetic variations and may lead to evolution. *Founder effects* result from establishment of a new population by individuals that do not contain all of the alleles that are present in the original population. *Bottleneck effects* result from reduction of the original population to a small remnant population whose members do not contain all of the alleles present in the original population. *Genetic drift* refers to random fluctuations in gene frequency which occur in small populations owing to the small number of individuals in the population. Changes in gene frequency that result from small population sizes are by definition evolution, and these changes result in changes in the average characteristics of small populations. Unlike natural selection, changes due to small populations are random and therefore do not necessarily result in better-adapted organisms.

Mechanisms of Evolution on a Large Scale (Macroevolution)

Some scientists have argued that mechanisms of *microevolution* (changes in gene frequency in a population, usually resulting in small or gradual changes in the average phenotypes of the organisms) do not provide a satisfactory explanation for *macroevolution* (larger-scale changes in gene frequency and phenotype frequency, including changes resulting in formation of new species). In particular, some of these scientists have pointed out that many macroevolutionary changes appear to occur during brief periods separated by long periods in which little macroevolutionary change occurs. Other scientists have argued that macroevolution usually occurs by the same mechanisms which cause microevolution but requires longer time periods. The detailed mechanisms by which most large-scale evolutionary changes occur is still unresolved, but probably involves natural selection (and probably other causes of genetic change such as genetic drift) acting on the genetic and developmental equilibrium in organisms. Multiple mechanisms for major evolutionary changes are quite likely.

Speciation

Speciation is probably the most dramatic example of macroevolution. A *species* is "biologically" defined as the largest group of organisms that can successfully sexually reproduce with each other. In cases in which use of the biological definition is impractical, a species is defined as a group of organisms that resemble each other more than they resemble other organisms.

The resemblances may be physical, chemical, or behavioral. *Speciation* (formation of new species) appears to occur by two major types of mechanisms (allopatric speciation, sympatric speciation) with intermediate mechanisms (parapatric speciation) possible.

Allopatric speciation involves reproductive isolation of two or more groups of organisms (derived from the same species) through mechanisms that require geographic isolation of the groups from each other followed by reproductive isolation.

Geographic isolation occurs whenever populations become spatially separated due to climatic changes, geological changes, migration, or other causes. While separated, different populations may undergo different changes in gene frequency and average phenotype, becoming progressively more different. If these differences become sufficiently large, allopatric speciation has occurred.

Reproductive isolation in most cases of allopatric speciation probably initially results from accumulated genetic differences, which result in no offspring or less fit offspring being produced if members of the isolated populations come in contact again. The inability to produce successful offspring is referred to as *postmating* or *postzygotic* reproductive isolation. If the different groups begin to come in contact frequently, they will probably evolve *premating* or *prezygotic* reproductive isolating mechanisms, simply because individuals that acquire those mechanisms through mutation or inheritance will not waste resources trying to mate with the "wrong" population and will therefore leave more offspring than will individuals that lack those mechanisms. Prezygotic isolating mechanisms could include temporal, behavioral, ecological, or mechanical isolation or inability of gametes to survive long enough after mating to allow fertilization. Postzygotic isolating mechanisms could include lethality, sterility, or low fitness in offspring.

Sympatric speciation involves reproductive isolation of two or more groups of organisms through mechanisms that do not require geographic isolation of the groups from each other. Sympatric speciation may occur through polyploidy, through disruptive natural selection, or through some types of mutations, and may occur through other as yet unknown mechanisms.

Polyploidy can result in sympatric speciation in organisms which can reproduce asexually and in which polyploidy (extra sets of chromosomes) is not lethal. Many plants and some animals appear to have formed new species by polyploidy without any geographic isolation. In the simplest case, one or both parents form gametes (sex cells) without doing meiosis to reduce the number of chromosomes. When these sex cells are involved in fertilization, the new offspring will have one or more extra sets of chromosomes, making it a polyploid. Alternatively, polyploidy may occur if the first cleavage division in the embryo is incomplete, resulting in chromosome duplication without cell division. Since a polyploid organism cannot produce fertile offspring when mated with a diploid organism because the chromosomes do not pair properly in the offspring, the polyploid organism is immediately reproductively isolated. Since polyploidy would not interfere with asexual reproduction, asexual reproduction could produce new individuals until enough organisms existed to begin sexually reproducing with each other. Polyploidy is also frequently involved in formation of new species after hybridization (interbreeding) between two existing species.

Other mechanisms such as *disruptive natural selection* may also be involved in sympatric speciation, since examples of apparent sympatric speciation without polyploidy have been described, but the detailed mechanisms have not been worked out. One suggested mechanism involves developmental timing mutations. Developmental timing mutations involving small changes in DNA sequence may result in large changes in phenotype. Mutations that alter the early stages in the formation of a structure usually result in a structure which is so abnormal that the change is lethal, but mutations which alter later stages in the development of the structure can result in altered but functional phenotypes. As an example, the developmental stages during which the body is being formed in vertebrate animals are relatively similar even though the adults are as different as fish and humans. In more closely related groups such as chimpanzees and humans, the embryos and the infants are very similar and the DNA sequence is at least 98% identical, but the growth patterns from infancy to adulthood are very different and result in distinctly different adult morphology. A human can be viewed as retaining many juvenile features (skull and head shape, lack of body hair) that are altered in adult chimps. Since the protein-coding parts of most genes in humans and chimpanzees are almost identical, the genetic changes that caused the differences between humans and chimpanzees probably occurred in genetic control elements that influence developmental timing.

Parapatric speciation involves reproductive isolation of two or more groups of organisms through mechanisms that create partial geographic isolation of the groups from each other. Species that occupy large geographic ranges frequently vary in their features at different points in their range and form multiple subspecies. A series of organisms of this type is frequently called a *cline*. As long as all of the subspecies are present, the organisms are still considered one species because all adjacent subspecies can interbreed, allowing gene flow among all of the populations. However, if some of the connecting subspecies become extinct because of climate changes or competition with other organisms, the subspecies at the extremes of the series of subspecies may have already become so different that they cannot interbreed successfully with each other. If this happens, the former subspecies are now different true species.

Other Patterns of Macroevolution

Scientists who study macroevolution use several terms to describe patterns seen in the fossil record.

Phyletic evolution indicates change in the average characteristics of a group (population or species) over time. This probably is nothing more than microevolution viewed over a much longer time frame. Rates of phyletic evolution vary from one group of organisms to another and within the same group at different times. Sometimes organisms appear unchanged (at least as far as the fossils indicate) over long periods, but sometimes changes appear to be relatively rapid.

Adaptive radiation refers to the rapid fragmentation of a group (usually a species) of organisms into multiple groups, usually occurring as a result of geographic isolation or immigration of the organisms into an area with numerous unoccupied ecological niches. This is basically a spectacular case of speciation, either allopatric or sympatric.

Extinction refers to the loss of a species from the fossil record or from the modern earth. Most species which can be identified from the fossil record no longer exist on the modern earth and are therefore extinct. Some of those species may have gradually changed into different species by phyletic evolution, but most apparently disappeared abruptly from the fossil record. In addition to loss of individual species, the fossil record indicates that periodic *mass extinctions* have occurred in which numerous species disappeared at the same time. Some of these mass extinctions may have resulted from climate changes such as ice ages, but some may have resulted from asteroid impacts with the earth or other rare catastrophic events.

Terms describing relative or interactive patterns of evolution include *divergent evolution*, *parallel evolution*, *convergent evolution*, and *co-evolution*.

Divergent evolution describes a pattern in which two or more groups from a single population or species become isolated from each other and become progressively less similar through accumulation of different changes. Speciation occurs when divergent evolution has progressed to the point that successful interbreeding is no longer possible. Structures that arose from a common ancestral structure are referred to as *homologous structures* even if they take on very different functions as a result of divergent evolution. The wing of a bird and the arm of a human are homologous structures.

Parallel evolution describes two groups that begin as a single species or population and that continue to evolve similar adaptations independently after they are separated.

Convergent evolution describes two groups which do not originate from a common group, but which evolve similar adaptations, usually as a result of exposure to similar environments. Structures that are derived from unrelated ancestral structures but that acquire similar features and functions through convergent evolution are referred to as *analogous structures*. The wing of a bird and the wing of a butterfly would be analogous structures.

Co-evolution describes the interlocking evolutionary changes occurring in two populations which interact through herbivory, predation, parasitism, commensalism, or mutualism.

The recent capability to analyze genetic and biochemical similarities/differences has greatly increased our ability to decipher evolutionary phenomena. All organisms use their DNA as the carrier for genetic material and all use ATP as the energy carrier. Amino acid sequence elucidation has confirmed a relation between all organisms to an extent. The amino acid sequences correspond closely to the evolutionary scheme worked out by comparative anatomists. An example is the closeness of chromosomes between the chimpanzee and the human being.

The Rate of Evolution

Evolution certainly does not proceed at a given and constant rate as well documented by the fossil record of a group. At times in relation to the earth's history, evolution has been slow or rapid; the fossil record of the horse definitely shows different rates. The horse started in stature resembling a fox terrier. Each period (from Eohippus, Mesohippus, Merichuppus, Pliochippus to Equus) is thought to have occupied about 7.5 million years, for example.

Artificial Selection

The best example in the literature is the domestic dog, which descended from a wolf (even today the two species are capable of cross-breeding), and the dog was specifically bred to achieve quite radical differences (Chihuahua vs. German Shepherd).

QUICK RECALL TEST QUESTIONS AND ANSWERS

Choose the Best Answer

1. Darwin's theory of evolution by means of natural selection proposes that:

   (A) organisms within a population vary in their characteristics and the most advantageous variations occur more frequently in the next generation.
   (B) organisms within a population vary in their characteristics, but these variations occur at the same frequency in subsequent generations.
   (C) all organisms within the population are very similar, so naturally occurring variations are not involved in evolution.

2. Natural selection may cause:

   (A) evolution of a population.
   (B) a change in gene frequency in a population.
   (C) adaptation of the population to the prevailing conditions.
   (D) all of the above are correct.

3. Natural selection will typically _____ the genetic diversity in a population.

   (A) increase
   (B) decrease
   (C) maintain (without increasing or decreasing)
   (D) have no effect on

4. Sexual reproduction will typically _____ the genetic diversity in a population.

   (A) increase
   (B) decrease
   (C) maintain (without increasing or decreasing)
   (D) have no effect on

5. Mutations will typically _____ the genetic diversity in a population.

   (A) increase greatly
   (B) increase slightly
   (C) maintain (without increasing or decreasing)
   (D) have no effect on

6. Natural selection would cause the most rapid adaptation in a population containing _____ phenotypes in each generation.

   (A) many similar
   (B) many different
   (C) a few similar

7. Adaptive radiation involves:

   (A) a slow change in group characteristics so that one species is gradually transformed into a new species.
   (B) formation of many new species from a single ancestral species, usually through adaptation to unoccupied ecological niches.
   (C) movement of a single species into an area to which it is already well adapted, so that little change in the species occurs.

8. Evolutionary _____ describes a pattern of evolution in which two or more groups of organisms that originated from a common ancestor gradually become more different from each other.

   (A) convergence
   (B) divergence
   (C) analogy
   (D) homology

9. Evolutionary _____ describes a pattern of evolution in which two or more groups of organisms that did not originate from a recent common ancestor and that were initially quite different from each other, gradually become more similar to each other.

   (A) convergence
   (B) divergence
   (C) analogy
   (D) homology

Answers

1. **(A)** Darwin believed that existing variations were selected among by natural selection, and the most advantageous variations became more frequent in subsequent generations.

2. **(D)** As described by Darwin and Wallace, natural selection may cause evolution. Modern biologists define evolution as a change in gene frequency in a population. Natural selection acts by causing differences in the chance of survival of organisms with different characteristics (differential survival of different phenotypes) and results in adaptation of the population to the current conditions. Therefore A, B, C, and D are all true.

3. **(B)** Natural selection will always decrease the genetic diversity in a population because it results in elimination of less advantageous phenotypes (and the genes responsible for them).

4. **(A)** Sexual reproduction creates new combinations of existing alleles (forms of genes) by combining genetic information from two parents at fertilization and reshuffling the genetic material in each parent through crossing over and independent assortment of homologous chromosomes during the first division of meiosis.

5. **(B)** Mutation increases genetic diversity by creating new alleles (forms of genes), but mutation is so infrequent (typically 1 mutation per million replications of a gene) that its quantitative effect is very small. However, mutation is the only mechanism that creates new alleles, so it is essential to the process of evolution.

6. **(B)** The most rapid evolutionary change should occur in a population containing many different phenotypes for natural selection to act upon.

7. **(B)** Adaptive radiation involves the splitting of one species into multiple species. This typically occurs most rapidly if vacant ecological niches (sets of ecological resources) are available to the organisms so that new variations do not have to compete with well-adapted organisms that are already using the ecological resources (occupying the niche).

8. **(B)** Divergence is the pattern in which related organisms become more different from each other.

9. **(A)** Convergence describes the pattern in which unrelated organisms become more similar.

Chemistry

CHAPTER 3

GENERAL CHEMISTRY

The Atom

John Dalton's theories—still accepted as fundamentally correct

    a. An element is composed of atoms. An atom is the smallest representative unit of an element that retains all the characteristics of that element. This is now known as the Law of Conservation of Matter. All atoms of an element possess the same chemical properties.

    b. Atoms of different elements have different properties.

    c. During a chemical reaction (nuclear reactions excepted, of course) atoms and elements are not created nor do they disappear.

    d. Atoms of more than one element may react to form compounds. In a pure compound the number of atoms of each element is constant.

Components of the Atom

   1. Nucleus: The nucleus—found at the center of an atom—contains neutrons and protons.

    a. Neutrons—no charge—mass of about 1 dalton

    b. Protons—relative charge of +1—mass of about 1 dalton. Number of protons in an atom determines the atomic number and the identity of the element.

   2. Electrons: Electrons—relative charge of −1—mass of about 0.0005 dalton. Number of electrons circling the nucleus is equal to the number of protons in the nucleus.

Placement of Electrons—Energy Levels

   1. Quantum numbers:

    a. Principal quantum number, n, determines the shell. It may be 1, 2, 3, 4, etc., in increasing distance from the nucleus and increasing energy. The K shell has a principal quantum number of 1.

    b. Angular momentum quantum number, l, determines the subshell. $l = 0, 1, 2, \ldots, (n-1)$.

    c. Magnetic quantum number, m_l, determines the orbital: $m_l = l, (l-1), \ldots, 0, \ldots, (1-l), -l$. The energies are virtually identical.

    d. Spin quantum number, m_s, describes the spin of an electron. Allowed values are $+\frac{1}{2}$ and $-\frac{1}{2}$.

   2. Pauli exclusion principle: No two electrons in an atom may have exactly the same set of four quantum numbers.

3. **Total number of electrons in a shell:** The total number of electrons in a shell is $2n^2$.

4. **Order of filling orbitals:** Orbitals are filled from lower to higher energy levels. They may be designated in shorthand form. For example, the following oxygen atom may be designated as $1s^2 2s^2 2p^4$. Within the 2p orbitals, it is possible for an electron to be in $2p_x$, $2p_y$, or $2p_z$. Hund's rule states that one electron of parallel spin will go into each of these until each has one electron; additional electrons of antiparallel spin will then be added as necessary until all are filled.

	1s	2s	$2p_x$	$2p_y$	$2p_z$
			\multicolumn{3}{c}{2p}		
Oxygen	(↑↓)	(↑↓)	(↑↓)	(↑)	(↑)

5. **The excited state:** The situation described above is that of the naturally occurring or ground state. By input of energy it is possible to raise electrons to higher energy levels. When electrons drop back from these higher energy levels (excited state) to the levels required by the ground state, there is an emission of radiation. (This phenomenon may be observed experimentally in the form of an emission spectrum.) To form an excited atom, an equivalent amount of energy must be supplied to the atom, which is then absorbed as the electron is promoted to a higher energy level (an absorption spectrum of this phenomenon may be recorded).

Periodic Table

The Periodic Table arranges the elements from left to right in order of increasing atomic number. The Periodic Law states that: The properties of the elements are periodic functions of their atomic numbers.

1. **Groups:** Vertical columns are called groups. All elements in the same group have the same number of valence electrons and, therefore, related chemical properties. For example, Group IA elements have only one electron in their outermost principal energy level. They tend to lose this electron readily to form cations with a +1 charge. Group VIIA elements have seven valence electrons. They tend to gain one electron to form anions with a −1 charge. At the extreme right of the table is the group known as the noble gases. These elements have complete outer shells and are essentially nonreactive. Properties of elements in other groups are now known to be related to placement of their electrons.

2. **Periods:** Horizontal rows of the table are called periods. Elements in the same period have the same number of principal energy levels. From left to right across a period, many properties exhibit periodicity (predictable variation in a property with changes in atomic structure). For example, from left to right, atomic radii and metallic characteristics decrease while ionization energy and electronegativity increase.

3. **Applications:** Just as an element in group IA loses a single electron in its outer shell to become a cation with a charge of +1, an element in group IIA can lose two electrons to become a cation with a charge of +2. Just as an element in group VIIA can gain one electron in its outer shell to become an anion with a charge of −1, an element in group VIA can gain two electrons to become an anion with a charge of −2.

Within any period, an increase in first ionization energy is seen with an increase in atomic number. Thus, the group IA elements (Li, Na, K, Rb, etc.) have a lower first ionization energy than group VIIA elements such as F, Cl, Br, etc. (The first ionization energy referred to here is for the removal of an electron from the outermost shell to form a cation with a +1 charge.) Although VIIA elements tend to form ions, they ordinarily do so by gaining an electron to form an anion with a −1 charge. This opposite but related phenomenon is known as electron affinity (EA). The noble gases of Group O have the highest first ionization energies. (This includes Ne, Ar, Kr, etc.)

Note also that group IA elements are the most metallic (Li, Na, K, etc.) and that the elements become progressively less metallic when proceeding to the right side of the table. The elements in group VIIA (F, Cl, Br, etc.) are not metallic, and group VIII (Ne, Ar, Kr, etc.) elements are virtually inert.

Gases

1. Ideal gas law: Although early laws were formulated by Boyle, by Charles, and by Gay-Lussac to explain parts of the interrelationships between temperature, pressure, and volume of a gas, one simple formula sums it up:

$$\frac{P_1 V_1}{T_1} = \frac{P_2 V_2}{T_2} = nR$$

$$PV = nRT$$

where P = pressure in atmospheres or torr
V = volume in liters (L)
T = absolute temperature in Kelvin (K)
n = moles of the gas
R = universal gas constant in appropriate units

Real gas behavior deviates from the ideal gas law at low temperature and high pressure. Because of the finite volume that atoms/molecules occupy, and because these particles collide not only with the walls of their container but also with each other, the following correction factors may be applied:

P is translated into $(P + n^2 a/V^2)$ and V is translated into $(V - nb)$

a and b are constants unique to each gaseous substance that must be obtained from the literature.

2. Partial pressures:

$$P_T = P_1 + P_2 + \ldots + P_n$$

(i.e., the total pressure of a mixture of gases is equal to the sum of the partial pressures). The partial pressure of each constituent gas in the mixture must be determined according to the number of moles of that gas present, i.e., $P_1 = n_1 P_T$; $P_2 = n_2 P_T$, ... , etc.

3. Diffusion—Graham's Law: Rate of diffusion is inversely proportional to the square root of the molecular weight.

$$\frac{v_1}{v_2} = \sqrt{\frac{M_2}{M_1}}$$

where v = velocity
M = molecular weight

Thus, a gas of twice the molecular weight of another gas will diffuse 0.71 as fast.

Liquids and Solids

Ideal gases are assumed to have negligible intermolecular interactions. Within a homologous series of organic compounds, the boiling point increases with increasing molecular weight. The same relationship may be seen within the halogens.

There are, however, forces in some compounds that cause them to be liquids or even solids at temperatures at which their molecular weights would suggest that they should be gases.

1. Dipole forces: In certain asymmetrical molecules the electrons become unevenly distributed between regions, and there results a partial positive charge in one region (and a partial negative charge in another). Molecules become arranged so that there is electrostatic attraction between adjacent molecules.

2. **Hydrogen bonds:** When a hydrogen atom in one molecule is covalently bonded to an atom of oxygen, nitrogen, or fluorine, there is a large difference in electronegativity, which results in strong partial charge character on each atom (positive on hydrogen and negative on oxygen, nitrogen, or fluorine). This results in an especially strong dipole-dipole attraction between adjacent molecules, which is called a *hydrogen bond*. The amount of energy necessary to break a hydrogen bond is in the range of 5–10 kcal/mole, which is approximately 5% of the strength of a typical covalent bond. This force is particularly significant in many biologically important molecules (amino acids and proteins, carbohydrates, nucleic acids, and others).

3. **London-van der Waals dispersion forces:** These forces involve interaction between molecules on the basis of their polarizability. The phenomenon of polarizability is also referred to as an *induced dipole* that is predicated on the repulsion of electrons that results from the oscillation of these bonding electrons in their orbitals within a molecule. They may be important in nonpolar compounds.

4. **Ionic forces:** Oppositely charged ions exhibit coulombic attraction. Because of the magnitude of the actual positive and negative charges on cations and anions, ionic forces of attraction are the strongest of the intermolecular forces. This results in ionic compounds having, in general, the highest melting and boiling points observed among chemical substances.

Phase Changes and Heat Capacity

1. **Nature of the solid, liquid, and gaseous phases:** $\text{Solid} \underset{B}{\overset{A}{\rightleftharpoons}} \text{Liquid} \underset{D}{\overset{C}{\rightleftharpoons}} \text{Gas}$

    where *A* is melting or fusion
       B is freezing
       C is vaporization or boiling
       D is condensation

2. **Energy of phase transition:**

    a. The energy involved in conversion from the solid to the liquid phase is H_f.
    b. The energy involved in conversion from the liquid to the gaseous phase is H_v.
    c. All molecules in one phase do not have the same energy—there is a range unique to each temperature that is governed by the Boltzmann distribution. This range of energies results from non-elastic collisions between atoms or molecules with each other, and with the walls of the container to which they are confined. A liquid at a temperature below its boiling point is subject to some of its molecules being vaporized by virtue of the fact that some molecules are sufficiently energetic to be converted into the gaseous state. The temperature of the liquid, however, is a measure of the average kinetic energy of the bulk liquid.

3. **Phase diagram:** The phase diagram allows the visualization of possible phases at particular temperatures and pressures.

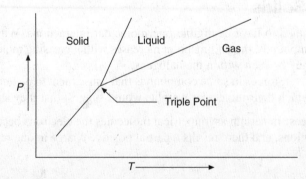

Note that the lines between phases in the phase diagram represent those conditions of pressure and temperature at which the phases indicated on the two sides of the lines may coexist. The point of intersection of the three lines is designated as *the triple point*; at this temperature and pressure all three phases may coexist.

4. Heat capacity: This is a measure of the energy required to increase the temperature of an object by a certain amount. Often, this quantity of energy is expressed as a specific heat capacity (c), which is unique for a particular substance. Specific heat capacity is defined in units such as $JK^{-1}mol^{-1}$ or $JK^{-1}g^{-1}$. The energy or heat (q) required to raise the temperature of a mass of a substance can be calculated as $q = mc\Delta T$, where ΔT is the change in temperature.

Chemical Compounds

1. Percent Weight and Empirical Formula: Chemical compounds are pure substances that may be broken down into two or more elements. A molecule is the smallest unit of a compound that still retains the properties of the compound; an atom is the smallest unit of an element.

A particular chemical compound will always have the same percentage composition by weight. This is known as the Law of Constant Composition. Considering the compound iron (III) oxide, it is found to consist of:

$$Fe = 69.94\%$$

$$O = 30.06\%$$

When this data is empirically determined, it is referred to as the percent composition data for the substance. It may be obtained by either decomposition of the compound, or, in the case of organic compounds, through combustion (burning in the presence of oxygen).

Since it is agreed that a molecule of a compound is made up of whole atoms of elements, we will try to find the lowest multiple(s) of whole numbers. We may do this in two steps:

(1) Divide each percentage by the atomic weight of that element.

$$Fe = \frac{69.94}{55.85} = 1.252$$

$$O = \frac{30.06}{16.00} = 1.879$$

(2) Convert these numbers to the lowest whole multiple(s).

$$\frac{1.252}{1.252} = 1.000 \text{ Iron} \qquad \frac{1.879}{1.252} = 1.501 \text{ Oxygen}$$

This would indicate 1.5 atoms of oxygen for each atom of iron. Since it is agreed that whole numbers of atoms are involved, the simplest formula would be Fe_2O_3. This is known as the empirical formula.

2. Molecular Formula: In some cases, however, the molecular weight of a compound does not agree with its empirical formula. (This is often true of organic compounds and sometimes true of inorganic ones.) The organic compound glucose may be used as an example. Its elemental composition would give an empirical formula of CH_2O. From molecular weight determination, however, it is found that glucose has a molecular weight of 180.15 g/mole. This may have been determined through any of the traditional colligative property measurements (freezing point depression, boiling point elevation, or vapor pressure lowering) or by determination of osmotic pressure of an aqueous solution of glucose. At any rate, the "apparent molecular weight" of only 30.03 g/mole for CH_2O clearly shows that the correct molecular formula for glucose must be an integral multiple of the empirical formula to reconcile with the molecular weight. Thus, $180.15/30.03 = 5.999 = 6$, so the correct molecular formula for glucose is $6(CH_2O) = C_6H_{12}O_6$.

3. Mole and Avogadro's Number: If the molecular weight is known, we may weigh that many grams of the compound and it has been shown that this mass will contain a chemically equivalent number of atoms or molecules that can be related to other chemical substances when reactions take place. This chemically equivalent number of particles is called a *mole*. A mole of any compound contains 6.023×10^{23} molecules of that compound. This is known as Avogadro's number.

Balanced Chemical Equations

Chemical equations may be written in unbalanced or balanced form, but to draw meaningful conclusions or predict reproducible outcomes, the equation must be balanced. Otherwise the equation is giving only the most rudimentary information about the chemical reaction or process, and it will not be clear that the Law of Conservation of Matter has been observed. The formulas for the **reactants** are those that appear to the left of the directional arrow in the equation, and the formulas for the **products** are those that appear to the right of the directional arrow. Sometimes the phase of the element/compound is also specified to give more detailed information about the reaction; i.e., (s) for solid, (l) for liquid, and (g) for gas may be included after the relevant formula.

1. Inorganic Chemistry:

$$H_2 + O_2 \rightarrow H_2O$$

This equation tells us that diatomic molecules of hydrogen and oxygen react to form water. Inspection indicates, however, that there are 2 atoms of oxygen on the left side but there is only 1 atom of oxygen on the right side. This does not agree with what we know about conservation of matter.

It is critically important to remember that an equation may **not** be balanced by changing the formulas for any of the elements or compounds depicted in the equation. This would alter the fundamental nature of the process being described! Rather, it **is** acceptable to manipulate the values of the coefficients **in front of** the formulas of the reactants and products. These are referred to as the stoichiometric coefficients of the equation. We could increase the atoms of oxygen on the right side by placing the coefficient 2 before H_2O, thus indicating 2 molecules of H_2O. This unbalances the hydrogen, however, with 2 atoms of hydrogen on the left and 4 on the right. We can correct this by placing the coefficient 2 before the H_2:

$$2H_2 + O_2 \rightarrow 2H_2O$$

Inspection indicates that there are now 4 atoms of hydrogen on each side and 2 atoms of oxygen on each side.

This is now a balanced equation. The coefficients tell us that 2 diatomic molecules of hydrogen will react with 1 diatomic molecule of oxygen to form 2 molecules of water. Since the same number of molecules (i.e., Avogadro's number) are required for a mole of any material, we can also say that 2 moles of hydrogen react with 1 mole of oxygen to produce 2 moles of water.

2. Organic Chemistry: The equation

$$C_3H_8 + O_2 \rightarrow CO_2 + H_2O$$

is not balanced. Since there are 3 atoms of carbon on the left and 1 atom on the right, we need to multiply the formula for carbon dioxide by 3. Similarly, we need to multiply the formula for water by 4 to balance the hydrogen. Then, however, there will be too few oxygens on the left. We need to multiply the formula for O_2 by 5. Our balanced equation is then:

$$C_3H_8 + 5O_2 \rightarrow 3CO_2 + 4H_2O$$

Check to see that this equation is balanced. It tells us that 1 mole of propane reacts with 5 moles of oxygen to produce 3 moles of carbon dioxide and 4 moles of water.

Solutions

1. **Concentration units:**

   a. Molarity

      moles/liter = (grams/molecular weight)/liters of solution

   b. Molality = moles of solute/kilograms of solvent
   c. Normality = equivalents of solute/liters of solution
   d. Equivalents = grams/equivalent weight

2. **Colligative properties:** Based on the number of dissolved particles, without regard to their nature.

   a. Boiling point elevation

      Boiling point elevation = $K_b m$
      where K_b is a constant for the specific solvent and m = molality of solute.

Note, however, that a 1 molal solution of NaCl would have twice the calculated effect since it would be 1 molal each in Na^+ and Cl^- (i.e., 2 molal total).

   b. Freezing point depression

      Freezing point depression = $K_f m$
      where K_f is a constant for the specific solvent and m = molality of solute particles (see comment above in 2.a. regarding ionizable solutes).

   c. Osmotic pressure. When an aqueous solution is placed on one side of a semipermeable membrane and pure water on the other side, there is net movement of water across the membrane. The applied pressure required to produce a net movement of zero is called the osmotic pressure.

$$\pi V = nRT$$

where π = osmotic pressure
   V = volume in liters (L)
   n = moles of particles in solution
   R = the universal gas constant R = 0.0821 L-atom/mole-K
   T = the temperature, kelvin units (K)

3. a. **Solubility:** A comparatively insoluble inorganic compound in water is in equilibrium with its soluble ions.

$$Al(OH)_3 \downarrow \rightleftharpoons Al^{3+} (aq) + 3OH^- (aq)$$

The solubility product constant is K_{sp}.

$$K_{sp} = 5 \times 10^{-33} = [Al^{3+}][OH^-]^3$$

Thus, in the specific case of $Al(OH)_3$, if the product of the molar concentration of OH^- raised to the third power and Al^{3+} exceeds 5×10^{-33}, precipitation will occur.

   b. **Gas Solubility:**

   1. Henry's law—the solubility of a gas in a liquid is directly proportional to the partial pressure of the gas in contact with the liquid.
   2. Gas solubility in a liquid decreases with increasing temperature.

Acids and Bases, pH, and Buffers

1. **Acids:**

   a. Brönsted-Lowry acid—a substance that donates a proton to an aqueous solution:

   $$HCl + H_2O \longrightarrow H_3O^+ + Cl^-$$
   (acid)

   b. Lewis acid—a substance that accepts an electron pair

2. **Base:**

   a. Brönsted-Lowry base—a substance that accepts a proton:

   $$H_3O^+ + NaOH \rightleftharpoons 2H_2O + Na^+$$
   (base)

   b. Lewis base—a substance that donates an electron pair

3. **Strength of acids and bases:**

   a. Strong acids and bases. A strong acid or base is assumed to be completely ionized. Therefore, the concentration of acid is equal to the concentration of hydrogen ions (or hydronium ions).

   $$HCl + H_2O \longrightarrow H_3O^+ + Cl^- \quad or \quad HCl \longrightarrow H^+ + Cl^-$$

   b. Weak acids and bases

   (1) $HF \rightleftharpoons H^+ + F^-$

   $$K_a = \frac{[H^+][F^-]}{[HF]} = 7 \times 10^{-4} \text{ (in this specific case)}$$

   Consider a $1M$ solution of HF for example:
   $[H^+] = [F^-]$
   So, $K_a[HF] = [H^+][F^-] = [H^+]^2$
   and $[H^+] = \sqrt{K_a[HF]} = \sqrt{7 \times 10^{-4}} = 2.6 \times 10^{-2}$
   In this example HF is called a conjugate acid, capable of releasing a proton. F^- is called a conjugate base, capable of combining with a proton.

   (2) Bases
   $NH_3 + H_2O \rightleftharpoons NH_4^+ + OH^-$
   $K_b[NH_3] = [NH_4^+][OH^-]$
   $K_b = 1.8 \times 10^{-5}$ for this particular base.
   Computation similar to that for acid would allow one to determine the $[OH^-]$ for a 1 molar NH_3 solution. H_2O is not included in the equilibrium expression because the concentration of water remains essentially constant.

4. **pH, pOH, and pK_w:**

   a. pH: A measure of the relative acidity of a solution. The pH of pure water is 7; acids have pH < 7, while bases have pH > 7.
   b. pOH: A measure of the relative basicity of a solution. The pOH of pure water is 7; acids have a pOH > 7, while bases have pOH < 7.
   c. pK_w: A constant relating pH and pOH according to the relationship $K_w = [H^+][OH^-]$. Taking the log of both sides gives the equation pK_w = pH + pOH = 14, which can be used to find the pH or pOH of a solution when the other quantity is known.
   d. Changes in pH and hydrogen ions. Remember that pH is a logarithmic scale. A decrease of one unit in pH (e.g., from 7 to 6) indicates an increase in the concentration of hydrogen ions by a factor of 10.

5. **Solution of salts:**

   a. A solution of the salt of a strong acid and a strong base is highly ionized and neutral.

   b. A solution of the salt of a strong acid and a weak base is acidic, because the conjugate acid of the weak base is sufficiently acidic that it undergoes a secondary ionization reaction that supplies hydrogen ions into solution.

For example: $HCl\ (aq) + NH_3\ (aq) \rightarrow NH_4^+\ (aq) + Cl^-\ (aq)$
Then in the secondary equilibrium: $NH_4^+\ (aq) \rightleftharpoons NH_3\ (aq) + H_2O\ (l)$

   c. A solution of the salt of a weak acid and a strong base is basic, because the conjugate base of the weak acid is sufficiently basic that it undergoes a secondary ionization reaction that supplies hydroxide ions into solution.

For example:

$$CH_3CH_2COOH\ (aq) + NaOH\ (aq) \rightarrow CH_3CH_2COO^-\ (aq) + Na^+ + H_2O\ (l)$$

Then in the secondary equilibrium:

$$CH_3CH_2COO^-\ (aq)\ +\ H_2O\ (l) \rightleftharpoons CH_3CH_2COOH\ (aq)\ +\ OH^-\ (aq)$$

6. **Buffers:** A buffer is a solution containing a weak acid or a weak base *and* a salt of that weak acid or weak base.

   a. The ionization of a weak acid, HA, may be shown as

$$HA \rightleftharpoons H^+ + A^-$$

   b. The ionization constant is defined as

$$K_a = \frac{[H^+][A^-]}{HA}$$

   c. The negative logarithm of K_a is defined as pK_a. It is then possible to define a useful relationship called the Henderson-Hasselbach equation:

$$pH = pK_a + \log\frac{[\text{conjugate base}]}{[\text{conjugate acid}]}$$

In the example we have already considered, of course, A^- would be the conjugate base and HA would be the conjugate acid in the buffer pair.

Although the conjugate acid is weakly ionized, it is assumed that the salt that produces the conjugate base is strongly ionized. Thus, the mixture of 500 ml each of $0.1M$ acetic acid and $0.1M$ sodium acetate would produce 1 liter of a solution that contains $0.05M$ acetic acid and $0.05M$ acetate ion. The Henderson-Hasselbach equation would provide us with

$$pH = pK_a + \log\frac{(0.05)}{(0.05)} = pK_a + \log 1 = pK_a$$

Thus, a mixture of equal concentrations of the conjugate base and the conjugate acid will produce a pH equal to the pK_a. From a practical standpoint it is usually considered that a buffer system is useful in the restraint of changes of pH only over the range of $pK_a \pm 1$ pH unit.

7. **Volumetric calculations with acids and bases:**

   a. Molarity = (grams acid or base/molecular weight)/liters
   b. Normality = (grams acid or base/equivalent weight)/liters

For a monoprotic acid such as HCl, the normality equals the molarity. For a diprotic acid such as H_2SO_4, the normality is twice the molarity.

   c.   Number of equivalents in neutralization:

$$L_{acid} \times N_{acid} = L_{base} \times N_{base} = \text{number of equivalents}$$

   d.   Neutralizations may be done using the experimental technique of titration, wherein a carefully measured and representative sample (an "aliquot") of the analyte, let's presume a base, is placed in a flask, diluted with solvent, and neutralized with an acidic solution whose concentration is precisely known. The acid is dispensed through a buret, which will allow for careful measurement of the volume of acid necessary to neutralize the base. The equivalence point (that is, when the number of moles of acid is equal to the number of moles of base) may be detected either by potentiometric means (such as with a pH meter) or with an added indicator, which changes color when all of the analyte has been consumed. Most indicators are weak organic acids whose color is sensitive to the pH environment. Hence a color change shows whether the indicator is protonated.

Electrochemistry

The electrolytic cell uses the flow of electrical current to cause a chemical reaction to occur. This type of chemical reaction is an oxidation-reduction (otherwise known as redox) reaction. In the electrolysis of molten NaCl, there is production of both Na and Cl_2. A convenient way in which to understand oxidation-reduction reactions, and to balance the equations describing them, is to separate the overall reaction into two half reactions, one for the oxidation process and the other for the reduction process. For the example given above, the half reactions involved are:

$$Na^+ + e^- \rightarrow Na^0 \qquad \text{(reduction)}$$

$$2Cl^- \rightarrow Cl_2^{\ 0} + 2e^- \quad \text{(oxidation)}$$

In balancing these half reactions, we must first balance one half reaction against the other to obtain the same number of electrons in each:

$$2[Na^+ + e^- \rightarrow Na^0] = 2Na^+ + 2e^- \rightarrow 2Na^0$$

$$1[2Cl^- \rightarrow Cl_2^{\ 0} + 2e^-] = 2Cl^- \rightarrow Cl_2^{\ 0} + 2e^-$$

When these balanced half reactions are added together, the electrons are canceled against each other to give a balanced equation for the net reaction:

$$2Na^+ + 2Cl^- \rightarrow 2Na^0 + Cl_2^{\ 0}$$

$$\text{or}$$

$$2NaCl \rightarrow 2Na^0 + Cl_2^{\ 0}$$

The reduction potential is an indication of the ease with which a chemical species is reduced (acquires electrons). Standard reduction potentials are listed as E° and give the potential associated with reducing a species at 25°C, 1 atm of pressure, and 1 M concentration of each ion. By definition:

$$2H^+(aq) + 2e- \rightarrow H_2(g) \qquad E° = 0.00 \text{ V}$$

Oxidation potentials are equal in magnitude to reduction potentials but opposite in sign. The cell potential for an electrolytic cell can be found by adding the oxidation and reduction potentials for each half-reaction:

$$E_{cell} = E_{reduction} + E_{oxidation}$$

Thermodynamics

1. **Laws:**

    a. *First law.* Energy can neither be created nor destroyed.
    b. *Second law.* The spontaneous flow of heat is always unidirectional from the higher to the lower temperature.
    c. *Third law.* The entropy of all pure crystalline solids may be taken as zero at the absolute zero of temperature.

2. **Change in enthalpy:** The change in enthalpy is ΔH. A negative ΔH for a reaction indicates that the products have a lower heat content than the reactants; therefore, heat is evolved into the surroundings. Such a reaction or process is known as an exothermic (or exergonic) reaction or process. Since enthalpy is independent of the route of a reaction, it is possible to algebraically add reactions to determine the overall enthalpy change for a complex series of reactions, including ones that may not be possible to determine experimentally. This statement is also known as Hess's Law.

$$Pb(s) + O_2(g) \longrightarrow PbO_2(s) \qquad \Delta H = -66.1 \text{ kcal/mole}$$
$$2H_2O(g) \longrightarrow 2H_2(g) + O_2(g) \qquad \Delta H = +115.6 \text{ kcal/mole}$$
$$\text{Sum} \quad Pb(s) + 2H_2O(g) \longrightarrow PbO_2(s) + 2H_2(g) \qquad \Delta H = +49.5 \text{ kcal/mole}$$

In this example the overall reaction would require input of heat. A reaction or process that requires additional heat from the surroundings is known as an endothermic (or endergonic) reaction or process.

3. **Change in entropy:** The change in entropy is ΔS. Entropy may be described as the degree of disorder of a system. It is also seen as unrecoverable energy. Without the addition of energy to a system, entropy increases to a maximum.

4. **Changes in Gibbs free energy:** Changes in Gibbs free energy are designated by ΔG. Some of the energy of a reaction is unavailable for useful work. The term ΔG indicates the energy that is available for useful work.

$$\Delta G = \Delta H - T\Delta S$$

where T = absolute temperature, K

A negative ΔG indicates a spontaneous reaction, that is, a reaction that will occur as written from left to right in the balanced equation. A positive ΔG indicates a reaction that would be spontaneous in the reverse direction. When $\Delta G = 0$, the system is at equilibrium.

Rate Processes in Chemical Reactions

1. **Rate-Controlling Step:** Although we sometimes write an equation in a simple way such as

$$A + B \rightarrow X + Z$$

it is not always so simple. There may be many intermediates in the process. For example, a product C could be formed, and then converted to D, etc. Somewhere along such a series of steps there would be a slowest or rate-controlling step. In spite of the other series of reactions, as the name implies, this rate-determining step would control or determine the rate of the overall reaction.

For the hypothetic reaction above, the rate equation would be written:

$$\text{Rate} = k[A]^1[B]^1$$

where k is referred to as the specific rate constant and the exponents indicate the **order** with respect to the concentration of each reactant. These orders are derived from the stoichiometric coefficients in the balanced equation for the reaction; when the numerical value of the coefficient is equal to one, the rate is said to have a first-order dependence on the concentration of that reactant. If the numerical value of the stoichiometric coefficient is equal to two, then the rate is said to have a second-order dependence on the concentration of that reactant.

The numerical value of k, the specific rate constant, is different for each reaction, and gives insight into the relative ease or difficulty with which that reaction will proceed. Its numerical value is a reflection of the collisional energy, frequency, and orientation that must exist in the rate-determining step to lead to successful formation of products.

2. Activation Energy, Catalysts, Enzymes: Although a reaction may be thermodynamically favorable, it will require a certain activation energy.

Activation energy (E_{act}) is defined as the minimum amount of energy necessary to transform reactants into products; the height of this activation barrier provides some insight into relative ease or difficulty involved for the reaction to proceed as written in the reaction equation. On the diagram below, it can be seen that the activation energy is indicated as the energy difference between the starting energy of the reactants and the top of the potential energy trajectory. This highest point on the potential energy pathway is referred to as the transition state, and reflects the most energetically demanding point in the course of the reaction, where partial bond-breaking and bond-forming has taken place.

Increasing the energy of the reaction system by increasing the temperature at which the reaction occurs will generally enhance formation of products, by shifting the Boltzmann distribution of energies, such that a higher percentage of reactant molecules will possess sufficient energy to traverse this activation barrier.

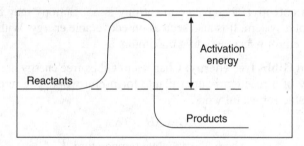

A catalyst or an enzyme (essentially a biological catalyst) may substantially increase the rate of a reaction by allowing the reaction to follow a lower-energy pathway that does not involve attaining the full energy of activation required by the uncatalyzed reaction.

3. Equilibrium Constant: Consider a reversible reaction:

$$^aA + {}^bB \rightleftharpoons {}^cC + {}^dD$$

We may calculate an *equilibrium constant*:

$$K_{eq} = \frac{[C]^c [D]^d}{[A]^a [B]^b}$$

4. Le Chatelier's Principle: Le Chatelier's principle states that when a system is at equilibrium, it will shift to relieve any stress placed on it. Thus, in the above example, addition of more C to the system would bring about the consumption of D and the production of more A and B (without changing the equilibrium constant).

GENERAL PRINCIPLES

Characteristics of Mixtures and Compounds

Mixture	Compound
1. Physical union	Chemical union
2. No new substances are formed	New substances are formed
3. Can be separated by physical means	Can be separated by chemical means
4. Elements form no definite proportions	Elements form definite proportions

Reactions

1. Single Replacement Reaction: In a single replacement reaction a more active element reacts with a compound to replace a less active one. A new element and a new compound are the result.

Examples: $Fe^0 + CuSO_4$ (aq) $\longrightarrow FeSO_4$ (aq) $+ Cu^0$

$Zn^0 + CuSO_4$ (aq) $\longrightarrow ZnSO_4$ (aq) $+ Cu^0$

2. Double Replacement Reaction: Double replacement reactions involve a double exchange; compounds react chemically to form two new compounds.

Examples: $NaCl$ (aq) $+ AgNO_3$ (aq) $\longrightarrow NaNO_3$ (aq) $+ AgCl$ (s)

HCl (aq) $+ NaOH$ (aq) $\longrightarrow NaCl$ (aq) $+ H_2O$ (l)

In the first example a precipitate ($AgCl$) is formed and in the second example a weakly ionized compound (H_2O) is formed. In the other cases (e.g., $NaCl + KNO_3$) a double replacement reaction could be written, but the equilibrium would involve all possible combinations of cations and anions since neither a precipitate, nor a gas, nor a weakly ionized compound is formed.

3. Synthesis Reaction: In a synthesis reaction two or more elements or compounds can unite to form a single compound.

Examples: Fe (s) $+ S$ (s) $\longrightarrow FeS$ (s)

CO_2 (g) $+ H_2O$ (l) $\xrightarrow{\Delta} H_2CO_3$ (aq)

4. Decomposition Reaction: In a decomposition reaction a compound is broken down into simpler compounds or into its elements.

Examples: $2KClO_3$ (aq) $\longrightarrow 2KCl$ (aq) $+ 3O_2$ (g)

$2HgO$ (s) $\longrightarrow 2Hg^0$ (s) $+ O_2$ (g)

Role of Enzymes in a Reaction

Consider the following reaction:

$$A + B + C \xrightarrow{\text{E (enzyme)}} ABCE \longrightarrow D + F + E$$
$$1 2 3 4 2$$

Substrate(s) or reactant(s) (1) react(s) with the enzyme (2) to form an enzyme-substrate complex (3). This complex breaks down into product(s) (4), and free enzyme (2) ready for the formation of a new enzyme-substrate complex is available again.

An enzyme speeds up the rate of the reaction but is not used up itself in the reaction.

Temperature Conversion Factors

On the Celsius scale (°C) the freezing point of water is 0°, and the boiling point is 100°. On the Fahrenheit scale (°F) they are respectively 32° and 212°.

The absolute Kelvin scale lists as absolute zero a temperature of −273°C, and therefore, the Kelvin and Celsius scales differ only in the choice of point zero. Kelvin temperature is, therefore, 273 plus the Celsius temperature. Let us illustrate and work two examples:

1. 104°F is what temperature on the Kelvin scale? The answer is 313 K and is obtained in the following manner:

First we must convert Fahrenheit to Celsius by using the following formulas:

$$\text{Celsius equals } \frac{5}{9} \times (\text{Fahrenheit} - 32)$$

$$\text{Fahrenheit equals } \frac{9}{5} C + 32$$

$$\text{Celsius} = \frac{5}{9} \times (104 - 32)$$

$$C = \frac{5}{9} \times 72$$

$$C = 40°$$

Now we take 273°, add 40°, and obtain a Kelvin temperature of 313 K.

2. 45°C will equal how many degrees F?
We utilize the conversion factors:

$$F = \frac{9}{5} C + 32$$

or

$$C = \frac{9}{5}(F - 32)$$

$$F = \frac{9}{5}(45) + 32$$

$$F = 81 + 32$$

$$F = 113°$$

Formulas and Laws

1. Specific Gravity: Specific gravity is usually expressed as the weight of an object in air divided by the loss of weight when weighed in water.

Example: A ball of steel weighs 300 grams in air and 250 grams when submerged in water; its specific gravity is 6.

$$\text{Specific Gravity} = \frac{\text{Weight in Air}}{\text{Loss of Weight}}$$

$$\text{Specific Gravity} = \frac{300}{50} = 6$$

2. **Density:** Density is expressed as $\dfrac{M(\text{mass})}{V(\text{volume})}$

For most substances, especially for liquids and solids, density is expressed in units of grams/mL. Because, on the other hand, gases are very diffuse, their densities are typically expressed in units of grams/L.

Determination of the mass of the object is relatively straightforward, regardless of the physical state, but there are a few different ways to evaluate the volume, particularly for solids. A regularly shaped solid can be measured and the volume calculated from the product of length × width × height; for an irregularly shaped solid, the volume can be determined by displacement. Because both liquids and gases are fluids, determination of their volume is technically similar.

Example: A piece of iron 60 inches long, 12 inches wide and 2 inches high has a mass of 2000 lb. The density of this piece is 1.39 lb/in^3 and was obtained as follows:

$$D = \frac{M}{V} = \frac{2000\,\text{lb}}{60\,\text{in.} \times 12\,\text{in.} \times 2\,\text{in.}}$$

$$D = \frac{2000\,\text{lb}}{1440\,\text{in}^3} = 1.39\,\text{lb/in}^3$$

ORGANIC CHEMISTRY

The field of organic chemistry covers a wide range of topics, and although space is limited, a review of the most important basic topics follows. It is important to review and recognize topics related to bonding and structural theory, correlation between structure and physical properties, stereochemistry, functional group identification, and spectroscopy. In addition, a survey of the most notable and biologically relevant reactions is undertaken, with some emphasis on mechanistic detail.

General Considerations

1. **Definition:** Organic chemistry is the chemistry of compounds of carbon. Historically, it has been the study of chemical compounds from living or dead organisms. Until 1828, it was believed that these compounds could not be synthesized from "inorganic" compounds outside living organisms. This theory was first breached by Friedrich Wöhler in 1828; he was successful in synthesizing urea from the inorganic compound, ammonium cyanate.

2. **Bonds:** In general, the bonds in the stable organic compounds are covalent bonds, formed by the sharing of electrons between atoms. If the electrons are shared unequally between two atoms, the bond is said to be a polar bond (e.g., C—Br or C—O).

Such a polar bond is a dipole, and the molecule possesses a dipole moment. The dipole moment is calculated by multiplying the charge by the distance of separation. Thus, methane (CH_4) has a dipole moment of zero. By comparison, CH_3Cl has a dipole moment of 1.87.

3. **Electronic Configuration of the Carbon Atom:** It is generally true that the orbital electrons in the outer unfilled shell are the most important in predicting the metal/nonmetal character of the compound as well as the expected valence. The carbon atom has two electrons in the K shell and four in the L shell ($1s^2 2s^2 2p_x^1 2p_y^1$). It might be expected to lose four electrons to produce the electronic configuration of the noble element helium, or gain four electrons to produce the electronic configuration of the noble element neon. For the most part it shares electrons to complete the L shell. Thus, it may be said to have a valence of 4 (see below).

4. **Bond Hybridization:** The orbital electrons of the carbon atom consist of two electrons in the $1s$ orbital, two electrons in the $2s$ orbital, and one electron each in the $2p_x$ and $2p_y$

orbital. (This may be written as $1s^2 2s^2 2p_x{}^1 2p_y{}^1$.) It exhibits a valence of 4. In simple compounds such as methane, four equivalent covalent bonds are formed. This may be considered to occur by raising one of the $2s$ orbital electrons to the $2p_z$ orbital and then forming four hybridized orbitals from the three $2p$ orbitals and the one remaining $2s$ orbital. These hybridized orbitals are sp^3 orbitals. The four covalent bonds in methane are the result of overlap of the one orbital electron of each of four hydrogen atoms with one sp^3 hybridized orbital electron of the carbon atom. These four bonds are called sigma bonds.

In a compound such as ethylene (ethene), however, there are pi as well as sigma bonds. Two of the three $2p$ orbital electrons are hybridized with the remaining $2s$ orbital electron. Thus, there are three equivalent sp^2 hybridized orbital electrons for each carbon atom. These participate in the covalent sigma bond between the two carbon atoms and in the covalent sigma bonds between the carbon atom and the hydrogen atoms. The remaining $2p$ orbital electron in each carbon atom participates in the weaker second bond between the two carbon atoms (a pi bond).

Compounds such as acetylene (ethyne) have a triple bond, consisting of one sigma bond and two pi bonds. In each carbon atom participating in a triple bond, there is contribution of two hybridized sp orbital electrons to produce two pi bonds. The stronger sigma bond between the carbon atoms is produced by the contribution of one $2p$ electron from each carbon atom. In acetylene itself there is another sigma bond between the carbon atom and a hydrogen atom; this bond is produced by the overlap of a $2p$ orbital from the carbon atom and the sole electron from the hydrogen atom.

5. Stereochemistry: Chemical compounds with the same molecular formula but different structural formulas are termed *isomers*. Those having atoms joined in a different order are *structural isomers* (e.g., 2-propanol and 1-propanol). Those having their atoms joined in the same order are termed *stereoisomers*. Stereoisomers that are mirror images of each other are termed *enantiomers*. Stereoisomers that are not enantiomers are called *diastereomers*.

```
   H—C=O            H—C=O            H—C=O
      |                |                |
   H—C—OH           H—C—OH          HO—C—H
      |                |                |
  HO—C—H           HO—C—H           H—C—OH
      |                |                |
   H—C—OH          HO—C—H            H—C—OH
      |                |                |
   H—C—OH           H—C—OH          HO—C—H
      |                |                |
    CH2OH            CH2OH            CH2OH
   D-glucose        D-galactose      L-galactose
```

D-Glucose and D-galactose are diastereomers. D-galactose and L-galactose are enantiomers.

To possess optical activity a compound must have a chiral center. A *chiral center* is a carbon atom that is attached to four different substituents. A compound possessing a chiral center may still not possess optical activity if there is a plane of symmetry in the molecule.

Light ordinarily oscillates in all planes. If it is passed through a polarizer, its oscillation is reduced to only one plane. If this plane-polarized light is allowed to pass through a solution of an optically active compound, the plane of the light will be rotated. If it is rotated to the right, the rotation is termed dextrorotatory or (+). If it is rotated to the left, the rotation is termed levorotatory or (−). The specific rotation $[\alpha]$ is characteristic of an optically active compound:

$$[\alpha] = \frac{\alpha}{(c)(l)}$$

where α = observed degrees of rotation

  c = concentration, grams per milliliter

  l = length of light path, decimeters

For comparison in the literature, the D line of sodium as the incident light and a temperature of 25°C have been agreed upon as standard.

  A mixture of equal amounts of two enantiomers (called a *racemic* mixture) will have a rotation of zero. The rotations are opposite in sign and equal in numerical value, canceling each other.

The Alkanes

Alkanes are saturated noncyclic compounds of carbon and hydrogen. If carbon atoms are arranged in a straight chain sequence

$$C—C—C—C$$

and hydrogen atoms are added to account for each carbon atom's valence of four, we produce a compound like this:

$$
\begin{array}{c}
\text{H} \quad \text{H} \quad \text{H} \quad \text{H} \\
| \quad\; | \quad\; | \quad\; | \\
\text{HC—C—C—CH} \\
| \quad\; | \quad\; | \quad\; | \\
\text{H} \quad \text{H} \quad \text{H} \quad \text{H}
\end{array}
$$

This compound is *n*-butane. The *n* designates the straight chain character. Another compound with the same numbers of carbon and hydrogen atoms is isobutane (or 2-methyl-propane).

$$
\begin{array}{c}
\text{H}_3\text{C—CH—CH}_3 \\
| \\
\text{CH}_3
\end{array}
$$

  It is useful to learn the names of many of the alkanes. With modification these names are an integral part of the names of the derivatives of alkanes.

Chain Length	Name	Chain Length	Name
1	Methane	11	Undecane
2	Ethane	12	Dodecane
3	Propane	13	Tridecane
4	Butane	14	Tetradecane
5	Pentane	15	Pentadecane
6	Hexane	16	Hexadecane
7	Heptane	17	Heptadecane
8	Octane	18	Octadecane
9	Nonane	19	Nonadecane
10	Decane	20	Eicosane

  The IUPAC rules for nomenclature require that a compound that is not a straight chain be named on the basis of its longest chain. Thus, the following compound is 2-methyl-4-ethyl-heptane:

$$
\begin{array}{c}
\text{H}_3\text{C—CH—CH}_2\text{—CH—CH}_2\text{—CH}_2\text{—CH}_3 \\
| \qquad\qquad\quad | \\
\text{CH}_3 \qquad\quad\;\; \text{CH}_2 \\
\qquad\qquad\qquad | \\
\qquad\qquad\qquad \text{CH}_3
\end{array}
$$

1. **Synthesis—Wurtz Reaction:**

$$2RBr + 2Na \longrightarrow RR + 2NaBr$$

(R will often be used to refer to an unspecified alkyl group.) More specifically:

$$2CH_3Br + 2Na \longrightarrow CH_3 - CH_3 + 2NaBr$$

If a mixture of two alkyl bromides is used, a mixture of three possible products is expected.

2. **Reactions:**

The alkanes are not very reactive, but they will undergo some reactions.

    a. *Halogenation*

$$
\mathrm{Cl_2} +
\begin{array}{cc}
H & H \\
| & | \\
HC & CH \\
| & | \\
H & H
\end{array}
\xrightarrow[\substack{\text{u.v.} \\ \text{light}}]{\text{heat}}
\begin{array}{cc}
H & H \\
| & | \\
HC & C-Cl \\
| & | \\
H & H
\end{array}
+ HCl
$$

Reaction may continue and produce a more highly chlorinated product.

    b. *Oxidation*

Alkanes may be oxidized to produce CO_2, water, and energy.

The Cycloalkanes

The small ring cycloalkanes (cyclopropane and cyclobutane) are strained and are more reactive. Cyclopropane is planar, and the bond angles must be 60°. The normal bond angle is 109° 28′. Five- and six-membered rings are not appreciably strained. Larger rings were once thought to be unstable because of the strain (Baeyer), but puckering allows relative freedom from strain.

    Example:

$$
\begin{array}{c}
CH_2 \\
\diagup \diagdown \\
CH_2 - CH_2
\end{array}
\qquad \text{cyclopropane}
$$

The Alkenes

The alkenes may be considered as alkanes from which hydrogen has been removed, producing a carbon-to-carbon double bond. The simplest example of this series is ethene (ethylene).

$$H_2C = CH_2 \qquad \text{ethene}$$

$$H_2C = CH - CH_2 - CH_3 \quad \text{1-butene}$$

$$
\begin{array}{c}
H \\
| \\
H_3C - C = C - CH_3 \\
| \\
H
\end{array}
\qquad \textit{trans}\text{-2-butene}
$$

$$
\begin{array}{c}
H \quad H \\
| \quad | \\
H_3C - C = C - CH_3
\end{array}
\qquad \textit{cis}\text{-2-butene}
$$

1. **Synthesis:**

   a. *Dehydrohalogenation*

   $$H_3C\!-\!CH_2Br + \text{alcoholic KOH} \longrightarrow H_2C\!=\!CH_2 + H_2O + KBr$$

   b. *Dehydration*

   $$H_3C\!-\!CH_2OH \xrightarrow[H_2SO_4]{\text{heat}} H_2C\!=\!CH_2 + H_2O$$

   c. *Dehalogenation*

   $$Br\!-\!CH_2\!-\!CH_2\!-\!Br + Zn \longrightarrow H_2C\!=\!CH_2 + ZnBr_2$$

   d. *Cracking* (relatively nonspecific decomposition reactions)

   $$H_3C\!-\!(CH_2)_4\!-\!CH_3 \xrightarrow[\text{cracking}]{\text{heat}} H_2C\!=\!CH_2 + H_3C\!-\!CH_2CH_2\!-\!CH_3$$

2. **Reactions:**

   a. *Addition of HX to the double bond*

   $$H_3C\!-\!CH\!=\!CH_2 + HBr \longrightarrow H_3C\!-\!\overset{\displaystyle H}{\underset{\displaystyle Br}{\overset{|}{\underset{|}{C}}}}\!-\!CH_3$$

   The Markownikoff Rule says that in the addition of an acid across a double bond, the double-bonded carbon having the most hydrogen will receive the H of HX. The above is true for ionic addition, but in the presence of peroxides we see a free radical anti-Markownikoff addition:

   $$H_3C\!-\!CH\!=\!CH_2 + HBr \xrightarrow{\text{peroxide}} H_3C\!-\!CH_2\!-\!CH_2Br$$

   b. *Hydrogenation* (catalyst such as Pt, Pd, or Ni):

   $$H_2C\!=\!CH_2 + H_2 \xrightarrow{Pt} H_3C\!-\!CH_3$$
   $$3H_2C\!=\!CH\!-\!CH\!=\!CH_2 + 4H_2 \xrightarrow{Pt} H_3C\!-\!CH\!=\!CH\!-\!CH_3$$
   $$+ H_2C\!=\!CH\!-\!CH_2\!-\!CH_3$$
   $$+ H_3C\!-\!CH_2\!-\!CH_2\!-\!CH_3$$

   c. $H_2C\!=\!CH_2 + Br2 \longrightarrow BrCH_2\!-\!CH_2Br$

   d. $H_2C\!=\!CH_2 \xrightarrow{\text{catalyst}}$ polymer (polyethylene in this case)

The Alkynes (derivatives of acetylene)

HC≡CH acetylene or ethyne

1. **Synthesis:**

   a. $CaC_2 + H_2O \longrightarrow C_2H_2 + CaO$

   b. *Dehydrohalogenation*

   $$H_3C\!-\!CHBr_2 + 2KOH \longrightarrow HC\!\equiv\!CH + 2H_2O + 2KBr$$

   c. *Dehalogenation*

   $$HCBr_2\!-\!CBr_2H + 2Zn \longrightarrow HC\!\equiv\!CH + 2ZnBr_2$$

2. Reactions:

a. *Hydrogenation*

$$HC\equiv CH + H_2 \xrightarrow{Pt} H_2C=CH_2 + H_2 \xrightarrow{Pt} CH_3-CH_3$$

b. *Hydrohalogenation—see reactions of alkenes*

c. *Halogenation—see reactions of alkenes*

d. *Reaction of active hydrogen*

$$H_3C-C\equiv CH + Ag^+ \longrightarrow H_3C-C\equiv CAg + H^+$$
$$H_3C-C\equiv CH + NaNH_2 \longrightarrow H_3C-C\equiv CNa + NH_3$$
$$H_3C-C\equiv CNa + CH_3Br \longrightarrow H_3C-C\equiv C-CH_3 + NaBr$$

Aromatic Compounds

Aromatic compounds consist of benzene and compounds whose chemical reactions are similar to those of benzene. Almost all aromatic compounds that you would be expected to recognize as such are derivatives of benzene; there are other unrelated aromatic compounds.

1. Nature of Benzene—Resonance: Although we may draw benzene as having three discrete double bonds and three discrete single bonds in conjugation, this does not adequately describe its structure. It may be shown as two structures in resonance.

In reality, however, it appears that each carbon atom has three discrete covalent bonds, and the fourth bonding electron of each carbon atom is delocalized in electron clouds around the ring.

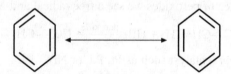

2. Synthesis of the Aromatic Ring: This is unusual; in general one will only be interested in reactions of compounds containing the benzene ring rather than in the synthesis of the aromatic ring.

3. Reactions: (ϕ is sometimes used as a shorthand designation for the phenyl group. Thus, benzene could be indicated as ϕ-H.)

a. *Monosubstitution*

$$\phi\text{-H} + HNO_3 \longrightarrow \phi\text{—}NO_2 + H_2O$$
$$\phi\text{-H} + H_2SO_4 \longrightarrow \phi\text{—}SO_3H + H_2O$$
$$\phi\text{-H} + Br_2 \xrightarrow{Fe} \phi\text{—}Br + HBr$$

b. *Friedel-Crafts reaction*

$$\phi\text{-H} + RCl \xrightarrow{AlCl_3} \phi\text{—}R + HCl$$

$$\phi\text{-H} + R\overset{O}{\overset{\|}{-C}}-Cl \xrightarrow{AlCl_3} \phi\overset{O}{\overset{\|}{-C}}-R + HCl$$

c. *Substitution in a benzene ring that already has one substituent*

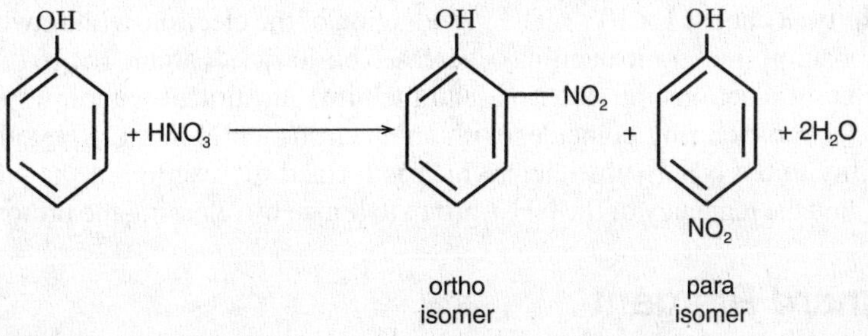

ortho
isomer

para
isomer

The placement of the second substituent is ordained by the first substituent. The OH substituent, as shown above, is an ortho, para-directing group. Other ortho, para-directing substituents include the CH_3 group and the halogens. The halogens deactivate the ring and also direct ortho, para. Many electrophilic substituents are said to be meta-directing: NO_2, CN, SO_3H, COOH, and so forth.

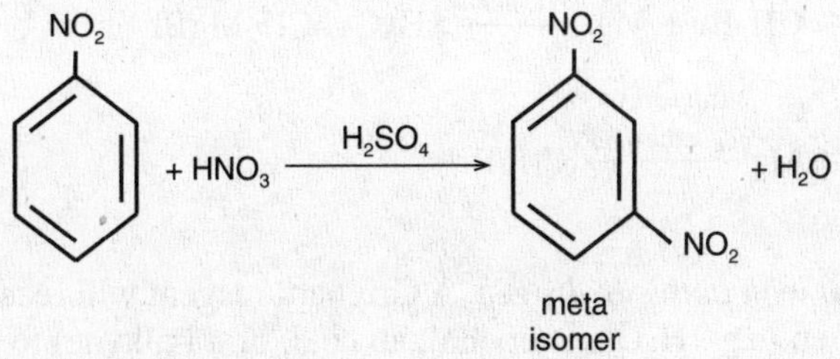

meta
isomer

The above meta-directing substituents also deactivate the ring.

Note that the reactions above *do* balance. In many cases below, we will write organic reactions that do not balance. This is done for the sake of simplicity and to emphasize the desired products.

d. *Diazotization of amines*

$$\phi-NH_2 + HNO_2 \longrightarrow \phi-N_2^+$$

e. *Reactions of diazonium salts* (see above)

$$\phi-N_2^+ + CuBr \longrightarrow \phi-Br$$

$$\phi-N_2^+ + CuCN \longrightarrow \phi-CN$$

$$\phi-N_2^+ + H_2O \xrightarrow{H+} \phi-OH$$

$$\phi-N_2^+ + \phi-OH \longrightarrow \phi-N{=}N-\phi-OH \text{ (Coupling)}$$

$$\phi-N_2^+ + H_2 \xrightarrow{Pt} \phi N\overset{\overset{\displaystyle H}{|}}{-}NH_2$$

4. Acidity and Basicity:

a. *Acidity*. Phenol will ionize as an acid with a K_a of about 1×10^{-10}. A methyl substituent in the ortho position will lower the K_a (and the acidity) to about 6×10^{-11}. The electron-releasing methyl substituent contributes electrons to the ring and depresses release of H^+. A nitro substituent in the ortho position, conversely, increases the acidity (K_a about 7×10^{-8}) by withdrawing electrons from the ring.

b. *Basicity*. Aniline (aminobenzene or phenylamine) has a K_a of about 4×10^{-10}. The introduction of an electron-releasing methyl group in the para position (i.e., *p*-methylaniline) increases basicity (K_b about 1×10^{-9}). The introduction of the electron-withdrawing nitro group into the para position (i.e., *p*-nitroaniline) decreases basicity (K_b about 1×10^{-13}). The methyl substituent releases electrons into the ring, and the nitro substituent withdraws electrons from the ring. An electron-rich ring coincides with an electron-rich N in the NH_2 substituent. This will add stability to the NH_3^+ substituent which is formed by reaction of the NH_2 substituent with a proton, and the tendency of the NH_3^+ group to ionize by releasing the proton is decreased.

The Grignard Reagent

The Grignard reagent is one of the most important and versatile in organic chemistry. We will try to outline only a few of its reactions.

1. **Synthesis:** The Grignard reagent is synthesized by the reaction of an alkyl halide with elemental magnesium in the presence of anhydrous ether.

Example:

$$H_3C-CH_2Br + Mg \xrightarrow[\text{ether}]{\text{anhydrous}} H_3C-CH_2MgBr$$

or

$$RBr + Mg \xrightarrow[\text{ether}]{\text{anhydrous}} RMgBr$$

2. **Reactions:**

a. *Reaction with active hydrogen*. A Grignard reagent will react with any compound having active hydrogen (e.g., H_2O, an alcohol, an acid, or a 1-alkyne) to form a hydrocarbon.

$$RMgBr + H_2O \longrightarrow RH + MgBrOH$$

b. *Reaction with aldehydes and ketones*

$$RMgBr + HCHO \xrightarrow[\text{ether}]{\text{anhydrous}} R-CH_2OM \xrightarrow{H^+} RCH_2OH \text{ (primary alcohol)}$$

$$RMgBr + R'CHO \xrightarrow[\text{ether}]{\text{anhydrous}} \underset{\underset{H}{|}}{RC}-OMgBr \xrightarrow{H^+} \underset{\underset{H}{|}}{RC}-OH$$

(secondary alcohol)

$$RMgBr + R'-C=O \xrightarrow[\text{ether}]{\text{anhydrous}} R'-COMgBr \xrightarrow{H^+} R'-C-OH$$

with R'' above and R below (tertiary alcohol)

c. *Reaction with CO_2*

$$RMgBr + CO_2 \xrightarrow[\text{ether}]{\text{anhydrous}} R-\overset{\overset{O}{\|}}{C}-OMgBr \xrightarrow{H^+} RCOOH$$

d. *Reaction with an ester or an acyl halide*

$$RMgBr + R'COOR'' \xrightarrow[\text{ether}]{\text{anhydrous}} R' \overset{\overset{\displaystyle O}{\|}}{-}C-R$$

$$RMgBr + R'COBr \xrightarrow[\text{ether}]{\text{anhydrous}} R' \overset{\overset{\displaystyle O}{\|}}{-}C-R$$

Alcohols

Alcohols may be designated as ROH. The simplest alcohol is CH_3OH and is named methanol (i.e., methan-ol) as a derivative of the one-carbon hydrocarbon, methane. Other alcohols are similarly named as derivatives of hydrocarbons. The compound below is named 2-pentanol or 2-hydroxypentane.

$$H_3C-CH_2-CH_2-CH-CH_3$$
$$|$$
$$OH$$

The alcohols are very weak acids, even weaker than water. Polarity and hydrogen bonding cause short chain alcohols to be soluble in water.

1. **Synthesis:**
   a. *Hydration of alkenes*

   $$H_2C=CH_2 + H_2O \overset{H^+}{\rightleftharpoons} H_3C-CH_2OH$$

   b. *Using Grignard reagents–discussed elsewhere*
   c. *Hydrolysis of alkyl halides*

   $$R-I + H_2O \overset{KOH}{\rightleftharpoons} ROH + I^-$$

   d. *Reduction of aldehydes and ketones*

   $$R-CHO + NaBH_4 \xrightarrow{H_2O} R-CH_2OH$$

2. **Reactions:**
   a. *Oxidation to form aldehydes or ketones*

   $$R-CH_2OH + K_2Cr_2O_7 \xrightarrow{H^+} R-CHO$$

This is useful only if the aldehyde may be removed (sometimes by distillation) before further oxidation to the carboxylic acid. A ketone may not be easily oxidized further, but chain rupture is possible.

   b. *Dehydration to form alkenes–discussed elsewhere*
   c. *Formation of esters*

   $$R-COOH + R-CH_2OH \overset{H^+}{\rightleftharpoons} R-COOCH_2-R$$

   d. *Conversion to halides*

   $$ROH + HI \rightleftharpoons RI + H_2O$$

Amines

Amines have the structure R—NH_2. The simplest example is methylamine (or aminomethane):

$$H_3CNH_2$$

1. **Synthesis:**
   a. $RX + NH_3 \longrightarrow R—NH_2$
   b. $RCN + LiAlH_4 \longrightarrow R—CH_2—NH_2$
   c. *Hofmann degradation*

$$R—CONH_2 \xrightarrow{Br_2,\ NaOH} RNH_2$$

2. **Reactions:**

   a. $R—NH_2 + HONO \xrightarrow{H_2O} ROH + N_2$

(This is the reaction for a primary alkyl amine)

   b. $R—NH_2 + HONO \longrightarrow RN_2^+$

(This is the reaction for a primary aromatic amine. The diazonium salt is stable at the temperatures of ice water. It is capable of numerous further reactions under appropriate conditions.)

   c. $R—NH_2 + R'—COOH + \text{dicyclohexylcarbodiimid} \longrightarrow R—NH—COR'$
   (an amide)

Amides

Amides have the structure R—NH—COR.
A simple example is acetanilide, ϕ—NH—CO—CH_3.

1. **Synthesis:**

   a. $R—NH_2 + R'—COCl$ (an acyl chloride) $\longrightarrow R—NH—\overset{\overset{\displaystyle O}{\|}}{C}—R'$

   b. $R—NH_2 + (R'—CO)_2O$ (an anhydride) $\longrightarrow R—NH—\overset{\overset{\displaystyle O}{\|}}{C}—R'$

   c. $R—NH_2 + R'—COOH + \text{dicyclohexylcarbodiimide} \longrightarrow R—NH—\overset{\overset{\displaystyle O}{\|}}{C}—R'$

(Primary amines are shown, but secondary amines may also be used.)

2. **Reaction:**

$$R—NH—COR' + H_2O \xrightarrow{H+} R—NH_3^+ + R'—COOH$$

(The reaction may also be accomplished in an aqueous base.)

Aldehydes and Ketones

1. **Synthesis:**

   a. *Reaction of a Grignard reagent with a carboxylic ester or an acyl halide to form a ketone* (outlined on page 246 under "Grignard Reagent")

   b. *Mild oxidation of an alcohol* (often feasible in the synthesis of ketones and sometimes in the synthesis of aldehydes)

$$RCH_2OH \longrightarrow R-CHO \text{ (aldehyde)}$$

$$\begin{array}{c} R' \\ | \\ R-COH \\ | \\ H \end{array} \longrightarrow \; > R-\overset{\displaystyle R'}{\underset{}{C}}=O \text{ (ketone)}$$

   c. *Friedel-Crafts acylation to produce aromatic ketones* (see "Aromatic Compounds," page 244)

   d. *Decarboxylation of acids to produce ketones*

$$2RCOOH \xrightarrow{ThO_2, \; \triangle} R-\overset{\displaystyle O}{\overset{\|}{C}}-R + CO_2$$

   e. *Oxidation of diols to form aldehydes*

$$R-\underset{|}{\overset{|}{C}}H-\underset{|}{\overset{|}{C}}H-R' \xrightarrow{HIO_4 \text{ or } Pb(OAc)_4} R-CHO + R'-CHO$$
$$\overset{OH}{}\;\;\overset{OH}{}$$

$$R-\underset{|}{\overset{OH}{C}}H-\underset{|}{\overset{OH}{C}}H-\underset{|}{\overset{OH}{C}}H-R' \xrightarrow{HIO_4 \text{ or } Pb(OAc)_4} R-CHO + R'-CHO + HCOOH$$

$$R-\underset{|}{\overset{OH}{C}}H-CH_2-\underset{|}{\overset{OH}{C}}H-R' \xrightarrow{HIO_4 \text{ or } Pb(OAc)_4} \text{No reaction}$$

2. **Reactions:**

   a. *Reaction with Grignard reagents*

$$R-\overset{\displaystyle O}{\overset{\|}{C}}-R' + R''MgBr \xrightarrow[\text{ether}]{\text{anhydrous}} R-\underset{|}{\overset{|}{C}}-R' \xrightarrow{H_2O} R-\underset{|}{\overset{|}{C}}-R'$$

with $OMgBr$ and R'' on the middle structure, and OH and R'' on the final structure.

$$R-CHO + R'MgBr \xrightarrow[\text{ether}]{\text{anhydrous}} R-\underset{|}{\overset{OMgBr}{C}}H-R' \xrightarrow{H_2O} R-\underset{|}{\overset{OH}{C}}H-R'$$

$$HCHO + RMgBr \xrightarrow[\text{ether}]{\text{anhydrous}} R-CH_2-OMgBr \xrightarrow{H_2O} R-CH_2OH$$

b. *Reaction of aldehydes or ketones with HCN*

$$R-CHO + HCN \longrightarrow R-\underset{\underset{H}{|}}{\overset{\overset{OH}{|}}{C}}-CN \xrightarrow{H_2O,\ H^+} R-\underset{\underset{H}{|}}{\overset{\overset{OH}{|}}{C}}-COOH$$

c. *Reaction of aldehydes or methyl ketones with NaHSO$_3$*

$$R-CHO + NaHSO_3 \longrightarrow R-\underset{\underset{H}{|}}{\overset{\overset{OH}{|}}{C}}-SO_3^-Na^+$$

d. *Reaction with alcohols*

$$R-CHO + R'-OH \xrightarrow{H^+} R-\underset{\underset{H}{|}}{\overset{\overset{OH}{|}}{C}}-OR' \xrightarrow{R'OH,\ H^+} R-\underset{\underset{H}{|}}{\overset{\overset{OR'}{|}}{C}}-OR'$$

$$\text{(a hemiacetal)} \qquad\qquad \text{(an acetal)}$$

$$R-\overset{\overset{O}{\|}}{C}-R' + R''OH \xrightarrow{H^+} R-\underset{\underset{OR''}{|}}{\overset{\overset{OH}{|}}{C}}-R' \xrightarrow{R''OH,\ H^+} R-\underset{\underset{OR''}{|}}{\overset{\overset{OR''}{|}}{C}}-R'$$

$$\text{(a hemiketal)} \qquad\qquad \text{(a ketal)}$$

e. *Reaction of ketones and aldehydes with hydroxylamine*

$$R-CHO + NH_2OH \xrightarrow{H^+} R-\overset{\overset{H}{|}}{C}=NOH$$

$$\text{(an oxime)}$$

f. *Reaction of ketones and aldehydes with hydrazine or hydrazine derivatives*

$$R-CHO + NH_2NH_2 \xrightarrow{H^+} R-\overset{\overset{H}{|}}{C}=N-NH_2$$

$$\text{(a hydrazone)}$$

g. *Oxidation of aldehydes*

$$R-CHO + Ag(NH_3)_2^+ \xrightarrow{OH^-} R-\overset{\overset{O}{\|}}{C}-O^- + Ag$$

$$\text{(Tollens' reagent)} \qquad\qquad \text{(silver mirror)}$$

$$R-CHO + Cu^{++} \xrightarrow{OH^-,\ citrate} R-\overset{\overset{O}{\|}}{C}-O^- + Cu_2O$$

$$\text{(Benedict's reagent)} \qquad\qquad \text{(red ppt.)}$$

h. *Haloform reaction with acetaldehyde or methyl ketones*

$$R-\underset{O}{\overset{O}{||}}C-CH_3 \xrightarrow{IO^-} RCO^- + CHI_3$$

i. *Aldol condensation* (requires alpha-hydrogen). Further reaction can also lead to polymers.

$$2CH_3-CHO \xrightarrow{OH^-} H_3C-\underset{H}{\overset{OH}{|}}C-CH_2-CHO$$

j. *Cannizzaro reaction* (for aldehydes having no alpha-hydrogen)

$$2\phi-CHO \xrightarrow{OH^-} \phi-CH_2OH + \phi-C-O^-$$

Carboxylic Acids

The carboxylic acids are organic compounds that ionize to produce free protons and carboxylate anions. The simplest example is formic acid, $H-C-OH$

1. **Synthesis:**

   a. *Addition of carbon dioxide to a Grignard reagent*

   $$R\,MgBr + CO_2 \longrightarrow R-C-OMgBr \xrightarrow{H^+} R-C-OH$$

   b. *Oxidation of alkene*

   $$R-C=C-R' + KMnO_4 \longrightarrow R-\underset{OH}{\overset{H}{|}}C-\underset{OH}{\overset{H}{|}}C-R'$$

   $$R-\underset{OH}{\overset{H}{|}}C-\underset{OH}{\overset{H}{|}}C-R' + KMnO_4 \longrightarrow RCOOH + R'COOH$$

   c. *Oxidation of primary alcohol*

   $$R-CH_2OH + KMnO_4 \longrightarrow RCOOH$$

   d. *Hydrolysis of nitrile*

   $$RCN \xrightarrow{H_2O,\,H^+} RCOOH$$

e. *Hydrolysis of esters*

$$R\overset{\displaystyle O}{\overset{\|}{-C}}-O-R' + H_2O \overset{H^+}{\rightleftharpoons} R-COOH + R'OH$$

f. *Saponification of esters*

$$R\overset{\displaystyle O}{\overset{\|}{-C}}-O-R' + NaOH \rightleftharpoons R'OH + R\overset{\displaystyle O}{\overset{\|}{-C}}-ONa \overset{H^+}{\longrightarrow} R-COOH$$

2. **Reactions:**
   a. *Neutralization of base*

   $$RCOOH + NaOH \longrightarrow R\overset{\displaystyle O}{\overset{\|}{C}}-O^- + Na^+ + H_2O$$

   b. *Esterification*

   $$RCOOH + R'OH \overset{H^+}{\rightleftharpoons} R\overset{\displaystyle O}{\overset{\|}{-C}}-OR' + H_2O$$

   c. *Formation of acylhalide*

   $$RCOOH \overset{PBr_3}{\longrightarrow} R\overset{\displaystyle O}{\overset{\|}{C}}-Br$$

   d. *Formation of anhydride*

   $$2RCOOH \longrightarrow R\overset{\displaystyle O}{\overset{\|}{-C}}-O\overset{\displaystyle O}{\overset{\|}{-C}}-R + H_2O$$

   e. *High-temperature decomposition*

   $$2RCOOH \overset{ThO_2,\ \Delta}{\longrightarrow} R\overset{\displaystyle O}{\overset{\|}{-C}}-R + CO_2 + H_2O$$

Esters

Esters may be formed from the reaction between an acid and an alcohol. Upon hydrolysis the products are an acid and an alcohol. We often think first of carboxylic acid esters, but they are not the only ones known. Phosphate esters are common in biochemistry.

The simplest carboxylic acid ester is methyl formate:

$$H\overset{\displaystyle O}{\overset{\|}{-C}}-O-CH_3$$

1. **Synthesis:**

   a. $R—COCl + R'—OH \longrightarrow R—\overset{\overset{\displaystyle O}{\|}}{C}—OR'$

   b. $(R—\overset{\overset{\displaystyle O}{\|}}{C})_2O + R'—OH \longrightarrow R—\overset{\overset{\displaystyle O}{\|}}{C}—OR'$

   c. $R—COOH + R'—OH \overset{H^+}{\rightleftharpoons} R—\overset{\overset{\displaystyle O}{\|}}{C}—OR' + H_2O$

   An equilibrium will be established. Removal of water by an appropriate method such as azeotropic separation will produce good yields. High yields based on one reactant can also be achieved by adding large quantities of the other reactant.

2. **Reactions:**

   a. *Acid hydrolysis*

   $$R—COOR' + H_2O \overset{H^+}{\longrightarrow} R—COOH + R'OH$$

   b. *Saponification*

   $$R—COOR' + H_2O \overset{OH^-}{\longrightarrow} R—COO^- + R'OH$$

Ethers

1. **Synthesis:**

   a. *Dehydration. (Remember that the choice of conditions determines whether the ether or the unsaturated hydrocarbon, in this case ethylene, is the major product.)*

   $$2CH_3—CH_2OH \overset{H_2SO_4, \Delta}{\longrightarrow} CH_3—CH_2—O—CH_2CH_3$$

   b. *Williamson synthesis.* Much more useful than the dehydration method if an unsymmetrical ether is desired.

   $$RONa + R'Br \longrightarrow ROR'$$

2. **Reactions:** Ethers are generally unreactive compounds. They are often useful as solvents in organic reactions because of their unreactive nature. They may be cleaved by heated halogen acids:

   $$ROR + HI \overset{heat}{\longrightarrow} RI + ROH$$

The ROH which is formed may react with HI to form an additional RI.

Final Remarks

As stated earlier, you cannot learn organic chemistry from a brief presentation such as this. We recognize that we have been able to present only some of the more important points. It is our intent that you use this material (and the questions and answers in the practice tests) to review the organic chemistry you have learned in your coursework. If you find areas of weakness in your preparation, we would recommend that you study those areas in your organic chemistry textbook.

Spectroscopic Instrumentation

Several different kinds of spectroscopy are used in determining structure of chemicals and in determining the amount of a particular chemical.

1. Visible and ultraviolet spectroscopy: *Visible spectroscopy* uses light of about 400–800 nm passing through a solution. The amount of light that is absorbed is a measure of the amount of a solute that is in solution. It is used primarily to quantitate a particular solute rather than to identify an unknown structure.

$$A = \varepsilon cl$$

(A is absorbance; ε is the extinction coefficient; c is the concentration in moles per liter; and l is the length of the light path through the solution.)

Ultraviolet spectroscopy may be used in determination of structure as well as in quantitation of solutes. In quantitation the same formula as in visible spectroscopy is applied.

$$A = \varepsilon cl$$

Thus, if the absorbance at a particular wavelength decreases from 1.0 to 0.5, the concentration has decreased by the same 50%. (The extinction coefficient [ε] does not change at a particular wavelength, and we would not have changed the length of the light path.)

Ultraviolet spectra also give an indication of conjugated double bonds. Increasing the conjugation in a series of compounds will increase the wavelength at which peak (maximum) absorption occurs.

$CH_2=CH-CH=CH_2$ has an absorption maximum at 220 nm

$CH_2=CH-CH=CH-CH=CH_2$ has an absorption maximum of 257 nm

With aromatic compounds

 has an absorption maximum at 215 nm

benzene

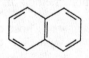 has an absorption maximum at 314 nm

naphthalene

2. Infrared spectroscopy: Infrared (IR) spectroscopy is sometimes used for quantitation, but it is more often used for determination of molecular structure. Absorption in the IR range of about 650 to 4000 waves/cm is usually of interest. The range from about 1500–4000 has absorption bands that are fairly specific for particular bonds and functional groups. (For example, carbon-to-oxygen double bonds in aldehydes, ketones, esters, and acids absorb at about 1650–1780 waves/cm.) By contrast, the range of the spectrum from about 650–1500 waves/cm is looked upon as the fingerprint region.

Thus two compounds might be known to be aldehydes by various tests, known synthetic route, or IR absorption around 1650–1780 waves/cm. Absorption in the fingerprint area would enable the chemist to distinguish between them and often to identify them.

3. Nuclear Magnetic Resonance (NMR) Spectroscopy: This refers to study of molecules in a magnetic field during radiofrequency irradiation. (Ordinarily the spectrum is obtained during constant radiofrequency irradiation and varying magnetic strength.)

The spectrum is displayed with high field at the right and low field at the left. The trimethylsilane peak (at the right) is given a value of zero. The distance of another peak from trimethylsilane is indicated as δ. Each peak represents one kind of hydrogen atoms. Thus benzene would have only one peak, since the hydrogens are all equivalent. Toluene, in contrast, would have two peaks. One peak would be for the hydrogens of the methyl substituent, and one peak would be for the ring hydrogens. Since there are 5 ring hydrogens and 3 hydrogens in the methyl substituent, the ratio of areas of one peak to the other would be 5/3 or about 1.67.

Toluene

We have concentrated on NMR with only the ^1H atoms. NMR with ^{13}C is also done, but consideration is beyond the scope of this book.

4. Mass spectrometry: A small sample is introduced into a mass spectrometer at high vacuum. The sample is vaporized and bombarded with electrons, leading to loss of an electron from the sample molecule. The result is a positively charged ion of the same mass as the beginning sample. (This is referred to as the molecular ion.) The ions pass through a magnetic field in which they are separated according to their mass/charge ratios. As stated to this point, the technique would have modest interest in the chemical laboratory. But it turns out that there is further breakdown to produce daughter ions. The entire mass/charge spectrum is very useful in determining molecular weight and assists in the determination of structure.

BIOCHEMISTRY

Biochemistry or biological chemistry may be seen as an attempt to better understand life by studying the chemicals that are important in living cells and organisms. One must consider the amounts and identities of a variety of chemicals, as well as the ways in which they are transformed during different life processes. Perhaps it should not be surprising that biochemistry calls upon the background of other areas of chemistry, including organic chemistry, analytical chemistry, inorganic chemistry, and physical chemistry.

In these few pages we can only touch lightly on a few concepts in biochemistry. Those of you who continue in the life sciences, such as medicine, dentistry, or pharmacy, will be taught a great deal more about this fascinating area. Here we can only begin to delineate the forest, leaving you to study the trees at a later time. For those who have had little or no exposure to biochemistry, this brief introduction will help to prepare you for the Medical College Admission Test and will also lay the groundwork for your course in professional school. For those who have already taken a course in biochemistry, this material will assist in consolidating the information you already possess.

Areas of Biochemistry

Although there are a number of ways of subdividing biochemistry, there are substantial similarities among them. The subdivision is done according to similarities in the properties of the compounds within each subdivision. A biochemist usually specializes in the study of one of these subdivisions:

pH and Buffers

The concepts of pH and buffers presented on pages 232–234 under acids and bases are used also in biochemistry. The biochemist applies these principles in the context of the human body.

The human body (and other animal bodies) requires that the pH be maintained over a rather small range. The pH of human blood is ordinarily maintained from 7.36 to 7.42. Buffers prevent greater fluctuation, which could occur in response to loss or gain of acid or base.

The buffer pairs used in human blood include HCO_3^-/H_2CO_3; base/acid species of oxygenated hemoglobin; and base/acid species of deoxygenated hemoglobin. The phosphate pair $HPO_4^{2-}/H_2PO_4^-$ would offer a possible buffer, but little is present in the blood.

Amino Acids, Peptides, and Proteins

Amino Acids: The naturally occurring amino acids are primarily α-amino acids of the general structure

$$
\begin{array}{c}
NH_2 \\
| \\
R-C-COOH \\
| \\
H
\end{array}
$$

If R does not represent H, then it will be noted that an asymmetric center exists, allowing for L and D isomers. The ones commonly found in nature, especially in higher animals, are usually of the L series. (The amino acid having no asymmetric center, and thus devoid of optical activity, is glycine.)

Although approximately 300 amino acids are found in nature, some are relatively rare. About 20 amino acids occur in all organisms. Amino acids can serve as biologically active compounds in their own right (e.g., neurotransmitters), but we tend to think of them most often as the monomers of which the polymeric peptides and higher molecular weight proteins are composed.

Subdivisions of Amino Acids. It is possible to subdivide the amino acids based on their R groups. This is useful in predicting such things as the folding of a protein in a lipoprotein membrane; it is also helpful in remembering the different amino acids. Thus, they may be subdivided into aliphatic, hydroxy, sulfur, aromatic, dicarboxy (or dicarboxy with one carboxyl as an amide), diamino, and imino on the basis of the R groups.

They may also be subdivided into acidic, basic, and neutral. Those having a second amino function are basic (two basic functional groups and only one carboxyl). Those having a second proton-releasing functional group are acidic. (This second group could be a carboxyl. It could also be the more weakly ionized phenolic or sulfhydryl group.) The neutral amino acids contain only a single acidic and a single basic group, thus canceling each other.

Essential Amino Acids. Although many amino acids may be synthesized in the animal body, certain animals are unable to synthesize sufficient quantities of particular amino acids, called *essential amino acids*. (The term indicates no judgment of the importance of these amino acids compared to that of the other amino acids. It simply indicates that for optimal health these amino acids must be supplied in the diet.) In humans, ten amino acids are usually called essential: phenylalanine, valine, tryptophan, threonine, isoleucine, methionine, histidine, arginine, leucine, and lysine. Of these, histidine and arginine may be required in the diet only of infants or under special circumstances.

Forms of an Amino Acid. A simple amino acid such as glycine can exist in three forms. At a low pH such as 1, the amino group is protonated (and carrying a charge of +1); the carboxyl is not ionized or charged; and the net charge is +1. At an intermediate pH such as 7, the amino function and the carboxyl function carry equal and opposite charges of +1 and –1, and the net is a charge of zero. At a still higher pH such as 12, the carboxyl is ionized and the amino not ionized, resulting in a net charge of –1. The mean of the pK_a of these two ionizable groups is the pH at which the amino has no net charge and will not move in an electrical field. This pH is defined as the *isoionic point* and designated as pI.

Peptides and Proteins: Peptides are linear chains of amino acids with the carboxyl group of one amino acid attached in amide (specifically peptide) linkage to the amino group of the next amino acid.

$$\begin{array}{c} R_3 \quad\; O \quad\;\; H \quad R_2 \quad\; O \quad\;\; H \quad\;\; R \\ | \quad\;\; \| \quad\;\; | \quad\;\; | \quad\;\; \| \quad\;\; | \quad\;\; | \\ H_3N^+\!-\!C\!-\!C\!-\!N\!-\!C\!-\!C\!-\!N\!-\!C\!-\!COO^- \\ | \qquad\qquad | \qquad\qquad | \\ H \qquad\qquad H \qquad\qquad H \end{array}$$

Proteins are larger assemblies of amino acids. The linear sequence of amino acids in a chain is called the *primary structure*. The orientation of the peptide chain (e.g., the alpha helix) is called the *secondary structure*. The relationship of portions of the polypeptide chains to one another is called the *tertiary structure*. In some cases there are dimers, trimers, tetramers, etc., of the polypeptide chains. This is called the *quaternary structure*. Sometimes the units are identical, sometimes not. In the enzyme lactate dehydrogenase, two different monomers are assembled into an active tetramer. Five different active lactate dehydrogenase tetramers are possible and are separable by electrophoresis.

The primary structure of a peptide or protein may be determined by a combination of procedures. The carboxy terminal amino acid may be determined by its enzymatic release by carboxypeptidases. The rate of release allows determination of the sequence of a small number of amino acids at the carboxy terminal end. Another method, the Edman degradation, utilizes reaction of the amino terminus with phenylisothiocyanate, hydrolysis of the derivative of this amino acid from the peptide chain, and identification of the amino acid derivative. This Edman degradation allows determination of a number of amino acids in sequence at the amino terminal end.

Determination of a number of amino acids at each end of a peptide chain would not allow determination of the sequence of a long peptide chain. Fortunately there are also other enzymes (endopeptidases) that perform internal cleavage with a high degree of specificity. The smaller peptides thus formed may be separated and sequenced. By utilizing different endopeptidases, it is possible to prepare a series of overlapping peptides. When they are sequenced, it is possible to determine the sequence of the intact peptide.

By other methodology it is also possible to synthesize peptides. This procedure, referred to as the Merrifield synthesis, utilizes a solid material with a functional group to which the peptide chain is attached.

Enzymes

In 1926 Sumner isolated the enzyme urease from jack beans and claimed the enzyme to be a protein. Few believed this initially, and the claim was not accepted until about 1935.

Now, over 2600 enzymes have been isolated. Although biological in origin and protein in structure, enzymes are simply catalysts, serving to increase the rate of reactions in which they are involved.

Nomenclature: Some enzymes are given trivial names, such as the proteolytic enzymes trypsin or pepsin, names that provide no information about their function unless one is familiar with these specific enzymes. Others have names that identify the substrate and type of reaction; examples are histidine decarboxylase (decarboxylating histidine to produce CO_2 and histamine), urease (breaking down urea to produce CO_2 and NH_3), and alcohol dehydrogenase (removing hydrogen and electrons from an alcohol to produce a reduced coenzyme and an aldehyde).

Since about 1965 (with a revision in 1972), there has been an attempt to confer more systematic nomenclature and classification on enzymes. An enzyme commission (EC) number is given as four numbers separated by periods. The first of these numbers indicates the main class.

1. Oxidoreductases—oxidation-reduction reactions
2. Transferases—transfer intact groups of atoms from donors to acceptors
3. Hydrolases—cleave by hydrolysis
4. Lyases—cleave C—C, C—O, C—N, and other bonds without hydrolysis or oxidation. (Hydration and dehydration reactions are included in this class.)
5. Isomerases—interconvert isomers, such as cis → *trans*; D⟶L
6. Ligases—form bonds as a result of condensation of two different substances with energy provided by ATP.

An example of EC nomenclature and numbering is alcohol: NAD^+ oxidoreductase (EC1.1.1.1). The first number identifies it as an oxidoreductase; the second number identifies its subclass; the third number identifies its sub-subclass; and the final number is a serial listing within the sub-subclass. EC1.1.1.1 is more commonly known as alcohol dehydrogenase.

Cofactors: In addition to the protein portion, many enzymes need cofactors or coenzymes. The protein enzyme without cofactor is known as an *apoenzyme*; the complete enzyme with cofactor or coenzyme is called a *holoenzyme*. The term coenzyme is usually given to an organic cofactor. A cofactor may serve by altering the three-dimensional structure of the enzyme and/or the bound substrate, or it may participate effectively as a second substrate. Thus, the enzyme lactate dehydrogenase catalyzes the oxidation of lactate to pyruvate as the coenzyme NAD^+ is reduced to $NADH + H^+$.

Energy: Enzymes are often looked upon as defying or contradicting the laws of chemistry. This is not true, of course. The free energy of the substrate initially must be higher than the free energy of the products or the reaction will not occur (without net input of energy). In this case we say that the reaction is thermodynamically unfavorable. Indeed, in this case, the reverse reaction would be thermodynamically favorable.

In the case of a thermodynamically favorable reaction, however, input of energy may still be necessary. This energy input, called the *energy of activation*, will be released again as the energy of the system proceeds to the lower energy level of the final products. (This is sometimes compared to a large stone being rolled from one valley into a valley of lower elevation. The energy expended in rolling the stone to the crest of the intervening hill will be released as the stone proceeds downhill. In addition to the release of energy equal to the input of energy to reach the crest, there is also release of energy related to the difference in elevation of the starting and the ending positions.) The role of the enzyme or of other catalysts is seen as lowering the activation energy of the reaction, thus increasing the rate.

Velocity and Inhibition: In the study of enzymes several relationships must be considered: (1) the rate of the reaction will increase with temperature until there is partial denaturation of the enzyme; (2) rates of reactions of enzymes are affected by pH and will ordinarily exhibit a pH range over which maximal activity is seen; (3) reaction rates ordinarily increase linearly with substrate concentration up to the point of maximum velocity, where it is considered that all enzyme molecules have substrate bound at the same time; (4) reaction rates ordinarily increase linearly with enzyme concentration.

The determination of maximum velocity is somewhat difficult because a plot of velocity versus substrate only approaches the maximum velocity with a reasonable substrate concentration. A more accurate method for determining maximum velocity involves a double reciprocal plot:

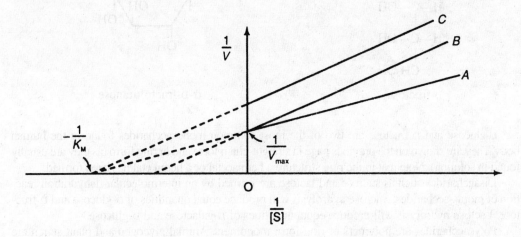

In this graph *A* is a plot of an uninhibited enzyme; *B* is a plot of the same enzyme in the presence of a competitive inhibitor; *C* is a plot of the enzyme in the presence of a noncompetitive inhibitor; *v* represents velocity and [S] represents substrate concentration. Note that the *y*-intercept is the reciprocal of maximal velocity, and the *x*-intercept is the negative of the reciprocal of the Michaelis constant, K_M, a characteristic of the individual enzyme. Note that the maximal velocity in the presence of a competitive inhibitor is the same as for the uninhibited enzyme. The maximal velocity in the presence of a noncompetitive inhibitor is lower (as noted by the fact that the reciprocal is higher).

Carbohydrates

Chemistry: Carbohydrates are a group of polyhydroxy aldehydes, polyhydroxy ketones, and closely related compounds. They may exist as monomers (monosaccharides), dimers (disaccharides), or polymers (polysaccharides).

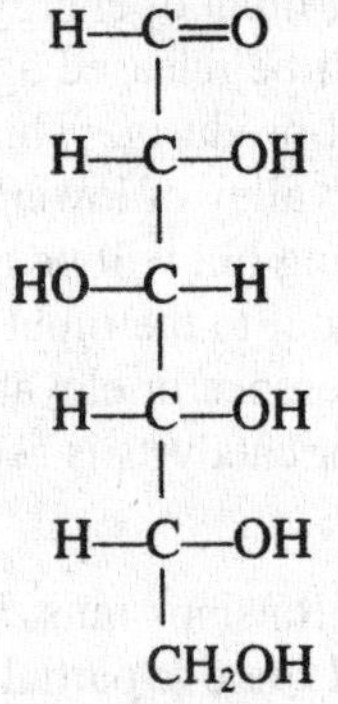

D-glucose

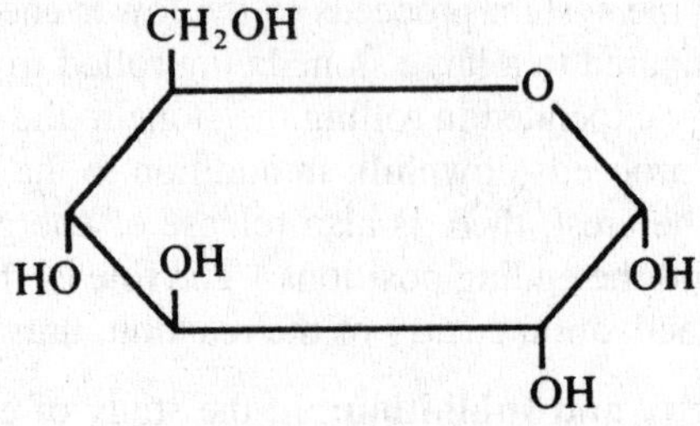

α-D-glucopyranose

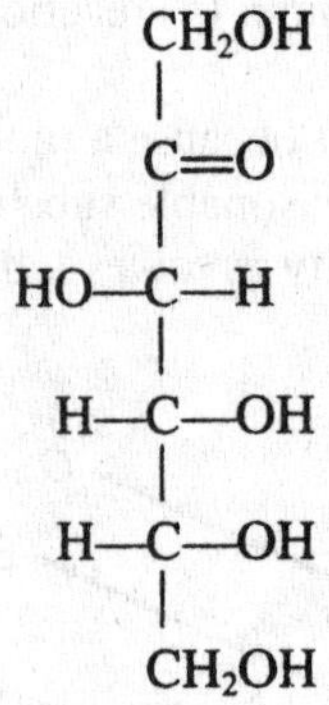

D-fructose

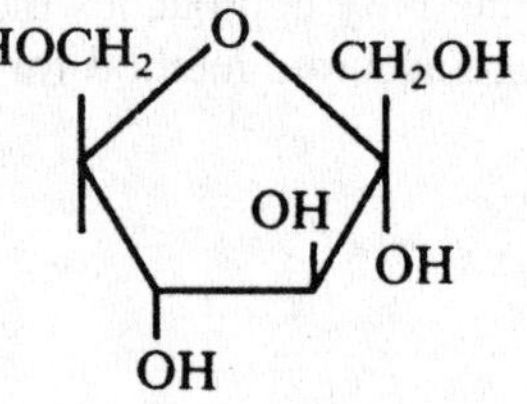

α-D-fructofuranose

D-glucose and D-fructose are two of the most common monosaccharides found in the human body. They are shown on the previous page in straight-chain form and in ring form (as they are usually found in solution). Note that in the ring structure a hemiacetal or a hemiketal has been formed.

Disaccharides such as sucrose and lactose are formed by an intermolecular dehydration reaction of monosaccharides. Sucrose hydrolysis will produce equal quantities of D-glucose and D-fructose. Lactose hydrolysis will produce equal quantities of D-galactose and D-glucose.

Polysaccharides are polymers of ring-form monomers. Animal glycogen and plant starch are polymers of α-D-glucopyranose. Cellulose is a polymer of β-D-glucopyranose.

Functions: Carbohydrates play a number of roles in nature. For example, they are metabolized for energy (4 kcal/g), metabolized for production of other required compounds such as certain amino acids, serve as components of nucleic acids (ribose in RNA and deoxyribose in DNA), serve as a structural element (cellulose of plants and cell walls of bacteria), serve as components of lubricants of bone joints, serve as cellular antigens, and are components of heparin.

Metabolism: Many pathways of carbohydrate metabolism could be considered here. We will confine ourselves to comments about glycolysis, the Krebs cycle (also known as the citric acid cycle or the tricarboxylic acid cycle), and the hexose monophosphate shunt (also known as the pentose phosphate pathway).

The complete metabolism of a molecule of glucose proceeds in a series of linked reactions, as shown on page 263. Energy associated with the bonds of glucose is eventually transferred to bonds of adenosine triphosphate (ATP) molecules, which are the molecules used most often to release this energy for work in the cell. Several of the steps shown in the diagram produce ATP directly; however, most ATPs made in the cell carry energy brought to them via "carrier" molecules, either NADH (reduced nicotinamide adenine dinucleotide) or $FADH_2$ (reduced flavin adenine dinucleotide), both of which are made in the reactions shown on page 263. Glycolysis occurs in the cytoplasm; the Krebs cycle, in the mitochondria.

Glycolysis. Glycolysis, in a series of reactions, converts glucose to pyruvic acid (or to lactic acid under conditions of oxygen deficiency). Thus, there is a net formation of 2 moles of ATP from the anaerobic glycolysis of 1 mole of glucose.

Krebs Cycle. Pyruvic acid may be converted to acetyl coenzyme A, producing 3 moles of ATP for each mole of pyruvate. The Krebs cycle may then metabolize the acetyl CoA through a series of reactions to produce 12 moles of ATP for each mole of acetyl CoA. Since the Krebs cycle is often studied with carbohydrate metabolism, many people unconsciously associate them. It should be recognized, however, that acetyl CoA is produced in metabolism of fatty acids and amino acids as well. Acetyl CoA from these other sources is also metabolized in the Krebs cycle.

The Krebs cycle, unlike glycolysis, cannot operate under anaerobic conditions. Oxygen and a functioning electron transport system are required for regeneration of oxidized FAD and NAD^+ (from reduced $FADH_2$ and NADH), but they are also required to produce and capture most of the energy that is realized from the Krebs cycle.

Hexose Monophosphate Shunt. The hexose monophosphate shunt is a series of reactions that serve primarily to produce NADPH and the pentoses (D-ribose and D-deoxyribose). NADPH is important in numerous biosynthetic reactions, including those for biosynthesis of fatty acids and cholesterol. As noted earlier, the pentoses are required for biosynthesis of the nucleic acids (DNA and RNA).

Lipids

Chemistry: Lipids are defined as compounds that may be extracted from biological materials with nonpolar solvents and that are insoluble in aqueous polar solvents. This includes the neutral glycerides (largely triglycerides), the phosphoglycerides, the sphingolipids, the steroids, the eicosanoids (particularly the prostaglandins), free fatty acids, and the lipid soluble vitamins (A, D, E, and K).

Fatty acids are components of many lipids, thus suggesting the need for a discussion of their structure. Fatty acids are generally long, unbranched hydrocarbons with a carboxyl group at one terminus. In the simplest case there are no carbon-to-carbon double bonds, but unsaturation (presence of double bonds) is common. When double bonds are present, they are usually in a *cis*-configuration and in a methylene-interrupted sequence (if more than one double bond is present).

Neutral Glycerides. Neutral glycerides, or acylglycerols, are simply glycerol in ester linkage with one to three fatty acid molecules. Esterification with one fatty acid molecule produces a monoglyceride (monoacylglycerol); esterification with two fatty acid molecules produces a diglyceride (diacylglycerol); and esterification with three molecules of fatty acid produces a triglyceride (triacylglycerol). As previously stated, the triglycerides represent the principal form of storage of excess food. This appears to be a wise arrangement because triglyceride produces 9 kcal/g during metabolism, compared with 4 kcal/g for either carbohydrate or protein, and triglyceride is stored in a substantially water-free state, compared with the hydrated carbohydrates and proteins.

triglyceride   a fatty acid (linoleic acid)

Phosphoglycerides. The phosphoglycerides are similar to the neutral glycerides, but a phosphate group is substituted for the fatty acid that would be found in the 3-position in a triglyceride. Various substituents may be attached to the phosphate group, thus forming other phosphoglycerides. Attachment of choline, for example, produces phosphatidylcholine; ethanolamine → phosphatidylethanolamine; serine → phosphatidylserine; inositol → phosphatidylinositol; and glycerol produces phosphatidylglycerol.

$$
\begin{array}{c}
O \\
\parallel \\
O \qquad H_2C-O-C-R_1 \\
\parallel \qquad\quad | \\
R_2-C-O-C-H \quad O \\
\qquad\qquad | \quad\ \parallel \\
\qquad H_2C-O-P-O^- \\
\qquad\qquad\qquad | \\
\qquad\qquad\qquad O^-
\end{array}
$$

phosphatidic acid

Sphingolipids. The sphingolipids are based on a long-chain amino alcohol, sphingosine, rather than on glycerol.

$$
\underset{\text{sphingosine}}{H_3C-(CH_2)_{12}-\overset{\displaystyle H}{\underset{\displaystyle H}{C}}=\overset{\displaystyle }{\underset{\displaystyle H}{C}}-\overset{\displaystyle OH}{\underset{\displaystyle H}{C}}-\overset{\displaystyle NH_2}{\underset{\displaystyle H}{C}}-CH_2OH}
$$

$$
\underset{\text{a sphingolipid}}{R-\overset{\displaystyle OH}{\underset{\displaystyle N}{C}}-\overset{\displaystyle H}{\underset{\displaystyle NH}{C}}-CH_2O-X}
$$

with
$$
\begin{array}{c}
| \\
C=O \\
| \\
R'
\end{array}
$$

In the preceding formula, R represents an unsaturated hydrocarbon chain, R′ represents another hydrocarbon chain (from an R′—COOH that has reacted with the NH_2 to form an amide linkage). X can represent phosphorylcholine in phosphodiester linkage, giving us sphingomyelin. It can also represent a simple glucose (giving us a glucocerebroside), or it can represent a more complex carbohydrate containing sialic acid (giving us a ganglioside).

Steroids. The term steroid is understood by the layperson to designate a natural or synthetic hormone. As used by the biochemist and other professionals in this field, however, it refers to the structure only and does not signify hormonal activity. The structure of a steroid is based on the cyclopentanoperhydrophenanthrene nucleus or steroid nucleus:

Some Major Steps in Glycolysis and the Citric Acid Cycle*

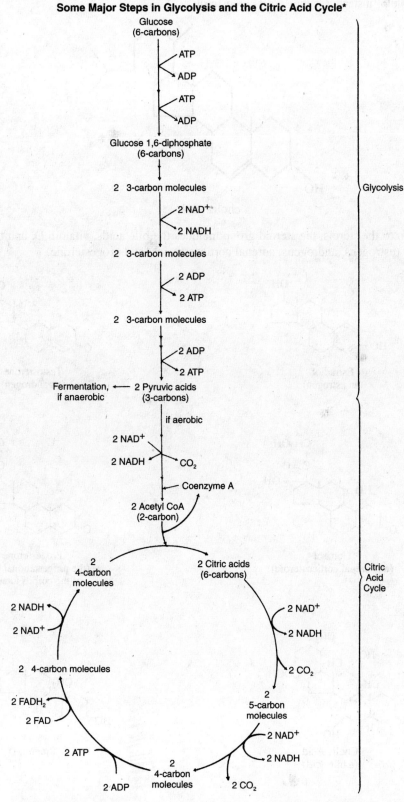

*Reprinted with permission from Barron's *How to Prepare for the Graduate Record Examination in Biology, Third Edition,* © 1989.

An example of a steroid is the sterol cholesterol:

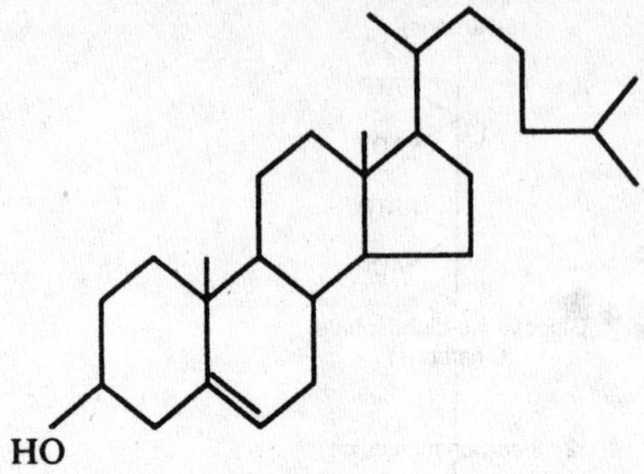

cholesterol

In addition to the sterols, the steroid group includes the bile acids, vitamin D, and the steroid hormones (estrogens, androgens, adrenal corticosteroids, and progesterone).

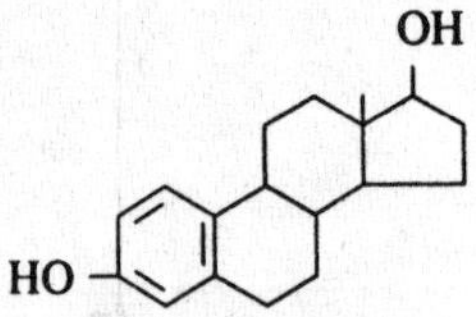

Estradiol
(an estrogen)

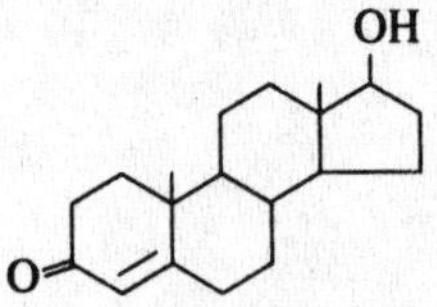

Testosterone
(an androgen)

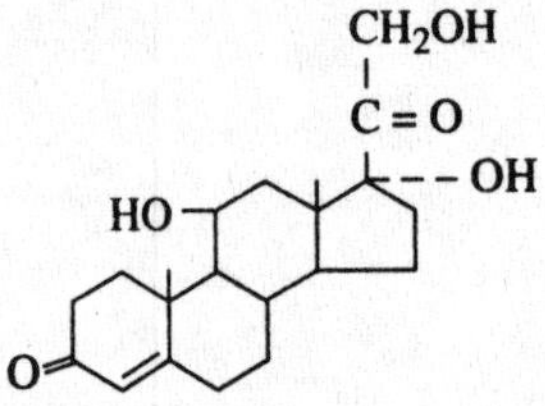

Cortisol
(an adrenal corticosteroid)

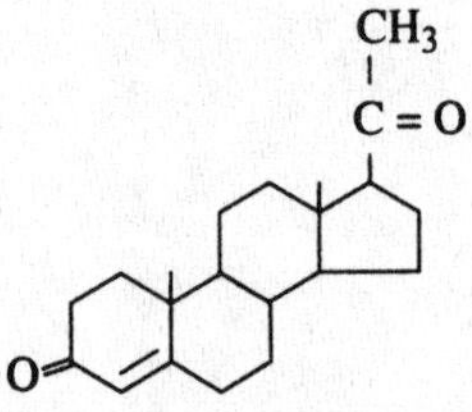

Progesterone
(the progestational agent
of the corpus luteum)

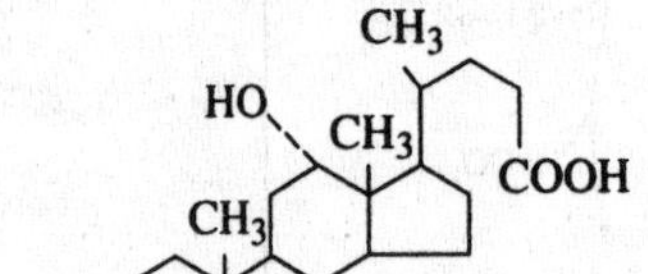

Cholic Acid
(a bile acid)

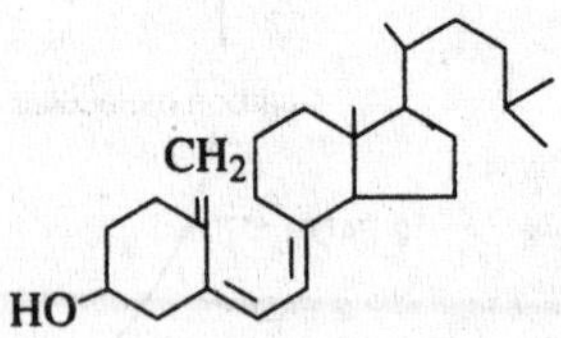

Vitamin D$_3$

Note that all of these compounds are derivatives of the steroid nucleus. Although we have shown only one representative of each class, some generalizations may be made if larger numbers of compounds are considered:

1. Total number of carbon atoms
   a. Sterols (e.g., cholesterol)—27–29
   b. Estrogens—18
   c. Androgens—19
   d. Adrenal corticosteroids—21
   e. Progesterone—21
   f. Bile acids—24
   g. Vitamin D_3—27

2. Other structural characteristics
   a. Sterols—β-hydroxyl in the A ring, ring double bond only in the B ring
   b. Estrogens—aromatic A ring, phenolic hydroxyl in the A ring
   c. Androgens—ketone in the A ring, ring double bond only in the A ring
   d. Adrenal corticosteroids—ketone in the A ring, ring double bond only in the A ring
   e. Progesterone—ketone in the A ring, ring double bond only in the A ring
   f. Bile acids—no double bonds in the ring system, only α-hydroxyls are attached to the rings, carboxyl group is present at the end of sidechain
   g. Vitamin D_3—incomplete B ring, double bonds in conjugation in "ring" B, methylene group rather than methyl at the point that is usually the junction of rings A and B, β-hydroxyl in the A ring

Eicosanoids. Some fatty acids, including linoleic acid, are very important to mammalian health, but cannot be synthesized in the body. These are therefore called *essential fatty acids*. Among the products of linoleic acid are the prostaglandins, 20-carbon fatty acids that include a 5-carbon ring. Prostaglandins are active in a variety of physiologically important ways and are sometimes used pharmacologically.

prostaglandin E_1
(PGE_1)

Two other important classes of eicosanoids are the leukotrienes and thromboxanes. Linoleic acid may be converted to arachidonic acid in the animal body (including humans). Arachidonic acid is a 20-carbon fatty acid with four *cis* double bonds. Arachidonic acid is stored in the 2-position of phosphoglycerides in membranes. The fatty acid in the 2-position is released by the enzyme phospholipase A_2. If it has the appropriate structure (such as arachidionic acid), it can be converted into prostaglandin, leukotriene, or thromboxane by appropriate enzymes.

Activity of phospholipase A_2 may be inhibited by aspirin and other nonsteroidal anti-inflammatory drugs (NSAIDs), leading to release of less polyunsaturated fatty acid from the membrane and ultimately less production of prostaglandins, leukotrienes, and thromboxanes. Inhibition of cyclooxygenase, however, by anti-inflammatory steroids leads to diminished production of prostaglandins but has no effect on leukotriene or thromboxane production.

Free Fatty Acids. Free fatty acids may sometimes be found in small amounts in various tissues. Fatty acids are also found in unesterified form in blood plasma, but in this case they are ordinarily bound noncovalently to plasma proteins, particularly albumin.

Lipid-soluble Vitamins. The lipid-soluble vitamins A, D, E, and K may also be classified as lipids, based on their solubility. They are stored in the body, and, in contrast to water-soluble vitamins, *steady* dietary intake of these vitamins is not vitally important.

Metabolism:

Hydrolysis to Produce Fatty Acids. Neutral glycerides may be hydrolyzed by lipases such as pancreatic lipase or hormone-sensitive lipase, thus releasing free fatty acids. Fatty acids may also be released from phosphoglycerides by hydrolysis that is catalyzed by phospholipase A_1 and phosopholipase A_2.

Oxidation to Fatty Acids in the Mitochondria. Fatty acids may then be oxidized via β-oxidation to produce acetyl CoA+ reduced flavin adenine dinucleotide ($FADH_2$) and reduced nicotinamide adenine dinucleotide ($NADH + H^+$). Thus, a molecule of fatty acid 16:0 would produce 8 molecules of acetyl CoA, 7 molecules of $FADH_2$, and 7 molecules of $NADH + H^+$. Each molecule of acetyl CoA can be metabolized in the Krebs cycle to produce 12 molecules of ATP. Each molecule of $FADH_2$ can produce 2 molecules of ATP when it is oxidized in the electron transport chain, and each molecule of $NADH + H^+$ can produce 3 molecules of ATP when oxidized in the electron transport chain.

Synthesis of Fatty Acids. Synthesis of fatty acids occurs in the nonparticulate cytoplasm. The pathway is not simply a reversal of β-oxidation; it requires biotin and carbon dioxide in addition to acetyl CoA. The carbon dioxide, however, is not incorporated into the fatty acid. Also the reducing equivalents required for the synthesis are derived from $NADPH + H^+$.

Synthesis of Glycerides. The neutral glycerides require L-3-glycerol phosphate in their biosynthesis. This glycerol phosphate may be formed by the enzymatic phosphorylation of glycerol or by the enzymatic reduction of dihydroxyacetone phosphate, which is produced in glycolysis.

Nucleotides and Nucleic Acids; Biosynthesis of Nucleic Acids and Proteins

Nucleotides: Both deoxyribonucleic acid (DNA) and ribonucleic acid (RNA) are polymers of nucleotides. A nucleotide consists of a nitrogen base (either a purine or a pyrimidine), a pentose (ribose or 2-deoyxribose), and a phosphate group. Deoxyribose is found in DNA; ribose, in RNA.

The nitrogen bases include the purines (adenine and guanine) in both DNA and RNA. The pyrimidines include cytosine and thymine in DNA; cytosine and uracil are present in RNA.

Other nitrogen bases are found in small quantities. Some synthetic nitrogen bases are used in the treatment of cancer and certain viral infections.

Nucleic Acids: As mentioned above, DNA and RNA are polymers of appropriate nucleotides. The attachment between nucleotides is phosphate–pentose-phosphate-pentose–, etc. This leaves the nitrogen base as an appendage from the linear chain. In double-stranded DNA there are two strands that are paired and linked (noncovalently) through their nitrogen bases. Adenine pairs with thymine, and cytosine pairs with guanine. Methods are available to allow determination of the primary structures of both DNA and RNA.

Biosynthesis of Nucleic Acids and Proteins: It is recognized that DNA codes for its own duplication, as well as for RNA synthesis. Messenger RNA, in turn, codes for the biosynthesis of polypeptide chains. Since there is a triplet code without commas, there are $4 \times 4 \times 4 = 64$ possibilities and sequences for specification of a single amino acid. Only about 21 amino acids, however, are known to have codes. It turns out that some codes give other instructions (e.g., initiation or termination of a peptide chain biosynthesis) and some amino acids have more than one code for their placement. Arginine, for example, has six different codons that can specify its placement.

Mutations in the DNA chain can occur, of course, as a result of errors in duplication, spontaneous changes in DNA, or changes resulting from radiation or mutagenic chemicals. A point mutation results in the presence of a different nitrogen base. This may, in turn, cause problems, or it may be a silent mutation. It would be silent if the base change resulted in no difference in the amino acid or if it resulted in the substitution of a very similar amino acid.

A frame shift mutation is likely to be more serious. Consider that insertion or deletion of a nitrogen base will change the sequence of bases following it in the chain. (Remember that there are no commas.) This may be a lethal mutation.

Mutations can be repaired by a number of mechanisms. For example, sometimes an affected area is removed and replaced by a strand that is duplicated again from the complementary DNA strand. Specific cellular enzymes exist to aid in identifying and repairing mutations.

Separation and Quantitation Techniques

1. Chromatography: One of the most important techniques for separation of compounds in biochemistry is *chromatography*. Although it may also be used in inorganic and organic chemistry, the usually smaller quantities involved in biochemistry make it even more popular and usevul there.

Chromatography may be considered to be a separation process in which a mobile phase passes across a stationary phase. Molecules that are in the mobile phase 100% of the time will elute from the chromatogram very quickly; those that are in the stationary phase 100% of the time will never elute. Those spending intermediate percentages of time in each phase will elute at intermediate times.

Different phases are used in various kinds of chromatography. Probably the most important ones are *gas-solid*, *gas-liquid*, *liquid-liquid*, and *liquid-solid*. (In the previous examples the first phase is the mobile one.)

The reason for the time spent in the mobile versus the stationary phase is influenced by properties such as size, charge, solubility, and volatility.

Gas-solid chromatography involves the passage of a mobile phase (gas) over a stationary phase (solid). Movement is increased (and elution time decreased) by high volatility and low affinity for the stationary phase.

Gas-liquid chromatography involves the passage of a mobile phase (gas) over a stationary phase (liquid). The stationary liquid phase needs to be stable at the temperature used for the chromatography. The compounds eluted most rapidly are those that are volatile and show little or no affinity for the stationary liquid phase.

Liquid-liquid chromatography involves the passage of a mobile phase (liquid) over a stationary phase (also liquid). The stationary phase must be bound to a surface and the two liquids must be essentially immiscible. The faster-eluting compounds are those that are quite soluble in the mobile phase and less soluble in the stationary phase.

Liquid-solid chromatography uses solid as the stationary phase. The faster-moving compounds are those that are quite soluble in the liquid phase and show little or no affinity for the solid phase.

One specialized form of liquid-solid chromatography is *affinity chromatography*. In this chromatography a specific compound is attached to the solid phase. This attached compound is one to which at least one component in a mixture has great affinity.

We will use the example of separation of enzymes by this method. Subjecting a mixture of enzymes to affinity chromatography allows one enzyme to be retarded or even stopped. (The solid has an attached compound for which one of the enzymes in the mixture has greater affinity. It could even be an antibody.) Then the retarded or bound enzyme (separated) can be eluted by a stronger salt solution.

2. Spectrophotometry: Spectrophotometry or colorimetry is an analytical tool that is used in the identification and quantification of light-absorbing compounds. Identification is based on the fact that different compounds absorb light to a greater or lesser extent at different wavelengths. Thus, identification of compounds may often be made by a plot of light absorption against wavelength.

Compounds may often be quantified without actually being separated. Either the compound itself or an appropriate derivative may absorb light at a characteristic wavelength. In that case, the absorbance at that wavelength may be used to measure the amount of the compound.

As an example, both NAD^+ and NADH absorb light at a peak of 260 nm. However, NADH (and not NAD^+) has another absorption peak at 340 nm. Thus the enzymatic conversion of NAD^+ to NADH may be followed by the increase in absorbance at 340 nm.

Spectrophotometry and colorimetry are terms that are often used synonymously. Actually, it is preferable to use colorimetry to refer to absorbance of light that is selected by a filter. The filter will usually produce light that is only somewhat pure (a range of wavelengths). A spectophotometer usually refers to a device in which the light of a particular wavelength is obtained from a prism or a diffraction grating.

If the transmitted light (I) is divided by the incident light striking a sample (I_0), the fraction I/I_0 is called transmittance (T). The Beer-Lambert equation is given as

$$-\log_{10}T = \varepsilon cl$$

where ε is the absorption coefficient, c is the concentration, and l is the path length.

CHAPTER 4

Physics

The MCAT physics problems are somewhat different from problems that you may have found on college physics tests. The physics questions are alternated with inorganic chemistry questions on the Physical Sciences test, instead of all being grouped together.

TEST-TAKING SUGGESTIONS FOR THE PHYSICS PORTION OF THE MCAT

A sometimes lengthy reading passage will contain information that you need in order to work the 4 or 5 problems that follow the passage. All of the information needed will not always be in the reading passage. Generally, you must understand the *concepts* of physics and the "conservation laws." Topics will encompass nearly all of physics: mechanics, simple harmonic motion, wave motion, heat and gas laws, electricity and magnetism, light and optics, modern physics, and nuclear physics, including radioactive decay. Memorizing hundreds of formulas will be of little benefit. You must practice making simple sketches, especially for problems in mechanics. Many are nearly impossible to work without a sketch to help you understand relationships. In addition to problems associated with specific passages, the test will have "independent" questions unrelated to any passage. The latter may be similar to end-of-chapter problems that you worked in your introductory physics classes. MCAT physics questions may be based on passages that seem to be "nonphysics." One recent set of test questions, involving novae composed of white dwarf stars and an ordinary star, required some understanding of gravitation. Another section included a passage about colliding continents and radioactive dating of rocks with questions on conservation of momentum and Newton's Third Law.

Look for *key words* in the questions. Words like "work," "potential energy," and "kinetic energy," especially when connected with the word "initial" or "final," might require you to use the conservation of mechanical energy principle. If you see the word "collide" or "collision," you will undoubtedly use the conservation of momentum principle and/or Newton's Third Law.

Because calculators are not permitted, you should practice problems like those in this book. Get practice in moving the decimal place in order to make the calculation easier. For example:

$$400 \text{ N} \times 0.35 \text{ millisec} = 0.4 \times 10^3 \text{ N} \times 0.35 \times 10^{-3} \text{ sec} = 0.4 \times 0.35 \text{ N sec}$$

You will probably benefit from using a college physics text to prepare. Your college or university library will have several on the shelves. Note: The words "University Physics" or "for Science and Engineering Students in a title," refer to textbooks that use the calculus.

In addition to study booklets like this one and MCAT preparation courses that you may take, it is important that you view and take actual previous MCAT tests. You can obtain one free practice test and purchase others at the AAMC online site: *http://www.aamc.org/students/ mcat/practicetests.htm* At the same *www.aamc.org/* site you can review frequently asked questions. There are forums where the tests are discussed. Try: *www.valuemd.com/premed-forum.* Knowing what to expect on the actual test will have you more confident and relaxed when you take the test.

You will notice that half or more of the physics questions are basically conceptual, often with no calculation required. In addition, there are several kinds of physics passages. One type describes experiments and will have data, perhaps in graphic form. This type may or may not require calculations, but should be read carefully at least once, since the questions might require you to use the data from the experiment directly. Another type is informational. Informational passages can be scanned quickly so that you can go to the questions and find out what is being asked of you. Do not assume that you must know everything in every passage. Note whether there are formulae in either type of passage, then go to the questions. Do not be concerned if the formula is new to you. A few MCAT questions deal with topics not in your college physics course. One passage described proportional counters used to detect charged particles in high-energy physics. Another dealt with the frequency of liquid sloshing in a tank, giving the formula for f. A third described "earthquake lights" caused by sonoluminescence. The questions that followed these passages could usually be answered using one's knowledge of basic physics, in spite of the unusual subject. Spend your time on the questions. Do not read and reread the passage before you go on to try to answer the questions. Questions will determine if a formula (or other formulae not in the passage) will be used. Ask yourself what concepts you need. "Conceptual" means that you understand how to *use* the concept, not that you know the name of the concept!

A conceptual question type that you may see on the MCAT may be a figure with an object arrow inside the focal length of a converging lens. The question asks what kind of image is formed. No calculation is needed. One need only remember the magnifying glass to answer that the image of the arrow is virtual and upright. A similar question might have a light ray entering a flat glass surface or a glass plate with parallel sides. You are to determine the direction(s) of the rays after refraction (bending) by the flat surface(s). The answer choices may not require number calculations. A passage may have many numerical values as well as a diagram but the questions related to the passage may be conceptual and perhaps none of the numbers are needed to answer the questions. Generally, you should scan the passage quickly to get the general meaning and read all the passage questions before attempting to answer the first question. This will determine how much you must refer back to the passage itself and will save time that may be better spent on the questions. Some passages will challenge you because you will not have seen the topics in your physics course. Rereading the passage will probably help here. Remembering that you can use your common sense and your reasoning ability to answer many of the MCAT questions will give you the confidence to handle unusual topics. The MCAT is designed to test your ability to think instead of your ability to memorize without really understanding.

Independent questions unrelated to any passage may be conceptual or may require calculations. A question may ask what quantities change when light passes from air to water. The four choices might be: velocity and frequency, frequency and wavelength, velocity and frequency, velocity and wavelength. However, you may be given the speed of light, c, and the index of refraction of water, n_w, and asked to calculate the speed of light in water. A Coulomb law question may ask what happens to the force between two charges when the separation doubles. You may be required to calculate a numerical answer or to answer that the force is smaller by a factor of 4. For either, you must understand the concept of the force law between the two charges.

Some examples of both conceptual questions and questions that require you to calculate a numerical result as you did in your physics class follow:

1. Two identical cars skid to a stop from speeds of 30 km/hr and 60 km/hr. How do the lengths of the skid marks compare?

    (A) They are the same length
    (B) The 60 km/hr mark is twice as long.
    (C) The 60 km/hr mark is four times as long.
    (D) The 60 km/hr mark is eight times as long.

    EXPLANATION: The work (force X distance) done by the *same* frictional force acting on both cars brings them to rest. The kinetic energy of the faster car is four times that of the slower car since KE depends on the square of the speed. The stopping distance for the faster car is four times that of the other.

    $$W = Fx = 1/2\ mv^2.\ \text{Answer: } \textbf{(C)}$$

2. One ball is dropped from a height of 10 meters. Another ball is projected horizontally with a speed of 20 m/s from the same height. Ignore air friction. How long does it take each ball to fall 2.0 meters?

    (A) 2.0 sec and 20.0 sec
    (B) 1.4 sec and 1.4 sec
    (C) 2.4 sec and 6.2 sec
    (D) 20.0 sec and 2.4 sec

    EXPLANATION: The concepts of projectile motion show that the vertical motion has acceleration g (independent of any horizontal motion). There is no horizontal acceleration. Since both balls start with zero initial vertical velocity, they both fall through 10 meters in the same time. The answers show that only **(B)** could be correct. You can save much time if you can bypass doing an actual calculation.

3. A simple pendulum has a period of 2.0 sec. If the mass is quadrupled, what is the period of oscillation?

    (A) 0.5 sec
    (B) 1.0 sec
    (C) 2.0 sec
    (D) 8.0 sec

    EXPLANATION: The period does not depend on the mass, only the length, *L*, and the value of *g* (use $g = 10$ m/s^2 on the MCAT). Answer: **(C)**

4. A light ray is incident at an angle of 40° from air onto a glass surface with an index of refraction of 1.6. The angle of refraction inside the glass is 23.7°. Suppose that instead the light ray were incident at the same angle of 40° from inside the glass. The refracted angle in air as the ray leaves the glass will be:

    (A) larger than 40°.
    (B) smaller than 40°.
    (C) equal to 23.7°.
    (D) between 23.7° and 40°.

EXPLANATION: Snell's Law, $n_1\sin\theta_1 = n_2\sin\theta_2$ applies here and $\sin\theta_2 = (n_1/n_2)\sin\theta_1$. If n_1 is greater than n_2, θ_2 will be larger than θ_1. Since $n_1 = 1.6$ when the ray is incident from inside the glass, the angle of refraction will be larger than $40°$. Again, you *can* calculate the angle but time is saved if you reason the solution as above. The question did not ask for the exact angle! Answer: **(A)**

5. Small spheres of aluminum and lead, each of radius 6.3 cm and of volume 0.001 m³ are lowered on strings into a container of pure water of density 1000 kg/m³. The density of aluminum is 2700 kg/m³ and that of lead is 11,300 kg/m³. The approximate buoyant forces exerted on the aluminum and lead spheres are, respectively:

(A) 1350 N and 5650 N
(B) 27,000 N and 113,000 N
(C) 10 N and 10 N
(D) 27 N and 113 N

EXPLANATION: A buoyant force on a completely submerged object equals the weight of the fluid displaced by the object and does not depend on the properties of the object (Archimedes principle). Only one answer has equal forces on the equal volume spheres. Answer: **(C)**

6. A proton and a singly ionized Li^7 ion are accelerated from rest through the same potential difference of 100,000 volts. What are the respective kinetic energies gained by the proton and the ion? Which has the higher speed? (Note: proton and ion both have the same charge $e = 1.6 \times 10^{-19}$ C)

(A) 1.6×10^{-14} J, 1.12×10^{-12} J; the ion
(B) 1.6×10^{-14} J, 1.12×10^{-12} J; the proton
(C) 1.12×10^{-14} J, 1.6×10^{-14} J; the ion
(D) 1.6×10^{-14} J, 1.6×10^{-14} J; the proton

EXPLANATION: There are two key points to note in the statement. (1) A proton and any *singly* ionized ion have the same magnitude charge, $+e$ (the basic unit of charge). (2) The work done is: $W_{net} = qV = eV =$ the change in KE. It is the same for both charges. Their final kinetic energies are the *same*. (If they started with unequal initial kinetic energies the correct answer would not change in *this* problem because they would both *gain* the same additional kinetic energy.) The question asked for the gain in kinetic energy. Answer: **(D)**. The proton is much lighter and has the higher speed at the same kinetic energy. It would not have mattered if the charges had opposite signs in *this* question as long as the magnitudes of the charges were the same.

The following question is of the type that requires that you calculate the answer:

7. A 100 megawatt nuclear power plant operates for 208.3 days. This is very nearly 18 million seconds. If all the mass that is converted to energy produced useful electrical energy, how much mass is consumed in the nuclear reaction?

   (A) 2.0 kg
   (B) 2.4 kg
   (C) 0.02 kg
   (D) 3 mg

   EXPLANATION: The mass converted to energy is given by the famous Einstein mass-energy equivalence expression: $E = m_o c^2$. Also, 1 watt = 1 J/s so 1 megawatt = 1.0×10^6 J/s. The plant operates for 18×10^6 s at 100×10^6 J/s. The total energy is: $E = (100 \times 10^6 \text{ J/s})(18 \times 10^6 \text{ s}) = 18.0 \times 10^{14}$ J $= m_o c^2$. Divide both sides by the square of the speed of light and we have:

   $$m_o = (18.0 \times 10^{14} \text{ J})/(9 \times 10^{16} \text{ m}^2/\text{s}^2) = 0.02 \text{ kg (20 grams)}$$

   Calculation is necessary to be certain of the answer. Answer: **(C)** (Actually more mass must be consumed because of heat losses.)

8. The speeds of longitudinal sound waves in air and aluminum are about 340 m/s and 5100 m/s, respectively. What are the wavelengths in air and aluminum of a 2000 Hz sound wave?

   (A) 0.37 m and 5.2 m
   (B) 0.82 m and 4.43 m
   (C) 0.17 m and 2.55 m
   (D) 1.1 m and 4.6 m

   EXPLANATION: The wave velocity = frequency × wavelength. A simple calculation ($\lambda = v/f$) gives answer **(C)**. Note that since all the answers differ you need do only one calculation (either for air or for aluminum).

9. A block of weight 10 N starts from rest at a height of 3.0 m and slides down a friction-less incline onto a rough horizontal table. The coefficient of friction of the table is 0.3. How far does the block slide horizontally before coming to rest?

   (A) 13 m
   (B) 10 m
   (C) 5 m
   (D) 2 m

   EXPLANATION: The gravitational potential energy, (mg)h, of the block is converted into kinetic energy at the bottom of the incline and then the energy is dissipated by the work done by friction. Conservation of mechanical energy shows that all these different forms of energy are equal. We can simply equate the initial PE at the top of the incline to the frictional work done to stop the block (we need not find the kinetic energy).

   Initial PE = final frictional work: $(mg)h = \mu(mg)x$

Now mg is the weight and $\mu = 0.3$. Cancel the weight mg.

Finally: $x = h/\mu = 3.0$ m/0.3 $= 10$ m. Answer: **(B)**

By using the conservation of energy principle wisely, we have saved much extra work. Because we did not need to know the kinetic energy we did not have to find the mass. Standing waves and resonance: Standing waves and resonant situations can often be analyzed by using simple sketches of the vibrating systems, often bypassing calculations. For example, longitudinal sound waves in both open-end pipes and pipes closed on one end as well as transverse waves on stretched strings involve standing waves that are harmonics. The harmonic overtones are integer multiples of the lowest natural frequency called the fundamental. Since each node and the adjacent antinode are always exactly one-quarter wavelength apart in a standing wave, the pipe length or string length will be some integer number of quarter wavelengths. Free ends such as the open ends of pipes will be antinodes and fixed ends where vibration cannot occur will be nodes. If both ends are the same (both free or both fixed) there are an even number of quarter wavelengths and *all* harmonic frequencies can occur. If the ends differ (one free and one fixed) there will be only odd numbers of quarter wavelengths and only the odd harmonics occur.

The following example will illustrate these concepts.

10. An pipe open on both ends is resonant at a lowest frequency of 340 Hz when the speed of sound is 340 m/sec. The pipe length is:

(A) 1.0 m
(B) 2.0 m
(C) 0.5 m
(D) 0.25 m

EXPLANATION: The fundamental occurs when the pipe is only 2 quarter wavelengths long.

A   N   A

Since the wavelength is 1.0 m ($\lambda = v/f = 340/340$) the pipe length is $2/4\lambda$ or 0.5 m. Answer: **(C)**

11. What is the wavelength of the second overtone for this pipe at 340 Hz?

(A) 6.0 m
(B) 3.0 m
(C) 2.0 m
(D) 0.33 m

EXPLANATION: If we sketch the pattern of antinodes and nodes for the fundamental and the first and second overtones we find:

A   N   A

A   N   A   N   A

A   N   A   N   A   N   A

Simply counting the number of quarter wavelengths the second overtone has:

$(6/4)\lambda = 0.5$ m or $\lambda = 0.33$ m. Answer: **(D)**

Of course, if you remember the rule that the standing wave on a "system" that has both ends the *same* is always an even number of quarter wavelengths you can skip the sketches, but they are good mnemonic devices. A stretched string has nodes at the ends and it also always has an even number of quarter wavelengths for standing waves. A pipe closed on one end vibrating in its lowest frequency has only one quarter wavelength of a standing wave in its length, A   N. The closed end is a node and the open end is an antinode. The frequency of its fundamental is then only half that of the same length open pipe. The first overtone will have a frequency three times that of the fundamental and the pipe will have three quarter wavelengths in its length and so on.

Fluids: Questions involving fluids are often conceptual on MCAT tests.

12. 10 liters of water are poured into an open cylindrical tank with a stopcock at the bottom. The stopcock is opened. As the water drains out of the stopcock, which statement is true concerning the water speed leaving the stopcock?

(A) The speed increases steadily.
(B) The speed decreases steadily
(C) The speed first increases then decreases.
(D) The speed first decreases then increases.

EXPLANATION: As the water level drops the water pressure at the stopcock drops steadily and the exit speed of the water decreases steadily. Answer: **(B)**

13. Smoothly flowing water fills a cylindrical pipe section, A, with a diameter of 10 cm and flows into a constricted section, B, with a smaller diameter of 6 cm. Which statement is correct?

(A) The pressure is greater in B than in A.
(B) The water speed is greater in B than in A.
(C) The volume flow rate is greater in B than in A.
(D) The water speed is greater in A than in B.

EXPLANATION: The Bernoulli equation will show that the pressure is greater in A where the water speed is slower, so answer A is not true. The volume flow rate is constant in both A and B so the water must speed up through the constricted B cross-section. Answer: **(B)**

14. Two putty balls have the same mass. Ball 1 has an initial velocity of 4 m/s in the positive *x* direction and Ball 2 is at rest. They collide inelastically and stick together. If they move off together at an angle of 15 degrees above the positive *x* direction, what is their speed?

(A) 2.0 m/s to the right
(B) 1.4 m/s to the right
(C) 0 m/s (they will stop)
(D) They do not move in the direction given in the question.

EXPLANATION: Ball 1 has a component of momentum *perpendicular* to the *x*-axis. The *total* vector momentum of the two-ball system will be conserved so the two balls will move together along the same original direction as the velocity vector of Ball 1. Answer: **(D)**

The remaining material in this Chapter 4 review assumes that you have previously reviewed mechanics topics covered in the first weeks of a physics course since mechanics is used in nearly all physics topics. Such problems as complex projectile problems will not be on the MCAT. Vector problems that require using sine, cosine, and tangent of angles from trigonometry will not plague you. You will not have to recall all the universal constants (such as the permittivity of a vacuum, ε_o). Needed values such as constants or density values will be given on the test. You will use many concepts from mechanics such as velocity, acceleration, force, Newton's Laws of motion, momentum, work, energy, conservation of mechanical energy, friction, and so forth. You might use mechanics in electric force problems, nuclear force problems, and other sometimes unique or unfamiliar problems.

The material in the rest of this physics review chapter consists of "standard" elementary physics problems such as one sees in college textbooks. Review of the material will aid in your recall of the concepts involved. Use of a "College Physics" textbook is strongly recommended. Recent textbook authors separate the end-of-chapter problems into the 3 categories of easiest, average difficulty, and most difficult (using a color code or 1, 2, or 3 dots, etc.) and usually offer many conceptual questions as well.

Preparing for the MCAT is somewhat different than when you prepared for your hour tests or final exams in your physics course. A student preparing for the MCAT should be able to solve nearly all of the easiest problems. Spending much time trying to solve difficult problems would be of little value. Always ask yourself first, which concept or idea is involved in the problem or question. Be prepared, be confident, and be well rested!

FREQUENTLY ENCOUNTERED PHYSICS PROBLEMS AND THEIR ANSWERS

Friction

$$\text{Formula } \mu = \frac{F}{N_p}$$

μ = coefficient of friction

F = frictional force

N_p = normal or perpendicular force

EXAMPLE: A 10,000 N force draws a 130,000 N railroad car at constant speed on level terrain.

1. Determine the coefficient of friction.

$$\mu = \frac{F}{N_p}$$

$$\mu = \frac{10,000 \text{ N}}{130,000 \text{ N}} = 0.077$$

(The coefficient of friction is the ratio of the frictional force to the perpendicular force N_p pressing the two surfaces together.)

2. The railroad car is pulled on a horizontal track at constant speed by a steel cable that makes a 30° angle above the horizontal. The tension in the cable is 1400 N. Determine the coefficient of friction.

$$
\begin{aligned}
F \text{ (parallel frictional force)} = F &= 1400 \text{ N} \times \cos 30° \\
&= 1400 \text{ N} \times 0.866 \\
&= 1212 \text{ N}
\end{aligned}
$$

The normal force N—which is the weight of the car—is 130,000 N. However, the vertical component of tension must be subtracted from it.

$$
\begin{aligned}
N &= 130,000 - 1400 \times \sin 30° \\
&= 130,000 \text{ N} - 700 \text{ N} \\
&= 129,300 \text{ N} \\
\mu &= \frac{F}{N} \\
\mu &= \frac{1212 \text{ N}}{129,300 \text{ N}} \\
\mu &= 0.009
\end{aligned}
$$

Work and Power

Work (W) equals the force (F) times the displacement (d) in the direction of the force, that is, $W = Fd$.

EXAMPLE: A machine is pushed 30 m on a level floor. The frictional force is determined as 10,000 N. Calculate the work performed.

$$W = Fd$$
$$W = (10,000 \text{ N})(30 \text{ m})$$
$$W = 300,000 \text{ N} \cdot \text{m}$$
$$= 300,000 \text{ J}$$

Recall: The work-energy unit, Joule is: $1 \text{ J} = 1 \text{ N} \cdot \text{m}$

EXAMPLE: Instead of being pushed, the above machine is dragged via a steel cable at an angle of 30° with the floor and with a force on the cable of 10,000 N. The work performed is?

$$W = (F \cos 30°)d$$
$$W = 10,000 \text{ N} \times 0.866 \times 30 \text{ m}$$
$$W = 259,800 \text{ J}$$

WORK AND ENERGY

EXAMPLE: A man pushes his snowblower with a constant force of 50 lb. The shaft makes an angle of 45° with the horizontal. The work done by the man in 150 ft is?

$$W = Fd \cos 45°$$
$$W = (50 \text{ lb})(150 \text{ ft})(0.707)$$
$$W = 5300 \text{ ft-lb}$$

POWER AND POWER UNITS

$$\text{Power} = \frac{\text{Work}}{\text{Time}} \text{ or } P = \frac{W}{t}$$

Units: $1 \text{ watt} = 10^7 \text{ ergs/sec} = 1 \text{ Joule/sec}$

         $1 \text{ horsepower (hp)} = 500 \text{ ft-lb/sec} = 746 \text{ watts}$

         $1 \text{ kilowatt} = 1000 \text{ watts} = 1.34 \text{ hp}$

EXAMPLE: By means of its steel pulleys, a crane raises a machine weighing 2200 N to a height of 30 m in 200 sec. The average horsepower necessary is?

$$P = \frac{W}{t}$$

$$P = \frac{\text{Force} \times \text{Distance}}{\text{Time}}$$

$$P = \frac{(2200 \text{ N})(30 \text{ m})}{200s} = 330 \text{ J/sec}$$

$$P = 330 \text{ watts}$$

$$P = 330 \text{ watts} \times \frac{1 \text{ hp}}{746 \text{ watts}}$$

$$P = 0.44 \text{ hp}$$

EXAMPLE: A man of mass 80 kg is taking a stress test. The test equals the activity of climbing stairs a vertical distance of 10 m in 5 sec. Calculate the horsepower he develops.

$$P = \frac{W}{t} = \frac{(mg)\,y}{t} = \frac{(80\ \text{kg})(9.8\ \text{m/sec}^2)(10\ \text{m})}{5\ \text{sec}}$$

$$P = 1568\ \text{kg} \cdot \frac{m^2}{\text{sec}^3}$$

$$P = 1568\ \text{watts}$$

$$P = 1568\ \text{watts} \times \frac{1\ \text{hp}}{746\ \text{watts}}$$

$$P = 2.1\ \text{hp}$$

EXAMPLE: To take the MCAT examination you must climb stairs to a height of 60 ft, and you weigh 180 lb. The work you do against the force of gravity is 10,800 ft-lb.

$$W = F \times D$$
$$W = 180\ \text{lb} \times 60\ \text{ft} = 10{,}800\ \text{ft-lb}$$

Energy

POTENTIAL ENERGY

Potential energy (PE)—or energy of position—is the product of the weight (w) of an object and the height (h) to which the object is elevated, or the work done in elevating it: $PE = wh$.

EXAMPLE: A machine weighing 23,000 N is raised onto the roof of a building 50 m high. Calculate the increase in potential energy or the work done in lifting the machine.

$$PE = wh$$
$$PE = (23{,}000\ \text{N})(50\ \text{m})$$
$$PE = 1{,}150{,}000\ \text{J}$$

KINETIC ENERGY

Kinetic energy = energy of motion.

Formulas: 1. $KE = \dfrac{1}{2}mu^2$ $KE = \text{J}$

2. $KE = \dfrac{1}{2}mv^2$

EXAMPLE: Determine the kinetic energy of a locomotive with mass of 110,000 kg and traveling at a speed of 50 km/hr (13.9 m/sec).

$$KE = \frac{1}{2}mu^2$$

$$KE = \frac{1}{2}(110{,}000\ \text{kg})(13.9\ \text{m/sec})^2$$

$$KE = 10{,}723{,}000\ \text{J}$$

Recall: The joule (J) is a unit of energy. It is a N · m, the work done by a force of 1 N through a distance of 1 m. It is the heat produced by an ampere flowing against an ohm for one second. One joule is equal to 10^7 ergs, and 4.185 J are equal to one calorie.

EXAMPLE: A rocket with a mass of 2000 kg is fired vertically upward with an initial velocity of 100 m/s.

1. Calculate the change in kinetic energy at maximum height reached.

$$\Delta K = K - K_0 \qquad K = \text{kinetic energy at maximum}$$
$$\text{height} = 0$$
$$-K_0 = -\frac{1}{2}mv_0^2 \qquad K_0 = \text{initial kinetic energy}$$
$$v_0 = \text{initial velocity}$$
$$-K_0 = -\frac{1}{2}(2000 \text{ kg})(100 \text{ m/sec})^2$$
$$\Delta K = -K_0 = -10,000,000 \text{ J}$$

Answer: At maximum height reached, the rocket has lost 10,000,000 J of kinetic energy.

2. Calculate the potential energy at maximum height, and the change in kinetic energy upon return to lift-off point.

a. $\quad v^2 = v_0^2 - 2gy \qquad\qquad v_0 = \text{initial velocity}$

$$y = \frac{v_0^2}{2g} \qquad\qquad y = \text{maximum height}$$
$$g = \text{gravitational acceleration}$$
$$y = \frac{(100 \text{ m/sec})^2}{2(9.8 \text{ m/sec}^2)}$$
$$y = \frac{10,000 \text{ m}^2/\text{sec}^2}{19.6 \text{ m/sec}^2}$$
$$y = 510 \text{ m}$$

b. $\quad PE = mgh$

$$PE = (2000 \text{ kg})(9.8 \text{ m/sec}^2)(510 \text{ m})$$
$$PE = 10,000,000 \text{ J}$$

The increase in potential energy, then, is 10,000,000 J, and one can deduce that the rocket returns to its lift-off point with the same velocity it had at the beginning. The rocket had lost 10,000,000 J of kinetic energy on the original flight, but gained this amount in potential energy and, therefore, the total change in energy was zero. The *KE* and *PE* balance each other and are constant; the principle of conservation of energy is demonstrated.

Momentum

Momentum is the product of the mass and velocity of an object:

$$p = mv \qquad p = \text{momentum}$$
$$m = \text{mass}$$
$$v = \text{velocity}$$

The change of momentum is equal to the force applied times time.

EXAMPLE: An 80-kg man is shot out of a cannon at the speed of 10 m/sec. What is his momentum?

$$p = mv$$
$$p = (80 \text{ kg})(10 \text{ m/sec})$$
$$p = 800 \text{ kg} \cdot \text{m/sec}$$

EXAMPLE: On landing, a plane is traveling at 100 km/hr. Brakes are applied, and the plane comes to a stop in 10 sec. Assuming the average mass to be 70 kg, what is the force of the seat belts on each passenger? (100 km/hr = 28 m/sec)

Step 1. Calculate the change in momentum.

$$p = -mv_0$$
$$p = -70 \text{ kg } (28 \text{ m/sec})$$
$$p = -1960 \text{ kg} \cdot \text{m/sec}$$

Step 2. Now calculate the force applied by the seat belt on a passenger.

$$F = \frac{p}{t}$$
$$F = -\frac{1960 \text{ kg m}}{(10 \text{ sec}) \text{ sec}}$$
$$F = -\frac{196 \text{ kgm}}{\text{sec}^2}$$
$$= -196 \text{ N}$$

Uniform Circular Motion

CENTRIPETAL ACCELERATION

EXAMPLE: A subway car traveling at a speed of 50 km/hr (14 m/sec) negotiates a curve whose radius is 200 m. What is its acceleration?

$$a = \frac{v^2}{r}$$

a = acceleration
v = velocity
r = radius

$$a = \frac{(14 \text{ m/sec})^2}{200 \text{ m}}$$
$$a = \frac{196 \text{ m}^2/\text{sec}^2}{200 \text{ m}}$$
$$a = 0.98 \text{ m/sec}^2$$

CIRCULAR MOTION

Recall: $\dfrac{360°}{2\pi} = 1 \text{ rad} = 57.3°$

$360° = 2\pi \text{ rad}; \ 180° = \pi \text{ rad}; \ 90° = \dfrac{\pi}{2}\text{ rad}$

The radian is a unit of measurement equal to the angle obtained at the center of a circle making an arc equal to the length of the radius.

EXAMPLE: An airplane has its automatic pilot fly a circular route at a constant speed of 100 km/hr. The route has a diameter of 3000 m.

1. Calculate the plane's angular speed.

$$\omega = \frac{v}{r}$$

$$\omega = \frac{27.8 \text{ m/sec}}{1500 \text{ m}}$$

$$\omega = 0.0186 \text{ rad/sec}$$

ω = angular speed

v = velocity = 100 km/hr = 27.8 m/sec

d = diameter = 3000 m

r = radius = $\dfrac{d}{2}$ = 1500 m

2. Calculate the angular distance and the arc length flown in 45 sec.

Angular distance $\theta = wt$

$$\theta = (0.0186 \text{ rad/sec})(45 \text{ sec})$$

$$\theta = 0.837 \text{ rad}$$

Arc length $s = r\theta$

$$s = (1500 \text{ m})(0.837)$$

$$s = 1256 \text{ m}$$

OR

$$s = vt$$

$$s = (27.8 \text{ m/sec})(45 \text{ sec})$$

$$s = 1251 \text{ m}$$

CENTRIPETAL FORCE

Centripetal force may be expressed as mass times velocity squared divided by the radius, that is, $F_c = \dfrac{mv^2}{r}$.

EXAMPLE: The previously cited subway car has a mass of 130,000 kg, travels at 50 km/hr (14 m/sec), and rounds the above radius of 200 m. Its centripetal force is?

$$F_c = \frac{mv^2}{r}$$

v = 14 m/sec

r = 200 m

$$F_c = 130,000 \text{ kg} \times \frac{(14 \text{ m/sec})^2}{200 \text{ m}}$$

$$F_c = 127,400 \text{ N}$$

EXAMPLE: A satellite is in circular orbit at an altitude of 5.0×10^2 km. One complete revolution takes 95 minutes.

1. Calculate the tangential velocity.

   Radius of earth = 6400 m

   Radius of orbit, r = 6400 km + 500 km = 6900 km, or 6.9×10^6 m

$$v = \frac{s}{t} = \frac{2\pi r}{t} = \frac{2\pi(6.9 \times 10^6 \text{ m})}{5700 \text{ s}} = 7600 \text{ m/s}$$

2. Calculate the angular speed

$$\omega = \frac{\theta}{t} = \frac{2\pi}{5700 \text{ s}} = 1.10 \times 10^{-3} \text{ rad/s}$$

   To get the tangential speed from this:

$$v = r\omega = (6.9 \times 10^6 \text{ m})(1.10 \times 10^{-3} \text{ rad/s}) = 7600 \text{ m/s}$$

3. Calculate the centripetal acceleration, due to gravity:

$$a_c = \frac{v^2}{r} = \frac{(7600 \text{ m/sec})^2}{6.9 \times 10^6 \text{ m}} = 8.4 \text{ m/sec}^2$$

EXAMPLE: An astronaut with a mass of 75 kg is being spun in a centrifuge with a radius of 40 m at a speed of 26 m/sec. What is the centripetal force on the astronaut?

$$F_c = \frac{mv^2}{r}$$

$$F = \frac{(75 \text{ kg})(26 \text{ m/sec})^2}{40 \text{ m}}$$

$$F = 1268 \text{ N}$$

   (Astronaut weights 735 N)

CENTRIFUGAL FORCE

$$F_r = \frac{mv^2}{r}$$

EXAMPLE: A 0.5-kg object is traveling in a circular orbit 20 m in diameter at a speed of 2 m/sec. The cord is subjected to a force of 0.2 N. What is the centrifugal force *on the cord*?

$$F_r = \frac{mv^2}{r} = \frac{(0.5 \text{ kg})(2 \text{ m/sec})^2}{10 \text{ m}} = 0.2 \text{ N}$$

Since the mass is expressed in kilograms, velocity in meters per second, and distance in meters, the unit of force will be the newton. Note that the diameter of the circle was given, but the radius is required in the equation.

Fluids at Rest

PRESSURE

$$P = \frac{F}{A}$$

P = Pressure
F = Force
A = Area

EXAMPLE: The end of a pillar of a building has an area of 400 in². The air hammer applies a force of 600 lb as the pillar is driven into the ground. What is the pressure under the pillar?

$$P = \frac{F}{A}$$

$$P = \frac{600 \text{ lb}}{400 \text{ in}^2}$$

$$P = 1.5 \text{ lb/in}^2$$

EXAMPLE: A man has a mass of 75 kg; his shoes have a surface area of 84 cm² (84 × 10⁻⁴ m²), and therefore, the pressure exerted because of his weight. The formula to be employed is:

$$P = \frac{mg}{A} = \frac{(75 \text{ kg})(9.8 \text{ m/sec}^2)}{84 \times 10^{-4} \text{ m}^2}$$

$$P = 87,500 \frac{\text{N}}{\text{m}^2}$$

DENSITY

Density is the mass per unit volume of a substance.

$$P = hdg$$

P = pressure

h = height

d = density

g = acceleration due to gravity

EXAMPLE: A tank 10 × 10 × 10 m is filled with gasoline (density of gasoline = 680 kg/m³).

1. Calculate the pressure at the bottom of the tank in N/m².

$$P = hdg$$

$$P = 10 \text{ m} \times 680 \text{ kg/m}^3 \times 9.8 \text{ m/sec}^2$$

$$P = 66,640 \text{ N/m}^2$$

2. Calculate the force at the bottom of the tank.

$$P = \frac{F}{A}$$
$$F = PA$$
$$F = (66{,}640 \text{ N/m}^2)(100 \text{ m}^2)$$
$$F = 6.66 \times 10^6 \text{ N}$$

EXAMPLE: Find the pressure due to a column of mercury 100 cm high.

$$P = hdg \qquad\qquad h = 100 \text{ cm} = 1.0 \text{ m}$$
$$P = (1.0 \text{ m})(13{,}600 \text{ kg/m}^3)(9.8 \text{ m/sec}^2) \qquad d = 13.6 \text{ g/cm}^3 \text{ (given)} = 13{,}600 \text{ kg/m}^3$$
$$P = 133{,}280 \frac{\text{Newtons}}{\text{m}^2} \qquad\qquad g = 9.8 \frac{\text{m}}{\text{sec}^2}$$

SPECIFIC GRAVITY

$$\text{Specific Gravity} = \frac{d}{d_?}$$

d = density of a substance

$d_?$ = density of standard substance, usually water (d_w)

EXAMPLE: A metal bar is suspended from a spring scale that reads 900 gm in air and 600 gm when submerged in water.

1. Calculate the specific gravity.

$$\text{Specific Gravity} = \frac{\text{Weight in Air}}{\text{Weight Lost in Water}} = \frac{900 \text{ gm}}{900 - 600 \text{ gm}}$$
$$\text{Specific Gravity} = \frac{900}{300} = 3$$
$$\text{Specific Gravity} = 3$$

2. Calculate the density of the metal.

$$d_w = \frac{1 \text{ gm}}{\text{cm}^3}$$

$$d = \text{Specific Gravity} \times d_w$$

$$d = 3\left(1\frac{\text{gm}}{\text{cm}^3}\right)$$

$$d = 3\frac{\text{gm}}{\text{cm}^3} = 3000\frac{\text{kg}}{\text{m}^3}$$

Buoyancy

EXAMPLE: A balloon on a transatlantic flight is operating where the density of air is 0.8 kg/m^3. It weighs 1300 N, has a volume of 225 m^3, and is filled with helium, with a d of 0.176 kg/m^3. What load can it support?

Step 1. $w = Vdg$ w = weight = mg

V = volume

d = density

Weight of Air Displaced = 225 m^3 × 0.8 kg/m^3 × 9.8 m/sec^2 = 1764 N

Weight of Helium = 225 m^3 × 0.176 kg/m^3 × 9.8 m/sec^2 = 388 N

Weight of Balloon = 1300 N

Step 2. $L = w_a - w_h - w_b$ L = load balloon can support

$L = 1764$ N $- 388$ N $- 1300$ N w_a = weight of air displaced

$L = 76$ N w_h = weight of helium

w_b = weight of balloon

The load the balloon can support is 76 N.

Gravity

All objects in the universe attract each other with a force equal to

$$F_{\text{grav}} = \frac{Gm_1 m_2}{r^2}$$

where m_1 and m_2 are the two masses, r is the distance between them, and G is the universal constant of gravitation, equal to 6.67×10^{-11} N · m^2/kg^2.

EXAMPLE: What is the force of attraction between a 10-metric-ton wrecking ball and a 50-kg man if they are 6 m apart?

$$F = \frac{(6.67 \times 10^{-11} \text{ N} \cdot \text{m}^2/\text{kg}^2)(10 \times 10^3 \text{ kg})(50 \text{ kg})}{(6 \text{ m})^2} = 9 \times 10^{-7} \text{ N}$$

EXAMPLE: What is the mass of the earth? The force on 1 kg at the surface (6400 km from the center) is 9.8 N.

$$m_2 = \frac{Fr^2}{Gm_1} = \frac{(9.8 \text{ N})(6.4 \times 10^6 \text{ m})^2}{(6.67 \times 10^{-11} \text{ N} \cdot \text{m}^2/\text{kg})(1 \text{ kg})} = 6.0 \times 10^{24} \text{ kg}$$

Temperature Calculations and Measurement

Recall:

	Freezing Point	Boiling Point of Water
Celsius	0°	100°
Fahrenheit	32°	212°
Kelvin	273	373

Formulas: $C = \dfrac{5}{9} \times (F - 32°)$

$F = \dfrac{9}{5} C + 32°$

EXAMPLE: A Celsius thermometer records a temperature of 37°C in a patient. What is the temperature on the Fahrenheit scale?

$$F = \frac{9}{5} \times 37° + 32°$$
$$F = 66.6° + 32°$$
$$F = 98.6°F$$

EXAMPLE: An indoor arena is kept at a temperature of 72°F. What is the corresponding reading on the Celsius scale?

$$C = \frac{5}{9} \times (72° - 32°)$$
$$C = \frac{5}{9} \times 40°$$
$$C = 22°C$$

Absolute Scale: Absolute zero (0 on the Kelvin scale) is the theoretical temperature at which all molecular motion ceases. The Kelvin scale, therefore, has no negative degrees. Celsius temperatures can be expressed on the Kelvin scale ($K = 273 + C$).

EXAMPLE: 40°C and −40°C can be expressed on the Kelvin scale as follows:

  a. $K = 273 + 40$
      $K = 313$ K

  b. $K = 273 + (-40)$
      $K = 233$ K

Heat

Heat is expressed in Joules, calories, or British thermal units. One British thermal unit is the heat required to raise the temperature of one pound of water one Fahrenheit degree. One calorie (cal) is the heat necessary to raise the temperature of one gram of water one Celsius degree. However, it requires 4186 J of heat to raise the temperature of 1 kg of water one Celsius degree. The "big" Calorie used in nutrition is a *kilocalorie*. (1 Cal = 4186 J and 1 "little" cal = 4.186 J.)

SPECIFIC HEAT

EXAMPLE: How much heat is required to raise the temperature of 5 kg of ethylene glycol (2200 J/Kg·°C) from 20 to 60°C?

$H = ms\Delta t$ where m = mass
s = specific heat
Δt = temperature change

$$H = (5 \text{ kg})(2200 \text{ J/kg} \cdot °C)(60° - 20°C)$$
$$= (5 \text{ kg})(2200 \text{ J/kg} \cdot °C)(40°C)$$
$$= 440.000 \text{ J}$$

HEAT LOST = HEAT GAINED

EXAMPLE: 15 kg of steel at 150°C are cooled in 22 kg of water at 40°C. The final temperature obtained in the water is 47°C. Calculate the specific heat of steel. (Remember that the heat lost by the steel equals the heat gained by the water.)

M_B = mass of first object (steel)

S_B = specific heat of first object

Δt_B = initial temperature of first of object − final temperature of first object

M_W = mass of second object (water)

S_W = specific heat of second object (4186 J/kg·°C)

Δt_W = final temperature of second object − initial temperature of second object

$$M_B S_B \Delta t_B = M_W S_W \Delta t_W$$

$$(15 \text{ kg}) S_B (150°C - 47°C) = (22 \text{ kg})(4186 \text{ J/kg} \cdot °C)(47° - 40°C)$$

$$S_B = (22 \text{ kg})(4186 \text{ J/kg} \cdot °C)(7°C)/(15 \text{ kg})(103°C)$$

$$= 420 \text{ J/kg} \cdot °C$$

HEAT OF VAPORIZATION

EXAMPLE: How much heat is necessary to change 200 gm of ice at −12°C to steam at 100°C? The specific heat of ice = 0.51 cal/gm · °C; the heat of fusion of ice = 80 cal/gm; specific heat of water = 1.0 cal/gm · °C; and heat of vaporization of water = 540 cal/gm.

Step 1. Heat required to raise the temperature of ice to the melting point

$$= M_i s_i (0°C - 12°C)$$

$$= 200 \text{ gm } (0.51 \text{ cal/gm} \cdot °C)(12°C)$$

$$= 1224 \text{ cal}$$

Step 2. Heat required to melt ice

$$= 200 \text{ gm } (80 \text{ cal/gm})$$

$$= 16,000 \text{ cal}$$

Step 3. Heat required to bring water to its boiling point

$$= (200 \text{ gm})\left(1 \frac{\text{cal}}{\text{gm} \, °C}\right)(100 - C°)$$

$$= 20,000 \text{ calories}$$

Step 4. Heat required to vaporize water

$$= 200 \text{ gm } (540 \text{ cal/gm})$$

$$= 108,000 \text{ cal}$$

Step 5. Total heat required:

$$1,224 \text{ cal}$$
$$16,000 \text{ cal}$$
$$20,000 \text{ cal}$$
$$\underline{108,000 \text{ cal}}$$
$$146,448 \text{ cal}$$

Thermodynamics

WORK AND HEAT

The following conversion values of mechanical energy to heat should be utilized:

$$4.18 \text{ J equals } 1 \text{ cal}$$
$$1 \text{ J equals } 0.239 \text{ cal}$$
$$778 \text{ ft-lb equals } 1 \text{ Btu}$$
$$1055 \text{ J equals } 1 \text{ Btu}$$

$$W = J \text{ (constant) } H \qquad W = \text{work}$$
$$J = \text{constant}$$
$$H = \text{heat}$$

EXAMPLE: Water drops 90 m over the horseshoe falls at Niagara. Calculate the rise in temperature of the water if its potential energy were converted into heat.

Step 1. Energy transformed per kg of water

$$w = \text{mgh}$$
$$= (1 \text{ kg})(9.8 \text{ m/sec}^2)(90 \text{ m})$$
$$= 882 \text{ J}$$

Step 2. Heat produced

$$= 882 \text{ J}$$

Step 3. Rise in temperature:

$\Delta t = $ rise (change) in temperature

$H = $ heat change in material

$M = $ mass (1 kg of water)

$S = $ energy or units of work (Btu), or the specific heat of a substance

(heat /unit mass -degree change in temperature)

$$= 4186 \frac{\text{J}}{\text{kg} \cdot \text{°C}}$$

$$= \Delta t = \frac{H}{MS}$$

$$= \Delta t = \frac{882 \text{ J}}{(1 \text{ kg})\left(4186 \dfrac{\text{J}}{\text{kg} \cdot \text{°C}} \right)}$$

$$\Delta t = 0.21 \text{°C}$$

EXAMPLE: A compressed gas at a constant pressure of 75 lb/in^2 enters a cylinder 2 in diameter and pushes a piston 5 in. The work done by the gas is?

$$W = P\Delta V \qquad\qquad P = 500,000 \text{ N/m}^2$$
$$W = (500,000 \text{ N/m}^2 \times 0.0016 \text{ m}^3) \qquad \Delta V = \pi r^2 s$$
$$= \pi (0.01 \text{ m})^2 \times 0.05 \text{ m}$$
$$= 0.0016 \text{ m}^3$$
$$= 800 \text{ Joules}$$

EFFICIENCY OF A BOILER

Recall: The maximum efficiency of a heat engine supplied with heat at temperature T_1 and delivering heat to a reservoir at temperature T_2 can be calculated as follows:

$$E = \frac{T_1 - T_2}{T_1} = 1 - \frac{T_2}{T_1}, \text{ where } T \text{ is in Kelvins.}$$

EXAMPLE: An engine driven by a boiler receives steam at 300°C. Its exhaust temperature is 100°C. Its efficiency is?

$$E = \frac{T_1 - T_2}{T_1}$$
$$E = \frac{(300 + 273)\text{K} - (100 + 273)\text{K}}{(300 + 273)\text{K}}$$
$$E = \frac{573 \text{ K} - 373 \text{ K}}{573 \text{ K}}$$
$$E = 0.349$$
$$E = 34.9\%$$

EXAMPLE: A heat engine removes 6000 J per cycle of heat energy from the heat chamber and exhausts 1000 J to a cold chamber.

1. What is the thermal efficiency of the engine?

$$E = 1 - \frac{T_{cold}}{T_{hot}} \text{ or } \frac{Q_{cold}}{Q_{hot}}$$
$$E = 1 - \frac{1000 \text{ J}}{6000 \text{ J}}$$
$$E = 1 - 0.17$$
$$E = 83\%$$

2. What is the work done by the engine?

$$W = Q_{hot} - Q_{cold}$$
$$W = 6000 \text{ J} - 1000 \text{ J}$$
$$W = 5000 \text{ J}$$

Electrostatics

THE ELECTRIC FORCE

A positive and a negative charge attract each other; two similar charges repel each other. The force is given by Coulomb's Law:

$$F_{\text{elec}} = \frac{kq_1q_2}{r^2}$$

where q_1 and q_2 are electric charges in coulombs (C), r is the distance between them, and k is the electric constant of free space, equal to 9.0×10^9 N · m²/C².

EXAMPLE: What is the electric force between two plastic spheres, carrying charges of 20 nC and 12 nC, respectively, if they are 15 cm apart? (1 nC $= 10^{-9}$ C)

$$F = \frac{(9.0 \times 10^9 \text{N} \cdot \text{m}^2/\text{C}^2)(20 \times 10^{-9}\text{C})(12 \times 10^{-9}\text{C})}{(0.15 \text{ m})^2} = 9.6 \times 10^{-5} \text{ N}$$

Since the charges are alike, the force is a force of repulsion.

THE QUANTUM OF CHARGE

All electric charges are integral multiples of the charge on an electron, 1.60×10^{-19} C.

EXAMPLE: How many electrons are there in a charge of 12 nC?

$$\frac{12 \times 10^{-9}\text{C}}{1.60 \times 10^{-19}\text{C}} = 7.5 \times 10^{10}$$

ELECTRIC FIELD

A positive charge in an electric field experiences a force in the direction of the field; a negative charge gets a force in the opposite direction. The magnitude of the force is

$$F_{\text{elec}} = \mathscr{E}q$$

where $\mathscr{E}$ is the electric field in newtons per coulomb.

EXAMPLE: How strong an electric field will exert a force of 2.0×10^{-16} N on the electron?

$$\mathscr{E} = \frac{F_{\text{elec}}}{q} = \frac{2.0 \times 10^{-16} \text{ N}}{1.60 \times 10^{-19} \text{ C}} = 1250 \text{ N/C}$$

EXAMPLE: How strong is the field at a distance of 3 cm from a point charge of 20 µC? The field is the force per coulomb of charge in the field. From Coulomb's law

$$\frac{F}{q} = \frac{kq_1}{r^2} = \frac{(9.0 \times 10^9 \text{ N} \cdot \text{m}^2/\text{C}^2)(20 \times 10^{-6}\text{C})}{(0.03 \text{ m})^2} = 2.0 \times 10^8 \text{ N/C}$$

which is the electric field strength.

ELECTRIC POTENTIAL DIFFERENCE

The electric potential difference between two points in an electric field is the energy change in moving a unit charge from one point to the other. The unit is the joule per coulomb, called a volt (V).

$$V = \frac{E_{elec}}{q}$$

EXAMPLE: The potential difference between the terminals of an automobile battery is 12 V. If the battery is charged using 1800 J of energy, how much charge is transferred from one terminal to the other?

$$q = \frac{E_{elec}}{V} = \frac{1800 \text{ J}}{12 \text{ V}} = 150 \text{ C}$$

EXAMPLE: In a uniform electric field of 650 N/C, what is the potential difference between two points that are 20 cm apart in the direction of the field?

1. Determine the force on a coulomb in the field.

$$F = \mathscr{E}q = (650 \text{ N/C})(1 \text{ C}) = 650 \text{ N}$$

2. Determine the work done in moving the charge.

$$W = Fs = (650 \text{ N})(0.20 \text{ m}) = 130 \text{ J}$$

This is the electric energy difference between the points.

3. Determine the potential difference.

$$V = \frac{E_{elec}}{q} = \frac{130 \text{ J}}{1 \text{ C}} = 130 \text{ V}$$

Electricity

OHM'S LAW

In a metal conductor at constant temperature, the ratio of the voltage to the current is a constant, that is,

$$R(\text{a constant}) = \frac{V}{I}$$

The constant is called resistance, measured in ohms = volts per ampere.

EXAMPLE: The difference in potential between two terminals is 10 volts. A current of 5 A passes; calculate the resistance.

$$R = \frac{V}{I}$$

$$R = \frac{10 \text{ volts}}{5 \text{ A}}$$

$$R = 2 \text{ ohms}$$

EXAMPLE: Increase the difference of the above potential to 20 volts. Calculate the current that passes. Remember that according to Ohm's Law, the resistance (*R*) will remain the same when the voltage is increased—it is constant.

$$R = \frac{V}{R}$$

$$I = \frac{20 \text{ volts}}{2 \text{ ohms}}$$

$$I = 10 \text{ A}$$

EXAMPLE: A motor needs a current of 8 A and has a resistance of 40 ohms. What voltage is necessary for the operation?

$$V = IR$$

$$V = 8 \text{ A} \times 40 \text{ ohms}$$

$$V = 320 \text{ volts}$$

EXAMPLE: A 150-watt bulb operates on a potential difference of 110 volts.

1. Calculate the current drawn.

$$P = IV$$

$$I = \frac{P}{V}$$

$$I = \frac{150 \text{ watts}}{110 \text{ volts}}$$

$$I = 1.36 \text{ A}$$

2. Calculate the resistance.

$$V = IR$$

$$R = \frac{V}{I}$$

$$R = \frac{110 \text{ volts}}{1.36 \text{ A}}$$

$$R = 81 \text{ ohms}$$

EXAMPLE: A current of 10 A flows through a wire for 45 min. The charge that passes through a cross section of the wire may be calculated as follows:

$$I = \frac{q}{t}$$

$$q = It$$

$$q = (10 \text{ A})(2700 \text{ sec})$$

$$q = 27,000 \text{ A} \cdot \text{sec or coulombs}$$

Electric Circuits

ELECTROMOTIVE FORCE (emf) AND INTERNAL RESISTANCE

$$V = E - Ir$$

V = terminal potential difference

E = no-load potential difference or emf

r = internal resistance

I = current

EXAMPLE: A battery powering a portable television has an emf of 10 volts and an internal resistance of 0.20 ohm. It supplies a current of 6 A. Calculate the terminal potential difference.

$$V = E - IR$$

$$V = 10 \text{ volts} - (6 \text{ A} \times 0.20 \text{ ohm})$$

$$V = 10 \text{ volts} - 1.2 \text{ volts}$$

$$V = 8.8 \text{ volts}$$

RESISTORS IN SERIES

EXAMPLE: A direct-current circuit is wired with resistances of 3 ohms, 6 ohms, and 2 ohms in series. These resistances could be replaced by one resistor of 11 ohms to produce equivalent resistance.

EXAMPLE: Three lamps are connected in series and exhibit a resistance of 15, 10, and 5 ohms, respectively. How much current is produced by a potential difference of 100 volts across its terminals?

1. Determine the current in the lamp.

$$R = (15 + 10 + 5) \text{ ohms}$$

$$R = 30 \text{ ohms}$$

$$I = \frac{V}{R}$$

$$I = \frac{100 \text{ volts}}{30 \text{ ohms}}$$

$$I = 3.33 \text{ A}$$

2. Determine the voltage across each lamp; it is the product of its resistance and the current.

$$V_1 = (3.33 \text{ A})(15 \text{ ohms}) = 50 \text{ volts}$$

$$V_2 = (3.33 \text{ A})(10 \text{ ohms}) = 33 \text{ volts}$$

$$V_3 = (3.33 \text{ A})(5 \text{ ohms}) = 17 \text{ volts}$$

RESISTORS IN PARALLEL

$$\frac{1}{R} = \frac{1}{R_1} + \frac{1}{R_2} + \frac{1}{R_3}$$

Recall that addition to a circuit of resistors in series increases the resistance while addition to a circuit of resistors in parallel decreases the resistance.

EXAMPLE: Using the example of 3, 6, and 2 ohms, the equivalent resistance can be calculated as follows:

$$\frac{1}{R_{eq}} = \frac{1}{R_1} + \frac{1}{R_2} + \frac{1}{R_3}$$

$$\frac{1}{R_{eq}} = \frac{1}{3 \text{ ohms}} + \frac{1}{6 \text{ ohms}} + \frac{1}{2 \text{ ohms}}$$

$$= \frac{2}{6 \text{ ohms}} + \frac{1}{6 \text{ ohms}} + \frac{3}{6 \text{ ohms}} = \frac{6}{6 \text{ ohms}}$$

$$\frac{1}{R_{eq}} = 1 \text{ ohm, OR, } R_{eq} = 1 \text{ ohm}$$

EXAMPLE: A circuit has resistances of 15, 10, and 5 ohms. If these are wired in parallel what is their combined resistance?

$$\frac{1}{R} = \frac{1}{R_1} + \frac{1}{R_2} + \frac{1}{R_3}$$

$$\frac{1}{R} = \frac{1}{15 \text{ ohms}} + \frac{1}{10 \text{ ohms}} + \frac{1}{5 \text{ ohms}}$$

$$\frac{1}{R} = (0.07 + 0.1 + 0.2) \text{ ohm}$$

$$\frac{1}{R} = 0.37 \text{ ohm}$$

$$R = \frac{1}{0.37} \text{ ohm}$$

$$R = 2.7 \text{ ohms}$$

EXAMPLE: Find the current in a series circuit with two energy sources ($E_1 = 12$ volts, $E_2 = -4$ volt) and two resistors ($R_1 = 15$ ohms, $R_2 = 10$ ohms).

$$E_1 + E_2 = I_1(R_1 + R_2) \text{ or } V_1 + V_2 = I_1(R_1 + R_2)$$

$$I_1 = \frac{E_1 + E_2}{R_1 + R_2} \text{ or } \frac{V_1 + V_2}{R_1 + R_2}$$

$$I_1 \frac{(12 - 4) \text{ volts}}{(15 + 10) \text{ ohms}}$$

$$I_1 = \frac{8 \text{ volts}}{25 \text{ ohms}} = 0.32 \text{ A}$$

EXAMPLE: A circuit has three resistors—of 2 ohms, 4 ohms, and 8 ohms.

1. What is the resistance of these three resistors when connected in series?

$$R_s = R_1 + R_2 + R_3$$

$$R_s = (2 + 4 + 8) \text{ ohms}$$

$$R_s = 14 \text{ ohms}$$

2. What is their resistance when connected in parallel?

$$\frac{1}{R_p} = \frac{1}{R_1} + \frac{1}{R_2} + \frac{1}{R_3}$$

$$\frac{1}{R_p} = \frac{1}{2 \text{ ohms}} + \frac{1}{4 \text{ ohms}} + \frac{1}{8 \text{ ohms}}$$

$$\frac{1}{R_p} = \frac{4}{8 \text{ ohms}} + \frac{2}{8 \text{ ohms}} + \frac{1}{8 \text{ ohms}}$$

$$\frac{1}{R_p} = \frac{7}{8 \text{ ohms}}$$

$$R_p = \frac{8}{7} \text{ ohms}$$

3. How much current would be drawn from a 12-volt battery?

SERIES

$$I = \frac{V}{R_s} = \frac{12 \text{ volts}}{14 \text{ ohms}} = 0.857 \text{ A}$$

Potential drop in each resistor:

$$V_1 = IR_1 = (0.857 \text{ A})(2 \text{ ohms})$$
$$= 1.7 \text{ volts}$$

$$V_2 = IR_2 = (0.857 \text{ A})(4 \text{ ohms})$$
$$= 3.4 \text{ volts}$$

$$V_3 = IR_3 = (0.857 \text{ A})(8 \text{ ohms})$$
$$= 6.9 \text{ volts}$$

The drop equals the voltage rise in the battery:

$$V_i = V_1 + V_2 + V_3$$

$$V_i = 12 \text{ volts}$$

PARALLEL

$$I = \frac{V}{R_p} = \frac{12 \text{ ohms}}{8/7 \text{ ohms}} = 10.5 \text{ A}$$

Current in each resistor:

$$I_1 = \frac{V}{R_1} = \frac{12 \text{ volts}}{2 \text{ ohms}} = 6 \text{ A}$$

$$I_2 = \frac{V}{R_2} = \frac{12 \text{ volts}}{4 \text{ ohms}} = 3 \text{ A}$$

$$I_3 = \frac{V}{R_3} = \frac{12 \text{ volts}}{8 \text{ ohms}} = 1.5 \text{ A}$$

$$I_i \text{ and } I_1 + I_2 + I_3 = 10.5 \text{ A}$$

CELLS IN SERIES

EXAMPLE: Three cells are connected in series; each has an emf of 10 volts and a resistance of 2 ohms. Calculate the current after the combination is connected to an external resistance of 20 ohms.

$$\text{Total emf} = 10 \text{ volts} + 10 \text{ volts} + 10 \text{ volts}$$
$$= 30 \text{ volts}$$
$$\text{Total Resistance } (R) = 2 \text{ ohms} + 2 \text{ ohms} + 2 \text{ ohms} + 20 \text{ ohms}$$
$$= 26 \text{ ohms}$$
$$\text{Total Current} = \frac{\text{Total emf}}{\text{Total Resistance}}$$
$$\text{Total Current} = \frac{30 \text{ volts}}{26 \text{ ohms}}$$
$$\text{Total Current} = 1.15 \text{ A}$$

CELLS IN PARALLEL

EXAMPLE: Consider the following three arrangements:

    a. A single cell
    b. Two cells in series
    c. Two cells in parallel

Compare the currents maintained in a 5-ohm resistor under each condition. Each cell has an emf of 3 volts and negligible internal resistance. The emf of (a) is 3 volts, of (b) 6 volts, and of (c) 3 volts.

$$\text{(a):} \ I_{\text{total}} = \frac{E_{\text{total}}}{R_{\text{total}}}$$
$$I_a = \frac{3 \text{ volts}}{5 \text{ ohms}}$$
$$I_a = 0.6 \text{ A}$$
$$\text{(b):} \ I_b = \frac{6 \text{ volts}}{5 \text{ ohms}}$$
$$I_b = 1.2 \text{ A}$$
$$\text{(c):} \ I_c = \frac{3 \text{ volts}}{5 \text{ ohms}}$$
$$I_c = 0.6 \text{ A}$$

In each cell, however, the current is 0.3 A (in part c).

Electric Energy

JOULE'S LAW

$$\text{Voltage} = \frac{\text{Energy}}{\text{Charge}} \qquad V = \text{volts}$$

$$V = \frac{W}{Q} \qquad W = \text{usually in joules}$$

$$\text{OR } VIt = I^2Rt \qquad Q = \text{usually in coulombs}$$

Rewriting $W = VQ$, we can make the substitutions $Q = It$ and $V = IR$. Then, the basic equation for electric energy may be $W = VQ = VIt = I^2Rt$. This equation indicates that one joule must be expended in maintaining for one second a current of one ampere in a circuit of one-ohm resistance.

EXAMPLE: A motor is used for 45 min to drive a conveyor belt. It uses 35 A at 110 volts. Calculate the electric energy used.

$$W = VIt$$

$$W = (110 \text{ volts})(35 \text{ A})(2700 \text{ sec})$$

$$W = 10{,}395{,}000 \text{ J}$$

$$W = 10.4 \times 10^6 \text{ J}$$

EXAMPLE: How many calories are produced in a central electric resistance heating system in 5 min as it draws 30 A connected to a 220-volt line?

Recall: 1 cal = 4.18 J

$$H = \frac{VIt}{J} \text{ or } H = \frac{W}{J}$$

$$H = \frac{(220 \text{ volts})(30 \text{ A})(300 \text{ sec})}{4.18 \text{ J/cal}}$$

$$H = \frac{1{,}980{,}000}{4.18 \text{ J/cal}}$$

$$H = 470{,}000 \text{ cal}$$

POWER AND RESISTANCE

EXAMPLE: The above furnace operating at 220 volts requires 2 hp. What are the current and the resistance of the unit?

1. Current

$$P = 2\text{hp} \times 746 \frac{\text{watts}}{\text{hp}}$$

$$P = 1492 \text{ watts}$$

$$P = VI$$

$$1492 \text{ watts} = 220 \text{ volts} \times I$$

$$I = 6.78 \text{ A}$$

2. Resistance

$$R = \frac{V}{I}$$

$$R = \frac{220 \text{ volts}}{6.78 \text{ A}}$$

$$R = 32 \text{ ohms}$$

Alternating Current

EFFECTIVE VALUES

In a sine-wave varying current, the average power is half the maximum power. The average power is $I_{rms}{}^2 R$, where I_{rms} is the root-mean-square, or effective, value of the current.

EXAMPLE: A sine-wave alternating current with a peak current of 60 A is passing through a resistance of 2.0 Ω. Find the peak power, average power, effective current, and effective potential difference.

1. The peak power is $I_{max}{}^2 R$:

$$P_{max} = (60 \text{ A})^2 (2.0 \ \Omega) = 7200 \text{ W}$$

2. The average power is half the maximum, 3600 W.
3. The effective current produces the average power:

$$I_{rms}{}^2 R = 3600 \text{ W}$$

$$I_{rms} = \sqrt{\frac{3600 \text{W}}{2.0 \ \Omega}} = 42 \text{ A}$$

4. Effective potential difference:

$$V_{rms} = I_{rms} R = (42 \text{ A})(2.0 \ \Omega) = 84 \text{ V}$$

EXAMPLE: An effective potential difference of 120 V supplies a resistance of 40 Ω. Find the maximum potential difference and current.

1. Maximum is RMS value times the square root of 2:

$$V_{max} = (120 \text{ V})\sqrt{2} = 170 \text{ V}$$

2. Effective current is

$$I_{rms} = \frac{V_{rms}}{R} \frac{120 \text{ V}}{40 \ \Omega} = 3.0 \text{ A}$$

3. Maximum current is

$$(3.0 \text{ A})\sqrt{2} = 4.2 \text{ A}$$

Machines and Mechanical Advantage

ACTUAL MECHANICAL ADVANTAGE (AMA) = F_O/F_I,

where F_o = output force and F_i = input force.

THEORETICAL MECHANICAL ADVANTAGE (TMA) = D_I/D_O,

$$Efficiency(E) = \frac{F_o/F_i}{d_i/d_o} = \frac{\text{AMA}}{\text{TMA}} = \frac{\text{Output Work}}{\text{Input Work}}$$

EXAMPLE: A man pushing down with a force of 200 N lifts a 800 N crate by utilizing a lever system. The lever arms are 2 m and 40 cm respectively.

1. Calculate the AMA.

$$\text{AMA} = \frac{F_o}{F_i}$$

$$\text{AMA} = \frac{800 \text{ N}}{200 \text{ N}}$$

$$\text{AMA} = 4$$

2. Calculate the TMA.

$$\text{TMA} = \frac{d_i}{d_o}$$

$$\text{TMA} = \frac{2 \text{ m}}{0.4 \text{ m}}$$

$$\text{TMA} = 5$$

3. What is the efficiency?

$$E = \frac{\text{AMA}}{\text{TMA}}$$

$$E = \frac{4}{5}(100\%)$$

$$E = 80\%$$

EXAMPLE: A car with a mass of 680 kg (weight = 6664 N) is pushed up a 30 m ramp exhibiting an incline of 30°. A parallel force of 4400 N is used to accomplish this task.

1. What is the AMA?

$$\text{AMA} = \frac{F_o}{F_i} = \frac{6664 \text{ N}}{4400} = 1.51$$

2. What is the efficiency of the system?

$$\text{TMA} = \frac{30 \text{ m}}{30 \sin 30°}$$

$$= \frac{1}{0.5} = 2$$

$$E = \frac{\text{AMA}}{\text{TMA}} = \frac{1.51}{2}$$

$$E = 76\%$$

Simple Harmonic Motion

PERIOD AND FREQUENCY

The motion of an oscillating object is described by its:

displacement—distance from central position
amplitude—maximum displacement
period (T)—time for one full cycle
frequency (f)—cycles per unit time. One cycle per second is called a hertz (Hz)

Frequency is the reciprocal of period.

EXAMPLE: What is the frequency of a vibrating rod that completes each cycle in 1/20 sec?

$$f = \frac{1}{T} \frac{1}{1/20 \text{ sec}} = 20/\text{sec} = 20 \text{ Hz}$$

PHASE

Phase is the time difference, in fractions of a cycle, between two objects oscillating with the same frequency. One cycle is 360°.

EXAMPLE: What is the phase difference between two identical pendulums with periods of 1.5 sec if one reaches its maximum displacement 0.2 sec before the other?

$$\text{Phase differnece} = \left(\frac{0.2 \text{ sec}}{1.5 \text{ sec}}\right)(360°) = 48°$$

Waves

A wave is a system of oscillating particles or fields, in which each point transmits energy to the next point in turn. The next point follows with a slight time delay, so the phase varies continuously.

crest—a point of maximum displacement that appears to travel through the medium
trough—a traveling point of negative maximum displacement
wave velocity—speed of travel of crests and troughs
wavelength (λ, Greek lambda)—distance between successive points in phase

FREQUENCY, WAVELENGTH, AND PHASE

Wavelength depends on frequency and velocity:

$$v = \lambda f$$

EXAMPLE: If a wave in a rope travels at 4.6 m/sec and the rope is shaken at one end with a frequency of 2.0 Hz, what is the wavelength of the wave in the rope?

$$\lambda = \frac{v}{f} = \frac{4.6 \text{ m/sec}}{2.0/\text{sec}} = 2.3 \text{ m}$$

EXAMPLE: If a 120-Hz wave of vibration in a steel rail travels at 840 m/sec, how far apart are two points that are 90° out of phase?

1. Find the wavelength.

$$\lambda = \frac{v}{f} = \frac{840 \text{ m/sec}}{120/\text{sec}} = 7.0 \text{ m}$$

2. Each phase cycle corresponds to a wavelength, so

$$\frac{90°}{360°} \times 7.0 \text{ m} = 1.75 \text{ m}$$

INTERFERENCE

When two identical waves arrive simultaneously at a point, their displacements add. If they arrive out of phase, the interference is *destructive*, and a *node*, a point of no vibration, is formed. If they arrive in phase, the interference is *constructive*, and an *antinode*, a point of maximum vibration, develops.

STANDING WAVES

A standing wave in a string has alternate nodes and antinodes, spaced ¼ wavelength apart.

EXAMPLE: In the fundamental mode, a string vibrates with a node at each end and an antinode in the middle. What is the frequency of vibration if the string is 25 cm long and the wave in it travels at 390 m/sec?

1. Find the wavelength. Since there is a node at each end, the string is a half-wavelength long.

$$\lambda = 2 \times 25 \text{ cm} = 0.50 \text{ m}$$

2. Now find the frequency.

$$f = \frac{v}{\lambda} = \frac{390 \text{ m/sec}}{0.50 \text{ m}} = 780 \text{ Hz}$$

EXAMPLE: At a higher mode, there are 5 antinodes in the string of the preceding problem. What is the frequency at this mode?

1. Find the wavelength. Since there are 2 antinodes in each wavelength, there are $2\frac{1}{2}$ wavelengths in the string.

$$\lambda = \frac{25 \text{ cm}}{2.5} = 10 \text{ cm}$$

2. Find the frequency.

$$f = \frac{v}{\lambda} = \frac{390 \text{ m/sec}}{0.10 \text{ m}} = 3900 \text{ Hz}$$

Sound Waves

A vibrating object sets the adjacent air into vibration. This starts a longitudinal wave traveling through the air, a sound wave.

PITCH AND FREQUENCY

The *pitch* of the sound is its apparent tonal level, as defined by musical scales. An increase of 1 octave represents doubling the frequency.

> EXAMPLE: When the oboe sounds 440-A, what is the frequency of the tuba, sounding A two octaves lower? One octave lower is 220 Hz, the next octave below is 110 Hz.

In the equal-tempered chromatic scale, each increase of a half tone represents a frequency increase by a factor of $2^{1/12} = 1.05946$.

> EXAMPLE: What is the frequency of high C, which is 3 halftones above A?

$$\text{Frequency} = 440 \text{ Hz} \times 1.05946^3 = 523.2 \text{ Hz}$$

INTENSITY

The intensity, or loudness, of a sound in bels is the order of magnitude of its energy as compared with the softest audible sound. Thus, 3 bels (B), or 30 decibels (dB), has 10^3 times the zero level.

> EXAMPLE: If a rock band produces sound at 80 dB, how does the intensity of this sound compare with that of the softest audible sound?

The value of 80 dB is 8 B, so the loudest sound has 10^8 times the intensity of 0 B.

SPEED OF SOUND

The speed of a sound wave depends on the nature of the medium in which it travels. It travels faster in liquids than in gases, and much faster in elastic solids. In air, the speed of sound depends on the temperature and can be calculated from the following formula:

$$v_{\text{air}} = 331 \frac{\text{m}}{\text{sec}} + 0.6\, T \frac{\text{m}}{\text{s} \cdot {}^\circ\text{C}}$$

> EXAMPLE: How far away is a wall if an echo is received from it 3.9 sec after the sound is produced when the temperature is 26°C?

1. Find the speed of sound.

$$v_{\text{air}} = 331 \frac{\text{m}}{\text{sec}} + \left(0.6\, \frac{\text{m}}{\text{s} \cdot {}^\circ\text{C}} \right)(26\,^\circ\text{C}) = 346.6 \text{ m/sec}$$

2. Calculate the distance the sound traveled:

$$s = vt = (346.6 \text{ m/sec})(3.9 \text{ sec}) = 1352 \text{ m}$$

3. Since the sound had to travel both ways, the distance of the wall is half this distance, or 676 m.

BEATS

Two sound waves of different frequencies arriving at a point will interfere, alternating constructive and destructive interference. The beat frequency is the difference between the frequencies of the two sounds.

> EXAMPLE: As an orchestra tunes up, the oboe sounds 440-A. If the clarinetist hears 3 beats per second when he plays A, what is the frequency of the clarinet's A?

> It could be either 443 Hz or 437 Hz.

DOPPLER EFFECT

If a sound source is moving away from an observer, the frequency heard is lower than the frequency emitted, and conversely.

$$f = f_s \frac{v}{v + v_s}$$

where f is the observed frequency, f_s is the frequency of the source, v is the speed of sound, and v_s is the speed of the source as it moves away from the observer.

> EXAMPLE: With the temperature at $-10°C$, a train moving toward the observer at 32 m/sec sounds its horn at 380 Hz. What frequency does the observer hear?

> 1. Find the speed of sound.

$$v = 331\frac{m}{sec} + \left(0.6\frac{m}{s \cdot °C} \right)(-10°C) = 325 \text{ m/sec}$$

> 2. Apply the formula; v_s is negative because the source is moving toward the observer:

$$f = (380 \text{ Hz})\frac{325 \text{ m/sec}}{(325 - 32)\text{m/sec}} = 421 \text{ Hz}$$

Light Rays

Light travels in straight lines (rays) unless deflected by reflection or refraction.

REFLECTION

In specular reflection, the angle of reflection is equal to angle of incidence. Angles are measured with respect to the perpendicular to the surface (the normal).

> EXAMPLE: If a light ray strikes a mirror at an angle of incidence of 22°, what is the angle between the incident and reflected rays?

> Since the angles are measured from the normal, there are 44° between the incident and reflected rays.

REFRACTION

When a light ray goes from one medium into another, it will bend. The speeds of light in the two media are proportional to the sines of the angles the rays make with the normal.

EXAMPLE: A light ray in air enters a piece of glass, in which light travels at 2.20×10^6 m/sec. If the angle of incidence is $25°$, which is the angle of refraction?

$$\frac{\sin \theta_{glass}}{\sin 25°} = \frac{2.20 \times 10^8 \text{ m/sec}}{3.00 \times 10^8 \text{ m/sec}}$$

$$\theta_{glass} = 18°$$

INDEX OF REFRACTION

The index of refraction (n) of a medium is the ratio between the speed of light in vacuum and the speed in the medium.

EXAMPLE: What is the index of refraction of the glass in the preceding example?

$$n_{glass} = \frac{c}{v_{glass}} = \frac{3.00 \times 10^8 \text{ m/sec}}{2.20 \times 10^8 \text{ m/sec}} = 1.36$$

REFRACTION BETWEEN TWO MEDIA

If light passes from medium A to B, or vice versa,

$$\frac{\sin \theta_A}{\sin \theta_B} = \frac{n_B}{n_A}$$

EXAMPLE: A ray of light passes from crown glass ($n = 1.62$) into water ($n = 1.33$), making an angle of incidence of $40°$. What is the angle of refraction?

$$\frac{\sin \theta_{glass}}{\sin \theta_{water}} = \frac{n_{water}}{n_{glass}}$$

$$\sin \theta_{water} = \sin 40° \left(\frac{1.62}{1.33}\right)$$

$$\theta_{water} = 52°$$

TOTAL INTERNAL REFLECTION

If a ray passes into a medium of lower index of refraction, the calculated angle of refraction may exceed $90°$. Then the ray is totally reflected.

EXAMPLE: What is the largest angle of incidence (the critical angle) at which a ray of light can pass from crown glass into water (constants given above)?

$$\frac{\sin i_c}{\sin 90°} = \frac{n_{water}}{n_{glass}} = \frac{1.33}{1.62}$$

$$i_c = 55°$$

Mirrors

PLANE MIRRORS

In a plane mirror, the image is virtual, erect, the same size as the object, and just as far behind the mirror as the object is in front of it.

> EXAMPLE: The image in a plane mirror of a book is 25 cm high when the book is 50 cm from the mirror. How high is the image if the book is moved to 150 cm?

The answer is 25 cm; the size of the image is always the same as the size of the object.

CONVEX MIRRORS

In a convex mirror, the focal length is half the radius of curvature and the image distance obeys the rule

$$\frac{1}{f} = \frac{1}{D_o} + \frac{1}{D_i}$$

where f is focal length, D_o is object distance, and D_i is image distance. The focal length is negative. The image is always erect, virtual, smaller than the object, and behind the mirror.

> EXAMPLE: A convex mirror has a radius of curvature of 60 cm. Where is the image of a lamp that is 180 cm from the mirror?

1. Find the focal length; it is half the radius of curvature, 30 cm, and is negative.

2. Use the formula to find the image distance.

$$\frac{1}{-30 \text{ cm}} = \frac{1}{180 \text{ cm}} + \frac{1}{D_i}$$

$$\frac{1}{D_i} = \frac{-180 \text{ cm} - 30 \text{ cm}}{(180 \text{ cm})(30 \text{ cm})}$$

$$D_i = -26 \text{ cm}$$

A negative sign indicates that the image is behind the lens. The sizes of the object (S_o) and of the image (S_i) are in the same ratio as the respective distances.

> EXAMPLE: If the lamp in the preceding example is 40 cm tall, how tall is the image?

$$S_i = S_o \left(\frac{-D_i}{D_o} \right) = 40 \text{ cm} \left(\frac{+26 \text{ cm}}{180 \text{ cm}} \right) = +5.8 \text{ cm}$$

The image is virtual.

CONCAVE MIRRORS

Focal length is half the radius of curvature and positive. Image is either real, inverted, and in front of the lens, or virtual, erect, and behind the lens.

> EXAMPLE: (Object distance greater than focal length) A concave mirror has a radius of curvature of 80 cm. Find the size and location of the image of a lamp that is 60 cm high and 180 cm from the mirror.

1. Find the focal length; it is half the radius of curvature, +40 cm.

2. Apply the formula to find the image distance.

$$\frac{1}{D_i} = \frac{1}{f} - \frac{1}{D_o} = +\left(\frac{1}{40 \text{ cm}}\right) - \frac{1}{180 \text{ cm}}$$

$$D_i = +\left(\frac{(40 \text{ cm})(180 \text{ cm})}{180 \text{ cm} - 40 \text{ cm}}\right) = +51.4 \text{ cm}$$

3. Set the sizes proportional to the distances.

$$S_i = (60 \text{ cm})\left(\frac{51.4 \text{ cm}}{180 \text{ cm}}\right) = 17 \text{ cm}$$

EXAMPLE: (Object distance less than focal length) A can 15 cm high is placed 25 cm in front of the same mirror as above. Find the size and location of the image.

1. Find the image distance.

$$\frac{1}{D_i} = \frac{1}{f} - \frac{1}{D_o} = \left(\frac{1}{40 \text{ cm}}\right) - \frac{1}{25 \text{ cm}}$$

$$D_i = -\left(\frac{(25 \text{ cm})(40 \text{ cm})}{25 \text{ cm} + 40 \text{ cm}}\right) = -66.7 \text{ cm}$$

The image is behind the mirror.

2. Solve for the size.

$$S_i = (15 \text{ cm})\left(\frac{66.7 \text{ cm}}{25 \text{ cm}}\right) = 40 \text{ cm}$$

The image is virtual.

Lenses

CONCAVE LENSES

Lenses that are thinner in the middle than at the edges form the same kinds of images as convex mirrors. They obey the same equations, and the focal length is negative.

EXAMPLE: Find the size and location of the image formed in a lens of focal length −40 cm of a book 25 cm high placed 30 cm from the lens.

1. Find the image distance:

$$\frac{1}{D_i} = \frac{1}{f} - \frac{1}{D_o} = \frac{1}{-40 \text{ cm}} - \frac{1}{30 \text{ cm}}$$

$$D_i = \frac{(-40 \text{ cm})(30 \text{ cm})}{(30 \text{ cm}) - (-40 \text{ cm})} = -17 \text{ cm}$$

The negative sign shows that the image is behind the mirror.

2. Find the image size.

$$S_i = S_o\left(\frac{-D_i}{D_o}\right) = (25 \text{ cm})\left(\frac{17 \text{ cm}}{30 \text{ cm}}\right) = 14 \text{ cm}$$

The image is virtual.

CONVEX LENSES

Lenses that are thicker in the middle than at the edges form the same kinds of images as concave mirrors. They obey the same equations, and the focal length is positive.

EXAMPLE: (Object distance less than focal length) Find the size and position of the image formed in a +12.0-cm lens of a postage stamp 2.4 cm high placed 10.0 cm from the lens.

1. Find the image position.

$$\frac{1}{D_i} = \frac{1}{f} - \frac{1}{D_o} = \frac{1}{12.0 \text{ cm}} - \frac{1}{10.0 \text{ cm}}$$

$$D_i = \frac{(10.0 \text{ cm})(12.0 \text{ cm})}{(10.0 \text{ cm}) - (12.0 \text{ cm})} = -60 \text{ cm}$$

The negative sign shows that the image is in front of the lens.

2. Find the image size.

$$S_i = S_o \left(\frac{-D_i}{D_o} \right) = 2.4 \text{ cm} \left(\frac{60 \text{ cm}}{10.0 \text{ cm}} \right) = 14 \text{ cm}$$

The image is enlarged and virtual.

EXAMPLE: (Object distance greater than focal length) What focal-length lens is needed to form a real image 35 mm high of a man 2.0 m tall when the man is 1.7 m from the lens?

1. Find the image distance in centimeters.

$$D_i = D_o \left(\frac{S_i}{S_o} \right) = 170 \text{ cm} \left(\frac{3.5 \text{ cm}}{200 \text{ cm}} \right) = 3.0 \text{ cm}$$

The image is real.

2. Find the focal length.

$$\frac{1}{f} = \frac{1}{D_o} + \frac{1}{D_i} = \frac{1}{170 \text{ cm}} + \frac{1}{3.0 \text{ cm}}$$

$$f = \frac{(170 \text{ cm})(3.0 \text{ cm})}{170 \text{ cm} + 3.0 \text{ cm}} = 2.9 \text{ cm}$$

The image is real and small.

COMBINATIONS OF LENSES

The power of a lens, in diopters, is the reciprocal of its focal length in meters. When lenses are combined, their powers add.

EXAMPLE: What is the focal length of a combination of a +50-cm convex lens and a −20-cm concave lens?

1. Find the powers of the two lenses.

$$\frac{1}{+0.50 \text{ m}} = +2.0 \text{ diopters}, \quad \frac{1}{-0.20 \text{ m}} = -5.0 \text{ diopters}$$

2. Add the powers.

$$2.0 - 5.0 = -3.0 \text{ diopter}$$

3. Find the focal length.

$$\frac{1}{-3.0 \text{ diopter}} = -0.33 \text{ m, or } -33 \text{ cm}$$

Any number of lenses can be combined in this way.

Composition of the Atom

SUBATOMIC PARTICLES

Recall that the nucleus of an atom is composed of neutrons (no charge) and protons (positive electric charge). The total number of particles equals the mass number; the number of protons equals the atomic number. In an atom, the number of protons equals the number of electrons. The number of neutrons can be found by subtracting the atomic number from the mass number.

EXAMPLE: How many particles of each type are there in an atom of $^{35}_{17}\text{Cl}$?

The atomic number is 17, so the element is chlorine (Cl). There are 17 protons in the nucleus and 17 electrons outside it. The number of neutrons in the nucleus is $(35 - 17) = 18$.

ISOTOPES

Isotopes of the same element have the same atomic number, but different mass numbers (because of different numbers of neutrons).

EXAMPLE: Of the following, which are isotopes of the same element?

$$^{65}_{29}\text{Cu} \qquad ^{65}_{30}\text{Zn} \qquad ^{60}_{29}\text{Cu} \qquad ^{60}_{28}\text{Ni}$$

There are two isotopes of copper (Cu), both with atomic number 29.

NUCLEAR REACTIONS

In any nuclear reaction, the mass numbers and the electric charges must be the same on both sides of the equation.

EXAMPLE: When aluminum atoms are bombarded with helium nuclei, which isotope is produced along with a neutron?

$$^{27}_{13}\text{Al} + ^{4}_{2}\text{He} \rightarrow ^{30}_{15}\text{P} + ^{1}_{0}\text{n}$$

An isotope of phosphorus is produced along with the neutron. The mass numbers are $27 + 4 = 30 + 1$. The electric charge (on the protons) is $13 + 2 = 15 + 0$.

Radioactivity

Large nuclei are unstable and break down, releasing particles and energy. There are two kinds of radioactivity in nature: alpha and beta.

ALPHA DECAY

In alpha decay, the nucleus releases an alpha particle, which is a nucleus of helium, $^4_2$He.

EXAMPLE: What nucleus results from the alpha decay of a nucleus of radon-210?

$$^{210}_{86}\text{Rn} \rightarrow {}^4_2\text{He} + {}^{206}_{84}\text{Po} + \gamma$$

The γ (gamma ray) is a high-energy photon, which always accompanies alpha decay. The mass numbers agree: $210 = 4 + 206$. The electric charges agree: $86 = 2 + 84$.

BETA DECAY

In beta decay, a neutron emits an electron, turning into a proton. It also produces a chargeless, massless particle called a neutrino.

EXAMPLE: What is the result of the beta decay of radium-227?

$$^{277}_{88}\text{Ra} \rightarrow {}^{227}_{89}\text{Ac} + {}^{\,0}_{-1}\text{e} + \nu$$

Because the electron and the neutrino have negligible mass, there is no change in the mass number; $227 = 227 + 0$. The atomic number increases by 1, and the electric charge balance is $88 = 89 - 1$.

HALF-LIFE

The half-life of a nucleus is the time required for half of any given sample to undergo radioactive decay.

EXAMPLE: The half-life of radon-214 is 2.5 sec. If a sample of this gas contains 200 g, how much will be left at the end of 10 sec?

Ten seconds is 4 half-lives, so the mass drops to half 4 times. The amount left will be

$$(200 \text{ g})(0.5)^4 = 13 \text{ g}$$

EXAMPLE: What is the half-life of a radioactive nucleus if it takes 4 billion years for 40 g to decay down to 10 g?

The mass of the sample has dropped to half twice, so the half-life is 2 billion years.

Nuclear Energy

The mass of a nucleus is less than the sum of the masses of the protons and neutrons that compose it. The difference is called the mass defect of the nucleus, which corresponds to the binding energy ($E = mc^2$).

UNITS OF MEASURE

The mass of nuclei is measured in unified mass units, or u.

$$1 \text{ u} = 1.66 \times 10^{-27} \text{ kg}$$
$$1 \text{ kg} = 6.02 \times 10^{26} \text{ u}$$
$$1 \text{ u} \leftrightarrow 931 \text{ MeV}$$

EXAMPLE: If the mass defect of a nucleus is 0.0067 u, how much energy will be needed to separate it into protons and neutrons?

$$0.0067 \text{ u} \times \frac{931 \text{ MeV}}{\text{u}} = 6.2 \text{ MeV}$$

EXAMPLE: If a nuclear reaction yields 6.5×10^{12} J of energy, how much mass disappears?

$$m = \frac{E}{c^2} = \frac{6.5 \times 10^{12} \text{ J}}{(3.0 \times 10^8 \text{ m/sec})^2} = 7.2 \times 10^{-5} \text{ kg, or 72 mg}$$

FUSION REACTIONS

When two small nuclei combine, their binding energy must be released.

EXAMPLE: How much energy is released when lithium-6 combines with deuterium to form two helium nuclei (deuterium is hydrogen-2)?

1. Write the equation.

$$^6_3\text{Li} + ^2_1\text{H} \rightarrow 2^4_2\text{He}$$

The mass numbers are $6 + 2 = 2 \times 4$. The electric charge numbers are $3 + 1 = 2 \times 2$.

2. Add the nuclear masses on each side of the equation to find the mass deficit.

Li - 6:	6.01512 u
H - 2:	2.0140 u
	8.02912 u
He - 4:	2×4.00260 u = 8.00520 u

The mass deficit is $8.0912 - 8.00520 = 0.0239$ u.

3. Determine the energy equivalent of the mass deficit:

$$0.0239 \text{ u} \left(\frac{931 \text{ MeV}}{\text{u}} \right) = 22 \text{ MeV}$$

NUCLEAR FISSION

When a very large nucleus splits into two medium-sized nuclei, the combined mass of the two fragments is less than the mass of the original nucleus. Thus, energy is released.

EXAMPLE: When Uranium-235 is split by impact with a slow neutron, how many neutrons are produced?

$$^{235}_{92}\text{U} + ^1_0\text{n} \rightarrow ^{92}_{36}\text{Kr} + ^{141}_{56}\text{Ba} + ?^1_0\text{n}$$

Barium and krypton result. To balance the mass numbers, three neutrons must be produced. These neutrons can split additional uranium nuclei, producing a chain reaction.

Photons

Light has a dual nature; it can be described as a wave or a stream of particles (photons).

WAVE PROPERTY OF LIGHT

As a wave, light obeys the equation

$$c = \lambda f$$

where c is the speed of the wave (3.00×10^8 m/sec); λ (lambda) is the wavelength, and f (nu) is the frequency.

> EXAMPLE: What is the frequency of yellow light of wavelength 570 nm (nanometers)?

$$f = \frac{c}{\lambda} = \frac{3.00 \times 10^8 \text{ m/sec}}{570 \times 10^{-9} \text{ m}} = 5.26 \times 10^{14}/\text{sec} = 5.26 \times 10^{14} \text{ Hz}$$

PHOTON ENERGY

The energy of a photon obeys the equation

$$E = hf = \frac{hc}{\lambda}$$

where h is Planck's constant, 4.14×10^{-15} eV·s.

> EXAMPLE: What is the energy of a photon of red light with wavelength 730 nm?

$$E = \frac{hc}{\lambda} = \frac{(4.14 \times 10^{-15} \text{ eV} \cdot \text{sec})(3.00 \times 10^8 \text{ m/sec})}{730 \times 10^{-9} \text{ m}} = 1.70 \text{ eV}$$

PHOTOELECTRIC EFFECT

A photon may release an electron from a metal surface. The energy of the electron is equal to the energy of the photon minus the work function of the metal.

> EXAMPLE: What is the maximum energy of an electron emitted by a metal whose work function is 2.60 eV if the incident light is ultraviolet with a wavelength of 370 nm?

1. Find the energy of the photon.

$$E = hf = h\frac{c}{\lambda} = \frac{(4.14 \times 10^{-15} \text{eV} \cdot \text{sec})(3.00 \times 10^8 \text{m/sec})}{370 \times 10^{-9} \text{ m}} = 3.36 \text{ eV}$$

2. Subtract the work function of the metal.

$$3.36 \text{ eV} - 2.60 \text{ eV} = 0.76 \text{ eV}$$

> EXAMPLE: What is the longest wavelength of light that will release an electron from a metal whose work function is 3.61 eV?

The minimum energy of the photon is the work function of the metal, so

$$\lambda = \frac{hc}{E} = \frac{(4.14 \times 10^{-15} \text{ev} \cdot \text{sec})(3.00 \times 10^8 \text{ m/sec})}{3.61 \text{ eV}} = 3.4 \times 10^{-7} \text{ m}$$

or 340 nm, in the ultraviolet.

Atomic Energy Levels

The electrons in the outer shells of an atom can be raised from ground state to excited states in quantized steps.

SPECTRA

When an electron falls to a lower energy state, it loses a definite amount of energy by emitting a photon having that energy. The spectrum of the light emitted by a substance contains only photons of certain definite energies.

> EXAMPLE: What is the wavelength of the light emitted when an electron drops from a 4.70-eV excited state to a 3.22-eV state?

1. The energy of the photon is 4.70 eV − 3.22 eV = 1.48 eV.

2. The wavelength of the photon is

$$\lambda = \frac{hc}{E} = \frac{(4.14 \times 10^{-15} \text{ eV} \cdot \text{sec})(3.00 \times 10^8 \text{ m/sec})}{1.48 \text{ eV}} = 8.39 \times 10^{-7} \text{ m}$$

which is the wavelength of an infrared photon, at 839 nm.

SPECTRUM OF ATOMIC HYDROGEN

The single electron of a hydrogen atom occupies quantum states which can be represented by the expression $-13.6 \text{ eV}/n^2$, where n is any whole number.

> EXAMPLE: What is the wavelength of a photon that is emitted when a hydrogen electron drops from the fifth to the second state?

1. Find the energy levels of the two states:

$$\frac{-13.6 \text{ eV}}{2^2} = -3.40 \text{ eV} \qquad \frac{-13.6 \text{ eV}}{5^2} = -0.54 \text{ eV}$$

2. Subtract to get the energy of the photon:

$$-0.54 \text{ eV} - (-3.40 \text{ eV}) = 2.86 \text{ eV}$$

3. Find the wavelength of the photon:

$$\lambda = \frac{hc}{E} = \frac{(4.14 \times 10^{-15} \text{ eV} \cdot \text{sec})(3 \times 10^8 \text{ m/sec})}{2.86 \text{ eV}} = 4.34 \times 10^{-7} \text{ m or 434 nm}$$

> EXAMPLE: What is the wavelength of a photon that will ionize a hydrogen atom in its ground state?

1. The energy needed is enough to raise the total energy level to zero:

$$0 - \frac{(-13.6 \text{ eV})}{1^2} = 13.6 \text{ eV}$$

2. Calculate the wavelength of this photon:

$$\lambda = \frac{hc}{E} = \frac{(4.14 \times 10^{-15} \text{ eV} \cdot \text{sec})(3.00 \times 10^8 \text{ m/sec})}{13.6 \text{ eV}} = 9.1 \times 10^{-8} \text{ m or 91 nm}$$

PART 2

MATHEMATICS, VERBAL SKILLS, AND ESSAY WRITING

Mathematics Review

A n understanding of basic mathematical skills is essential for the science and quantitative skills test questions. This section reviews the most important mathematical concepts that may be present in these tests. This presentation does not attempt to cover all areas in great depth. Rather, it should be used in conjunction with texts so that the student will be prepared for mathematically oriented test questions.

ARITHMETIC

Operations on Numbers

Whole numbers are the counting numbers, 1, 2, 3, 4, 5, . . . *Integers* are the positive and negative whole numbers and zero: . . . , −3, −2, −1, 0, 1, 2, 3, . . . A *mixed number* consists of an integer combined with a fraction, for example, $3^1/8$. Many questions call for rounding off an answer "to the nearest integer." To round off a mixed number to the nearest integer, drop the fraction part of the number; if the fraction part is $^1/2$ or more than $^1/2$, increase the integer by 1; if the fraction part is less than $^1/2$, keep the original integer. For example, $4^7/8$ rounded off to the nearest integer is 5, but $3^1/3$ rounded off to the nearest integer is 3.

Questions often require that decimal answers be rounded off to some specified degree of precision, for example, to the nearest tenth, or the nearest hundredth, or to the nearest thousandth. To answer such a question, drop all digits in the decimal that are to the right of the specified digit; if the first digit dropped is 5 or more, increase the last digit retained by 1; if the first digit dropped is less than 5, keep the last digit retained at its present value. As examples, 81.698 rounded to the nearest tenth is 81.7; 81.698 rounded to the nearest hundredth is 81.70 (note that the zero is retained to show a hundredths place); 45.639 rounded to the nearest tenth is 45.6.

The rules for rounding off decimals also apply to rounding off whole numbers to a specified degree of precision. For example, 102,681 rounded off to the nearest thousand is 103,000; 102,681 rounded off to the nearest hundred is 102,700; 49,294 rounded off to the nearest thousand is 49,000.

Precision and Significant Digits

All measurements are approximate. Consider a measurement said to be 43 grams to the nearest gram. The unit of measure is the smallest unit indicated by the number and is the unit which was applied in the measurement. In the illustration, the unit is the gram and the maximum possible error is one-half that unit. Thus, 43 grams to the nearest gram means the true measure is between 43 ± 0.5 grams. A measure of $28^1/2$ feet means that the unit of measure is $^1/2$ foot and the maximum error is therefore $^1/4$ foot. A measure of $28^1/2$ feet could represent a true measure of anywhere between $28^1/4$ feet and $28^3/4$ feet. A measurement of 2.05 inches means that the unit of measure is 0.01 inch (that is, $^1/100$ of an inch), and the 2.05 may represent a true measure anywhere between 2.045 and 2.055 inches.

If an approximate number is multiplied by some number greater than 1, the precision of the result is reduced since the maximum error is also multiplied by that number. If the approximate measure of $28^1/_2$ feet, which has a maximum error of $^1/_4$ foot, is multipled by 5, the result is $5 \times 28^1/_2$ or $142^1/_2$ feet with a maximum error of $5 \times ^1/_4$ or $1^1/_4$ feet. Thus, the $142^1/_2$ foot approximation really represents a measure anywhere between $141^1/_4$ feet and $143^3/_4$ feet.

If an approximate number is represented as a decimal, every digit starting from the left-most non-zero digit and extending through the digit which represents the unit of measure is a *significant digit*. Thus, 2345 has 4 significant digits, 23.45 also has 4 significant digits, 0.00023 has 2 significant digits, and 2300 may have either 2, 3 or 4 significant digits depending on whether the two zeroes represent accurate measures in the tenths and units places or are merely used as "fillers" to locate the decimal point. Note that the position of the decimal point has nothing to do with the number of significant digits. The speed of light is 186,272 mi/sec; this figure has 6 significant digits; if we talk about the speed of light being 186,000 mi/sec., the figure has only 3 significant digits.

Performing mathematical operations on approximate numbers cannot increase the number of significant digits. If two approximate numbers are multiplied together or divided, you should carry out the multiplication or division and then round off your answer to the number of significant digits in the number with the *fewest* significant digits. Note that in the case of multiplication and division, the position of the decimal point has nothing to do with the number of significant digits in the answer. The situation in addition and subtraction is very different. If 231.2 is added to 15.623, the sum becomes 246.823, but digits beyond 246.8 are not significant since 231.2 was accurate to the nearest tenth only. Thus, in adding or subtracting approxi-mate numbers, you should first carry out the operation and then round the answer to the first place where the *last* significant digit of any of the numbers is found. Note also that if 231.2 had been added to 15.673, the sum would first be 246.873, which would be rounded off to 246.9.

Percent and Percentage

Problems involving percent actually involve three quantities: the base, the percent (or rate), and the percentage. The *percent* (expressed as a decimal such as .20 or as a part of 100 such as 20%) is the ratio of one quantity (the percentage) to another (the base). The number of which the percent is taken is the *base*; the result after the percent of the base is taken is the *percentage*. For example, if we say that 40% of the 2000 bacteria in a certain culture are spirochetes, then there are 800 spirochetes present in the culture. 40% or .40 is the percent or rate, 2000 is the base, and 800 is the percentage. The best way to solve any problem involving percent or percentage is with an equation based on the formula $p = br$, that is, percentage equals base times rate. Thus, if asked to find what percent of the 2000 bacteria in a culture is represented by the 800 spirochetes, the equation $800 = 2000r$ is solved. If asked to find the number of bacteria in a culture in which 800 spirochetes are known to represent 40%, the equation $800 = b(.40)$ is solved. If asked to find how many spirochetes there are in a culture containing 2000 bacteria of which 40% are spirochetes, the equation $p = 2000(.40)$ is used.

ALGEBRA

Ratio and Proportion

RATIO

A comparison of two values that are expressed in the same units. It may be expressed as an indicated division or as two numbers separated by a colon.

EXAMPLE: A comparison of the length of two insects might be expressed as $2\,cm:3\,cm$, that is, as $2:3$ or as $\dfrac{2\ cm}{3\ cm}$, that is, as $\dfrac{2}{3}$. Note that in each case, the name of the units cancels and the ratio consists of two pure numbers, $2:3$ or $\dfrac{2}{3}$. The units involved must be the same, however; the ratio of 3 inches to 2 yards is not $3:2$, but 3 inches to 72 inches, that is $3:72$ or $\dfrac{3}{72}$ or $\dfrac{1}{24}$.

PROPORTION

A statement that two ratios are equal. For example, $1:2\ =\ 4:8$ or $\dfrac{1}{2}=\dfrac{4}{8}$ represents a proportion.

The first and last terms of a proportion are called the *extremes* and the second and third terms of a proportion are called the *means*. In the proportion $\dfrac{1}{2}=\dfrac{4}{8}$, 1 and 8 are the extremes and 2 and 4 are the means. A most important relation used to solve problems involving proportions is this: In any proportion, the product of the means equals the product of the extremes.

EXAMPLE: If two substances, A and B, are to be mixed in the ratio of 2 parts of A to 3 parts of B, how many milliliters of A must be mixed with 15 milliliters of B to make the proper mixture?

Let $x =$ the number of milliliters of A.
Since the ratio of A to B equals the ratio $2:3$, a proportion is formed:

$$\frac{x}{15}=\frac{2}{3}$$

In a proportion, the product of the means equals the product of the extremes (cross multiply):

$$3x = 2(15)$$
$$3x = 30$$
$$x = 10$$

If the means in a proportion are equal, either of the means is called the *mean proportional* between the two extremes. Thus, in the proportion $\dfrac{1}{3}=\dfrac{3}{9}$, 3 is the mean proportional between 1 and 9.

EXAMPLE: Find the mean proportional between 4 and 16.

If x is the mean proportional, then:

$$\frac{4}{x}=\frac{x}{16}$$

In a proportion, the product of the means equals the product of the extremes (cross multiply):

$$x^2 = 4(16)$$
$$x^2 = 64$$

Take the square root of both sides of the equation: $x = \pm 8$.

Note that every positive number has two square roots, one positive and one negative. In a practical problem, one of the roots (usually the negative one) may have to be rejected as meaningless (for example, if x represents a length).

Equations

EQUATIONS CONTAINING FRACTIONS

These are solved by multiplying all terms on both sides of the equation by the Least Common Denominator of all the fractions.

EXAMPLE: Find a if $\dfrac{a}{4} - \dfrac{a}{6} = \dfrac{1}{2}$.

The least common denominator for 4, 6, and 2 is 12. Multiply all terms on both sides of the equation by 12:

$$12\left(\frac{a}{4}\right) - 12\left(\frac{a}{6}\right) = 12\left(\frac{1}{2}\right)$$
$$3a - 2a = 6$$
$$a = 6$$

QUADRATIC EQUATIONS

Second-degree equations may often be solved by factoring.

EXAMPLE: Solve $2x^2 + 5x = 3$.

Rewrite the equation so that all terms are on one side in descending order of exponents, equal to 0:

$$2x^2 + 5x - 3 = 0$$

The quadratic trinomial on the left factors into two binomials. The factors of the first term, $2x^2$, become the first terms of the binomials:

$$(2x \quad)(x \quad) = 0$$

The factors of the last terms, −3, become the second terms of the binomials, but they must be chosen in such a way that the product of the inner terms added to the product of the outer terms equals the middle term of the original trinomial, $+5x$. Try −1 and +3 as the factors of −3:

$$-x = \text{inner product}$$
$$(2x - 1)(x + 3) = 0$$
$$6x = \text{outer product}$$

Since $(-x) + (6x) = +5x$, these are the correct factors:

$$(2x - 1)(x + 3) = 0$$

Set each factor equal to zero:

$$2x - 1 = 0 \quad \text{OR} \quad x + 3 = 0$$
$$2x = 1 \qquad\qquad x = -3$$
$$x = \frac{1}{2}$$

The solution is $x = \dfrac{1}{2}$ or −3.

If a quadratic equation cannot be solved by factoring, the *quadratic formula* may be used: In a quadratic equation of the form $ax^2 + bx + c = 0$,

$$x = \frac{-b \pm \sqrt{b^2 - 4ac}}{2a}$$

EXAMPLE: Solve $x^2 - 4x - 3 = 0$

Here $a = 1$, $b = -4$ and $c = -3$:

$$x = \frac{-(-4) \pm \sqrt{(-4)^2 - 4(1)(-3)}}{2(1)}$$

$$x = \frac{4 \pm \sqrt{16 + 12}}{2}$$

$$x = \frac{4 \pm \sqrt{28}}{2}$$

$$x = \frac{4 \pm \sqrt{(4)(7)}}{2}$$

$$x = \frac{4 \pm 2\sqrt{7}}{2}$$

$$x = 2 \pm \sqrt{7}$$

RADICAL EQUATIONS

Equations in which the variable appears under a radical sign. They may be solved by isolating the radical on one side of the equation and then squaring both sides.

EXAMPLE: Solve $\sqrt{x^2 - 8} - x = 4$

Isolate the radical on one side of the equation:

$$\sqrt{x^2 - 8} = x + 4$$

Square both sides of the equation:

$$x^2 - 8 = (x + 4)^2$$
$$x^2 - 8 = x^2 + 8x + 16$$
$$-8 - 16 = 8x$$
$$-24 = 8x$$
$$-3 = x$$

The process of squaring may introduce an *extraneous root*; therefore, radical equations solved by squaring must always have the solution(s) checked to see if any are extraneous; checking must be done by substituting in the *original* equation:

$$\sqrt{(-3)^2 - 8} - (-3) \stackrel{?}{=} 4$$
$$\sqrt{9 - 8} + 3 \stackrel{?}{=} 4$$
$$1 + 3 \stackrel{?}{=} 4$$
$$4 \: ? \: 4 \: \sqrt{}$$

-3 is a true root.

EQUATIONS CONTAINING DECIMALS

Such equations are best solved by removing all decimals by multiplying each term in the equation by the highest power of 10 that will remove all the decimals:

EXAMPLE: Solve $153 + 0.085x = 0.85x$

Multiply each term by 1000:

$$153,000 + 85x = 850x$$
$$153,000 = 850x - 85x$$
$$153,000 = 765x$$
$$200 = x$$

Formulas

Questions may be asked requiring you to transform a given formula so that it is solved for a specified variable in terms of the others. This is accomplished in the same manner as the solution of a literal equation; the specified variable must be isolated on one side of the equation with all terms not containing this variable on the other side.

EXAMPLE: The formula for obtaining the Fahrenheit temperature, F, when the Celsius temperature, C, is known is $F = \dfrac{9}{5}C + 32$. Find an expression for C in terms of F.

To solve for C, first multiply both sides by 5:

$$5F = 9C + 160$$

Isolate the term containing C on the right side:

$$5F - 160 = 9C$$

Divide both sides by 9:

$$\frac{5F - 160}{9} = C$$

Factor out a 5 in the numerator:

$$\frac{5(F - 32)}{9} = C$$

In another form:

$$C = \frac{5}{9}(F - 32)$$

Scientific Notation

Scientific notation is a method of writing a number as the product of a power of 10 and a decimal number whose whole number part is between 1 and 10. For example, 3.6903×10^4 is in scientific notation. Scientific notation is a convenient method for designating very large or very small numbers. It is particularly useful when only a small number of significant digits are used in the number. For example, the speed of light is said to be 186,000 mi/sec. The only significant digits are "186" since the three zeros are merely used to indicate the placement of the decimal point. The speed of light is expressed more meaningfully in scientific notation as 1.86

$\times 10^5$ mi/sec. Scientific notation makes the number easier to handle and also makes it clear that the zeros are not significant digits.

Questions may involve conversion from scientific notation to ordinary notation or vice versa. Since multiplication by 10 results in moving the decimal point one digit to the right, the number 1.25×10^4 becomes 12,500 in ordinary notation (the decimal point is moved 4 places to the right). Similarly, 10 raised to a negative exponent indicates division by 10 that many times. Division by 10 results in moving the decimal point to the left one place. Thus, 1.25×10^{-2} is equivalent to 0.0125 in ordinary notation. 81,250 in ordinary notation becomes 8.125 $\times 10^4$ in scientific notation, and 0.002728 becomes 2.728×10^{-3}.

Exponents and Logarithms

POSITIVE EXPONENTS

A positive exponent is a number which indicates the number of times a quantity is to be used as a factor in a power. For example, 2^4 means (2)(2)(2)(2) or 16.

ZERO EXPONENTS

By definition $x^0 = 1$ for all values of x except $x = 0$, which is undefined. Thus, $5^0 = 1$ and $(-3)^0 = 1$.

NEGATIVE EXPONENTS

By definition, $x^{-n} = \dfrac{1}{x^n}$ provided $x \neq 0$. Thus, $3^{-2} = \dfrac{1}{3^2} = \dfrac{1}{9}$.

FRACTIONAL EXPONENTS

By definition $x^{m/n} = \sqrt[n]{x^m}$ or $(\sqrt[n]{x})^m$ provided $n \neq 0$. Thus, $x^{1/2} = \sqrt{x}$, and $8^{2/3} = (\sqrt[3]{8})^2 = 2^2 = 4$.

LAW OF EXPONENTS

For multiplication: $(x^a)(x^b) = x^{a+b}$ Example: $y^3 \cdot y^4 = y^7$

For division: $x^a \div x^b = x^{a-b}$ Example: $y^6 \div y^2 = y^4$

For powers: $(x^a)^b = x^{ab}$ Example: $(y^2)^3 = y^6$

For roots: $\sqrt[b]{x^a} = x^{a/b}$ Example: $\sqrt{y^6} = y^3$

EXPONENTIAL EQUATIONS

An exponential equation is an equation in which the variable appears in an exponent. Simple exponential equations may be solved by expressing both sides of the equation as powers of the same base.

EXAMPLE: Solve $3^{x-1} = 9$

Express both sides of the equation as powers of the same base, in this case, 3:

$$3^{x-1} = 3^2$$

Since the bases are the same, the exponents must be equal:

$$x - 1 = 2$$
$$x = 2 + 1$$
$$x = 3$$

If it is impossible to express both sides of the equation as powers of the same base, logarithms must be used to solve an exponential equation (see next section).

LOGARITHMS

The logarithm of a number is the exponent to which a given base must be raised to produce the number. The given base for *common logarithms* is 10.

Thus, $\log_{10} 100 = 2$ since $10^2 = 100$
$\log_{10} 10,000 = 4$ since $10^4 = 10,000$
$\log_{10} 50 = 1.6990$ since $10^{1.6990} = 50$
$\log_{10} 10 = 1$ since $10^1 = 10$

In writing common logarithms, the base, 10, is generally omitted. Thus, we say log 100 = 2, log 10,000 = 4, log 50 = 1.6990, and log 10 = 1.

Of course, log 50 = 1.6990 cannot be found readily. Like all common logarithms, it consists of two parts. The whole number part, or *characteristic*, is positive and is 1 less than the number of digits before the decimal point if the number is 1 or greater. Thus, the characteristic for log 839 would be 2. If the number is a positive number less than 1, the characteristic is negative and its absolute value is 1 more than the number of zeroes between the decimal point and the first significant digit. Thus, the characteristic for log 0.0072 would be −3.

The *mantissa*, or decimal part of the logarithm, is found in the Table of Common Logarithms. The mantissa is always positive and is the same for the same sequence of significant digits. Thus, the mantissas for 365, 36.5, and 0.0365 are the same. The mantissa for log 50 is found by looking for the sequence of digits, 500; the table shows the mantissa for this sequence to be .6990. The characteristic for log 50 is 1, so log 50 = 1.6990. Since the mantissa is always positive and the characteristic may be negative, the log for a number such as 0.00372 must be written as 7.5705 − 10.

INTERPOLATION

If we have a Table of Common Logarithms that provides entries for numbers with a sequence of only 3 digits, we must interpolate to find a mantissa of a number having 4 significant digits. To find the mantissa for log 183.6, we look for the mantissa for the sequence 183 (it is .2625) and for the mantissa for the sequence 184 (it is .2648). Since 1836 lies between 1830 and 1840, its mantissa will lie at a proportionate distance between their mantissas.

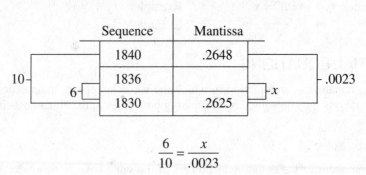

$$\frac{6}{10} = \frac{x}{.0023}$$

The product of the means equals the product of the extremes (cross multiply):

$$10x = 6(.0023)$$
$$10x = .0138$$
$$x = .00138 \text{ or } .0014$$

Mantissa for log 1836 is .2625 + .0014 = .2639

Log 183.6 is 2.2639 since the characteristic for 183.6 is 2.

LAWS OF LOGARITHMS

Since logarithms are exponents, they obey the same laws of exponents:

For multiplication: $\log (ab) = \log a + \log b$

EXAMPLE: $\log 8 = \log (4 \cdot 2) = \log 4 + \log 2$

For division: $\log \left(\dfrac{a}{b} \right) = \log a - \log b$

EXAMPLE: $\log \left(\dfrac{12}{4} \right) = \log 12 - \log 4$

For powers: $\log a^n = n \log a$

EXAMPLE: $\log 2^3 = 3 \log 2$

For roots: $\log \sqrt[n]{a} = \dfrac{1}{n} \log a$

EXAMPLE: $\log \sqrt{5} = \dfrac{1}{2} \log 5$

SOLVING EXPONENTIAL EQUATIONS BY LOGARITHMS

EXAMPLE: Solve for x: $3^x = 17$.

Since both sides cannot be written as powers of the same base, take logarithms of both sides of the equation:

$$x \log 3 = \log 17$$
$$x(0.4771) = 1.2304$$
$$x = \frac{1.2304}{0.4771}$$

The solution is completed by dividing 1.2304 by 0.4771.

NATURAL OR NAPERIAN LOGARITHMS

Common logarithms use the base 10. In more advanced mathematics and in many scientific applications, it is more effective to use logarithms with a base called the natural number and represented by e; e is approximately 2.718. Logarithms using the base e are called natural or Naperian logarithms and are designated by ln. Thus, ln 100 = 4.605 since $e^{4.605} = 100$

$$\ln 100,000 = 9.210 \quad \text{since } e^{9.210} = 10,000$$
$$\ln e = 1.000 \quad \text{since } e^1 = e$$
$$\ln 1 = 0 \quad \text{since } e^0 = 1$$

Using either base 10 or base e, a negative logarithm indicates a number between 0 and 1. There are no logarithms for negative numbers.

Natural logarithms obey the same laws as common logarithms since both are exponents. For example, $\ln 65 = \ln (5 \cdot 13) = \ln 5 + \ln 13$.

Variation

DIRECT VARIATION

Many physical variables are so related that an increase in one will produce an increase in the other. For example, the pressure of a confined gas will increase as the temperature of the gas is increased. If the values of two variables bear a constant ratio to each other, they are said to be in direct variation; sometimes it is said that "y varies as x" or "y varies directly with x." Direct variation can be expressed in symbols as $\frac{y}{x} = k$ or $y = kx$, where k is called the constant of variation.

> EXAMPLE: If the work done, y, by a constant force varies directly as the distance, d, through which the force acts, and if $y = 16$ when $x = 3$, find y when $x = 9$.

Use the formula $y = kx$. Substitute 16 for y and 3 for x:

$$16 = 3k$$

Solve for k, the constant of variation:

$$\frac{16}{3} = k$$

Since k is a constant, substitute the new value of x in $y = \frac{16}{3}x$:

$$y = \frac{16}{3}(9)$$
$$y = 48$$

INVERSE VARIATION

In many sciences, two variables are related so that their product is constant; when one gets larger, the other gets smaller. In an electrical circuit of constant voltage, for example, the product of the current and the resistance is constant. Current and resistance are said to vary inversely. Inverse variation involves a relationship of the form $xy = k$ or $y = \frac{k}{x}$, where k is the constant of variation.

> EXAMPLE: The volume, y, of a gas at a constant temperature is inversely proportional to the pressure, x. If $y = 30$ when $x = 2$, find y when $x = 12$.

Substitute in $xy = k$ to find the constant, k:

$$(2)(30) = k$$
$$60 = k$$

Since k is a constant and equal to 60, now substitute 12 for x in $xy = 60$:

$$12y = 50$$
$$y = 5$$

JOINT VARIATION

Some physical phenomena involve the variation of more than two variables. If y varies directly with both x and z, then the basic relationship may be expressed as $y = kxz$. If y varies directly with x but inversely as the square of z, then the basic relationship may be expressed as $y = \frac{kx}{z^2}$.

TRIGONOMETRY AND THE RIGHT TRIANGLE

The Pythagorean Theorem

Many problems involving right triangles can be solved by use of the Pythagorean Theorem, which states that in any right triangle, the square of the length of the hypotenuse equals the sum of the squares of the lengths of the legs. In the diagram shown, where a and b are the lengths of the legs and c is the length of the hypotenuse, $a^2 + b^2 = c^2$. Thus, if the lengths of any two sides of a right triangle are known, the length of the third side can be found.

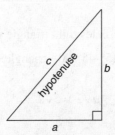

EXAMPLE: If the hypotenuse of a right triangle is 7 feet, and the length of one leg is 4 feet, find the length of the other leg.

If b is the length of the other leg, apply the Pythagorean Theorem:

$$4^2 + b^2 = 7^2$$
$$16 + b^2 = 49$$
$$b^2 = 49 - 16$$
$$b^2 = 33$$

Take the square root of both sides of the equation:

$$b = \pm\sqrt{33}$$

Reject the negative value as meaningless for a length:

$$b = \sqrt{33}$$

Pythagorean Triples

Certain special cases result in right triangles in which the ratio of the lengths of the sides can be represented by integers. They are the 3-4-5, 5-12-13, and 8-15-17 right triangles. Note that in every case the largest number in the triple represents the hypotenuse; the other two represent the legs. These triples should be committed to memory, as they make the solutions of many right triangles extremely easy.

EXAMPLE: Find the remaining leg of a right triangle whose hypotenuse is 15 and one of the whose legs is 12.

The hypotenuse, 15, is equal to 3 times 5 and the leg, 12, is equal to three times 4. Hence the triangle is a 3-4-5 right triangle with all the values multiplied by 3. The remaining leg is three times 3 or 9.

45°-45°-90° and 30°-60°-90° Triangles

The MCAT includes questions that may require knowledge of the relationships among the sides of two special right triangles, the 45°-45°-90° triangle and the 30°-60°-90° triangle. The relationships can all be determined by use of the Pythagorean Theorem and certain facts from plane geometry, but it is recommended that the student commit to memory the two diagrams below and use the values shown as formulas to apply in solving either of these special triangles.

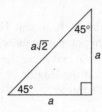 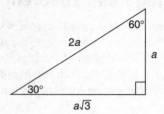

EXAMPLE: Find the leg of an isosceles right triangle whose hypotenuse is $5\sqrt{2}$.

An isosceles right triangle is a 45°-45°-90° triangle. Applying the formulas from the diagram above, the hypotenuse is $a\sqrt{2}$:

$$a\sqrt{2} = 5\sqrt{2}$$
$$a = 5$$

From the diagram above, the length of a leg is a:

$$\text{leg} = 5$$

EXAMPLE: If the hypotenuse of a 30°-60°-90° triangle is 6, find the length of the leg opposite the 30° angle and the length of the leg opposite the 60° angle.

The formula for the hypotenuse of a 30°-60°-90° triangle is $2a$:

$$2a = 6$$
$$a = 3$$

The formula for the leg opposite 30° is a:

$$a = 3$$

The formula for the leg opposite 60° is $a\sqrt{3}$:

$$a\sqrt{3} = 3\sqrt{3}$$

Trigonometric Functions

The three basic trigonometric functions are defined for acute angles from ratios in a right triangle:

$$\sin A = \frac{\text{opposite side}}{\text{hypotenuse}} = \frac{a}{c}$$

$$\cos A = \frac{\text{adjacent side}}{\text{hypotenuse}} = \frac{b}{c}$$

$$\tan A = \frac{\text{opposite side}}{\text{adjacent side}} = \frac{a}{b}$$

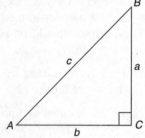

A convenient way to remember these definitions is by memorizing the mnemonic *soh-cahtoa*. Split into three parts, *soh,cah,toa*, where "*s*" stands for sine, "*o*" for opposite, "*h*" for hypotenuse, etc., the mnemonic gives all three definitions. Note that sin is an abbreviation for sine, cos for cosine, and tan for tangent. When any 2 parts from among the two acute angles and the three sides of a right triangle are known, any of the other parts can be found.

EXAMPLE: In the right triangle shown, find the length of side $\overline{EG}$.

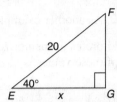

$\overline{EG}$ is the side adjacent to the 40° angle and 20 is the hypotenuse. Hence the cosine is used:

$$\cos 40° = \frac{\text{adjacent leg}}{\text{hypotenuse}}$$

From the Table of the Values of Trigonometric Functions, $\cos 40° = 0.7660$:

$$0.7660 = \frac{x}{20}$$

Multiply both sides of the equation by 20:

$$20(0.7660) = x$$
$$15.32 = x$$

A student taking the MCAT will be expected to know the sines and cosines of 0°, 90°, and 180°. These are shown in tabular form below:

	0°	90°	180°
sin	0	1	0
cos	1	0	−1
tan	0	∞	0

The sines, cosines, and tangents of 0° and 90° are deduced from consideration of what happens as angle A in the diagram of $\triangle ABC$ collapses toward 0°. $\overline{BC}$ will approach 0, and thus the $\sin 0°$ and the $\tan 0°$ will both be 0. As angle A collapses, the hypotenuse $\overline{AB}$ will approach $\overline{AC}$, and hence $\frac{AB}{AC}$ will equal 1 at 0°, or $\cos 0° = 1$. The values for 90° are deduced in a similar manner; those for 180° are the result of an extension of the definitions of the trigonometric functions to values beyond the acute angles found in a right triangle.

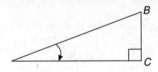

MCAT candidates are also expected to know the sines, cosines, and tangents of 30°, 45°, and 60°. If the candidate commits to memory the formulas for the sides as recommended in the section of this book on the 45°-45°-90° triangle and the 30°-60°-90° triangle, these values need not be memorized since they can be obtained by applying the definition of the sine, cosine, or tangent to the expressions in the formulas. For example, $\sin 45° = \frac{\text{opposite side}}{\text{hypotenuse}} = \frac{a}{a\sqrt{2}} = \frac{1}{\sqrt{2}}$.

The value $\dfrac{1}{\sqrt{2}}$ can be used for sin 45° or it can be changed to $\dfrac{1}{2}\sqrt{2}$, obtained by multiplying the numerator and denominator by $\sqrt{2}$. As another example, cos 60° $= \dfrac{a}{2a} = \dfrac{1}{2}$. For the convenience of those candidates who would prefer to memorize the values of the sine, cosine, and tangent of 30°, 45°, and 60°, a table of these values is also given here:

	30°	45°	60°
sin	$\dfrac{1}{2}$	$\dfrac{1}{2}\sqrt{2}$	$\dfrac{1}{2}\sqrt{3}$
cos	$\dfrac{1}{2}\sqrt{3}$	$\dfrac{1}{2}\sqrt{2}$	$\dfrac{1}{2}$
tan	$\dfrac{1}{3}\sqrt{3}$	1	$\sqrt{3}$

SYSTEMS OF MEASUREMENT

The MCAT candidate will be expected to understand and operate in either the metric system of measurement or in the system of common British units. It may be required to perform conversions from one system to the other, but in all such cases, the conversion factor will be supplied with the question.

The Common British System

The following equivalences and abbreviations should be known:

> 1 yard (yd) = 3 feet (ft) = 36 inches (in)
>
> 1 foot = 12 inches
>
> 1 mile (mi) = 5280 feet = 1760 yards
>
> 1 pound (1b) = 16 ounces (oz)
>
> 1 ton (T) = 2000 pounds
>
> 1 gallon (gal) = 4 quarts (qt) = 8 pints (pt)
>
> 1 quart = 2 pints
>
> 1 pint = 16 fluid ounces (oz)

This table of equivalences permits conversions within the British system.

EXAMPLE: How many ounces are there in 3 tons?

$$3 \text{ tons} \times \frac{2000 \text{ lbs}}{\text{ton}} \times \frac{16 \text{ oz}}{\text{lb}}$$

$$3 \times 2000 \times 16 \text{ oz} = 96,000 \text{ oz}$$

Note that names of units which appear once in a numerator and a denominator are cancelled. For example, tons ÷ tons = 1 and lbs ÷ lbs = 1. This leaves only the name of the units in which the answer is denoted.

BALANCING EQUATIONS CONTAINING PHYSICAL UNITS

The preceding comment on cancelling the names of units in an equation points up the importance of balancing the names of units on both sides of an equation that deals with physical units.

EXAMPLE: Given that the distance, d, that a body falls if dropped from rest is $\frac{1}{2}$ the acceleration due to gravity, a, times the time, squared, t^2, find the distance in meters that a body will drop in 3 minutes.

The given equation is:

$$d = \frac{1}{2}at^2$$

We cannot substitute $16\,\text{ft/sec}^2$ for a, or $3\,\text{min}$ for t and expect to get a distance in meters because the units involved will not balance:

$$d(\text{meters}) \neq \frac{1}{2} \cdot \frac{16\,\text{ft}}{\text{sec}^2}(3\,\text{min})^2$$

Since $1\,\text{min} = 60\,\text{sec}$, we can replace $(3\,\text{min})^2$ by $(3 \times 60)^2(\text{sec})^2$, and since $1\,\text{ft} = 0.3\,\text{meter}$, we can replace $16\,\text{ft}$ by $16(0.3\,\text{meter})$:

$$d(\text{meters}) = \frac{1}{2} \cdot \frac{16\,(0.3\,\text{meter})}{\text{sec}^2}(3 \times 60)^2\,(\text{sec})^2$$

Cancelling names of units wherever possible shows that both sides of the equation are in meters only:

$$d(\text{meters}) = \frac{1}{2} \cdot \frac{16\,(0.3\,\text{meter})}{\cancel{\text{sec}^2}}(3 \times 60)^2\,\cancel{(\text{sec})^2}$$

If the units in an equation cannot be balanced in this way, it is an indication that there is an error somewhere in the equation.

The Metric System

The basic units for the metric system are:

For length: meters (abbreviated m)
For volume: liters (abbreviated l or L)
For mass: grams (abbreviated g)

The following prefixes are attached to the names of the basic units to denote other units whose size equals the basic unit multiplied or divided by a power of 10:

$$\text{pico (p)} = 10^{-12}$$
$$\text{nano (n)} = 10^{-9}$$
$$\text{micro } (\mu) = 10^{-6}$$
$$\text{milli (m)} = 10^{-3}$$
$$\text{centi (c)} = 10^{-2}$$
$$\text{deci (d)} = 10^{-1}$$
$$\text{deka (da)} = 10$$
$$\text{hecto (h)} = 10^{2}$$
$$\text{kilo (k)} = 10^{3}$$
$$\text{mega (M)} = 10^{6}$$

Thus, a kilometer (km) is 10^3 or 1000 times as large as a meter. A centimeter (cm) is 10^{-2} times a meter or $\frac{1}{100}$ the size of a meter. A milligram (mg) is 10^{-3} times the size of a gram or $\frac{1}{1000}$ the size of a gram.

Conversions may be made within the metric system simply by moving the decimal point. Thus, $53\,cm = 0.53\,m$ (since a meter is 10^2 centimeters). Similarly, $8.3\,kg = 8300\,g$ (since a kilogram is 10^3 grams).

ELEMENTARY PROBABILITY

The probability of an event occurring $= \dfrac{\text{the number of favorable cases}}{\text{the total possible number of cases}}$.

For example, the chance of a tossed coin landing heads up is $\frac{1}{2}$ or 0.5, since there is 1 favorable case, heads, out of a total possible number of 2 cases, either heads or tails. The probability of drawing a king on a single draw from a pack of 52 cards is $\frac{1}{13}$. The number of favorable cases is 4 (there are 4 kings) and the total possible number of cases is 52; $\frac{4}{52} = \frac{1}{13}$.

The probability of two or more independent events occurring is the product of their separate probabilities. Thus, the probability of tossing 3 coins and having them all land heads up is $\left(\frac{1}{2}\right)\left(\frac{1}{2}\right)\left(\frac{1}{2}\right) = \left(\frac{1}{2}\right)^3 = \frac{1}{8}$ or 0.125.

If a coin has been tossed 3 times and has landed heads up each time, what is the probability that a fourth toss will result in a head? The answer is still $\frac{1}{2}$ since the fourth result is not affected by the three previous cases (it is said that "coins and cards have no memory"). The probability that all of four tossed coins will land heads up is $\left(\frac{1}{2}\right)\left(\frac{1}{2}\right)\left(\frac{1}{2}\right)\left(\frac{1}{2}\right) = \left(\frac{1}{2}\right)^4 = \frac{1}{1} = 0.0625$.

In a medical situation, suppose that a patient requires ear surgery for which the success rate is 90%. Note that this is equivalent to saying that the probability of success is $\frac{9}{10}$ or 0.9. If the patient requires surgery on both ears, what is the probability of a successful outcome for both?

$$(0.9)(0.9) = 0.81 = 81\%$$

Note that in these calculations, the assumption has been made that the events are independent, that is, that one event does not influence another. Thus, it is assumed that the surgical patient is a normal patient and that success of surgery on one ear does not make success on the other ear more or less probable.

In a compound probability situation, be sure to examine the number of favorable cases and the total possible number of cases for each of the separate situations.

Example: What is the probability of drawing 2 blue marbles from a bag containing 4 red and 6 blue marbles if the first marble is not replaced before the second one is drawn?

The probability of drawing a blue marble on the first draw is $\frac{6}{10}$. But since this first blue marble is not replaced, there are now only 5 blue marbles in the bag out of a total of only 9 marbles. Therefore, the probability of drawing a blue marble on the second draw is $\frac{5}{9}$. The probability of the two events occurring one after the others is $\frac{6}{10} \times \frac{5}{9}$ or $\frac{30}{90}$ or $\frac{1}{3}$.

STATISTICS

Some Measures of Central Tendency

Suppose you are asked to examine the fasting blood glucose concentrations of several patients in a hospital and obtain the results in mg/dl as 100, 80, 100, 90, 100, 120, and 125.

The *range* (the distance between the extreme values) is from 80 to 125, or 45.

The *mode* (the most common value in the series) is 100.

The *arithmetic mean* or *average* is the sum of all the values divided by the number of values:

$$\frac{100 + 80 + 100 + 90 + 100 + 120 + 125}{7} = 102.1$$

The *median* (the middle value when they are arranged in order of size) is 100 since arrangement in order of size gives 80, 90, 100, 100, 100, 120, 125, and the middle number is 100. If there were an even number of items in the series, there would be no single middle number; in such a case, the median is taken as the value halfway between the two middle values.

The Standard Deviation

The standard deviation is a statistical measure that indicates the dispersion or spread of the values in a set of data. You will not be expected to calculate it on the MCAT, but you must be able to interpret it. In the previous illustration, the standard deviation is 15.8. You should know that in a normal distribution, 68% of the values will fall within the arithmetic mean ±1 standard deviation and 96% of the values will fall within the arithmetic mean ±2 standard deviations. Thus, in the example shown, 68% of the values would be expected to lie between 102.1 − 15.8 or 86.3, and 102.1 + 15.8 or 117.9. The fact that only 4 out of the 7 values fall in this range $\left(\frac{4}{7} = 57.1\% \right)$ is due to the sample being so small. 96% of the values would be expected to fall between 102.1 − 31.6 or 70.5, and 102.1 + 31.6 or 133.7. Actually, all 7, that is 100% of them, do so.

Correlation

Suppose two variables change at random. The *coefficient of correlation* is a statistical measure of the degree to which the variation in one imitates the variation in the other. On the MCAT, you will not be expected to calculate a coefficient of correlation, but you will be expected to understand the nature of this measure.

The coefficient of correlation may have values between −1 and +1 inclusive; for example, values of +.86 or −.23 are typical. A correlation of +1 is a perfect positive correlation; the two variables involved move up and down together although they may be measured in different units and the moves may be of different magnitudes. A correlation of −1 is a perfect negative correlation; the variables involved move at the same times and to the same degree but in opposite directions (one decreases when the other increases). A correlation of 0 means that there is no relation between the variations in the two.

The output of a factory and its direct costs would tend to move together to some degree; hence the correlation between these two could be expected to be positive although not nearly as great as +1. It is usually true that the higher the price, the lower the sales; if there is a price increase, sales tend to drop; hence price and sales can be expected to be negatively correlated.

The three graphs below represent "scatter diagrams" obtained by plotting random readings of two variables, *x* and *y*. Graph *A* shows no association between *x* and *y* and hence the correlation would probably be close to 0. Graph *B* shows a generally negative correlation (*y* decreases when *x* increases), and Graph *C* shows a positive correlation.

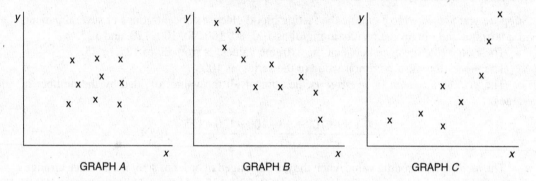

GRAPHIC REPRESENTATION OF DATA AND FUNCTIONS

Medical and other scientific publications use graphic representation of data and of algebraic functions to make relationships clear and also to deduce other information from such a representation.

The Rectangular or Cartesian Coordinate System

This system permits the location of any point on a plane with reference to two perpendicular axes whose point of intersection is called the *origin*. The horizontal axis is the *x*-axis, and the vertical axis is the *y*-axis. The position of a point is specified by an ordered pair of numbers in parentheses, for example, (4,3), which are called the *coordinates* of the point. The *x*-coordinate, also called the *abscissa*, is always written first, and the *y*-coordinate, also called the *ordinate*, is second. The abscissa is the distance measured horizontally from the *y*-axis and the ordinate is the distance measured vertically from the *x*-axis to the point. In the diagram, *P* is the point (4,3), *Q* is the point (−2,5), and *R* is the point (−3,−6).

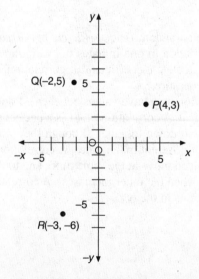

A first degree equation in two variables has an infinite number of pairs of values of x and y that satisfy it. These points may be plotted on a graph to represent the equation. A first degree equation always has a graph that is a straight line.

EXAMPLE: Draw the graph of $x + 4y = 8$.

Solve the equation for y in terms of x:

$$4y = -x + 8$$
$$y = -\frac{1}{4}x + 2$$

Choose some convenient values for x and calculate the corresponding values of y from the equation:

x	−4	0	8
y	3	2	0

Plot the points $(-4,3)$, $(0,2)$, and $(8,0)$ and draw a straight line through them. This line is the graph of $x + 4y = 8$.

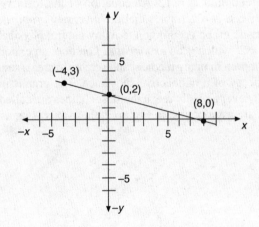

SLOPE OF A LINE

If Δy represents the change in the y-values from one point to another and Δx represents the change in the x-values of these two points, then the slope, m, of the line joining the two points is defined as $m = \dfrac{\Delta y}{\Delta x}$. If the coordinates of the two points are represented by (x_1, y_1) and (x_2, y_2), then the slope may also be defined as $m = \dfrac{y_2 - y_1}{x_2 - x_1}$. The slope is the rate of change of y with respect to x.

EXAMPLE: Find the slope of the first two points plotted to draw the graph of the line $x + 4y = 8$ in the section preceding this. These are the points $(-4,3)$ and $(0,2)$.

Let $(-4,3)$ be (x_1, y_1) and $(0,2)$ be (x_2, y_2). Then $y_2 - y_1$ or Δy is $2 - 3$ or -1, and $x_2 - x_1$ or Δ_x is $0 - (-4)$ or 4. $m = \dfrac{-1}{4}$: The slope is $-\dfrac{1}{4}$.

THE SLOPE-INTERCEPT FORM OF A STRAIGHT LINE

In the last example, notice that the slope of the line is $-\frac{1}{4}$ and that $-\frac{1}{4}$ (or m) is also the coefficient of x in the equation

$$y = -\frac{1}{4}x + 2$$

The constant term $+2$, which we denote by b, is the y-intercept, that is, the value of y where the graph crosses the y-axis. By solving the equation of a line for y, we can put it in the form $y = mx + b$, which tells us immediately the slope and y-intercept of the line. For example, the line $y = \frac{2}{3}x - 4$ has a slope of $\frac{2}{3}$ and a y-intercept of -4. This information can be used to draw the graph of the equation instead of plotting points. Begin with the y-intercept (at the point $[0,-4]$), and move 3 units to the right and 2 units up to locate the next point on the line; continue this process for more points on the line.

Graphs of equations other than first degree do not appear as straight lines. The graphs of such equations may be drawn by preparing a table of corresponding values of x and y (obtained by substitution in the equation). These values are used to plot points whose coordinates they are; joining the points with a smooth curve produces the graph representing the equation. Figure 1 shows the graph of the equation $xy = 12$. An equation of the form $xy = k$ where k is a constant is a relationship between two variables that are *inversely proportional*; this type of relationship and its characteristic graph is common to many natural physical phenomena. Figure 2 illustrates the graph of $y = 2^x$ which is an *exponential function*; an exponential function and its characteristic graph is common in many medical and scientific areas, such as the growth of bacteria in a culture or the decay of a radioactive substance. The graphs in both Figures 1 and 2 approach certain lines but never actually reach them; such lines are called *asymptotes*. In Figure 1, both the x- and y-axes are asymptotes; in Figure 2, the x-axis is an asymptote.

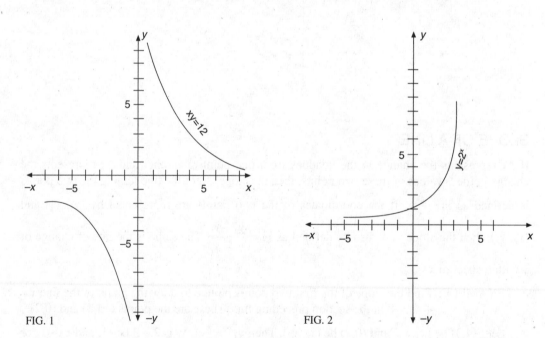

FIG. 1   FIG. 2

Finding the Equation from a Graph

Suppose that readings from experiments are taken on two variables, say blood clotting time and the quantity administered of a certain anti-clotting substance. If these data are used as coordinates of points plotted on a rectangular coordinate chart, and if the points turn out to lie in a straight line, then we know that we can represent the relationship between the two variables by a first degree algebraic equation. In fact, we can write the equation; all we need do is read the value of the y-intercept, b, from the graph and figure the slope, m, by noting the Δy and the Δx between two of the points; substituting the values of m and b in the slope-intercept form, $y = mx + b$, gives the equation.

But suppose that points plotted from experimental data readings do not lie in a straight line. Then the equation of the graph is not a first degree equation. To find out what it is, we use other types of coordinate systems. Two of those that are especially useful with the types of equations and graphs common in medicine and other sciences are the semi-log scale and the log-log scale.

SEMI-LOG GRAPHS

The rectangular coordinate system uses scales on the x- and y-axes that are arithmetic, that is, the distances on the scale from 0 to 1, from 1 to 2, from 2 to 3, etc., are always the same. The semi-log coordinate system uses an x-axis that has an arith-metic scale, but the distances from the origin along the y-axis represent the values of the logarithms of the numbers instead of the numbers themselves. Thus, the y-axis scale begins at 1 (since log 1 = 0). Since log 10 = 1 and log 100 = 2, the distance on the scale from 1 to 10 is the same as the distance from 10 to 100. It is also the same as the distance from 100 to 1000, etc.

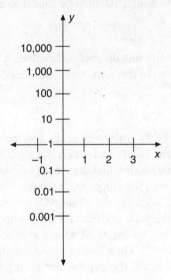

Now suppose that experimental data readings are plotted as points on a semi-log chart, and they turn out to lie in a straight line. Reading the slope, m, and the y-intercept, b, from the graph will enable us to write an equation, but the variable represented on the vertical scale will be log y instead of y and the intercept, b, will actually be log b. Note that log b is some constant. The equation will then be log $y = mx + \log b$. Since the common logarithm is defined as the exponent to which 10 must be raised to give the number, we can write $y = 10^{mx+\log b}$. Thus, we have found an exponential function from the data plotted on a graph.

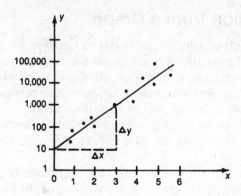

EXAMPLE: The graph above, drawn on semi-log coordinate paper, shows a line obtained by plotting a scattering of points from experimental data. Find the equation of the line.

Read the y-intercept, b, from the graph: $b = \log 10 = 1$. Calculate the slope, m:

$$m = \frac{\Delta y}{\Delta x} = \frac{\log 1000 - \log 10}{3 - 0} = \frac{3 - 1}{3} = \frac{2}{3}$$

Using the slope-intercept form of the straight line, $y = mx + b$:

$$\log y = \frac{2}{3}x + 1$$

Since $\log y$ is the exponent to which 10 must be raised to equal y:

$$y = 10^{2/3x+1}$$

Note that although for simplicity this discussion involves a y-axis scale that is for common logs (base 10), semi-log scales used in medicine could be scaled for natural logarithms (base e).

LOG-LOG GRAPHS

In semi-log graphs, the x-axis has an arithmetic scale and the y-axis has a scale that is logarithmic. In log-log graphs, both the x-axis and y-axis have scales that are logarithmic.

Suppose we plot points from experimental data and find that they lie in a straight line on a log-log chart. As before, we can read the slope, m, and the y-intercept, b, and use them in the $y = mx + b$ form of the straight line to write the equation. However, the variables are now $\log y$ and $\log x$ instead of y and x, and the value we read for the y-intercept is actually $\log b$. Thus, we can write an equation, $\log y = m \log x + \log b$. Making use of the laws of logarithms, $m \log x = \log x^m$, and $\log x^m + \log b = \log (bx^m)$. Thus, our equation becomes $\log y = \log (bx^m)$. Since we have the logs of two expressions equal, the expressions themselves are equal. Thus, our equation is $y = bx^m$. Since m may be any positive or negative integer or even a fraction, we have a powerful tool for converting data readings into complicated equations of degree greater than 1.

A first degree equation in two variables can always be rewritten in the form $y = mx + b$, and its graph is *always* a straight line on rectangular coordinate graph paper. The MCAT candidate should know that one type of exponential equation is of the form $y = a^{bx+c}$, where a, b, and c are constants, and that its graph is *always* a straight line when drawn on semi-log coordinate paper. In scientific work the "a" of $y = a^{bx+c}$ is frequently equal to e, the natural number, and c is frequently equal to 0, so that the most common form of an exponential equation in medicine or other sciences is $y = e^{bx}$.

MCAT candidates should also know that an equation of the form $y = ax^n$ where a and n are constants and n may be positive, negative, or a fraction, is known as a power law; its graph is *always* a straight line when drawn on log-log coordinate paper.

VECTOR ADDITION AND SUBTRACTION

Vectors

Most quantities are *scalar* quantities, that is, they have magnitude only. The length of a line, the number of pages in this book, or your bank balance are all scalar quantities. Some quantities have both a magnitude and a direction. They are called *vector* quantities. Examples are a wind velocity of 15 mph in an easterly direction, a downward (vertical) water pressure of 20 lb/in^2, or the motion of a ship sailing northeast at 23 knots. A directed line segment called a *vector* is used to represent such quantities; its length represents the magnitude of the quantity and its orientation represents the direction.

Vector Addition

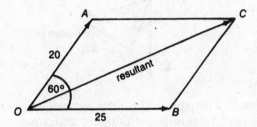

Suppose that two forces, one of 20 lb and one of 25 lb act simultaneously on a body at an angle of 60° to each other. We may represent the 20 lb force by vector $\overrightarrow{OA}$ and the 25 lb force by the vector $\overrightarrow{OB}$. Complete the parallelogram of which $\overrightarrow{OA}$ and $\overrightarrow{OB}$ are two sides. The diagonal of the parallelogram, $\overrightarrow{OC}$, is a vector that is called the sum of the vectors $\overrightarrow{OA}$ and $\overrightarrow{OB}$. $\overrightarrow{OC}$ is also called the *resultant* of the two vectors, $\overrightarrow{OA}$ and $\overrightarrow{OB}$, and $\overrightarrow{OA}$ and $\overrightarrow{OB}$ are the *components* of the force represented by $\overrightarrow{OC}$. If the object on which forces $\overrightarrow{OA}$ and $\overrightarrow{OB}$ are acting is free-moving, the object will move in the direction represented by $\overrightarrow{OC}$ and with a force whose magnitude is represented by the length of $\overrightarrow{OC}$.

If it is desired to compute the magnitude of $\overrightarrow{OC}$ in the above example, $\triangle OBC$ must be solved. Since $AOBC$ is a parallelogram, $BC = OA = 20$, and $\angle B \doteq 120°$. By the Law of Cosines, $(OC)^2 = (OB)^2 + (BC)^2 - 2(OB)(BC)\cos \angle B$. All the quantities on the right side of the equation are known, so $(OC)^2$, and hence $\overrightarrow{OC}$, can be calculated.

Questions on the MCAT involving vector addition could involve simpler cases than the above, usually those in which the two component forces are at right angles to each other.

> EXAMPLE: Find the resultant force and the angle it makes with the larger component, if two component forces, one of 10 lb and one of 20 lb, act at 90° to each other.

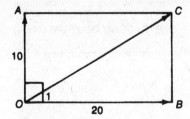

Draw vectors representing the two forces and complete the parallelogram of which they are sides. The diagonal of this parallelogram, which comes from their common origin, is the resultant or sum of the two forces. Vector $\overrightarrow{OC}$ is the resultant. In right $\triangle OBC$, $OB = 20$ and $CB = OA = 10$. By the Pythagorean Theorem, $(OC)^2 = 20^2 + 10^2$ or $(OC)^2 = 400 + 100$; since $(OC)^2 = 500$, $OC = \sqrt{500}$ or $10\sqrt{5}$. In right triangle OBC, $\tan \angle 1 = \dfrac{\text{opposite leg}}{\text{adjacent leg}} = \dfrac{10}{20} = \dfrac{1}{2} = 0.5000$. From the Tables of Trigonometric Functions, the angle whose tangent is 0.5000 is 27° to the nearest degree, so the resultant makes a 27° angle with the larger component.

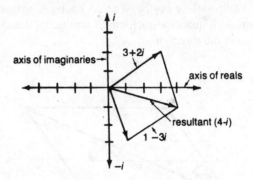

Vectors may also be added by representing them as complex numbers. The vector represented by the complex number $3 + 2i$ is the vector that extends from the origin to the point representing $3 + 2i$ graphically. Suppose we wish to add the vector represented by $3 + 2i$ to the vector represented by $1 - 3i$. As before, the resultant can be drawn as the diagonal of the parallelogram formed by using the two given vectors as sides. The complex number that is the end point of the resultant can be read from the graph; it represents the resultant vector. However, the sum can be obtained more simply by adding the two complex numbers algebraically:

$$\begin{array}{r} 3+2i \\ \underline{1-3i} \\ 4-i \end{array}$$

The resultant is $4 - i$.

Subtraction of Vectors

To subtract one vector from another, we simply add the additive inverse of the vector to be subtracted. If the complex number representation of the vectors is used, this simply means that the signs of the vector being subtracted are changed and the resulting complex number is then added to the other vector. If the parallelogram method is used, the vector being subtracted is replaced by a vector of the same magnitude but extending in the opposite direction. This new vector is then added to the other vector by forming a parallelogram and finding the diagonal that is the resultant (see diagram).

SUBTRACTING $\vec{OB}$ FROM $\vec{OA}$

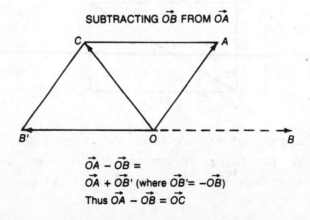

$\vec{OA} - \vec{OB} =$
$\vec{OA} + \vec{OB'}$ (where $\vec{OB'} = -\vec{OB}$)
Thus $\vec{OA} - \vec{OB} = \vec{OC}$

CHAPTER 6

Verbal Reasoning— Test-Taking Strategies

This portion of the book will focus on various techniques to help you get the most out of reading.

You can learn to read efficiently and effectively, and the more you read the better you will read. People who do not like to read generally do not read well, and most people who do not read well read too slowly. They read almost word by word and must consequently backtrack to capture the main idea. You should read as fast as you can think without the loss of comprehension, misreading, or losing facts or ideas.

Learning to read rapidly takes effort, willpower, and a plan. Success depends on your interest and the effectiveness of the techniques and habits you acquire. Find the time for the activities that are necessary for academic success: first things first!

A great deal of your success depends on your frame of mind. You must develop confidence in your own ability. Believe in yourself. You have been successful in the past, and will be successful in the future. Confidence comes with knowledge, experience, and practice.

In the MCAT Examination, reading skill or verbal reasoning is assessed by presenting to the examinee 7–9 selections, each of which is approximately 600 words long. Every selection is followed by a set of 5–7 questions pertaining to it. Subjects from a wide variety of areas are used to test the student's ability to analyze data accurately. The information necessary to answer the questions is in the selection, and no prior knowledge is necessary to arrive at a correct answer.

APPROACH TO THE READING QUESTIONS

There is no one correct way to handle this section. Some people routinely read the selection first, and some read the questions first. With either approach, rapid processing of information and maximum retention are key elements. The technique of highlighting central topics and key words and phrases (described later in this chapter) is useful here.

If you prefer to read the selection first, use the highlighting technique to emphasize the central topic and key words and phrases. When you finish the selection, you should immediately move on to the questions and answer them one by one while the information is still fresh in your mind.

Some people read the questions first since they feel that they have better attention to details when they know what to expect. If you choose this approach, you read the passage with specific questions in mind. Then you can either answer the questions as a group when you have finished the passage, or answer the questions as the answers appear in the selection. Whichever way you proceed, we still advocate the highlighting method.

Do not, however, leave questions blank in the hope of returning to them later, whether or not you have read and highlighted the passage. Your highlights in a passage are removed once you have left the passage and have gone to another. This could be costly since rereading the entire passage may require a great deal of time. Answer all questions as best you can, marking those you are not certain of for checking if you have time at the end. Please remember that you must base your answers on the material presented in the passage, not on your own knowledge or experience. Do not base your answer on information that isn't there.

Ways and Means

Reading experts seem to agree that the rapid reader's comprehension is usually excellent, and the slow reader's comprehension is usually poor. This does not mean that the rapid reader never slows down for difficult material or to note key words and phrases related to the central topic of the passage. It does mean that the rapid reader is able to find the right speed for the material, whereas the slow reader habitually reads more slowly than the occasion or subject matter demands.

WORD-BY-WORD READING

Word-by-word reading does not improve comprehension and makes concentration more difficult. Understanding and comprehension demand that you read groups of words, or ideas. As you read, you must analyze, think, group ideas and topics, spot relationships, and see similarities and differences in the passage. The word-by-word reader sees only the trees and misses the forest.

BACKTRACKING

Most readers backtrack occasionally. This technique is not only acceptable but also part of efficient reading. All of us look back and reread a word or several words now and then. The good reader, however, does it less frequently than the poor reader. The efficient reader basically looks back only when he needs to, whereas the slow reader does it mechanically and out of habit. The inefficient reader usually reads most words, phrases, sentences, and paragraphs more than once since he often misses the central idea or meaning the first time. The first time through, he has merely read the words and must therefore reread the selection to see how they are connected. The habit of reading single words rather than groups usually keeps you from grasping the central theme. Grouping words, sentences, and paragraphs as you go along allows you to make sense of the material and to focus on the theme and idea.

PAUSING AND STOPPING

Inefficient readers usually allow long and frequent pauses as they proceed. This not only hinders concentration but also makes it difficult to absorb the ideas presented. If you pause after reading only a few sentences, you lose track of the author's train of thought. You may remember certain details, but the connections get lost.

QUICK SKIMMING TO ELICIT THE GENERAL THEME

This technique involves reading rapidly and concentrating on the key words and phrases that develop and support the theme. One might think that in this approach, the main point could be missed; however, nothing could be further from the truth. This is purposeful reading for comprehension, since its object is to grasp the central point and carefully note the key elements that support that point.

Key Words That Announce Conditions and Should Be Kept in Focus!

1. again, also, accordingly, just as
2. therefore, thus, hence, henceforth
3. for example, for instance, in other words
4. nevertheless, however, notice, but
5. always, at all times, under all circumstances, every time
6. finally, in conclusion, in brief, at last
7. never, not, no, none
8. only, specifically, significantly, importantly, decidedly
9. first, another, and, likewise, as well as, besides
10. despite, although, regardless

How Is Material Usually Organized?

1. Most selections have a *central subject* (main idea) that could be used as the *title*. In many instances, the first sentence of a paragraph will tell you this main idea.
2. The material is usually presented in a fashion that answers a question, poses one, gives a solution, or gives a noncommittal statement of fact.
3. Key words and facts should substantiate and solidify the main idea of the reading. These are the details. Always look for key words. If you go back and read the key words, you should be able to get the essence of the passage.
4. The details are usually of two types. The main details are directly related to the central theme, and are used to develop it. The subordinate details break down and clarify the main details, to further develop the theme. Breaking the material down this way can help you to understand it.
5. Read in a questioning manner. This will ensure that you are actively involved. Ask *who*, *what*, *when*, and *where* to elicit key elements. Ask *how* and *why* to determine reasons.

Suggested Method for Efficient Analysis of Reading Material

1. Identify the topic or main theme, and highlight it with the cursor.
2. Find the main details about the topic, and highlight these also with the cursor.
3. The material not highlighted will be the subordinate details and the extraneous elements or qualifiers.
4. As you read, you will be thinking in terms of the relationship between central idea, key details that support the main idea, and those nonhighlighted minor details about the key details.

Don't go overboard! Focus on key elements only. This simple method will allow you to backtrack if needed, and will help you answer the questions at the end of a selection. Your information is now arranged to emphasize the interrelationships of facts. While you have read, you have been forced to think and organize the material. You have formed associations that will foster recall.

A PLAN FOR SELF-IMPROVEMENT

1. Set aside a time and place specifically for reading every day even if it is only 10 minutes. You know the conditions under which you function best. No one can set them for you.
2. Develop the habit of reading for ideas. After you have read a passage, ask yourself what the central theme was and verbalize it. The verbalization will quickly synthesize the material and draw upon relationships (similarities, differences) in the passage. The central idea will be not only highlighted but also substantiated and amplified by the highlighted key words and phrases. Picture yourself as a critic who is writing a review that will evaluate the material for a potential reader.
3. Read different material; become a versatile reader.
4. Keep a record of your progress and be optimistic. A positive attitude is half the battle. Don't be discouraged by plateaus; they are common.

The Do's and Don'ts

1. Even though *scientific* reading, unlike pleasure reading, often involves word-by-word reading, you should coordinate speed and thought processes, and you should read as fast as you think. Backtracking usually interferes with efficient assimilation and processing of information.
2. Even though close, word-by-word reading is slower and more tedious, eliminate irrelevant thoughts. You don't want them to intrude just because you believe you must have something to think about. Irrelevant thoughts make concentration impossible.
3. Usually, poor concentration will lead to poor comprehension, and unnecessarily slow reading can lead to poor concentration and poor comprehension. Read as rapidly as you can without losing comprehension. Adapt speed as necessary.
4. Don't hold back your thinking processes by unnecessarily slow reading. Do not create a gap between reading and thinking. In the same vein, do not stop and pause frequently since this also will allow gaps in your thinking to occur.
5. Remember, it's a poor reader who stops too often and pauses too long at each stop.
6. Apply the same concentration whether a selection is long or short.
7. Look for a general impression, main thoughts, and implications so that you may draw inferences. Read ideas rather than words. Identify your topics, the details about them, and the details about the details. Above all, don't fail to note the important ideas.
8. Whether you are the original writer or the reader of a selection, you must approach it with the thought of a distinct design and technique to present a specific subject matter and topic. Look for special effects and results.
9. You can usually identify the main topic of a paragraph by key words or phrases that could serve as possible titles. Concentrate on why certain words are used and how they are used. By concentrating on why and how, you can establish and follow the main idea. During your reading, you should realize that the paragraph is merely a sum of its parts. In turn, look at paragraphs as key elements in the development of the ideas of the passage. Don't let minor details or sentences overshadow paragraphs or the whole selection. Where there are paragraph headings, these usually lead you to main ideas.
10. Central thoughts are usually found in the lead sentence or in the summary sentence, but they may be located in other places and may, at times, be implied rather than stated. Read to understand by focusing on central ideas and units of thought.
11. Exhibit versatility, and adjust to the material. Don't use the same technique for all material; be pliable, adapt, use common sense.

12. Most of the material you confront will be familiar and understandable to you. Don't stick too closely to the particular selection; always associate present material with previous material. Nothing is ever completely new. In this context, you must focus on detail and read for specific comprehension and specific meanings to see what is new. Whether you read for general or specific ideas, use your previous knowledge. Read for meaning. Try to determine the meaning of unfamiliar words as you reason through a selection. Don't let an unfamiliar word stump you and worry you unduly; the context will often help you determine the meaning.

13. Do not decrease speed because of fear that you might miss something, and do not fall into the trap of reading each sentence twice before you proceed. Don't reread material unless necessary, but if you need to reread, do not hesitate to spend the time to clarify meaning.

14. Do not read each sentence as a distinct unit, but use each unit to build the paragraph and the selection to create the whole.

15. As you read a selection composed of several paragraphs, reflect whether succeeding paragraphs amplify the ideas or points raised in the preceding paragraphs or whether they provide an example or illustration of them. Is a qualifier of a point introduced, or is another aspect of the same subject considered?

16. Before you answer the whole battery of questions, quickly review your highlights to make sure you understood the point.

17. Under no circumstances should you get yourself involved more deeply than necessary with the reading selection and with the task. Don't read more into it than is there; answer the questions only on the basis of what is presented.

18. Be critical when you read; extract the important facts and see relationships and associations. Visualize descriptions accurately. Avoid misreading.

19. Avoid superficiality when you consider the selection. Don't come to a conclusion before you have read the whole passage and without sufficient thought. Don't jump to a conclusion.

PRACTICE READING EXERCISES

Exercise I

Identify the central theme or topic, details, and details about details.

Directions: Read the sample and highlight the topic, and the details about the topic. Do not highlight the details about the details.

EXAMPLE: Following the work of Chalmers and others, 831 geriatric and orthopedic patients in West London were reviewed for osteomalacia.

    (a) The topic deals with osteomalacia.
    (b) Details or key words are geriatric and orthopedic patients.
    (c) Details about details are 831 patients and West London.

> **Directions:** Read the sample paragraph and highlight the topic and the details about the topic.

EXAMPLE: Following the work of Chalmers and others, 831 geriatric and orthopedic patients in West London were reviewed for osteomalacia. History, relevant blood tests (calcium, phosphate, alkaline phosphatase, 24-hour urinary calcium) and radiology were assessed. Thirty-eight bone biopsies were performed. Thirty-three were positive (32 female, 1 male). Average age was 73.4 years. None had a history of gastric surgery. Twenty-eight were widows living alone. Three were sisters (spinsters) living together. Twenty-two lived on their own property. Average weekly income was $25.00. Average weekly food bill, $9.00 (mostly bread, canned meat, and canned fruit). The minimum for a balanced diet was thought to be $18.00. Average milk consumption was one pint per week. None of the patients cooked regularly. Twenty-six never cooked at all. None had sought the assistance of any of the welfare organizations, through either pride, ignorance, or apathy. All showed subjective and objective improvement following calcium and Vitamin D supplementation and dietary improvement.

Method: Following the work of Chalmers and others, 831 geriatric and orthopedic patients in West London were reviewed for osteomalacia. History, relevant blood tests (calcium, phosphate, alkaline phosphatase, 24-hour urinary calcium) and radiology were assessed. Thirty-eight bone biopsies were performed. Thirty-three were positive (32 female, 1 male). Average age was 73.4 years. None had a history of gastric surgery. Twenty-eight were widows living alone. Three were sisters (spinsters) living together. Twenty-two lived on their own property. Average weekly income was $25.00. Average weekly food bill, $9.00 (mostly bread, canned meat, and canned fruit). The minimum for a balanced diet was thought to be $18.00. Average milk consumption was one pint per week. None of the patients cooked regularly. Twenty-six never cooked at all. None had sought the assistance of any of the welfare organizations, through either pride, ignorance, or apathy. All showed subjective and objective improvement following calcium and Vitamin D supplementation and dietary improvement.

METHOD IN OUTLINE FORM

(a) The topic: osteomalacia

(b) Details or key words:

1. geriatric orthopedic patients
2. History, blood tests radiology bone biopsies
3. age milk consumption week
4. none cooked regularly none assistance
5. improvement calcium Vitamin D dietary

(c) Details about details:

1. 831
2. 33 positive
3. 73.4 years
4. twenty-eight widows
5. one pint
6. twenty-six never

(d) Extraneous material:

1. West London
2. 32 female
3. None gastric surgery
4. Twenty-two own property

Having used the highlighting technique, let us use this information to answer the type of questions used in the examination.

Directions: Choose the best answer.

---

1. Osteomalacia:

   (A) has a predilection for males.
   (B) occurs more frequently in females. —
   (C) can be diagnosed only by bone biopsy.
   (D) has a predilection for apartment dwellers.

2. The average weekly income did not allow these people to buy more food.

   (A) True
   (B) False
   (C) They needed to save for their old age.
   (D) They spend their money on the little luxuries of life.

3. From these data we may conclude that:

   (A) homeowners are more likely to develop osteomalacia than are renters.
   (B) spinsters will not develop osteomalacia if they live alone.
   (C) consumption of bread is a consistent factor in the development of osteomalacia.
   (D) there seems to be a correlation between an unbalanced diet, irregular meal consumption, and osteomalacia.

4. Given a greater income, these individuals would have:

   (A) eaten more nutritious meals.
   (B) cooked at least two meals a day.
   (C) spent a greater percentage of their income on food.
   (D) the passage does not give enough information to answer this question.

5. This study:

   (A) indicated that dietary supplementation is beneficial.
   (B) utilized every technique available.
   (C) utilized a great variety of patients.
   (D) showed that at least ten percent of the elderly suffer from osteomalacia.

Answers

1. Answer **(B)**

   Statement A: The numbers (32:1) clearly show that males are not prone to osteomalacia.

   Statement B: Explained above.

   Statement C: History, relevant blood tests, and radiological examination can be used to diagnose osteomalacia, as well as a bone biopsy.

   Statement D: Living in an apartment is not mentioned; however, the paragraph does mention that 22 of 33 lived on their own property.

2. Answer **(B)**

   Statement A: The average weekly income is stated as $25.00 and a minimum considered necessary for a balanced diet was $18.00.

   Statement B: Explained above.

   Statement C: These were elderly individuals and the issue of saving is not addressed.

   Statement D: The passage does not comment on the luxuries of life.

3. Answer **(D)**

   Statement A: There is no discussion of homeowners vs. renters in the passage as far as disease is concerned.

   Statement B: The paragraph does not differentiate between spinsters living alone or imply that widows are more prone to the disease because they might live alone.

   Statement C: Although bread was a high intake item, no relationship to the disease was implied.

   Statement D: An unbalanced diet and the irregular consumption of food are definite contributory factors.

4. Answer **(D)**

   Statement A: Income ($25.00) exceeded expenditures ($18.00) for a necessary balanced diet.

   Statement B: The passage states that most did not cook at all.

   Statement C: There is no issue of income and expenditure; income was adequate to live on a balanced diet.

   Statement D: This is the best answer since the passage truly does not discuss the issue of greater income and a person's spending habits.

5. Answer **(A)**

   Statement A: Improvement was noted after dietary supplementation.

   Statement B: Only three techniques were mentioned and no reference was made to limitations of techniques.

   Statement C: Only registered, orthopedic patients of West London were used; this is certainly not a great variety.

   Statement D: Of the 831 patients, 33 were diagnosed to have osteomalacia; this figure is not even 5 percent.

Exercise 2

Identify the central theme or topic, details, and details about details.

> **Directions:** Read the sample and highlight the topic, and the details about the topic. Do not highlight the details about the details.

EXAMPLE: James Berlin ends his discussion of "the New Rhetoric" with a list of four attitudes that work against social change.

    (a) The topic deals with attitudes that work against social change.
    (b) Details or key words are James Berlin, "the New Rhetoric."
    (c) Details about details are four.

EXAMPLE: James Berlin ends his discussion of "the New Rhetoric" with a list of four attitudes that work against social change. Reification occurs when the system is fortified by the attitude that nothing can ever be changed. Prescientific thinking trusts in luck or good fortune to bring about the needed social change, no action is necessary. Acceleration refers to the increasingly fast-paced, data-saturated lifestyle that keeps people from critically examining the world around them as they slip into a consumerist trance. Finally, mystification refers to responses to social ills based on racism, sexism, nationalism, or any form of bigotry. These four mentalities are roadblocks to progressive change, but they are roadblocks that can be dismantled with the dialectic of New Rhetoric.

    Students are told everywhere of the superior freedom that Americans enjoy yet they are ceaselessly faced with arbitrary authoritarian hierarchies which they must be empowered to examine and challenge. Berlin's "liberatory classroom" encourages self-autonomy and self-fulfillment in the students as they examine power structures and resist social influences that alienate and disempower. The development of this critical thinking process is worked out on paper in a nonhierarchical classroom where both student and teacher create the course together. The primary goal of this environment is to help students grow from being manipulated pawns to active, critical builders of an improving society. The best way to do this is to help them develop their rhetorical skills by examining these issues in writing.

Method: James Berlin ends his discussion of "the New Rhetoric" with a list of four attitudes that work against social change. Reification occurs when the system is fortified by the attitude that nothing can ever be changed. Prescientific thinking trusts in luck or good fortune to bring about the needed social change; no action is necessary. Acceleration refers to the increasingly fast-paced, data-saturated lifestyle that keeps people from critically examining the world around them as they slip into a consumerist trance. Finally, mystification refers to responses to social ills based on racism, sexism, nationalism, or any form of bigotry. These four mentalities are roadblocks to progressive change, but they are roadblocks that can be dismantled with the dialectic of New Rhetoric.

Students are told everywhere of the superior freedom that Americans enjoy yet they are ceaselessly faced with arbitrary authoritarian hierarchies which they must be empowered to examine and challenge. Berlin's "liberatory classroom" encourages self-autonomy and self-fulfillment in the students as they examine power structures and resist social influences that alienate and disempower. The development of this critical thinking process is worked out on paper in a nonhierarchical classroom where both student and teacher create the course together.

The primary goal of this environment is to help students grow from being manipulated pawns to active, critical builders of an improving society. The best way to do this is to help them develop their rhetorical skills by examining these issues in writing.

METHOD IN OUTLINE FORM

(a) The topic: attitudes that work against social change

(b) Details or key words:

1. James Berlin the "New Rhetoric"
2. Reification
3. Prescientific thinking
4. Acceleration
5. Mystification
6. roadblocks can be dismantled with dialectic of New Rhetoric
7. Students told of superior freedom Americans enjoy yet faced with arbitrary authoritarian hierarchies they must examine and challenge
8. "liberatory classroom" encourages self-autonomy and self-fulfillment examine power structures and resist social influences
9. critical thinking process on paper in nonhierarchical classroom student and teacher create the course together
10. goal to help students grow to active critical builders of improving society
11. develop rhetorical skills by examining issues in writing

(c) Details about details:

1. four
2. attitude that nothing can ever be changed
3. luck or good fortune, needed social change
4. fast-paced, data-saturated lifestyle keeps people from critically examining the world
5. responses to social ills
6. Berlin's
7. alienate and disempower
8. from being manipulated pawns

Having read the passage and used the highlighting technique, let us use this information to answer the type of questions used in the examination.

Directions: Choose the best answer.

---

1. Which of the following statements is neither supported nor contradicted by the information in the passage?

   (A) Students are told that Americans enjoy superior freedom.
   (B) The "liberatory classroom" is a nonhierarchical one in which the student and teacher create the course together.
   (C) An important component of the nonhierarchical classroom is the social hour in which members share ideas after the class is over.
   (D) The four attitudes that are roadblocks to social change can be dismantled by the dialectic of New Rhetoric.

2. According to the passage, which of the following concerning the four attitudes that work against social change is/are correct?

   (A) Prescientific thinking trusts that luck will bring about needed social change.
   (B) An increasingly fast-paced, data-saturated lifestyle keeps people from critically examining their world.
   (C) Both A and B are correct.
   (D) Neither A nor B is correct.

3. Concerning the creation of the nonhierarchical classroom, which of the following comes closest, according to the passage, to describing its purpose?

   (A) It allows students to see the teacher as a role model.
   (B) It is designed to help students grow into active members of a society that they are helping to improve.
   (C) It provides an environment where students can learn large amounts of information.
   (D) It will prepare students to become effective classroom teachers.

4. Concerning the role of the "New Rhetoric" regarding social change, which of the following is neither supported nor contradicted by the passage?

   (A) According to the passage, the "New Rhetoric" can dismantle the roadblocks to progressive change.
   (B) Part of the process involved in the "New Rhetoric," the passage implies, is to make students more socially aware, a process that involves the examining of issues and writing about them.
   (C) The passage indicates that the "New Rhetoric" approaches writing by having students revise drafts of their work-in-progress.
   (D) The "liberatory classroom," the passage implies, serves as a kind a laboratory for practicing the "New Rhetoric."

Answers

1. Answer **(C)**
Statement A: According to the first sentence of paragraph two, students are told that Americans enjoy superior freedom.
Statement B: The passage states that students and teachers create the course together in the "liberatory classroom," which is nonhierarchical.
Statement C: There is no mention of a social hour in connection with a nonhierarchical classroom.
Statement D: The final sentence of paragraph one asserts that the "roadblocks to social change can be dismantled with the dialectic of New Rhetoric."

2. Answer **(C)**
Statement A: According to sentence two of paragraph one, prescientific thinking places its trust in luck or good fortune.
Statement B: Under the rubric "acceleration," the passage asserts that our fast-paced, data-saturated lifestyle prevents people from critically examining the world around them.
Statement C: Since both A and B are correct according to the passage, C is the correct response.
Statement D: Refer to C above.

3. Answer **(B)**
   Statement A: One feature of a nonhierarchical classroom as it is described in the passage is to encourage self-autonomy and by implication to deemphasize the role of authority of the teacher. There is, in any case, no mention in the passage of the teacher as role model.
   Statement B: The next-to-last sentence in paragraph two identifies this as the "primary goal" of the "liberatory classroom."
   Statement C: This is not mentioned in the passage.
   Statement D: This is not mentioned in the passage.

4. Answer **(C)**
   Statement A: The passage does assert that roadblocks to social change can be dismantled with the dialectic of New Rhetoric.
   Statement B: A main goal of the "New Rhetoric" as it is explained throughout the passage is to raise the students' level of social awareness, and to make them "critical builders of an improving society." Part of the process is to have them examine "these issues in writing."
   Statement C: The passage does not address the processes involved in the actual writing, which might, indeed, include the production and revision of drafts. Since this is not included in the passage, C is correct.
   Statement D: Though no formal definition of "liberatory classroom" is given, the reader must infer from the details provided in paragraph two that it is, in fact, a kind of laboratory in which principles of the "New Rhetoric" are practiced. This is clearly a logical inference.

Exercise 3

Identify the central theme or topic, details, and details about details.

> **Directions:** Read the sample and highlight the topic, and the details about the topic. Do not highlight the details about the details.

EXAMPLE: Just about anyone you talk to nowadays complains about the cost of his automobile insurance. It's about time that someone came to the defense of the insurance companies.

   (a) The topic deals with automobile insurance.
   (b) Details or key words are complains cost defense companies.

> **Directions:** Read the sample and highlight the topic, and the details about the topic. Do not highlight the details about the details.

EXAMPLE: Just about anyone you talk to nowadays complains about the cost of his automobile insurance. It's about time that someone came to the defense of the insurance companies.

   We are all familiar with the effects of inflation, but most people forget that the insurance companies are affected too. An interesting point should be noted. Even though the total costs of producing a policy have been increasing because of increased salaries, paper cost, equipment replacement, etc., the insurance companies' expense ratios have been going down.

   If expenses are reduced, then why are premiums going up? Let's look at what makes up the rates that the insurance companies must charge. Automobile repair rates for labor have risen about 20 percent in the last year and a half. In addition, it has been shown that a new automobile costing $5000 would cost $20,000 if it were to be repaired with replacement parts (not including the engine). During this same period, a semiprivate hospital room has increased in cost over 22 percent and physicians' and surgeons' fees have increased 20 percent. Lawyers continue to ask for larger awards, and the courts are granting them. How can insurance companies continue to pay amounts inflated in this manner without reflecting the increase in their rates?

It is a real shame that the insurance companies don't make these facts known more widely to their customers. A widespread advertising campaign would help to explain their position and make it more tolerable when that next bill comes and has once again increased.

Method: Just about anyone you talk to nowadays complains about the cost of his automobile insurance. It's about time that someone came to the defense of the insurance companies.

We are all familiar with the effects of inflation, but most people forget that the insurance companies are affected too. An interesting point should be noted. Even though the total costs of producing a policy have been increasing because of increased salaries, paper cost, equipment replacement, etc. the insurance companies' expense ratios have been going down.

If expenses are reduced, then why are premiums going up? Let's look at what makes up the rates that the insurance companies must charge. Automobile repair rates for labor have risen about 20 percent in the last year and a half. In addition, it has been shown that a new automobile costing $5000 would cost $20,000 if it were to be repaired with replacement parts (not including the engine). During this same period, a semiprivate hospital room has increased in cost over 22 percent and physicians' and surgeons' fees have increased 20 percent. Lawyers continue to ask for large awards, and the courts are granting them. How can insurance companies continue to pay amounts inflated in this manner without reflecting the increase in their rates?

It is a real shame that the insurance companies don't make these facts known more widely to their customers. A widespread advertising campaign would help to explain their position and make it more tolerable when the next bill comes and has once again increased.

METHOD IN OUTLINE FORM

(a) The topic: automobile insurance

(b) Details or key words:

1. complains cost
2. defense companies
3. inflation policy increasing
4. expense ratios down
5. premiums up
6. repair risen replacement parts
7. hospital physicians increased
8. lawyers awards courts granting
9. advertising campaign tolerable next bill increased

(c) Details about details:

1. 20 percent
2. $5000, $20,000
3. 22 percent, 20 percent

Having read the passage and used the highlighting technique, let us use this information to answer the type of questions used in the examination.

Directions: Choose the best answer.

---

1. The main point of the passage is to

   (A) come to the aid of the insurance companies.
   (B) write your representatives to curb the rise of insurance rates.
   (C) start a widespread advertising campaign to curtail insurance costs.
   (D) imply that insurance premiums are based on many factors and are a complex issue.

2. Which of the following is contradicted by the passage?

   (A) Many people complain about their insurance rates.
   (B) Insurance companies' expense ratios are continuing to rise with inflation.
   (C) Insurance companies are affected by the inflationary features of the economy.
   (D) Salaries affect policy costs.

3. The main topic of the passage is

   (A) public awareness.
   (B) advertising strategy.
   (C) automobile insurance rates.
   (D) expense ratios.

4. Which of the following is supported by the passages?

   (A) A car repaired with replacement parts would cost four (4) times as much as a new car.
   (B) The public is fully aware of why their insurance premiums are increasing.
   (C) Insurance premiums have risen mainly because of larger awards in lawsuits.
   (D) Inflation has little effect on insurance rates.

5. Factor(s) affecting the overall pricing structure of rates could be considered as

   (A) paper costs.
   (B) equipment replacement.
   (C) hospitalization costs.
   (D) all of the above.

Answers

1. Answer **(D)**
   Statement A: No aid to insurance companies is advised, but it is suggested that the companies communicate to the public how rates are derived and what affects them.
   Statement B: No campaign is suggested that involves elected officials.
   Statement C: It is suggested that insurance companies explain their position on rates, but that certainly is not the main thread of the passage.
   Statement D: This is the best answer since it addresses the complex factors upon which rates are based.

2. Answer (**B**)

Statement A: The passage implies that a lot of people comment on the high cost of insurance.

Statement B: It clearly is stated in the passage that insurance companies' expense ratios have been dropping and so the statement is contradicted by the passage.

Statement C: The key element of the passage is that insurance companies, just like the public, are affected by many economic parameters.

Statement D: Salaries are mentioned as one factor playing a role in rate determination.

3. Answer (**C**)

Statement A: The point of public awareness concerning factors affecting premiums is expressed; however, the issue is more specific.

Statement B: Insurance companies are advised to inform the public about rate determinants, but that certainly is not the key element or topic.

Statement C: Rates and what affects the rates and their impact on the public generally are addressed.

Statement D: Expense ratios were commented on specifically and were made the key issue.

4. Answer (**A**)

Statement A: The passage mentions that a car costing $5000 new would cost $20,000 if it were repaired with replacement parts.

Statement B: Although public awareness is an issue, the passage neither implies nor states the level of awareness.

Statement C: Awards due to legal procedures are clearly only one factor of this complex issue.

Statement D: Inflation is an important factor and greatly influences the rate structure.

5. Answer (**D**)

The passage clearly identifies paper costs, equipment replacement costs, and hospitalization costs as factors that affect premiums.

Exercise 4

Identify the central theme or topic, details, and details about details.

Directions: Read the sample and highlight the topic, and the details about the topic. Do not highlight the details about the details.

EXAMPLE: Anthropologists call such ceremonies as weddings, funerals, and bar mitzvahs, "rites of passage."

(a) The topic deals with ceremonies "rites of passage."
(b) Details of key words are weddings funerals bar mitzvahs.
(c) Details about details are Anthropologists.

EXAMPLE: Anthropologists call such ceremonies as weddings, funerals, and bar mitzvahs, "rites of passage." They are crucial to us as human beings, and in every culture they evolve to mark those crucial and critical times when our individual communal lives go through events that are both difficult and dangerous: death, life, union, separation. They are necessary features of our various traditions and cultures, crucially important in making our cultures what they are. Polish Catholic weddings and Irish Catholic funerals are famously important in defining what those two traditions truly are, and the baptisms and funerals of Protestant African Americans are just as crucial in defining those traditions. When we participate in and with those events as experienced by our neighbors and friends, we both add something and get something. We add our respect for the difference that makes our neighbor special, and we get a renewed respect for our own traditions and for what makes them unique.

Method: Anthropologists call such ceremonies as weddings, funerals, and bar mitzvahs, "rites of passage." They are crucial to us as human beings, and in every culture they evolve to mark those crucial and critical times when our individual communal lives go through events that are both difficult and dangerous: death, life, union, separation. They are necessary features of our various traditions and cultures, crucially important in making our cultures what they are. Polish Catholic weddings and Irish Catholic funerals are famously important in defining what those two traditions truly are, and the baptisms and funerals of Protestant African Americans are just as crucial in defining those traditions. When we participate in and with those events as experienced by our neighbors and friends, we both add something and get something. We add our respect for the difference that makes our neighbor special, and we get a renewed respect for our own traditions and for what makes them unique.

METHOD IN OUTLINE FORM

(a) Topic: ceremonies, "rites of passage"

(b) Details or key words:

1. weddings, funerals, bar mitzvahs
2. crucial to human beings
3. mark crucial and critical times
4. necessary features of various traditions
5. crucially important in making cultures
6. we participate in events experienced by neighbors friends
7. we add respect for difference
8. get renewed respect for own traditions unique

(c) Details about details:

1. Anthropologists
2. death, life, union, separation
3. Polish Catholic weddings, Irish Catholic funerals, defining traditions
4. Protestant African Americans, traditions
5. neighbors and friends, traditions unique

Having read and used the highlighting technique let us use this information to answer the type of questions used in the examination.

Directions: Choose the best answer.

---

1. This passage implies that

    (A) rituals in cultures different from our own are often so complex that we should not try to participate in them.

    (B) virtually any communal ceremony, whether a wedding, funeral, or bar mitzvah, would qualify to anthropologists as a "rite of passage."

    (C) rituals in the modern world have become so diluted that they rarely have the substance of the original rite.

    (D) Irish Catholics would probably not welcome Polish Catholics at their wedding ceremonies.

2. Which of the following is contradicted by the information in the passage?

    (A) Rites of passage in various traditions and cultures are interesting to observers because they are often colorful, but they rarely actually make the culture what it is.

    (B) Union and death are two events that might qualify as events marked by communal ceremonies.

    (C) Baptism in Baptist churches involves immersion, whereas Presbyterian baptism requires only the sprinkling of water.

    (D) Food is usually a major component of communal rituals.

3. According to the passage, what is one by-product of our participating in important events of our friends and neighbors, particularly when these events originate in traditions different from our own?

    (A) We come to realize that our own traditions are usually more appealing than those of diverse cultures.

    (B) We learn to deal with the discomfort that often accompanies new experiences.

    (C) We both add our respect for them, and gain renewed respect for the uniqueness of our own rituals.

    (D) We can often pick up bits and pieces of other languages by participating in rituals of those whose language differs from our own.

4. A Protestant christening ceremony is one of those "rites of passage" referred to in the passage that serve to mark an important event in our culture.

    (A) This particular ritual, though not mentioned specifically in the passage, would qualify as one of those "rites of passage."

    (B) Protestant christening ceremonies are mentioned in the passage, but they do not qualify as "rites of passage."

    (C) There is not enough information provided by the passage to allow the reader to conclude that the ceremony mentioned would qualify as a "rite of passage."

    (D) The statement is contradicted by the passage.

Answers

1. Answer **(B)**

   Statement A: Although rituals in cultures different from our own culture may seem, or actually be, more complex than rituals with which we are quite familiar, the passage does not deal with these complexities; instead it suggests that we should participate in rituals that are a part of cultures different from our own.

   Statement B: The passage clearly states in the first sentence that anthropologists include the ceremonies mentioned in this response as "rites of passage."

   Statement C: Though many rituals have, no doubt, become diluted in the modern world, this passage does not address this issue overtly or implicitly.

   Statement D: The passage mentions Irish Catholic weddings and Polish Catholic weddings to make a point about famously defining rituals, but nowhere does it indicate who would welcome whom at a wedding ceremony.

2. Answer **(A)**

   Statement A: The passage clearly states that rites of passage do, in fact, make the culture what it is. This response is therefore clearly contradicted by the passage.

   Statement B: Union and death are referred to in sentence two as among those events that mark crucial times in communal lives.

   Statement C: The difference between Baptist and Presbyterian baptismal rites is not discussed in the passage, which therefore neither confirms nor contradicts the information in this response.

   Statement D: Specific components of various communal rituals are not mentioned in the passage. The presence or absence of food in rituals is neither contradicted nor confirmed.

3. Answer **(C)**

   Perhaps the main point of the passage is to suggest that we both give respect to a culture different from our own by participating in its rituals, and gain an appreciation for what is unique in our own rituals from our participation. Responses A, B, and D are not mentioned in the passage.

4. Answer **(A)**

   Statement A: Protestant christening ceremonies are not named specifically in the passage. However, they fit the implied definition provided in sentence one, and they fit the spirit of the definition extended through the passage for a defining cultural ritual.

   Statement B: In fact Protestant christening ceremonies are not mentioned specifically in the passage in any context, and they do, in fact, fit the implied definition of a "rite of passage" developed in the passage.

   Statement C: See explanation of statement A, which indicates that the passage supports the inference that a Protestant christening ceremony is a "rite of passage."

   Statement D: The passage does not deal with the issue explicitly and does not contradict it by implication.

Exercise 5

Identify the central theme or topic, details, and details about details.

> **Directions:** Read the sample and highlight the topic, and the details about the topic. Do not highlight the details about the details.

EXAMPLE: In the first half of the 1600s, during the British Civil War, ten Puritan families, Roundheads as their critics called them, came up from Virginia to Maryland, where religious diversity was more greatly tolerated, and established Providence, the original settlement on the Severn River.

(a) The topic deals with the original settlement on the Severn River.
(b) Details or key words are Puritan families came to Maryland, religious diversity tolerated, established Providence.
(c) Details about details are Roundheads from Virginia.

> **Directions:** Read the sample selection and highlight the topic and the details about the topic. Do not highlight the details about the details.

EXAMPLE: In the first half of the 1600s, during the British Civil War, ten Puritan families, Roundheads as their critics called them, came up from Virginia to Maryland, where religious diversity was more greatly tolerated, and established Providence, the original settlement on the Severn River. In 1650 Providence was "erected" into a county named Annarundell after the wife of Cecil Calvert, Lord Baltimore, the Lady Anne Arundel. Annapolis, also on the Severn River and named after Lord Baltimore's wife, was originally Anne Arundel Town, a small town but one of the new country's most important because of its extensive population of impressive lawyers, Francis Scott Key and William Pinkney to name two, and because it was the site of one of the country's earliest colleges, St. John's College, chartered in 1784 and opened in the fall of 1789. From early settlement on, the Chesapeake never went untouched by the many wars England involved herself in, but the Severn, unlike some of its sister rivers, remained mostly uninvolved, perhaps because it led to no important harbors, perhaps because its banks gave no rapid access to cities. Its role has been mostly to provide homes and spawning and nesting grounds for the rich web of plant and animal life. The river has long been a sanctuary, an estuary yawning wide into the Chesapeake where Annapolis reigns and the waters are salt.

Method: In the first half of the 1600s, during the British Civil War, ten Puritan families, Roundheads as their critics called them, came up from Virginia to Maryland, where religious diversity was more greatly tolerated, and established Providence, the original settlement on the Severn River. In 1650 Providence was "erected" into a county named Annarundell after the wife of Cecil Calvert, Lord Baltimore, the Lady Anne Arundel. Annapolis, also on the Severn River and named after Lord Baltimore's wife, was originally Anne Arundel Town, a small town but one of the new country's most important because of its extensive population of impressive lawyers, Francis Scott Key and William Pinkney to name two, and because it was the site of one of the country's earliest colleges, St. John's College, chartered in 1784 and opened in the fall of 1789. From early settlement on, the Chesapeake never went untouched by the many wars England involved herself in, but the Severn, unlike some of its sister rivers, remained mostly uninvolved, perhaps because it led to no important harbors, perhaps because its banks gave no rapid access to cities. Its role has been mostly to provide homes and spawning and nesting grounds for the rich web of plant and animal life. The river has long been a sanctuary, an estuary yawning wide into the Chesapeake where Annapolis reigns and the waters are salt.

METHOD IN OUTLINE FORM

(a) Topic: original settlement on the Severn River

(b) Details or key words:

1. Puritan families came to Maryland, religious diversity tolerated, established Providence
2. Providence "erected" into county named Annarundell after wife of Lord Baltimore, Lady Anne Arundel
3. Annapolis originally Anne Arundel Town, small town but important because of impressive lawyers and one of country's earliest colleges
4. Chesapeake never untouched by wars but Severn mostly uninvolved no important harbors, no rapid access to cities
5. role to provide homes and spawning and nesting grounds for plant and animal life
6. river a sanctuary where Annapolis reigns and waters salt

(c) Details about details:

1. Roundheads from Virginia
2. Annapolis, on Severn River, named after Lord Baltimore's wife
3. Francis Scott Key, William Pinkney
4. St. John's College
5. England involved in

Having read the passage and used the highlighting technique, let us use this information to answer the type of questions used in the examination.

Directions: Choose the best answer.

---

1. Concerning the original settlement on the Severn River,

    (A) one can assume that it was formed by Virginians who were attempting to escape higher taxes.
    (B) it is clear that those who made it were searching for fertile land and abundant wildlife.
    (C) it appears from the passage that it was formed by people in search of greater religious freedom.
    (D) the passage indicates that its inhabitants shared no particular religious or political beliefs.

2. The passage suggests that Annapolis was

    (A) almost from the beginning a heavily populated port.
    (B) in its early years an important small town, known for its impressive lawyers and one of the country's earliest colleges.
    (C) not especially important until the establishment of the Naval Academy.
    (D) a summer retreat for wealthy families from Baltimore.

3. Which of the following statement(s) is/are contradicted by the passage?

    (A) Puritans are also referred to as Roundheads.
    (B) Settlements along the Severn River generally remained uninvolved in wars in which England was involved.
    (C) St. John's College is one of the country's oldest colleges.
    (D) Anne Arundel was a sister of Cecil Calvert, Lord Baltimore.

4. Which of the following is neither supported nor contradicted by the passage?

    (A) Many inhabitants of settlements on the banks of the Severn traditionally earned their living from oystering and fishing.
    (B) Annapolis attracted some of the country's most impressive lawyers, among them Francis Scott Key and William Pinkney.
    (C) The earliest settlement on the Severn was called Providence.
    (D) The Severn River provided no rapid access to cities.

5. What body of water, according to the passage, does the Severn River lead into?

    (A) The Potomac River
    (B) The Atlantic Ocean
    (C) The Rappahannock River
    (D) The Chesapeake Bay

Answers

1. Answer **(C)**

    Statement A: There is no mention of taxes either in Virginia or Maryland in the passage.

    Statement B: Though it is implied that the land on the banks of the Severn is fertile and that the wildlife is abundant, there is no suggestion in the passage that this played a role in the settlement of the land.

    Statement C: The passage does, in fact, indicate that the tolerance of religious diversity, in effect greater religious freedom, was the main reason that early settlers moved from Virginia to Maryland.

    Statement D: This is contradicted by the fact that the original ten families who first settled Providence were Puritans, and they were therefore united by their shared religious beliefs.

2. Answer **(B)**

    Statement A: This statement is contradicted by the passage.

    Statement B: This passage indicated in its third sentence that Annapolis was small, that it was known for its impressive lawyers, and that is was the site of one of the country's earliest colleges.

    Statement C: The Naval Academy is not mentioned in the passage.

    Statement D: There is no reference to wealthy families from Baltimore in the passage.

3. Answer **(D)**

    Statement A: Sentence one indicates that Puritans were known as Roundheads by their critics.

    Statement B: The passage notes specifically that the Severn, unlike some of its sister rivers, was "mostly uninvolved" in England's many wars.

    Statement C: St. John's College, chartered in 1784, is identified in the passage as one of America's oldest colleges.

    Statement D: The Lady Anne Arundel is identified in the passage as the wife of Lord Baltimore, not as his sister; the passage, therefore, contradicts this statement.

4. Answer **(A)**

    Statement A: There is no suggestion in the passage that people along the Severn made or make money fishing and oystering. All three of the remaining statements appear in the passage.

5. Answer **(D)**

    Statement A: It is not mentioned in the passage.
    Statement B: It is not mentioned in the passage.
    Statement C: It is not mentioned in the passage.
    Statement D: The Chesapeake Bay is the only body of water other than the Severn River mentioned in the passage, and the Severn is described as "yawning wide into the Chesapeake."

Writing the Essay

Since 1985, the Association of American Medical Colleges (AAMC) has been trial-testing an essay topic on the MCAT. This project was in response to a study about the professional preparation of the physician. The 1989 administrations of the MCAT included 60 minutes for the writing of two essays. In 1991 the writing sample (WS) became a permanent part of the MCAT. The writing of the essay on the new computer-based MCAT differs from that of the paper-based form only in that the essay is composed on-screen rather than on paper. You will be able, within the writing sample response screen, to edit and to move text by cutting and pasting. At the present time, there is no spell-check function for the writing of the essay.

Medical school faculties have long felt that writing skills are essential for a physician. Many have expressed the opinion that present-day students are somewhat weak in these skills. The goal of the writing sample is to see if the student has the ability and skill to write under standardized conditions. The students should be able to:

1. develop a central theme
2. synthesize material
3. separate major from minor issues
4. propose alternative solutions
5. present a theme in a flowing and logical manner
6. write in correct English, timed, at a first-draft composition level

The AAMC suggests that the best way for students to prepare generally for writing the essays in the Writing Sample part of the MCAT is to take courses in composition or expository writing, which will raise their awareness of the components of a well-written essay. Classes in all disciplines that contain an intensive writing component can also be helpful. Clearly, students should familiarize themselves with the topics that have been subjects for previous MCAT examination essays as well as the standard response format that is typically indicated by the MCAT essay prompts. This introductory section and the practice test essay that follow address both of these areas. The topics for the essays in the Writing Sample will not attempt to gauge the student's knowledge in the subject areas of physics, biology, or chemistry, nor will they deal with the student's reasons for wishing to pursue a career in medicine.

SCORING METHOD

All essays will be scored by an experienced group of readers. A minimum of four readers will rate each essay on a six-point scale, two readers for the first essay and two different readers for the second. For reporting purposes, the scores will be averaged and converted to an alphabetical score, with the scale ranging from J to T.

An essay that *exhibits* the major characteristics of logical analysis and presentation would fall in the range from J to Q, with J representing a percentile score between 0–8 and Q representing a range of 54–65. Essays in the Q and above range clearly should display a *grasp* of the material under discussion. The T range will represent the 91–100 percentile. Papers falling into this range definitely must *demonstrate* facets essential to good writing such as purpose, goal, and conviction.

Medical schools will receive the alphabetical score, but may also obtain writing samples. Both the examinee and the schools will receive percentile data, score distribution characteristics, and confidence bands.

CHARACTERISTICS OF GOOD WRITING

E. B. White, one of America's finest writers, once observed that there is "no infallible guide to good writing." There are, however, some principles of good writing that can be learned and that, when learned, can improve virtually everyone's writing. A first requirement is that one find something of interest, preferably something original, to say about the subject at hand. Having satisfied the first requirement, the writer's second goal is to communicate his or her ideas with absolute clarity. To communicate clearly in an essay of the kind required on the MCAT one must focus on the three major components of written communication: (1) unity and coherence, (2) support of the main idea with concrete details and examples, and (3) mechanical concerns.

Unity in an essay results from having a sharply focused central idea, often referred to as a thesis. This thesis typically includes the subject about which one is writing and a predicate, which consists of the major point or points that the writer is making about the subject. The body of the essay will develop this thesis in detail, and the essay will have unity or lack of it to the degree that the writer maintains focus on the central idea. If, for example, the thesis of an essay is that justice (the subject) is blind (the predicate), the essay will be unified in direct proportion to the skill with which the writer maintains focus on this thesis—in other words, the success he or she has in avoiding excursions into subjects unrelated, or related only tangentially, to the main idea.

Closely related to unity in an essay is coherence, which refers to the integration of the various parts. When ideas in a composition flow smoothly from one idea to another and thus create the sense that each idea follows logically from the one preceding it, the essay is said to have coherence. A primary way that one achieves coherence is by using transitional words and phrases such as "moreover," "however," "therefore," "in other words," and "for example." In a good essay each sentence flows smoothly into the next, and each paragraph grows logically from the one that precedes it.

If an essay, therefore, contains those ingredients mentioned above—unity, typically resulting from a thoughtful, original thesis that runs through the essay much the way the spinal column runs through the body, and coherence, which results from the use of devices that hold sentence to sentence and paragraph to paragraph, much the way glue holds clippings on the page of a scrapbook—it will very likely be a good, strong essay. To make a good essay better and a very good one excellent requires attention to the two remaining aspects of written communication: (1) supporting, concrete details and examples, and (2) mechanics. For an essay to convey a sense of authority, general or abstract statements must be anchored in specific details. If one asserts, for example, that the American dollar is strong in the world market, he or she might observe that it is worth $1.30 in Canada. Or if one is writing about the dangers of horseback riding and jumping, he or she might cite the paralysis from the neck down of the experienced equestrian Christopher Reeve.

The final area for concern for this discussion is mechanics, which covers such things as grammar, spelling, and punctuation. Because many mechanical errors result from carelessness, all writers should proofread as carefully as time permits. There is little disagreement among writing teachers as to the importance of revision, but in a timed essay such as that on the MCAT, there will be a minimum amount of time to devote to revision. You should, however, proofread your essay at least once, looking for such things as misspellings, faulty punctuation, and subject–verb disagreement.

PREPARING FOR THE MCAT ESSAY

Although the specific essay questions for the MCAT change from test to test, the general type of question remains the same. By becoming acquainted with the format of the kind of questions that have been asked in the past, you can better prepare yourself to deal with whatever specific question you get on your examination. Typically the question begins with a directive to write a *unified* essay in response to the question that follows. You are then given a statement, usually one that could be characterized as an aphorism, which is an assertion that has the ring of truth. You are then asked to explain what you think the statement means, after which you are to describe a circumstance in which the statement might not be true. Finally, in what is probably the central part of your essay, you are to discuss the conditions that must prevail in order for the statement to be considered true.

There are several underlying principles involved in this kind of question. The first is the principle of unity, referred to in the general discussion of good writing on page 364, and discussed below in the section on specific ways in which you can unify your response to the MCAT question itself. The second principle involves your ability to explain clearly what a statement means. Keep in mind that explanation involves a straightforward amplification of the statement, and it will often require that you clarify terms or stipulate definitions of words that might be open to interpretation. Explanation does not require you to analyze (to address questions of "why" the statement says what it says); that will come later in the discussion section of your essay. A third principle is a bit more subtle. You are asked to describe a situation in which the given statement may not be true. Although this may appear to be an oblique way of approaching an actual discussion of the statement's truth, it is based on the principle that we often understand what something *is* by understanding, first, what it is not. In this case it is a call to consider the truth of a statement by understanding the conditions under which it is *not* true. This is actually a very useful exercise, and rather than seeing it as a hurdle to cross before you begin your discussion, take advantage of the opportunity afforded by this part to open your mind to the reality that the truth of any statement is dependent, to a certain extent, on the circumstances surrounding it.

The final part of the question, which calls on you to discuss the circumstances in which the statement *is* true, is asking you to rigorously analyze the statement by presenting conditions that appear to confirm its essential truth. The key concept here is "analysis." The question may not use the word "analyze" as a stated directive, but keep in mind the principle that when you are asked to discuss, often you are actually being asked to analyze. Analysis can use the rhetorical modes mentioned above, such as definition, description, and explanation; but analysis uses these modes finally to communicate to the reader *why* something is as it is. In what will probably be a part of your strategy in the essay, you may go a step beyond analysis into persuasion, which is the use of analysis to convince the reader that your central thesis is correct. Unless you find yourself in violent disagreement with the statement presented in the question, however, the persuasive component of your essay will be what could be referred to as "soft sell." Though there are occasions in writing when strong persuasion is called for, it is not a good idea to allow your essay for the MCAT to be dominated by an argumentative tone, if for no other reason than that the question itself begs for an objective, open-minded, and carefully reasoned response.

With the general principles discussed above in mind, examine them in the following question, which resembles the questions given before on the essay part of the MCAT:

Consider This Statement

All that is necessary for the triumph of evil is that good men do nothing.

Write a unified essay in which you perform the following tasks. Explain what you think the above statement means. Describe a specific situation in which good men were, in fact, doing something, but evil triumphed nonetheless. Discuss what you think determines when the triumph of evil is dependent on the fact that good men are doing nothing.

Explain What the Statement Means

Clearly in order to explain what the statement in question means you should stipulate possible definitions for "evil" and for "good men," both of which are open to interpretation. You might, for example, equate evil with forces that bring about destruction—of life, of liberty, and of those virtues that have traditionally been held sacred in our society. Good men, in this context, would be those who believe in these virtues. The statement itself seems to rest on an unspoken acceptance among most people of these stipulated definitions. With the meaning of the key terms of this statement now understood, you could explain that the statement means that when good men—those who hold those values that promote the survival and well-being of human beings—do not actively protect those values, destructive human impulses will subvert the human race. In short, the statement is a strong warning against apathy to those who value life, liberty, and the pursuit of happiness. The strong warning comes in the form of an all-or-nothing plea: if well-meaning individuals do nothing to resist destructive forces, they will lose all; evil will triumph in spite of the good intentions of those individuals.

When Might the Statement NOT Be True?

The second part of the question asks you to describe a situation in which good men were doing something (i.e., not doing "nothing") and yet evil triumphed nonetheless. Many illustrations of such a conceivable circumstance will come to your mind. In war-torn countries where invaders are attempting to overthrow the existing order, perhaps an order in which peaceful citizens were coexisting and enjoying life, the revolutionists may simply outnumber those who wish to uphold the status quo. These latter "good men" may, in fact, risk their lives fighting for the principles in which they believe; but "evil," in the form of the invaders, could triumph in spite of their efforts. One could also imagine a situation in which the balance between forces of good and those of evil is delicate. In such a situation, some natural disaster such as an earthquake could destabilize conditions; the evil forces could take advantage of the chaos and upset the delicate balance in favor of evil. Imagine, for example, a largely peaceful town in which order prevails. An earthquake strikes the town, and looters take over privately owned businesses and appropriate money and goods, perhaps including guns and ammunition, that belong to good people. This might enable chaos, or evil, to triumph over good. The weakness of an all-or-none statement like the one with which you are concerned is that there are exceptions to virtually every rule, and with a little imagination you are certain to discover some of these exceptions. In this case, all that you would need to do is to find a circumstance in which good men are not doing enough. They may be doing *something*, but it simply may not be sufficient. If you establish such a circumstance, you have found a flaw in the statement that *all* that is necessary for the triumph of evil is that good men do nothing.

Circumstances Where the Statement IS True

The final part of the question asks you to discuss what you think determines when all that is necessary for the triumph of evil is that good men do nothing. Here, for the sake of unity and coherence, you should find a transition that acknowledges that in spite of the exceptions described above, the statement contains a strong element of truth. You might acknowledge that all-or-none statements like the one in question typically are employed to jar the reader into considering a worst-case scenario. You are then in a position to discuss the statement in terms of its implications or of the essential truth conveyed by the spirit of the statement. The main section of your essay, therefore, will be concerned with the consequences of apathy. What happens when people do not actively promote the values in which they believe? You could begin with the institution of the family and argue that well-meaning parents, in failing to be an active part of their children's lives, leave children vulnerable to influences that they may be unable to deal with effectively. Life and literature are full of examples that support this point, and you should cite some of these examples. Joyce Carol Oates's story, "Where Are You Going, Where Have You Been?" tells of a young girl whose parents ask their daughter superficial questions, but they fail to become involved in a meaningful way in her life. She seeks attention from casual strangers and ultimately winds up being lured from her home by the diabolical villain ironically named Arnold Friend. You could next move to examples involving social issues or conditions within our country and then within the world in which "good men" are doing little to actively promote peace or to preserve our environment. Good men and women were simply not doing enough in Dunblane, Scotland, to prevent the senseless murder of innocent schoolchildren by a deranged sociopath some time ago. By all accounts the village is filled with good, peace-loving men and women. But there was also ample evidence that the man who opened fire on the children was known to be a potential threat. One must ask if these good people so took their peaceful lives for granted that they failed to act and, through their apathy, left open the gate, if not for the triumph of evil, then at least for its intrusion into their lives.

Remember that the question will call for a unified essay in which you are to perform several tasks. The simplest way to unify your essay is to construct an introductory paragraph in which you blueprint your essay and state your main idea or thesis. This will be helpful both for the reader and for yourself. In the time allotted you will probably be able to write an essay of approximately 500 words or less. This means that you will likely have no more than four or five well-developed paragraphs. Use transitions between paragraphs to alert the reader to the fact that you are moving on to another topic, and then be sure that you link each topic of each paragraph to the main idea in the introductory paragraph. There are, of course, many subtler ways of unifying an essay and of giving it coherence. But on this essay you will be pressed for time and will have less time to formulate elaborate rhetorical strategies. Organizing the essay around a thesis and presenting a blueprint in the introductory paragraph will help assure the essay's unity, and it will help guarantee that you do not neglect any aspect of the question. Remember, your essay will be scored as a draft. You can go back and polish it if time permits, but the most important ingredients are: (1) the quality of the essay's ideas; (2) the unity and coherence of the various parts; and (3) the appropriateness of supporting examples.

Two final questions often arise when students are preparing for the MCAT essay: one is that of whether or not to outline the essay before writing it; the other is whether or not there is a need for a concluding paragraph. The fact is that it is virtually always helpful to outline an essay, and it is usually hazardous not to do so. Writers compose in different ways, and they outline in different ways. Some require a comprehensive outline with details, and details about details enumerated; others need only a skeletal outline including only the main topics. Your purpose in writing this essay is to produce a final product that is organized and unified, which is precisely what an outline helps guarantee that you will do. Keep in mind the method of outlining that has worked best for you in the past, and use it for this essay. If you have not outlined your essays before writing them in the past, learn to do so now. Practice picking the main points that you would cover for the sample essay topics below, and jot them down on the scratch paper provided, experimenting with various levels of detail that will be helpful for you to include. You can, of course, outline your essay in your head if this method works best for you.

As for the matter of a concluding paragraph for your essay, there is disagreement among experts on this subject. The traditional viewpoint is that a final paragraph which restates your main ideas and finally opens the subject for more general application can be desirable. Another viewpoint is that if you have fully and clearly explored your subject in the essay, a formal conclusion is redundant. You should be guided in your MCAT essay by two factors. The first of these is time: if you are pressed for time, the concluding paragraph is the most dispensable part of the essay. The second factor has to do with your own perception of how well you have presented your points in the rest of the essay. If, after rereading your essay, you sense that the organization has been weak, try to strengthen it with a conclusion that summarizes and restates your main points. If you decide that you do not have time for, or do not need, a concluding paragraph, at least clinch your essay with a strong sentence, one that brings it to closure. The endpoint of each unit of writing—a sentence, a paragraph, or an entire essay—is strategically the most emphatic point of that unit. You want to leave the reader of your MCAT essay with the sense that you have squarely confronted the issues raised by the question.

SAMPLE ESSAYS

The following two topics, essays, and analyses (from Practice Tests A and B) may be helpful to you in considering what constitutes a superb Writing Sample essay.

Consider This Statement

It is no wise man that will quit a certainty for an uncertainty.

Samuel Johnson

Write a unified essay in which you perform the following tasks. Explain what you think the above statement means. Describe a specific situation in which a wise person would quit a certainty for an uncertainty. Discuss the circumstances that you think determine whether or not one should or should not give up certainty for uncertainty.

Writing Sample Essay

A wise person, according to Johnson, is one who knows that dreams and hopes are no substitute for reality. Though it may not always be pleasant or exciting to know what the next day will bring, there is no wisdom in reaching out for something exciting or pleasant when one cannot be sure that it is there. A realist has more hope to find happiness if he takes his reality and alters it than one who casts about in the dark hoping to find a pot of gold. A person may take his last dollar and buy a lottery ticket, hoping to win a jackpot, but the wise individual will take his last dollar and use it to buy food. Though the foolish person may think that because he is desperate, good, and deserving and that God or fate will intervene on his behalf, the wise one knows that fate and God will do little to even the odds. The wise person knows he needs food more than he needs a one-in-seven-million chance of becoming rich.

But what courage does it take to face each day that is the same as the last? Is it wise to keep one's feet firmly planted on the ground, taking no risks? To stay with what is certain out of fear of the unknown is certainly safe, but it may be unwise. Imagine a shoe retailer is approached by a partner who has developed a new last and leather that will make women's shoes more comfortable to wear, but they will appear just as stylish. The partner asks the store owner to place the new shoes in his front window, and for this favor the two will share whatever profits come from the venture in half. The shoe salesperson refuses, knowing that the shoes he has shown in his window for the last five years have brought in a steady stream of customers. Though he is not getting rich, at least he is certain that his current display works. The partner sets off to find another store owner, discovering one only three doors down from the first shop he visited. The second owner takes the risk, for he knows that nothing great is achieved without some peril. For days the first shoe salesperson sees streams of people walking by his store, and wondering where they are going, peeks outside to see them entering his competitor's shop. Word has spread, and even the first shop-keeper's regular male customers desert him for the shop down the street. Though women buy the new shoes for themselves, men pick them up for their wives; and while they are in the shop, they find it convenient to buy their own shoes there, too. The first shopkeeper goes out of business, blaming himself for not having the wisdom to have faith in a good, albeit unproved, idea.

Had the shopkeeper been wiser, perhaps what he would have seen was that this was not a matter of uncertainty. It is possible that had he been thinking, he would have recognized that it was a certainty that women would want to wear a more comfortable shoe, and that though it seemed new and risky to stock the new shoes, there was no risk involved at all. The wisdom is not in an unwill-ingness to make a change, it is in the unwillingness to make a change without considering the realistic possibilities of it. The chances involved in buying a lottery ticket make it such an impossible odd that the wise individual will reject the notion of spending his last dollar on it. The chances that women will prefer comfortable and stylish shoes over uncomfortable and stylish shoes, however, is not a chance at all. It is reasonable to assume that given the choice between discomfort and comfort the customer will choose comfort. A wise person knows a certainty when he sees it, and he knows that sometimes what appears to be a risk is not a risk at all. By the same token, a wise person knows when a safe offer is really a risk, and no matter how often he says, "I need this money, surely fate will let me have it. It is only fair that one who is as deserv-ing as I should win" will not change the odds in a lottery. So the wise individ-ual is indeed one who will not quit certainty for uncertainty, but it is the same wise individual who knows the difference.

Explanation of Response: 6

This essay focuses clearly on Johnson's statement and addresses each of the three writing tasks. Paragraph one explains what the statement means and gives a specific situation in which one would not be wise to give up a certainty for an uncertainty. Paragraphs two and three explore cir-cumstances that determine whether it is wise or unwise to give up a certainty for an uncertainty.

The paper provides an explanation of the quotation by introducing "reality" as a qualifier for "certainty" and "dreams and hopes" for "uncertainty." This allows the author to cite concrete examples like the one that refers to the lottery to complete the explanation by referring to real-istic and unrealistic acts. Through an effective example in paragraph two, the paper illustrates that safety, contrary to the implication of the quotation, may sometimes be unwise, as the first owner discovers. Finally the passage provides a balanced analysis of the things that determine whether quitting certainty for uncertainty is wise or unwise.

The writing in this essay is clear and controlled. The writer's use of concrete examples is one of the strongest features of the passage. They grow logically out of the main ideas of each paragraph and illustrate the ideas very effectively. The lottery ticket example is easy to relate to as an example of the uncertainty of taking a long shot, whereas the shoe shop example provides a clear example of a time when acting on at least mild uncertainty can be wise indeed. There is variety in the sentence structure, and the paper flows smoothly from one sentence to the next.

Consider This Statement

Men are dependent on circumstances, not circumstances on men.

Herodotus

Write a unified essay in which you perform the following tasks. Explain the meaning of the above statement. Describe a specific situation where circumstances might be dependent on individuals. Discuss what you think determines whether or not individuals are dependent on circumstances or vice versa.

Writing Sample Essay

Herodotus's viewpoint here is clearly a fatalistic one. It is easy to see the logic behind it. Because mankind does not exist separately from either the rest of existence or the past, then every time that a person acts, she is in some ways also reacting to that surrounding existence and to the history that preceded that act. It is a frustrating point of view; and, in spite of its strange truth, it is probably a viewpoint best left without too much rumination. It is the given in life and the unchangeable. A resignation to this point of view would in some ways also be a voluntary denial of one's autonomy, of one's existence.

I say "voluntary" because I believe that the opposite viewpoint is, paradoxically, just as true. If I turn my head while driving in order to check my radio dial and in doing so also slightly turn my steering wheel causing an accident with an oncoming school bus, did not my act of turning my head create a circumstance whereby that accident occurred? Of course, it did. If I had not turned my head, then I would have not turned the wheel; and if I had not turned the wheel then the bus would not have hit my car. However, from Herodotus's viewpoint, my act did not exist by itself. Had the radio not been in the car, had a different song even been on the station, then I would perhaps not have turned my head to adjust the dial. Had the bus driver waited longer at her last stop or had she not stopped for a cup of coffee on her way to work, then perhaps she would not have been at that place at that specific time. The issue is as puzzling as the issue of whether the chicken appeared first or the egg. It is the question of the identification of an original cause in a long line of causes.

What a thinking person is most likely to conclude is that individuals and their circumstances are mutually interdependent rather than mutually exclusive and that therefore a statement like that of Herodotus is, in a sense, meaningless. His is only a statement of perspective and, further, a rather negative one. But to say the opposite, that circumstances are dependent on individuals and not vice versa, would be naive and ignorant. A rational person would have to accept interdependence of individuals and circumstances in order to live realistically and effectively in the world. She would then act carefully, remaining aware both that there are circumstances over which she has no control and that her act will be part of the circumstances to come.

Explanation of Response: 6

The paper focuses sharply on the statement and addresses each of the three writing tasks. Paragraph one explains what the statement means, paragraph two gives a specific situation in which individuals do, in fact, determine circumstances (a reversal of the assertion that "men are dependent on circumstances, not circumstances on men"), and paragraph three reconciles the statement and the situation that illustrates that the opposite of the statement may also be true.

The paper provides an analysis of the potential dangers of all-or-none statements like the one in question. It does so by examining the logical extension of the idea that individuals are dependent on circumstances and by characterizing the implications of this assertion as "fatalistic." The logic of the paper's argument is sophisticated, on the one hand agreeing with the "strange truth" of Herodotus's point in paragraph one, but in paragraph two illustrating with a series of circumstances "dependent on individuals" that the reverse is also true. The final paragraph presents a balanced consideration of the interdependent relationship between individuals and the circumstances that they create and by which they are shaped.

The writing is clear and nicely controlled. The sentences are varied, containing simple (e.g., sentence one), compound (e.g., sentence four), and complex structures (e.g., sentence three). The first sentence of each paragraph serves as a topic sentence and gives unity to the paragraph that follows. Transitions, such as "however" in sentence five of paragraph two, provide coherence within the paragraph.

PRACTICE TOPICS

Use the questions below to practice your skills at outlining. After you outline the individual essays, choose at least one of the questions and, using your outline, write a full essay in response to the question. Time yourself at 30 minutes per essay.

1. Consider this statement:

   Too great haste in paying off an obligation is a kind of ingratitude.

   Write a unified essay in which you perform the following tasks. Explain what you think the above statement means. Describe a specific situation in which paying off an obligation quickly or hastily would not be a form of ingratitude. Discuss what you think determines when paying off an obligation with great haste is a kind of ingratitude.

2. Consider this statement:

   They who are in highest places, and have the most power, have the least liberty....

   Write a unified essay in which you perform the following tasks. Explain what you think the above statement means. Describe a specific situation in which those who are in the highest places and have the most power, in fact, manage to have at least a fair amount of liberty. Discuss what you think determines whether those in high places who possess much power have liberty.

3. Consider this statement:

   A soft answer turneth away wrath.

   Write a unified essay in which you perform the following tasks. Explain what you think the above statement means. Describe a specific situation in which a soft answer might *not* turn away wrath. Discuss what you think determines the circumstance in which a soft answer does turn away wrath.

4. Consider this statement:

**Revenge is a kind of wild justice, which the more man's nature runs to,
the more ought law to weed it out.**

Write a unified essay in which you perform the following tasks. Explain what you think the above statement means. Describe a specific situation in which revenge is a kind of justice that law ought not prohibit. Discuss what you think determines the point at which law ought to weed out revenge.

Additional Topics

You might find it helpful in understanding the format of the MCAT essay to take the statements below and form questions like the ones above and like those in the sample essay questions in the Model Examination sections.

1. Wise men say nothing in dangerous times.
2. Never tell your resolution beforehand.
3. They that endeavor to abolish vice, destroy also virtue; for contraries, though they destroy one another, are yet the life of one another.
4. A service beyond recompense weighs so heavy that it almost gives offense.
5. All evils are equal when they are extreme.
6. Quarrels would not last long if the fault were on only one side.

PART 3

MODEL EXAMINATIONS

Answer Sheet

MODEL EXAMINATION A

Directions: After locating the number of the question to which you are responding, fill in the circle containing the letter of the answer you have selected. Use pencil (not a ballpoint pen) to completely blacken the circle.

PHYSICAL SCIENCES

1 Ⓐ Ⓑ Ⓒ Ⓓ
2 Ⓐ Ⓑ Ⓒ Ⓓ
3 Ⓐ Ⓑ Ⓒ Ⓓ
4 Ⓐ Ⓑ Ⓒ Ⓓ
5 Ⓐ Ⓑ Ⓒ Ⓓ
6 Ⓐ Ⓑ Ⓒ Ⓓ
7 Ⓐ Ⓑ Ⓒ Ⓓ
8 Ⓐ Ⓑ Ⓒ Ⓓ
9 Ⓐ Ⓑ Ⓒ Ⓓ
10 Ⓐ Ⓑ Ⓒ Ⓓ
11 Ⓐ Ⓑ Ⓒ Ⓓ
12 Ⓐ Ⓑ Ⓒ Ⓓ
13 Ⓐ Ⓑ Ⓒ Ⓓ
14 Ⓐ Ⓑ Ⓒ Ⓓ
15 Ⓐ Ⓑ Ⓒ Ⓓ
16 Ⓐ Ⓑ Ⓒ Ⓓ
17 Ⓐ Ⓑ Ⓒ Ⓓ
18 Ⓐ Ⓑ Ⓒ Ⓓ
19 Ⓐ Ⓑ Ⓒ Ⓓ
20 Ⓐ Ⓑ Ⓒ Ⓓ
21 Ⓐ Ⓑ Ⓒ Ⓓ
22 Ⓐ Ⓑ Ⓒ Ⓓ
23 Ⓐ Ⓑ Ⓒ Ⓓ
24 Ⓐ Ⓑ Ⓒ Ⓓ
25 Ⓐ Ⓑ Ⓒ Ⓓ
26 Ⓐ Ⓑ Ⓒ Ⓓ

27 Ⓐ Ⓑ Ⓒ Ⓓ
28 Ⓐ Ⓑ Ⓒ Ⓓ
29 Ⓐ Ⓑ Ⓒ Ⓓ
30 Ⓐ Ⓑ Ⓒ Ⓓ
31 Ⓐ Ⓑ Ⓒ Ⓓ
32 Ⓐ Ⓑ Ⓒ Ⓓ
33 Ⓐ Ⓑ Ⓒ Ⓓ
34 Ⓐ Ⓑ Ⓒ Ⓓ
35 Ⓐ Ⓑ Ⓒ Ⓓ
36 Ⓐ Ⓑ Ⓒ Ⓓ
37 Ⓐ Ⓑ Ⓒ Ⓓ
38 Ⓐ Ⓑ Ⓒ Ⓓ
39 Ⓐ Ⓑ Ⓒ Ⓓ
40 Ⓐ Ⓑ Ⓒ Ⓓ
41 Ⓐ Ⓑ Ⓒ Ⓓ
42 Ⓐ Ⓑ Ⓒ Ⓓ
43 Ⓐ Ⓑ Ⓒ Ⓓ
44 Ⓐ Ⓑ Ⓒ Ⓓ
45 Ⓐ Ⓑ Ⓒ Ⓓ
46 Ⓐ Ⓑ Ⓒ Ⓓ
47 Ⓐ Ⓑ Ⓒ Ⓓ
48 Ⓐ Ⓑ Ⓒ Ⓓ
49 Ⓐ Ⓑ Ⓒ Ⓓ
50 Ⓐ Ⓑ Ⓒ Ⓓ
51 Ⓐ Ⓑ Ⓒ Ⓓ
52 Ⓐ Ⓑ Ⓒ Ⓓ

VERBAL REASONING

53 Ⓐ Ⓑ Ⓒ Ⓓ
54 Ⓐ Ⓑ Ⓒ Ⓓ
55 Ⓐ Ⓑ Ⓒ Ⓓ
56 Ⓐ Ⓑ Ⓒ Ⓓ
57 Ⓐ Ⓑ Ⓒ Ⓓ
58 Ⓐ Ⓑ Ⓒ Ⓓ
59 Ⓐ Ⓑ Ⓒ Ⓓ
60 Ⓐ Ⓑ Ⓒ Ⓓ
61 Ⓐ Ⓑ Ⓒ Ⓓ
62 Ⓐ Ⓑ Ⓒ Ⓓ
63 Ⓐ Ⓑ Ⓒ Ⓓ
64 Ⓐ Ⓑ Ⓒ Ⓓ
65 Ⓐ Ⓑ Ⓒ Ⓓ
66 Ⓐ Ⓑ Ⓒ Ⓓ
67 Ⓐ Ⓑ Ⓒ Ⓓ
68 Ⓐ Ⓑ Ⓒ Ⓓ
69 Ⓐ Ⓑ Ⓒ Ⓓ
70 Ⓐ Ⓑ Ⓒ Ⓓ
71 Ⓐ Ⓑ Ⓒ Ⓓ
72 Ⓐ Ⓑ Ⓒ Ⓓ

73 Ⓐ Ⓑ Ⓒ Ⓓ
74 Ⓐ Ⓑ Ⓒ Ⓓ
75 Ⓐ Ⓑ Ⓒ Ⓓ
76 Ⓐ Ⓑ Ⓒ Ⓓ
77 Ⓐ Ⓑ Ⓒ Ⓓ
78 Ⓐ Ⓑ Ⓒ Ⓓ
79 Ⓐ Ⓑ Ⓒ Ⓓ
80 Ⓐ Ⓑ Ⓒ Ⓓ
81 Ⓐ Ⓑ Ⓒ Ⓓ
82 Ⓐ Ⓑ Ⓒ Ⓓ
83 Ⓐ Ⓑ Ⓒ Ⓓ
84 Ⓐ Ⓑ Ⓒ Ⓓ
85 Ⓐ Ⓑ Ⓒ Ⓓ
86 Ⓐ Ⓑ Ⓒ Ⓓ
87 Ⓐ Ⓑ Ⓒ Ⓓ
88 Ⓐ Ⓑ Ⓒ Ⓓ
89 Ⓐ Ⓑ Ⓒ Ⓓ
90 Ⓐ Ⓑ Ⓒ Ⓓ
91 Ⓐ Ⓑ Ⓒ Ⓓ
92 Ⓐ Ⓑ Ⓒ Ⓓ

Answer Sheet

MODEL EXAMINATION A

WRITING SAMPLE

Use separate ruled
sheets of paper.

93

94

BIOLOGICAL SCIENCES

95 Ⓐ Ⓑ Ⓒ Ⓓ	121 Ⓐ Ⓑ Ⓒ Ⓓ
96 Ⓐ Ⓑ Ⓒ Ⓓ	122 Ⓐ Ⓑ Ⓒ Ⓓ
97 Ⓐ Ⓑ Ⓒ Ⓓ	123 Ⓐ Ⓑ Ⓒ Ⓓ
98 Ⓐ Ⓑ Ⓒ Ⓓ	124 Ⓐ Ⓑ Ⓒ Ⓓ
99 Ⓐ Ⓑ Ⓒ Ⓓ	125 Ⓐ Ⓑ Ⓒ Ⓓ
100 Ⓐ Ⓑ Ⓒ Ⓓ	126 Ⓐ Ⓑ Ⓒ Ⓓ
101 Ⓐ Ⓑ Ⓒ Ⓓ	127 Ⓐ Ⓑ Ⓒ Ⓓ
102 Ⓐ Ⓑ Ⓒ Ⓓ	128 Ⓐ Ⓑ Ⓒ Ⓓ
103 Ⓐ Ⓑ Ⓒ Ⓓ	129 Ⓐ Ⓑ Ⓒ Ⓓ
104 Ⓐ Ⓑ Ⓒ Ⓓ	130 Ⓐ Ⓑ Ⓒ Ⓓ
105 Ⓐ Ⓑ Ⓒ Ⓓ	131 Ⓐ Ⓑ Ⓒ Ⓓ
106 Ⓐ Ⓑ Ⓒ Ⓓ	132 Ⓐ Ⓑ Ⓒ Ⓓ
107 Ⓐ Ⓑ Ⓒ Ⓓ	133 Ⓐ Ⓑ Ⓒ Ⓓ
108 Ⓐ Ⓑ Ⓒ Ⓓ	134 Ⓐ Ⓑ Ⓒ Ⓓ
109 Ⓐ Ⓑ Ⓒ Ⓓ	135 Ⓐ Ⓑ Ⓒ Ⓓ
110 Ⓐ Ⓑ Ⓒ Ⓓ	136 Ⓐ Ⓑ Ⓒ Ⓓ
111 Ⓐ Ⓑ Ⓒ Ⓓ	137 Ⓐ Ⓑ Ⓒ Ⓓ
112 Ⓐ Ⓑ Ⓒ Ⓓ	138 Ⓐ Ⓑ Ⓒ Ⓓ
113 Ⓐ Ⓑ Ⓒ Ⓓ	139 Ⓐ Ⓑ Ⓒ Ⓓ
114 Ⓐ Ⓑ Ⓒ Ⓓ	140 Ⓐ Ⓑ Ⓒ Ⓓ
115 Ⓐ Ⓑ Ⓒ Ⓓ	141 Ⓐ Ⓑ Ⓒ Ⓓ
116 Ⓐ Ⓑ Ⓒ Ⓓ	142 Ⓐ Ⓑ Ⓒ Ⓓ
117 Ⓐ Ⓑ Ⓒ Ⓓ	143 Ⓐ Ⓑ Ⓒ Ⓓ
118 Ⓐ Ⓑ Ⓒ Ⓓ	144 Ⓐ Ⓑ Ⓒ Ⓓ
119 Ⓐ Ⓑ Ⓒ Ⓓ	145 Ⓐ Ⓑ Ⓒ Ⓓ
120 Ⓐ Ⓑ Ⓒ Ⓓ	146 Ⓐ Ⓑ Ⓒ Ⓓ

The MCAT Model Examination A

PHYSICAL SCIENCES

TIME—70 MINUTES FOR 52 QUESTIONS

Directions: The following questions or incomplete statements are in groups. Preceding each series of questions or statements is a paragraph or a short explanatory statement, a formula or set of formulas, or a definition. Read the written material and then answer the questions or complete the statements. Select the ONE BEST ANSWER for each question and indicate your selection by marking the corresponding letter of your choice on the Answer Form. Eliminate those alternatives you know to be incorrect and then select an answer from among the remaining alternatives. A periodic table is provided (see p. 563). You may consult it whenever you wish to do so.

Passage I (Questions 1–5)

An X-ray tube consists of two metal electrodes, a heated filament cathode, and an anode containing the metal target sealed under high vacuum in a glass envelope. The heated filament in the cathode emits electrons which are accelerated by a high DC voltage and collide with the positive anode target. Two different types of X-ray spectra may be seen. The continuous or "bremsstrahlung" spectrum that is always present is produced when the electron penetrates through the outer electron cloud and is abruptly accelerated by the large positive charge on the nucleus of a heavy atom. The production of X-rays increases with increasing atomic number but is typically no more than 1% efficient, the remaining energy appearing as heat in the target metal. The sharp line spectra that can be seen at higher voltages occur when the incident electrons eject an inner shell electron, such as an $n = 1$ shell electron. The spectral line is produced when an electron, say from $n = 2$, fills the vacancy in the $n = 1$ shell, emitting an x-ray photon whose energy corresponds to the energy difference between the $n = 2$ and $n = 1$ shells. The intensity of X-rays is proportional to the number of photons created. The photon energy $E = hf = hc/\lambda$ where h is Planck's constant and c is the speed of light. Figure 1 is a sketch of intensity versus wavelength for a molybdenum target with an accelerating voltage of 35,000 V.

1. Figure 1 shows that the continuous X-ray spectrum has a minimum (cut-off) wavelength. No shorter wavelengths are emitted from the tube. This minimum wavelength corresponds to:

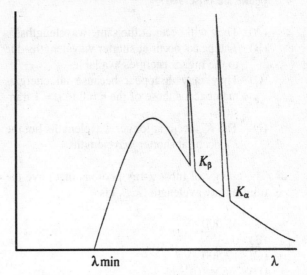

Figure 1. X-ray intensity versus wavelength

(A) the smallest number of emitted photons.
(B) the highest energy photons emitted.
(C) the type of cathode used.
(D) the type of anode material used.

2. The sharp K_α peak in Figure 1 corresponds to an electron transition from state $n = 2$ to $n = 1$, whereas K_β corresponds to a transition from state $n = 3$ to $n = 1$. The K_α peak is higher than the K_β peak. Which peak corresponds to higher-energy X-ray photons? Which transition is more probable?

(A) K_α is higher energy; K_α is more probable.
(B) K_α is higher energy; K_β is more probable.
(C) K_β is higher energy; K_β is more probable.
(D) K_β is higher energy; K_α is more probable.

3. The current to the heated filament in the cathode is increased while the accelerating voltage is kept constant. This increased current increases the number of electrons striking the target increasing the overall intensity. What effect does this have on the minimum wavelength value?

(A) The minimum value will move to shorter wavelength values.
(B) It will move to longer wavelength values.
(C) There will no longer be a cutoff wavelength.
(D) The minimum wavelength will remain the same.

4. If the accelerating voltage, V_o, is increased while keeping the filament current constant, the overall intensity will also increase. What effect will this have on the wavelength position where the two peaks are observed?

(A) They will occur at the same wavelengths.
(B) The peaks occur at shorter wavelengths due to the higher energies available.
(C) They may disappear because all energies may exceed those of the $n = 3$ to $n = 1$ transition.
(D) The K_α occur at longer wavelengths but the K_β occur at shorter wavelengths.

5. The energy of those x-ray photons that have the minimum wavelength (λ_{min}) is:

(A) 35,000 eV
(B) 0 eV
(C) 17,500 eV
(D) 5.6×10^{-15} eV

Passage II (Questions 6–11)

A safety engineering firm is producing a film for high school driver education classes. The firm uses skilled test drivers driving both small cars and larger vans. The vans weigh three times as much as the cars and have larger tires with twice the tread width. In a demonstration that tests reaction times and skid-to-stop distances and shows them on the film, three guns that fire a yellow paint onto the road are mounted on the bumpers and fired electrically. When the driver hears the report of the first gun, he locks the brakes, and the touch of his foot on the brake pedal fires a second yellow pellet. The third pellet is fired when the car stops. The safety engineers also design several remote controlled cars and vans in order to film crash results.

6. Drivers of a car and a van brake hard and skid to a stop from 50 mph. The skid marks are measured to be the same length for both. Why are the stopping distances the same length?

(A) The mechanical work done by friction to stop both is the same.
(B) The frictional force between tires and road is three times greater for the heavier van so it slides the same distance as the car.
(C) The frictional force for the car and van are the same.
(D) The wider tires on the van require less friction force than the narrow tires on the car.

7. Two drivers in identical cars skid to a stop from speeds of 20 mph and 40 mph. How do the lengths of the skid marks compare?

(A) They are the same length.
(B) The 40 mph mark is twice as long.
(C) The 40 mph mark is four times as long.
(D) The 40 mph mark is eight times as long.

8. A remote-controlled car and van are crashed head-on at the same speed. Why does the car suffer more damage in the collision?

(A) The car and van had the same momentum.
(B) The forces during collision are equal and opposite, so the smaller and weaker car suffers more damage.
(C) The van exerts a larger force on the car.
(D) The mechanical work done in stopping the car is greater.

9. The van going at a speed of 15 mph collides head-on with a car going at a speed of 45 mph. Because the van weighs three times as much, their vector momenta are equal and opposite. However, examination shows that the car suffers more damage than the van. Why?

(A) The massive van exerts a larger force on the car.
(B) The lighter car exerts a smaller force on the van.
(C) The forces exerted during the collision are equal and opposite, so the weaker car suffers more damage.
(D) The mechanical work required to stop the van is smaller.

10. For the reaction time test, one driver is tested at 20 mph and 60 mph. It is noted that the distance between the first two paint marks is three times farther for the 60 mph test than the 20 mph test. How do his reaction times compare at 20 mph and 60 mph?

(A) His reaction time at 60 mph is three times faster.
(B) His reaction times remain the same.
(C) His reaction time at 20 mph is three times faster.
(D) His reaction time at 20 mph is one-third as long as at 60 mph.

Passage III (Questions 11–16)

Calcium carbonate reacts with water and carbon dioxide to produce soluble calcium bicarbonate according to the reaction:

$$CaCO_3(s) + CO_2(g) + H_2O(l) \rightarrow Ca(HCO_3)_2(aq)$$

This reaction is responsible for the erosion of caves containing large deposits of calcium carbonate. Calcium carbonate reacts with hydrochloric acid to produce calcium chloride, according to the reaction:

$$CaCO_3(s) + 2HCl(aq) \rightarrow CaCl_2(aq) + CO_2(g) + H_2O(l)$$

Heating calcium carbonate at high temperatures produces calcium oxide, which is used to neutralize acidic soils, as follows:

$$CaCO_3(s) \rightarrow CaO(s) + CO_2(g)$$

11. A chemist places a sample of calcium carbonate into a sealed container under pure carbon dioxide gas. Will the sample react to form calcium bicarbonate?

(A) Yes, because carbon dioxide is present.
(B) Yes, because calcium carbonate is present.
(C) No, because water is absent.
(D) No, because hydrochloric acid is absent.

12. A sample of calcium oxide is placed into water. What is the approximate pH of the solution:

(A) 2
(B) 6
(C) 7
(D) 9

13. Which of the following is a strong electrolyte?

(A) $CO_2(g)$
(B) $H_2O(l)$
(C) $CaCl_2(aq)$
(D) $Ca(s)$

14. A lake contains runoff from a mountain that has large deposits of calcium carbonate and freezes at a point 1.6°C lower than other lakes at similar altitude. What is the most likely explanation for this?

(A) Dissolved calcium bicarbonate lowers the freezing point.
(B) Dissolved calcium carbonate lowers the freezing point.
(C) Dissolved calcium bicarbonate raises the freezing point.
(D) Dissolved calcium carbonate raises the freezing point.

15. What is the charge of the calcium ion in calcium chloride?

(A) –1
(B) –2
(C) +1
(D) +2

16. Decomposition of a sample of calcium carbonate produced 56.1 g CaO. How much carbon dioxide is produced at STP?

(A) 11.2 L
(B) 22.4 L
(C) 33.4 L
(D) 40.6 L

Passage IV (Questions 17–20)

A large cylindrical tank 5 meters in radius is filled to the top with water. A small amount of water is then added until it mounds up slightly above the edges of the tank (because of surface tension). The tank is 3 meters high. A stopcock 2 meters below the top edge can be opened to allow water to flow out horizontally. The tank sits in a catch basin to catch any water that flows over the top edge. If the stopcock is opened, the water will flow out in a smooth jet that lands on the floor beyond the edge of the catch basin. A closed top can be clamped onto the top of the tank and connected to an air pump so that the air pressure on the top surface of the water can be increased above one atmosphere. Wooden cubes that are 10 cm on an edge and have a mass density of 700 kg/m^3 are available.

The mass density of water is 1000 kg/m^3.

1 atmosphere pressure = 1.03×10^5 N/m^2.

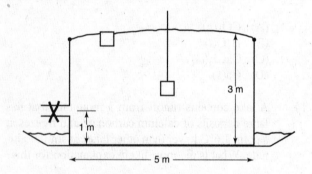

17.   A single cube of wood is placed carefully on the mounded water surface, causing water to overflow into the catch basin. How much water overflows into the catch basin?

(A)   A volume of water equal to 30% of the volume of the wood block.

(B)   A mass of water equal to 70% of the mass of the wood block.

(C)   A volume of water equal to the volume of the wood block.

(D)   A volume of water the weight of which equals the weight of the block.

18.   The block of wood is now submerged completely under the water surface by pushing down on it with a very thin rigid rod, and some more water overflows into the catch basin. How much *total* water is now in the catch basin?

(A)   A mass of water equal to the mass of the block of wood.

(B)   A weight of water equal to the weight of the block of wood.

(C)   A volume of water equal to the volume of the wood block.

(D)   A weight of water equal to 70% of the weight of the wood block.

19.   The buoyant force the water exerts on the submerged block is:

(A)   equal to the weight of the block.

(B)   smaller than the weight of the block by 30%.

(C)   equal to the weight of the water in the catch basin.

(D)   equal to 70% of the weight of the block.

20.   The blocks are removed and the water in the tank is adjusted until the water surface is level with the top edge of the tank. A smaller tank is only 2 m in radius but is filled to the same height with water as the large tank and also has a stopcock 2 m below its top edge. How do the speeds of water exiting through the two stopcocks compare?

(A)   The water from the large tank is 67% faster.

(B)   The water from the small tank is 33% slower.

(C)   The water from the large tank is about 6 times faster because it has 6 times the volume of the small tank.

(D)   The speeds are the same.

Passage V (Questions 21–25)

A pendulum system consists of a bob of mass 2 kg on the end of a cord that is 80 cm long from the cord support to the center of the bob. The system behaves as a simple pendulum if one displaces the pendulum through a small angle (less than about 10°) from the vertical. The period is given by:

$$T = 2\pi\sqrt{L/g}$$

Other masses and cord lengths are available.

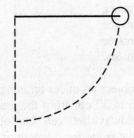

21. The bob is raised to the position where the cord is horizontal (90°) and then released. What is the speed of the bob as it passes through the lowest point of its swing?

    (A) 2.0 m/s
    (B) 4.0 m/s
    (C) 5.1 m/s
    (D) 5.9 m/s

22. The bob is now raised until the cord makes an angle of 4° with the vertical. What is the period of oscillation when the bob is released?

    (A) 1.8 s
    (B) 2.8 s
    (C) 1.4 s
    (D) 2.6 s

23. The bob is raised higher so that the cord makes the angle of 8° with the vertical. What is the period of oscillation now?

    (A) 3.6 s
    (B) 3.2 s
    (C) 1.8 s
    (D) 0.9 s

24. The bob is replaced with a bob of 3 kg. A new cord is of unknown length. When the period is timed, it is found to be 2.0 s for small angles. What is the length of the new pendulum?

    (A) 1.0 m
    (B) 2.0 m
    (C) 1.8 m
    (D) 2.4 m

25. NASA, upon renewing the moon landing program in preparation for sending men and women to Mars, sends the 2.0-second pendulum system to the moon. What happens to the measured period of the pendulum when used on the moon?

    (A) T increases.
    (B) T decreases.
    (C) T hardly changes at all.
    (D) The pendulum will not work on the moon where there is no gravity.

Questions 26–32 are independent of any passage and of each other.

26. Water flows without friction through a water-filled pipe of cross-sectional area 3.0 m² at a speed of 2.0 m/s. The pipe's cross-sectional area first constricts to 1.0 m² and then expands to 2.0 m². What is the water speed in the 2.0 m² cross section of the pipe?

    (A) 9.0 m/s
    (B) 4.0 m/s
    (C) 3.0 m/s
    (D) 1.0 m/s

27. Rutherford first observed nuclear transmutation when ^{14}N was bombarded with alpha particles (^{4}He nuclei). The reaction is written as:

    $$^4_2\text{He} + ^{14}_7\text{N} \rightarrow ^{17}_8\text{O} + ?$$

    What is the missing particle ?

    (A) $^4_2$He (alpha particle)

    (B) $^1_1$H (proton)

    (C) $^1_0$n (neutron)

    (D) $^0_{-1}$e (electron)

28. Two charged particles, A and B, are a distance *r* apart so that a certain force exists between them. The charge on A is tripled while the distance between the charges is also tripled. How does the force between the particles change?

(A) It does not change.
(B) It increases by a factor of 3.
(C) It decreases by a factor of 9.
(D) It decreases by a factor of 3.

29. A 3-ohm resistor and a 6-ohm resistor are connected in parallel and a 2-ohm resistor is connected in series with this combination as shown. If a current of 3 amperes is sent through the 2-ohm resistor, the currents through the 3- and 6-ohm resistors are, respectively:

(A) 3 and 2 amperes
(B) 1 and 2 amperes
(C) 2 and 1 amperes
(D) 0.5 and 2.5 amperes

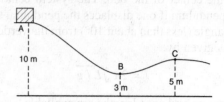

30. A golf ball is dropped from the top of a very tall building. (Air friction is present.) Which graph below correctly shows the velocity of the ball as a function of time?

(A)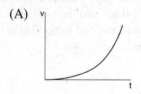

(B)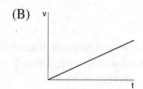

(C)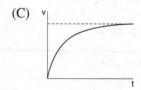

(D)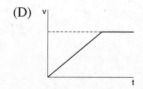

31. A box slides on a frictionless surface from rest at point A, which is 10 m above the ground, to point C at 5 m above the ground. What is the speed of the box at point C?

(A) 4.95 m/sec
(B) 9.90 m/sec
(C) 19.6 m/sec
(D) 98.0 m/sec

32. A lighted object produces an image on a screen. The screen is 30 cm from the lens. The lens is exactly midway between the object and the screen. What is the focal length of the lens?

(A) +30 cm
(B) +15 cm
(C) +60 cm
(D) −30 cm

Passage VI (Questions 33–38)

The colorimeter is a device for measuring the amount of light that passes through a solution. When the color (wavelength) of light is selected properly, the colorimeter is a useful tool for determining the amount of a particular light-absorbing material in solution.

A colorimeter is equipped with a meter that responds in linear fashion to the amount of light reaching it. The meter is set to zero with no light and it is found that a cuvette containing pure water gives a reading of 81 for light of a particular wavelength. When the same cuvette with an aqueous solution is placed in the light path, a reading of 72 is obtained.

33. The transmittance of the solution is:

(A) 0.811.
(B) 81.1.
(C) 0.889.
(D) 0.722.

34. The absorbance of the solution is:

(A) 0.189.
(B) 0.111.
(C) 0.278.
(D) 0.051.

35. If the light is of a particular wavelength that is specifically absorbed by the solute (or one of its functional groups), dilution of the solution with an equal volume of water will produce a new solution whose absorbance will be:

   (A) 0.026.
   (B) 0.095.
   (C) 0.282.
   (D) greater than 0.5.

36. If the path length through which light travels in the above solution is halved, the absorbance will be:

   (A) 0.013.
   (B) 0.052.
   (C) 0.041.
   (D) 0.190.

37. If the solute concentration for the first reading in this question set is doubled, the reading for this higher concentration will be:

   (A) 64.
   (B) 51.
   (C) 18.
   (D) 5.

38. If the wavelength of the light in this previous question is doubled, the reading will:

   (A) be doubled.
   (B) be halved.
   (C) show no change.
   (D) change by an amount that cannot be predicted.

Passage VII (Questions 39–45)

A 0.01 mole sample of HCl is diluted to 1000 mL with water and mixed in a beaker to produce solution A. To this is added 1000 mL of water. After mixing, the resulting solution is solution B. To this is added 0.02 moles sodium propionate. After mixing, the resulting solution is solution C. To this is added 0.01 mole sodium propionate and 0.01 mole propionic acid. After mixing, the resulting solution is solution D. To this is added 1000 mL more water. After mixing, the resulting solution is solution E. To another beaker is added 0.005 mole of pyruvic acid. Water is added to a total volume of 500 mL. After mixing, the resulting solution is solution F. To solution F is added 0.005 mole of sodium pyruvate. After mixing, the resulting solution is solution G. K_a values are 1.3×10^{-5} for propionic acid, 1.4×10^{-4} for pyruvic acid, and 5.9×10^{-10} for boric acid. pK_a values are 4.89 for propionic acid, 3.85 for pyruvic acid, and 9.23 for boric acid. (For the purpose of this problem, assume no volume change occurs after the addition of small quantities of liquid or solid.)

39. The pH of solution A is:

   (A) 2.0.
   (B) 3.0.
   (C) 4.0.
   (D) 6.0.

40. The pH of solution B is:

   (A) less than 2.
   (B) between 2 and 3
   (C) between 3 and 4.
   (D) between 4 and 7.

41. The pH of solution C is equal to the pK_a of the weak acid, propionic acid, because:

   (A) there are equal quantities of HCl and propionic acid.
   (B) the quantity of sodium propionate is twice that of propionic acid.
   (C) the quantity of sodium propionate equals that of propionic acid.
   (D) all the sodium propionate has been converted to propionic acid.

42. The strongest acid used in the sample preparations was:

   (A) hydrochloric acid.
   (B) propionic acid.
   (C) boric acid.
   (D) pyruvic acid.

43. The pH of solution E is:

   (A) between 2 and 3.
   (B) between 4 and 5.
   (C) between 5 and 6.
   (D) greater than 6.5.

44. Among pyruvic acid, propionic acid, and boric acid:

   (A) pyruvic acid is most acidic because it has the lowest pK_a.
   (B) propionic acid is most acidic because it has the lowest pK_a.
   (C) boric acid is most acidic because it has the lowest pK_a.
   (D) boric acid is most acidic because it has the highest pK_a.

45. The percent of ionization of pyruvic acid is:

   (A) 0.12.
   (B) 1.2.
   (C) 12.
   (D) greater than 20.

Questions 46–52 are independent of any passage and of each other.

46. Compound A is known to have a molecular weight of 20. The molecular weight of Compound B is not known. Upon observing that gaseous Compound B will diffuse half as fast as gaseous Compound A, we can calculate the molecular weight of Compound B as:

   (A) 10.
   (B) 20.
   (C) 40.
   (D) 80.

47. In the titration of a 0.100 N solution of NaOH, it is found that 20.0 ml of a 0.200 N solution of an unknown acid will neutralize 40.0 ml of the 0.100 N NaOH. This indicates that the unknown acid is:

   (A) monoprotic
   (B) diprotic
   (C) triprotic.
   (D) none of the above.

48. If it is known that the pH of a solution is 4.5, we can calculate that the pOH is:

   (A) 4.5.
   (B) 7.5.
   (C) 9.5.
   (D) 12.5.

49. The pK_a of an acid HA is 4.2. The pH at which equal concentrations of A^- and HA are present in solution is:

   (A) 2.4.
   (B) 4.2.
   (C) 7.0.
   (D) 9.8.

50. A buffer is made of a weak acid ($pK_a = 5.9$) and its salt. Such a buffer functions best to suppress changes of pH on addition of acid when the pH of the solution is:

   (A) 3.9.
   (B) 5.9.
   (C) 7.0.
   (D) 8.9.

51. One liter of a gas is held at a pressure of 1 atm. If there is no change in temperature, increasing the pressure to 2 atm will result in a volume change to:

   (A) 2.0 liters.
   (B) 0.95 liter.
   (C) 0.50 liter.
   (D) 0.20 liter.

52. In recovery of silver from photographic film, you have decided to dissolve the silver ion with dilute nitric acid. Addition of dilute HCl to precipitate AgCl seems to result in unacceptable losses. You might improve recovery by addition of _____ in the latter step.

   (A) $NaNO_3$
   (B) NaCl
   (C) Ag_2SO_4
   (D) sodium acetate

VERBAL REASONING

TIME—60 MINUTES FOR 40 QUESTIONS

Directions: The questions are based on the accompanying seven passages. Read each passage carefully, then answer the following questions. Consider only the material within the passage. For each question, select the ONE BEST ANSWER and indicate your selection by marking the corresponding letter on the Answer Form.

Passage I (Questions 53–58)

Periodic demands for educational reform, in conjunction with the corresponding efforts of the nation's public school systems to improve their instructional programs, are not an unusual phenomenon in the annals of this country's history. The most recent reform movement, however, which is viewed by many as a demand on the part of legislatures and the public for more effective schools, might be classified as unique. During the last 20 years, monumental amounts of research and discussion have been generated regarding all facets of public education.

The outcry was created in part by declining economic conditions and by the publication of such exhaustive studies of school resources and their impact as the Coleman et al., (1966) report on the *Equality of Educational Opportunity* and others (Jensen, 1969; Jenks et al. 1970; Rist, 1970; Avech, 1974), which seemed to point out the failure of the American educational system. The results of their findings caused considerable dismay in the educational community and the population at large, since they suggested that schools make little, if any, difference in the lives of the children who attend them. The socio-economic status of the individual's family (Hodgson, 1975) as well as a measure of "pure luck" (ERIC Action Brief, 1981) were credited with influencing student achievement and other educational outcomes to a much greater degree than a pupil's school experiences.

After the initial reaction of shock, neither researchers nor practitioners were content to stand by and accept the pessimistic picture that had been painted for them as a final verdict. In response, literally hundreds of studies have been conducted in schools across the country that focus on every aspect of public education.

Researchers have gone into the field in great numbers to obtain a firsthand view of the educational process in action. One early example of a now classic study that

Adapted from E. E. Seibel, "Principal Change Facilitator Style: Its Relationship to School Climate and Student Achievement." Doctoral Dissertation, Virginia Commonwealth University, 1986.

made an attempt to overcome the existing attitude of fatalism was that conducted by Weber (1971) in four Washington, D.C., schools. The results indicated that by placing a consistent school-wide emphasis on the teaching of basic skills, school leaders could be influential in improving the reading achievement of disadvantaged inner-city youngsters.

Many other research efforts, both ethnographic and quantitative in nature, have produced positive results and have infused practitioners with a new hope and a renewed belief that what takes place in schools can indeed make a significant difference in both the academic lives and the personal development of the pupils that they serve.

Although the negative effects of the early findings have been lessened, they have not been wiped away. The call for further reform continues, as evidenced by the continuing wave of national, state, and public demands contained in such reports as *A Nation at Risk* (Goldberg & James, 1983) and *Making the Grade* (Graham, 1983). Consequently, the research effort has intensified and has resulted in the translation of many of its findings into positive plans of action.

53. The central thesis of the passage is:

(A) schools do not make a difference in the lives of the students who attend them.

(B) instructional programs must always be improved and updated so that educational critics will be satisfied.

(C) although the call for educational reform in the United States has been an ongoing process, the past 20-year period has been an extremely research-oriented time in the public education arena.

(D) middle class parents should consider providing academic instruction for their children in the home setting.

54. According to this passage, what factors were partially responsible for triggering the educational reform movement that is discussed therein?

   (A) The fact that the majority of citizens in the United States have attended the public schools themselves and therefore knew that instructional programs needed to be changed.
   (B) The fact that many people wanted to teach their children at home and did not want to pay taxes to support the public school system.
   (C) Anger over the implication that the amount of money a family has, as well as the amount of "luck" they encounter, can make a difference in a child's education.
   (D) A decline in the national economy and the publication of exhaustive school resource studies.

55. The demand for educational reform and the resulting research that has been conducted over the past 20 years has been centered on:

   (A) public schools.
   (B) private schools.
   (C) home education.
   (D) correspondence courses.

56. The fourth paragraph states: "Researchers have gone into the field in great numbers to gain a first-hand view of the educational process in action." Which of the following statements would be reasonable assumptions to make as a result of that sentence?

   I. Many studies have been conducted in school settings.
   II. The people conducting the research are not simply basing their results on educational theories.
   III. There appears to be a great deal of interest in the educational process.

   (A) I only
   (B) II only
   (C) I and II only
   (D) I, II, and III

57. What groups might the word "practitioners," used in paragraph three, stand for?

   (A) doctors, dentists, lawyers
   (B) educators
   (C) superintendents, principals, teachers
   (D) both B and C

58. The author of this passage gives the impression that:

   (A) there is little hope for the successful future of public education in the United States.
   (B) although serious problems exist in the educational arena, progress is being made, partially, as a result of the hands-on involvement of researchers.
   (C) the field of education is so large that effective change cannot occur.
   (D) too many people are involved in doing educational research.

Passage II (Questions 59–64)

The fairy tale of Cinderella is one of the most widely known folk stories in the world. In its various versions it captures the struggle for the young girl's passage into womanhood. It covers, in its scope, several of Karen Horney's ideas, as well as the trials, totems, and family patterns found in primitive cultures. The Cinderella story chronicles the transformation of the girl into the woman, the profane into the spiritual; ending in the heroine's resolution of her feminine powers.

The Cinderella story goes back as far as seventh-century China. It is classified among the most well-known folktales in the world, and there is a version in nearly every language. The plot is universal: Cinderella, a beautiful, kind, and loving girl, suffers within her family, and is aided by some form of magic through which she meets the man she is destined to marry. After the initial meetings with this man, she loses some article symbolic of the womb, and the man uses this article to find and betroth her.

Several of Karen Horney's theories from "The Distrust Between the Sexes" are evident in this folktale. One of the main ideas in Cinderella is the concept of the evil stepmother or foster mother. Even in instances where Cinderella's father is still living, the stepmother is allowed to abuse her. Her elder sisters are also given this privilege. This is because the mother and sisters are older and less attractive than the heroine. Cinderella's persecution is permitted because, as Horney says, ". . . it

Adapted from Heather Tuttle "If the Shoe Fits," VCU, 1990.

is only the sexually attractive woman of whom [man] is afraid and who . . . has to be kept in bondage." In the cultures from which the story derives, old women are not sexually threatening to men and so the stepmother is given the power (by the father) to make the heroine submissive. Horney continues: "Old women, on the other hand, are held in high esteem, even by cultures in which the young woman is dreaded and therefore suppressed." Not only is the stepmother granted more power over Cinderella due to her position, but she feels her power potentially jeopardized by the sway that Cinderella's beauty may have over men. The sisters also feel jeopardized by the heroine's sexual attractiveness, which leads to greater resentment and cruelty on their part.

Another of Horney's theories prevalent in the story is the duality of motherhood. There are two aspects of motherhood, the virgin mother who is self-sacrificing, nurturing, and selfless, and the mother goddess, warm, earthy, sensual, and fertile. Both aspects are visible in the heroine. Cinderella, as she is first seen, sleeps in the cold, empty hearth, reflective of the virgin's womb, empty until acted upon by some outside force. She is covered in ashes, dressed in rags; in general a picture of self-effacing humility. Despite the hardships put upon her by her family, she is kind to them and even tries her best to beautify her stepsisters for the ball. She is virtuous, in contrast to her stepsisters and stepmother. After marriage to the prince, in the end, the heroine does not seek any revenge on her persecutors. In some renditions, she actually invites her family to come live with her and her new husband. Further evidence of this virginal mother aspect is the part that the prince plays in her life at this point. Like the ultimate example of nurturing motherhood, Mother Mary, who waits for the male god to act upon her, Cinderella lies in wait for the prince to come and save her. He is the aid she needs to be freed of her harsh life.

The other aspect of motherhood is revealed in her when magic help arrives from the outside. She is bestowed with sensual, material things: beautiful clothes, ornaments, cosmetics; things to make her desirable to men. The heroine is also gifted with the famous shoes, reflective of the womb. This prince is usually attracted to her for her physical appearance. She is displaying her sensual, seductive, earthy side and the prince is a reward for her power to act on him with her seductive ability. This dichotomy provides some confusion to the heroine, her family, and her suitor. The journey to resolve the puzzle of her twofold womanhood is a main theme in this folklore.

The passage from a girl to a woman is only one of the several transitions that take place within our heroine. She also undergoes a spiritual transformation. In the beginning of every account, the heroine is dirty and ragged. In at least three versions, she is made to wear animal skins. These things are representative of the material, animalistic, profane world. As she is put through the trials for entering into adulthood, she is also put through trials to test her spirituality. In spite of hardships, she manages to remain pious, loving, and kind. These trials come to an end and she becomes clean and well dressed. She is described as radiant, angelic, and fairylike. The heroine is then presented to the prince. The image of the prince embracing the servant girl is heavily laden with religious meaning, especially during the period when this story became popular. This analogy was very often used by the convents of the Middle Ages to relate the relationship of the nuns to Jesus Christ. Cinderella's spiritual ascent is completed with her royal wedding.

The heroine's time of testing is not completely at an end until the two sides of her femininity merge. They have been in the process of merging since the time of her totem's arrival. Since the arrival of the totem, she has actively struggled with her two female aspects, the virginal/nurturing and the earthy/seductive. The heroine in each version of the tale is given a womb symbol: either a shoe or a ring. This symbol accompanies her when she meets the prince in her state of beauty and sensuality. She then loses this article with the prince, who uses it to find her. When he sees her again, she is once more virginal, modest; covered in dirt and ashes, yet she is missing this symbol of her womanhood. The prince is confused; this is not quite the girl he thought he came for. After he places the shoe on her foot (or the ring on her finger, as the case may be) he sees her as whole: sensual, earthy, yet loving and virginal. She no longer runs from him as she did in earlier encounters, when things became too intimate with the prince.

This is also a moment of recognition for Cinderella. She has discovered a unity of both female forces within her. There were clues previously as to the wholeness of her nature, but she ignored them. She managed to overlook the times when she was sensual, at the ball, and was still kind to her family, generously giving them jewelry. She failed to see her true nature when she was beautiful and yet very humble in the presence of nobility. Now she can no longer hide herself. The prince has seen her spiritual, virginal, and sensual facets and her true nature is revealed to all, including her astonished family. She has found strength in her wholeness, and the prince is both her aid in discovering herself and her reward for being discovered.

59. This passage asserts that:

 I. only those versions of the story that are American can be used to illustrate Horney's theories.
 II. regardless of the version of the Cinderella tale, the story tells of a young girl's passage into womanhood.
 III. the concept of the evil stepmother or foster mother is a main ingredient in the Cinderella story.
 IV. Cinderella's sisters typically are older than she and less attractive.
 V. the prince finally sees only one facet of Cinderella.

 (A) I, II, and III
 (B) I and IV
 (C) II, III, and IV
 (D) IV only

60. According to this passage, Cinderella:

 (A) contemplates revenge on her sisters and mother but doesn't carry through with it.
 (B) does not seek revenge at all.
 (C) gives up her need for revenge after she marries the prince.
 (D) cannot bring herself to completely forgive her persecutors.

61. The author of this passage concludes the following from the fact that in at least three versions of the story, Cinderella is made to wear animal skins.

 (A) She needs the warmth that these skins provide.
 (B) The animal skins have nothing to do with the rites of passage that she is going through.
 (C) The animal skins symbolize the profane animal world that she figuratively is leaving.
 (D) She may decide to keep the animal skins.

62. Throughout the essay, but especially in the concluding paragraphs, the author suggests that Cinderella:

 (A) is less complex than she had originally thought herself to be.
 (B) is moving psychologically toward a condition of wholeness.
 (C) intentionally exploits the prince to bring about her own growth.
 (D) is weakened by her newly discovered wholeness.

63. One might draw the following conclusions from this passage:

 (A) Horney probably had the Cinderella story in mind when she formulated her theories.
 (B) Folktales and fairy tales such as Cinderella can be useful in illustrating aspects of psychological theories such as those of Horney.
 (C) Horney's theories are valid because the plots of the various versions of the Cinderella story bear them out.
 (D) Horney altered the story to make it fit her theories.

64. An appropriate title for this essay would be:

 (A) "If the Shoe Fits": Horney's Theories and the Cinderella Story.
 (B) The Narcissism of Cinderella.
 (C) The Stepmother as Heroine.
 (D) The Varieties of Magical Experience: The Shoe that Fits.

Passage III (Questions 65–69)

Probably most people enter medical school driven in large measure by their desire to help their fellow humankind. Although the prospects of achieving substantial wealth and reasonably high public esteem may be related motives, most consider that the search to live some form of the Golden Rule is an important reason for entering medical school. There is a growing perception among the general public, however, that many physicians are more interested in themselves and their families than in their patients. An understanding of the role conflicts experienced in medical school, residency training, and professional practice must begin in the earliest days of medical education.

The sociologist, Wendy Carlton, studied the development of medical students and concluded that three rather distinct perspectives, the moral, clinical, and legal, directly affect decision making by physicians. Her extensive observation suggested to her that "medical students are being socialized into using the clinical perspective to resolve clinical problems with little or no regard for the ethical aspects of their professional behavior. In particular there is a striking absence of both discussion of and concern with ethical issues, despite a growing body of literature that argues for the relevance of training in ethics for physicians in an age of technological medicine." The clinical perspective, to Carlton,

Adapted from addresses of Dr. Stephen M. Ayres, Dean, School of Medicine, Medical College of Virginia, Virginia Commonwealth University, 1990.

meant the traditional evaluation of the patient to create a "clinical picture" and, indeed, she entitled her book *In Our Professional Opinion.*

Carlton found that medical students upon entering medical school use the moral, clinical, and legal perspectives in that order. After acquiring clinical experience they apply the ranking used by physicians: clinical, legal, and then the moral. Hospital administrators invoke the legal, the clinical, and then the moral. "Laypersons," she contended, "use the moral perspective and depend on professionals to provide the clinical and legal perspectives, though they may use information from the media in an attempt to address the clinical and legal aspects of problem solution."

There is considerable concern on the part of many that the clinical perspective described by Carlton can degenerate into a callous disregard for patient interest. Shem, in 1978, presented a satirical view of the brutal world of the intern in his book, *The House of God.* Terry Mizrahi, a sociologist who observed medical house staff behavior in a large urban teaching center, felt that Dr. Shem's book "verified the overall detachment and dehumanizing resulting from the training process." Her book, *Getting Rid of Patients,* "substantiated a world of contradictions wherein the patient was oppressed while being characterized as the oppressor."

Melvin Konner, an anthropologist who entered medical school in his mid-thirties after a variety of experiences (including a two-year stint with faith healers from the hunter-gatherers of the Kalahari desert in Africa), described his educational experiences in *Becoming A Doctor.* He characterized physicians as "tough, brilliant, knowledgable, hardworking, and hard on themselves. They are reliable and competent in situations ranging from 18-month-long management of cancer chemotherapy through 18-hour-long brain surgery to emergencies in which life may hinge on what they can do in 18 seconds. They have experienced many things that are closed to others. With very few exceptions, they are professionals."

"Perhaps they have earned the right to arrogance; they certainly feel that they have. But one wonders if they can see the self-serving aspects of their behavior." Konner goes on to emphasize the importance of "a nonphysical aspect to healing, which I am prepared to call spiritual. It relates to heart and mind, hope and will, love and courage, values and ideas, social and cultural—including religious—life. In the hospital, I learned to keep my thoughts to myself about all such matters. There, the pretense is that everyone knows about them, and it is unnecessary to talk of them. In reality, everyone 'knows' about them but practically nobody cares, except insofar as finding them the source of a good laugh. Such cynicism, which increases during the medical school years, deeply affects the young physicians' view of life—not just of illness but of the whole human experience. They have trained themselves to participate just so far and no farther with, say, a terminal cancer patient in his or her search for personal meaning; but then they cannot simply slough off this habit of diffidence when it comes to their own search for meaning, when they contemplate the course of their own lives. It is less than appealing, what this makes of them; yet I love them in some crazy way . . . I would not want my daughter or son to be one or to marry one . . . Yet of course, when I am in trouble—and notice that I do not say 'if'—I will go to them, and they will improve my chances."

The life of the medical student is challenging and at times frustrating. Although intelligence and good undergraduate preparation are essential, they are not enough. Medicine is really the study of the human condition. What was once called "bedside manner" or "attitude" really means an understanding of the ingredients of human happiness. Although good health seems essential for the enjoyment of life, it is clearly not enough. And the advantages of good health frequently must be tempered by the need for reasonable diet, reasonable shelter, and love and understanding. The practice of medicine is a calling, not a business. Physician-healers must know the science of health and disease but must also know what comprises the total experience that generally is called "being human." The first year of medical education, and part of the second, emphasizes the science of medicine. The patient experience toward the end of the first year of medical education, and the remaining years of education, are designed to help the student internalize the view that the practice of medicine must be based on the broadest possible understanding of the human condition. "The secret of the care of the patient is in caring for the patient."

65. The author could have chosen as a title for this passage:

 (A) Professional Growth of the Practicing Physician.
 (B) The Development of Medical Students.
 (C) The Life of the Medical Student.
 (D) The Development of the Physician.

66. The medical student of today:

 (A) is greatly concerned with achieving high public esteem.
 (B) needs only superior intelligence and good undergraduate education to succeed.
 (C) hopes to marry a classmate in order to have a more congenial marriage.
 (D) is concerned and wants to serve humanity.

67.   Carlton suggests that as medical students undergo their training:

(A)   the ethical and moral issues predominate their decision-making process.

(B)   socialization elevates clinical decision making as a predominant force.

(C)   they are greatly influenced by hospital administrators who concentrate on legal issues.

(D)   they soon feel that they have earned the right to arrogance because of their thorough training.

68.   In its discussion of the balance between the science of medical practice and what could be termed the art of dealing with patients, the passage implies that:

(A)   good health is enough for the enjoyment of life.

(B)   love and understanding of human emotions are not serious considerations in the overall scheme of a human being.

(C)   bedside manner can be learned.

(D)   medicine must use as its basis for practice a broad appreciation of life and humankind.

69.   Which of the following statement(s) is/are *contradicted by* the passage?

(A)   Medical education should not consider the role conflicts experienced by students of medicine.

(B)   Laypersons focus quickly on the clinical and legal perspectives.

(C)   Physicians concentrate on their own happiness and are not hard on themselves.

(D)   All of the above.

Passage IV (Questions 70–75)

Throughout the various phyla of the plant and animal kingdom, numerous species have evolved. It is apparent that sexual reproduction plays an important role in the continuation of the species and in the expression of different phenotypes within the species. This mode of reproduction is accomplished by the fusion of two gametes that will give rise to a zygote. In order for future generations to maintain the same number of chromosomes as their parents, the gametes must undergo a reduction in chromosome number. If the offspring express phenotypic traits that are different from those of their parents, there must be a rearrangement of the DNA within the chromosomes. The reduction of the number of chromosomes and mixing of the gene pool are accomplished by the process of meiosis.

The process of meiosis is characterized by a naturally occurring sequence of events that are usually artificially subdivided into ten different stages. The first five stages constitute the first or reductional division of meiosis. At the end of the reductional division, the chromosomes are reduced to one-half their original number (haploid). The last five stages constitute the second or equatorial division of meiosis. Germ cells undergoing meiosis give rise to haploid gametes that contain one representative of each type of chromosome. The chromosomes of the gametes may also demonstrate variations in genetic composition due to crossing over that takes place during the first prophase.

Replication of DNA occurs during interphase before the process of meiosis begins. The condensation and coiling of chromatin to form chromosomes marks the beginning of prophase 1, the first stage of meiosis. Homologous chromosomes pair with one another to form a structure called a bivalent. Next, each chromosome splits lengthwise to form two chromatids. The homologous pairs of chromosomes are now composed of four chromatids that are referred to as a tetrad. The chromatids of tetrads become short and thick and breaks may occur in them. The breaks are eventually repaired but segments of different chromatids may be joined together. This process, referred to as crossing-over, enables segments of two different chromatids to be joined together. This enables the gametes to receive chromosomes derived from segments of both homologous chromosomes. In the second stage of meiosis or metaphase 1, the nuclear membrane disappears, a spindle apparatus forms, and the homologous pairs align along the equatorial plate of the cell. In anaphase 1, the homologous chromosomes migrate to opposite poles of the cell. Telophase 1 is characterized by the complete separation of the homologous pairs, and the spindle apparatus disappears. The nuclear membrane begins to reform and in many organisms a cytoplasmic division may occur at this stage.

After a brief interphase, prophase II begins. Prophase II is the first stage in the second or equatorial division of meiosis. It is characterized by the condensing of chromatin to form the chromosomes. During metaphase II, the spindle apparatus forms and the chromosomes line up along the equatorial plate. In anaphase II, the daughter chromosomes migrate to opposite poles of the cell. Anaphase II differs from the first anaphase in that the centromere divides and the two chromatids now become

From Hugo R. Seibel and Kenneth E. Guyer. *How to Prepare for the Medical College Admission Test*, 6th ed. Hauppauge. New York: Barron's Educational Series. Inc., 1990.

the daughter chromosomes. The daughter chromosomes separate completely and reach opposite poles of the cell in telophase II. Subsequent divisions of the cytoplasm result in the formation of two daughter cells that have a haploid number of chromosomes.

The two divisions of the germ cell during meiosis produce four gametes with one-half the original number of chromosomes.

70. According to this passage, at the end of the reductional division of meiosis:

    (A) four haploid sets of chromosomes are produced.
    (B) the homologous pairs of chromosomes are completely separated.
    (C) the chromatin duplicates and coils.
    (D) the centromeres divide and daughter chromosomes move to opposite poles of the cell.

71. At which state or phase does the process known as "crossing-over" occur?

    (A) during the equatorial division
    (B) before the tetrad separates
    (C) during anaphase I
    (D) during prophase II

72. The phase during which there is a duplication of the chromatin is known as:

    (A) metaphase I.
    (B) anaphase II.
    (C) telophase I.
    (D) interphase.

73. Which process from the list below makes variation in genetic composition possible?

    (A) the formation of homologous pairs
    (B) mitotic division of germ cells
    (C) crossing over
    (D) random mutations

74. Using information provided in the passage, one could reasonably conclude that:

    (A) all species in both the plant and animal kingdom are capable of sexual reproduction.
    (B) haploid cells are found only in animals.
    (C) four functional gametes are always formed by the process of meiosis.
    (D) zygote formation may produce an offspring that has the same number of chromosomes as its parents.

75. Which of the following statement(s) is/are *supported by* the passage?

    (A) Meiosis is artificially subdivided into ten stages.
    (B) Reproduction results in phenotypic expression.
    (C) DNA duplicates before meiosis starts.
    (D) All of the above.

Passage V (Questions 76–80)

Does the order of a child's birth in a family have a bearing on the type of adult he/she will grow up to be, or is the theory of ordinal position simply an interesting topic of cocktail party conversation? Although it has been the highlight of numerous debates and the subject of various studies, ordinal position remains a little-understood personality variable.

Consider the oldest child in a family of three children. Parents often claim that their firstborn has a solid head on his/her shoulders, behaves in a mature manner, and is capable of getting along with adults. This important family member often exhibits a quiet front, yet is able to take the lead, care for his/her siblings, and act like a miniature adult. Parents view the firstborn as an intelligent individual who will grow up to be a pillar of the community. A perfect illustration of the importance of being firstborn can be seen in the old custom of primogeniture that was particularly popular during the feudal period in Europe.

Primogeniture allowed the oldest member of a family, in most situations oldest male, to inherit all lands and possessions of his parents, to the exclusion of his siblings. The ordinal position of being the firstborn male therefore carried much power, as the firstborn was considered to be intelligent, level-headed, and capable of taking over as family protector and landlord once the father died. Theoretically the oldest would be unselfish and see to the care of the younger family members, but in actuality this was often not the case. Outlawed in the United States and no longer the mode of inheritance in Europe for today's population as a whole, primogeniture was in evidence as late as the 1920s and can still be seen in degree with some of Europe's royal families.

The second-born child in a family of three is pictured quite differently from the oldest. This child is much more lively, less willing to take orders, does not show the same interest in adults, and often has difficulty communicating with them. He/she may even become a "problem" child in school. Teachers have been heard to complain that "B is not in the least like A was . . . ."

From Hugo R. Seibel and Kenneth E. Guyer. *How to Prepare for the Medical College Admission Test*, 6th ed. Hauppauge. New York: Barron's Educational Series. Inc., 1990.

Could it be that the second born is striking out in an attempt to find his/her own place? The problems of the second child in a family seem to intensify even more when the "baby" comes along and moves him/her into the "middle child" position. Now he/she has to contend not only with a successful older brother or sister, but also with the youngest who seems to be the favorite.

The youngest child appears not to feel the need to measure up to anyone and goes along his/her own way to develop into an often exuberant, well-rounded individual. Because he/she is the baby, the mother doesn't expect this third sibling to function like a miniature adult, and she considers "cute" a great number of the actions that were viewed as unsatisfactory in the case of the other children.

Personality traits are not the only topic of interest in the ordinal position arena. The academic ability of children in various birth positions has also received attention. One interesting study reported a comparison of mathematics grades between women who were separated into three groups: (1) firstborn, (2) at least second born but not last born, and (3) last born in a family. Women without siblings were excluded from the study. The results indicate a statistical difference in mathematics grades between groups (1) and (3) but no other significant differences. Group (1) achieved higher mathematics grades than group (3).

Theories of motivation and anxiety have been advanced to explain the difference in achievement. The motivation theory states that the oldest child receives more encouragement from the parents than is given to other children. For a time, the first child is the only child, an experience not shared by the other children. Particularly during this early period the parents may try very hard to help the child, thus striving to experience vicariously their own unfulfilled expectations. The anxiety theory adds another factor to try to explain the lower achievement of the youngest child. Not only is the youngest child not pushed, as was the case with his/her older siblings, but this lack of parental pushing may be interpreted as lack of parental interest. The youngest child may develop feelings of anxiety, and these may interfere with performance. Thus, the youngest child may suffer as a result of less parental pressure and expectations as well as suffering from self-imposed anxiety, both contributing to lower performance.

76. The central thesis of the passage is that:

(A) the motivational drive (as well as the anxiety level of children) is directly linked to the order in which they are born.

(B) the development of a child's personality may be affected by the ordinal position he/she holds in his/her family.

(C) primogeniture, which is the custom of passing on property to the oldest male member of a family, is the vehicle used by the royal families of Europe to ensure that their fortunes will remain intact.

(D) ordinal position remains a little understood personality variable despite the fact that it is a popular topic both at the research and at the debate level.

77. Based on the information given in the passage, it is reasonable to conclude that:

(A) the oldest child in a family is the child best equipped to handle stressful situations.

(B) more research needs to be conducted before any concrete judgments can be made regarding the effect that birth order has on an individual's personality.

(C) academically, the youngest child tends to be lazy because he/she has been babied by parents and siblings.

(D) married couples should become well versed in ordinal position literature so that they will have a guide to follow when they are ready to have children.

78. What is the probable reason that the author used the paragraph on primogeniture in this passage?

(A) As a means of making the passage more interesting for the reader by introducing a historical topic.

(B) In order to make the reader aware of the fact that the firstborn was expected to share his inheritance with his younger siblings.

(C) To make the reader aware of the fact that the custom was outlawed in the United States around 1920.

(D) As a means of illustrating that ordinal position, especially the place of the firstborn, has been a topic of interest for a long period of time.

79.   Which of the following statements is/are *supported by* the information in the passage?

   I.   Parents often claim that firstborn children behave in a more mature manner than later-born.

   II.   The "baby" of the family is often a child with an outgoing personality.

   III.   By the time the third child comes along, mothers no longer seem to put the same emphasis on certain aspects of behavior that they did when raising their first.

   (A)   I only
   (B)   II only
   (C)   I and II only
   (D)   I, II, and III

80.   Which of the following statements is *contradicted by* the information given in the passage?

   (A)   Comparison to older siblings, by teachers and other adults, is the best method for stimulating the middle child to work harder.
   (B)   Second-born children who later move into the "middle child" position achieve on a higher plane in school than do second born who remain in the same position.
   (C)   The youngest child does not feel the need to measure up to anyone.
   (D)   The second-born child sometimes has a problem communicating with adults.

Passage VI (Questions 81–87)

Performance appraisals—"Who needs them? I'm doing a good job, so why does someone need to sit and put it in writing, then waste my time and theirs talking about it? If I'm doing something that they don't like, let them tell me about it when it happens." This is a typical comment heard from many employees.

The performance appraisal, if completed properly, can be one of the most useful tools a manager can use in developing and training subordinates regardless of what some employees may express. It is a compilation of the employee's strengths and weakness in one concise form. It serves to show the employee the areas in which a good job is being done and also indicates which areas need improvement. The appraisal serves as a permanent record that documents the employee's growth and progress or shows why a promotion is not offered. A performance appraisal forces a manager to discuss an employee's performance on a one-to-one basis and find out more about what the employee's opinions and aspirations might be. This area is often overlooked in the busy day-in and day-out routine of business. It gives the employee a chance to see what the boss really thinks about his or her work.

An interesting and often very beneficial way of handling a performance appraisal is to give employees a blank evaluation form a few days before the appraisal interview and ask that they rate themselves. When the appraisal takes place, the manager and employee compare their evaluations and work out the areas of disagreement so that each understands the other's position. An unusual result often takes place. Not only do the manager and employee end up with a better knowledge of each other, but they often find that their evaluations are very close to being in agreement If anything, the employees usually find that they have underrated themselves. An exception to this result, which the manager must be alert to recognize, is that an unsatisfactory performer may evaluate his or her performance higher than does the manager. The appraisal interview in this situation can often be more valuable than that of the satisfactory performer. It gives the manager an opportunity to counsel an already trained employee and turn around the performance rather than having to seek out and train a replacement. The manager must evaluate the time expense, and attitude of the present employee against the time and expense of hiring and training a new employee.

Performance appraisals, properly administered, can cut down on turnover and greatly increase the morale of a department. The result is increased productivity, which is really what we are all striving to accomplish.

Although standard procedure in industry for many years, performance appraisals have also reached higher education. In recent years college students have come to see themselves as purchasing a service, specifically that of education. They have demanded greater accountability, asking that the remuneration of faculty members be tied to teaching effectiveness. Many faculty members agree with the concept in theory but feel that measurement of teaching effectiveness is flawed.

Teaching effectiveness is often determined through evaluations by administrators, faculty colleagues, or students, or by a combination of two or more of these evaluations. Students are usually most interested in evaluations by students, believing that they are the "consumers" who are most directly affected by the quality of the "product" called teaching. Faculty members counter that evaluations by students are flawed, in that they are affected by the charisma (or lack of it) of the instructor, the level of difficulty of the subject matter, and the grades given in the course.

A more objective method has been suggested by various groups—the student performance at the end of the course.

From Hugo R. Seibel and Kenneth E. Guyer. *How to Prepare for the Medical College Admission Test,* 6th ed. Hauppauge, New York: Barron's Educational Series, Inc., 1990.

All students taking a particular course could be given a standard test; mean scores in sections taught by different instructors could then be compared and related to each instructor's teaching effectiveness. The results could be affected, of course, by the students' IQs, motivation, and prior instruction in the material covered by the course.

81. Of the positive aspects pertaining to the use of performance appraisals, which of those listed below is/are directly alluded to in the passage?

   (A) The performance appraisal gives the employee and the manager a time to discuss the employee's future in private.
   (B) Employees and managers usually can work out their differences during the appraisal interview.
   (C) Performance appraisals often lead to a better understanding between managers and employees and eventually can lead to increased productivity.
   (D) All of the above.

82. Which of the following statement(s) is/are NOT *supported nor contradicted by* the information in the passage?

   (A) Most large companies are now using the performance appraisal method because it has been proven a highly effective tool for dismissing unsatisfactory employees.
   (B) All performance appraisals are preceded by giving employees blank forms to rate themselves.
   (C) Managers feel that performance appraisals are a waste of time.
   (D) All of the above.

83. Which of the following statements is/are *contradicted by* the information in the passage?

   (A) A satisfactorily performing employee will rate himself or herself higher than the manager.
   (B) A performance appraisal points out only the weak areas of performance.
   (C) A performance appraisal is the most useful tool a manager uses in developing and training subordinates.
   (D) All of the above.

84. Some faculty members, addressing concerns about the accuracy and validity of student evaluations of teaching, caution that:

   (A) all suggested methods of evaluation of teaching effectiveness are quite subjective.
   (B) the charisma of the instructor is a factor in evaluation of teaching effectiveness.
   (C) evaluations of an instructor's teaching effectiveness are unaffected by student grades.
   (D) evaluations of an instructor's teaching effectiveness are affected by the time of day when lectures are given.

85. According to the passage, greater difficulty of the course would have what effect on student ratings of teacher effectiveness?

   (A) lower ratings
   (B) higher ratings
   (C) no effect
   (D) the passage does not say

86. The author indicates that students are most interested in ratings of teaching effectiveness when determined by:

   (A) evaluation by faculty colleagues.
   (B) evaluation by administrators.
   (C) evaluation by students.
   (D) objectively determined progress of the performance of the class.

87. Regarding performance appraisals in industry and student evaluations of teaching, the passage asserts that:

   (A) students view themselves as consumers.
   (B) performance evaluations benefit the parties involved.
   (C) performance appraisals can lead to increased productivity.
   (D) all of the above are true statements.

Passage VII (Questions 88–92)

Paul Tillich, in his article "The Lost Dimension in Religion," asserts that in contemporary Western society there is an absence of spirituality; moreover, that in spite of a growing interest in religion, and because of it, the religious element as Tillich defines it has all but vanished. The popularity of "go-to-church-every-Sunday" and the televangelism of the '80s belong to the "concrete religion" of literal hermeneutics (the science of interpreting an author's words or scriptures), rituals, and institutions.

The lost dimension as Tillich describes it is the loss of each individual's asking himself or herself basic and important existential questions such as: "What is the meaning of life? Where do we come from, where do we go to? What shall we do, what should we become in the short stretch between birth and death?" This spiritual "dimension of depth" is lost to modern man, he says, and "religion as the state of being grasped by an infinite concern" is absent.

Though written 30 years ago, this observation is still insightful today, perhaps even more so. Tillich explains how spiritual depth has become lost to contemporary Man. He traces the causes to Man's relationship with Nature and with himself, a relationship in which Nature is "subjected scientifically and technically" by the whims of Man, and self-knowledge is nearly nonexistent.

But, Tillich claims that, though today's generations lack the courage to ask themselves weighty eschatological questions (dealing with final matters, such as death), previous generations had the courage to do so. On this point, Tillich is slightly evasive. Does he mean that, say, a rise in materialism and technology parallels a drop in spirituality, and that previous generations who were less materialistic and technologically oriented were more spiritual? Perhaps, but he seems to rely heavily on our technologically oriented lives as evidence of a decline in spirituality. One might agree with him on this point but still believe that the roots go much deeper, and that our technology-based living and subsequent relationship with Nature is indeed an effect of something else as much as it is a cause of a loss of spirituality. Might not the dualistic perspective implicit in our own philosophical heritage, which seeks to divide the whole into parts, be called into question, along with the scientific method and "value-free" science? The present-day relationship between Man and Nature may well be a cause of the "loss of the dimension of depth"; but one could also argue that the seeds were sown a long time ago, so long ago that a more appropriate discussion of the loss of spiritual depth would include Man's relationship to technology as well.

The true religion, according to Tillich, moves vertically, hence "depth." It involves a personal dimension as well; personal existential questions ask for personal existential answers. And what Tillich sees in present-day religion (institutional and literalistic) is a horizontal aspect, a dimension that denies itself "basic and universal meaning" and the symbolic interpretation of sacred texts. This "horizontal" religion goes hand-in-hand with contemporary horizontal living, where technological/industrial society makes things " 'better and better,' 'bigger and bigger,' " there is "movement ahead without end," and "every moment is filled with something" whether it be television or a 40-hour-a-week job. In the horizontal dimension, "no one can experience depth . . . [or start] becoming aware of himself." Symptomatic of this kind of life is the question of whether or not God exists, a "discussion in which both sides are wrong, because the discussion itself is wrong and possible only after the loss of the dimension of depth."

Tillich advocates a kind of personal inquiry, a soul-searching "in spite of the loss of the dimension of depth"; an asking of questions such as "What is the meaning of Life?" But Tillich, for all his discussion of spirituality, makes no reference to the intuitive side of Man's nature. Tillich seems to imply that existential questions and any answers they might find are rational in their relationship to one another, and that the latter follows logically from the former; that there is indeed an answer that can be articulated. I suspect that this perspective is still inside the cultural context that gave rise to the loss of the dimension of depth in the first place—perhaps Tillich needs to step out of that context and into a context that is intuitive and in which personal existential questions are acknowledged from a source much deeper than the rational mind. It is perhaps the intuitive/spiritual that is the true religious character that, as Tillich says, "in spite of the loss of dimension of depth, its power is present, and is most present in those who are aware of the loss . . . ."

88.   The author of this passage observes that according to Tillich, contemporary society:

(A) is no longer interested in religion.
(B) suffers from a loss of spirituality.
(C) is more than willing to ask itself weighty existential questions.
(D) none of the above.

89. Which of the following, according to the passage, accurately reflects Tillich's view?

    (A) True religion moves vertically.
    (B) True religion is the same as present-day (institutional and literalistic) religion.
    (C) Present-day society encourages individuals to ask deep questions about human existence.
    (D) True religion asks questions addressing whether or not God exists.

90. Although the passage reflects general agreement with Tillich on many points, the author disagrees with Tillich on which of the following?

    (A) his assertion that modern man lacks true religion
    (B) his belief that people are more materialistic today than in the past
    (C) his definition of spirituality
    (D) his failure to take into account the intuitive side of human nature in discussing ways by which individuals can find answers to spiritual questions

91. The author finds Tillich's ideas about the lost dimension in religion:

    (A) less valid than they were when Tillich wrote them 30 years ago.
    (B) at least as insightful as they were 30 years ago.
    (C) interesting but too theoretical to be applied to actual human beings.
    (D) illustrative of T.S. Eliot's idea that modern man lives in a spiritual wasteland.

92. An appropriate title for this essay might be:

    (A) The Relevance of Tillich's Ideas Thirty Years Later.
    (B) The Optimism of Paul Tillich.
    (C) Tillich as Champion of Man's Intuition.
    (D) The Tillich that No One Knows.

WRITING SAMPLE

TIME—2 ESSAYS
60 MINUTES (30 MINUTES/TOPIC)

Directions: This is a test of your writing skills. The test consists of two parts. You will have 30 minutes to complete each part. Use your time efficiently. Before you begin writing each of your responses, read the assignment carefully to understand exactly what you are being asked to do. Because this is a test of your writing skills, your response to each part should be as well organized and clearly written as you can make it in the time allotted.

93. Consider this statement:

   Men are dependent on circumstances, not circumstances on men.

   Herodotus

   Write a unified essay in which you perform the following tasks. Explain the meaning of the above statement. Describe a specific situation where circumstances might be dependent on individuals. Discuss what you think determines whether or not individuals are dependent on circumstances or vice versa.

94. Consider this statement:

   The voluntary death by which a man puts an end to intolerable suffering is really an act of redemption.

   Ernst Heinrich Haeckel
   (German biologist)

   Write a unified essay in which you perform the following tasks. Explain what you think the above statement means. Describe a specific situation in which the voluntary death by which a person put an end to intolerable suffering would not be an act of redemption. Discuss what you think determines the choice of voluntary death in the face of human suffering.

BIOLOGICAL SCIENCES

TIME—70 MINUTES FOR 52 QUESTIONS

Directions: The following questions or incomplete statements are in groups. Preceding each series of questions or statements is a paragraph or a short explanatory statement, a formula or set of formulas, or a definition. Read the written material and then answer the questions or complete the statements. Select the ONE BEST ANSWER for each question and indicate your selection by marking the corresponding letter of your choice on the Answer Form. Eliminate those alternatives you know to be incorrect and then select an answer from among the remaining alternatives.

Passage I (Questions 95–99)

The function of the thyroid gland is to produce colloidal material containing the thyroid hormones T_3 (triiodothyronine) and T_4 (thyroxin), which affect the rate of metabolism of all tissues.

The iodides consumed by the body are absorbed and carried to the iodide pool in the extracellular fluid via the circulatory system. Five basic events occur during the production of thyroid hormone: (a) trapping iodide; (b) oxidation of iodide to iodine; (c) synthesis of hormone; (d) storage of hormone in the thyroid follicle; and (e) release of hormone into the circulation. TSH (thyroid stimulating hormone) from the anterior pituitary influences the trapping mechanism. It can be stated that thyroid hormone: (a) controls the rate of metabolism; (b) controls growth, maturation, and differentiation of the organism; and (c) influences nervous system activity.

Problems associated with thyroid function are:

1. **Cretinism**—a congenital failure of proper development. The cretin is a dwarf physically and mentally.

2. **Myxedema**—an acquired thyroid deficiency in the adult. This deficiency can be due to thyroidectomy, neoplasms, or a pituitary deficiency in TSH secretion. The clinical picture is the presentation of a patient who is fairly heavy, phlegmatic, and devoid of expression; the skin is rough and dry and sensitive to cold. The patient is sluggish mentally and physically. Laboratory tests show a low basal metabolic rate, low protein-bound iodine, and a high serum cholesterol level.

3. **Graves' disease**—an increased activity of the thyroid gland. The patient exhibits loss of weight, nervousness, irritability, increased metabolic rate, rapid heart rate, and sweating.

A patient is brought into the emergency room and, upon examination, a thyroid goiter is discovered. You suspect that he is suffering from a thyroid disorder, and you ask the intern for a definition of *hypothyroidism.*

95. He responds that *hypothyroidism* is the general term for syndromes that reflect:

   (A) increased secretion of thyroid hormones.
   (B) decreased secretion of thyroid hormones.
   (C) no change in secretion of thyroid hormones.
   (D) increased secretion of thyroid stimulating hormone releasing factor.

96. A basal metabolism rate test is ordered that measures the rate of oxidative metabolism. In hypothyroidism, this rate is:

   (A) above normal.
   (B) normal.
   (C) below normal.
   (D) not significant in your diagnosis.

97. Because of the hypothyroidism that you suspect, you would also consider that this patient:

   I.   has gained weight.
   II. converts less food into energy.
   III. stores more food as fat.
   IV. has an accelerated metabolic rate.

   (A) I, III, and IV only
   (B) II, III, and IV only
   (C) I, II, and III only
   (D) all of the above

98. The physical examination in this patient would also yield the following:

   (A) The patient is mentally sluggish.
   (B) The patient's skin is rough and dry.
   (C) The patient's serum cholesterol level would be elevated.
   (D) All of the above.

99. If hyperthyroidism were the diagnosis you would reason and find:

   (A) a pituitary deficiency in TSH.
   (B) a block in the oxidation of iodide to iodine.
   (C) a phlegmatic patient.
   (D) irritability.

Passage II (Questions 100–107)

The ABO blood grouping system is explained on the basis of a single triallelic system with genes A, B, and O operating at a single genetic locus. Phenotypic and genotypic characteristics may be expressed as follows:

Phenotype	Genotype
A	A/A; A/O
B	B/B; B/O
O	O/O
AB	A/B

The A and B genes appear to be codominant; they are dominant over O, which is recessive.

Paternity will be excluded if the child (a) has an antigen that is present in neither the mother nor the putative father, and (b) does not have an antigen that the putative father has and would have had to give to his progeny (e.g., a type O child and a type AB putative father).

Correct reassignment of infants misassigned to parents in a hospital is often achieved by looking for any of the following kinds of incompatibilities between the infants and the couples and then assigning each infant to a couple with which only compatibilities exist:

1. The child has an antigen that is present in neither spouse.
2. The child lacks one or more antigens that either spouse or both spouses would have had to give him/her.

Increased probability of exclusion of alleged paternity or of a correct parental reassignment of misassigned infants results in several kinds of blood groups, HLA, and the following kinds of genetically determined proteins are also included in the studies: hemoglobin, serum proteins, red cell enzymes, and several other enzymes.

The ABO blood group is transmitted in humans as alleles A and B that are codominant, occurring at the same autosomal locus as a recessive allele O. In some cases it may be utilized to assist in determining paternity or in reuniting a lost child with his or her biological parents.

100. A woman of blood type O claims a child of blood type AB, and alleges that the father is a man of blood type B. The most likely explanation is that:

   (A) these are the biological parents.
   (B) she is the mother but the man is not the father.
   (C) neither is a possible parent of the child.
   (D) she is not the mother but the man's blood type does not rule him out as the father.

101. If the man in question 100 is found to have previously fathered a child of blood type O, the chance that a child of the man and the woman in this question would be blood type O is:

   (A) zero.
   (B) 25%.
   (C) 33%.
   (D) 50%.

102. With the information from the above question, the chance that any child of the man and woman would be a girl with blood type B is

   (A) zero.
   (B) 25%.
   (C) 33%.
   (D) 50%.

103. The above man with a phenotype B will possess which of the following genotypes?

   (A) A/O
   (B) B/O
   (C) O/O
   (D) A/B

104. Phenotype may be defined as:

   (A) genetic makeup of an individual.
   (B) hidden traits of an individual.
   (C) unrelated characteristics.
   (D) visible expression of genotype.

105. Alleles are genes that:

    (A) arise during the cross-over process.
    (B) are linked to one chromosome only.
    (C) are always sex-linked and are transmitted from mothers to their sons.
    (D) occupy corresponding positions on homologous chromosomes.

106. Rh-related hemolytic anemia of the newborn (erythroblastosis foetalis) may result when the:

    (A) father, mother, and fetus are all Rh negative.
    (B) father and mother are Rh positive, but the fetus is Rh negative.
    (C) mother is Rh negative and the fetus is Rh positive.
    (D) mother is Rh positive and the fetus is Rh negative.

107. The czarina of Russia and Queen Victoria of England were normal women who produced sons suffering from hemophilia, a disease that is caused by a sex-linked recessive gene, h. The more common dominant gene, H, produces normal blood clotting. The genotype of these women must have been:

    (A) HH.
    (B) Hh.
    (C) hh.
    (D) none of the above.

Questions 108–112 are NOT based on a descriptive passage.

108. Which of the following catalyzes synthesis of messenger RNA in eukaryotes?

    (A) RNA polymerase I
    (B) RNA polymerase II
    (C) RNA polymerase III
    (D) RNA polymerase IV

109. Which of the following organelles are involved in the synthesis of proteins that will be secreted from a eukaryotic cell?

    (A) free ribosomes
    (B) mitochondria
    (C) ribosomes on rough endoplasmic reticulum
    (D) Golgi bodies

110. A normal vertebrate skeletal muscle fiber (cell) is:

    (A) uninucleate and striated.
    (B) multinucleate and striated.
    (C) uninucleate and nonstriated (or unstriated).
    (D) multincleate and nonstriated (or unstriated).

111. The proximal convoluted tubule in the human kidney is primarily involved in:

    (A) filtration of material from blood to urine.
    (B) establishment of a high salt concentration in the kidney.
    (C) reabsorption of useful solutes from urine.
    (D) hormonally controlled water reabsorption from urine.

112. The two cerebral hemispheres in the mammalian brain are connected by the:

    (A) corpus callosum.
    (B) pons.
    (C) medulla oblongata.
    (D) cerebellum.

Passage III (Questions 113–119)

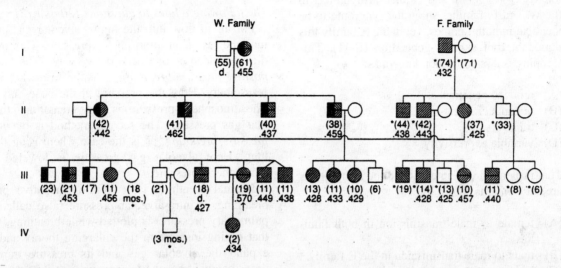

Study of *W* and *F* families showing presence of syncope, electrocardiographic evidence of prolonged Q-T interval and abnormal audiogram. The propositus (Case 1) is III-10 (**arrow**). Case 2 is her cousin (III-2). Figures in parentheses indicate subject's age. Intervals (in hundredths of a second) appear directly below each subject's age. **Black** symbols indicate abnormal audiogram; hatched symbols indicate prolonged QTc interval (0.425 second) (////) or syncope (\\\\); d = died. A history, physical examination and one or more electrocardiograms were obtained in all patients. An audiogram was obtained in all cases, except those marked by a star, in which hearing was only examined clinically.

Inheritance of Q-T prolongation (≥ 0.425 sec) and cardiac arrhythmias in the W. and F. families is shown in the above pedigree, which was ascertained through the proposita, III-10, who suffered cardiac arrest and had to be resuscitated 12 hours after her first delivery following an uneventful pregnancy. A major objective of the study was the determination of whether prolonged Q-T interval in these families was (1) the autosomal recessive form, Jervell, Lang-Nielsen syndrome, also characterized by high-frequency perceptive deafness, (2) Ward-Romano syndrome, an autosomal dominant form, not associated with deafness, or (3) perhaps a third type, inherited in some other fashion.*

113.   Prolonged Q-T interval and cardiac arrhythmias appear to be phenotypic manifestations of the same allele, a phenomenon known as:

(A)   genetic heterogeneity.
(B)   genetic polymorphism.
(C)   pleiotropism.
(D)   phenocopies.

114.   The pedigree clearly shows that the arrhythmias in the W. family are dominant because they:

(A)   affect both monozygotic twins in the third generation.
(B)   are sometimes associated with deafness.
(C)   show unbroken lineal descent.
(D)   are transmitted by both sexes.

115.   Likewise, the pedigree clearly shows that deafness in the W. family is also dominant, but the arrhythmias are the result of an allele at a different locus because:

(A)   nondisjunction occurs among the progeny of couple II- I @ 2.
(B)   disjunction occurs among the progeny of couple II-1 @ 2.
(C)   independent assortment occurs among the children of couple II-1 @ 2.
(D)   meiotic drive occurs among the children of couple II-1 @ 2.

*Adapted by Dr. J. I. Townsend, Virginia Commonwealth University, from "Q-T Prolongation and Ventricular Arrhythmias With and Without Deafness in the Same Family;" E.C. Mathews, A. W. Blount, and J.I. Townsend. *The American Journal of Cardiology*, (1972): 29:702.

116. Careful comparative diagnostic studies of prolonged Q-T interval and cardiac arrhythmias in the W. and F. families show the syndrome to be identical in both families, yet in the F. family this dominant trait skips a generation (II-11). This skipping is a phenomenon known as:

    (A) reduced penetrance.
    (B) unequal crossing-over.
    (C) transversion.
    (D) variable expressivity.

117. That prolonged Q-T interval and the arrhythmias are autosomal is shown by:

    (A) female to male transmission in both families.
    (B) male to male transmission in the F. family.
    (C) lack of male to male transmission.
    (D) male to female transmission.

118. That deafness is autosomal is shown by:

    (A) male to male transmission.
    (B) lack of male to male transmission.
    (C) two affected males (II-3 and II-5) have daughters whose hearing is normal.
    (D) an affected female (II-2) has a daughter whose hearing is normal.

119. The proposita (III-10) has by far the greatest prolonged Q-T interval (0:570 sec) in this extended pedigree. The likely explanation is that she:

    (A) is an example of genetic anticipation.
    (B) has a deletion of the locus on one chromosome.
    (C) has a duplication of the locus on one chromosome.
    (D) is homozygous for the mutant allele.

Passage IV (Questions 120–123)

The following relates to questions 120 and 121:

For air to flow into the lungs, alveolar gas pressure must be less than atmospheric pressure. This pressure difference can be produced in two ways. The first is by *positive pressure breathing*, as is the case when using a resuscitator. Here the pressure at the nose and mouth (the atmospheric pressure) is made greater than the alveolar gas pressure. The second method is by *negative pressure breathing*, as is the case when using the iron lung. Here alveolar gas pressure is lowered below atmospheric pressure.

Normal breathing is a form of negative pressure breathing. If intra-alveolar pressure (also called intra-pulmonary pressure) is plotted while breathing, we see that during inspiration the enlarging thorax and lungs expand the alveolar gas and its pressure transiently drops below atmospheric pressure (i.e., it becomes negative). This pressure difference causes air to flow into the lungs. Expiration involves transiently elevating the intra-alveolar pressure above atmospheric pressure. This occurs as the collapsing chest-lung system compresses the alveolar gas. Gas then flows out of the lungs.

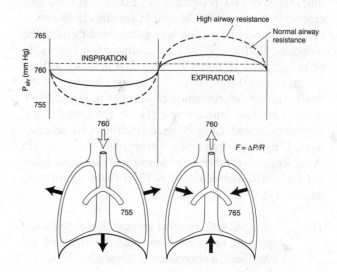

Air flow is directly proportional to the pressure difference between alveolar gas and the atmosphere, and inversely proportional to airway resistance:

$$Flow\ (F) = \frac{P_{atm} - P_{alv}}{\text{Airway Resistance (R)}}$$

Thus, the greater the airway resistance, the greater the pressure difference required to produce any given flow. High airway resistance will produce greater fluctuations in intra-alveolar pressure during inspiration and expiration.

The severity of airway resistance is reflected in the *intrapleural pressure* as well as the intra-alveolar pressure during the breathing cycle. Before inspiration begins, the intrapleural pressure reflects the elastic strength with which the lungs are tending to collapse. Of course, at this volume (the FRC) the elastic force of the lungs is balanced by the elastic strength of the chest wall tending to expand. The intrapleural pressure is slightly negative (i.e., below atmospheric pressure).

During inspiration, the elastic recoil strength of the lungs progressively increases as the lungs are stretched. This alone would lower the intrapleural pressure (i.e., make it more negative). In addition, the lowered intra-alveolar pressure (reflecting airway resistance during inspiration) and tissue viscous resistance (which opposes the inflation effort) lower the intrapleural pressure even more. Thus, during inspiration the intrapleural pressure becomes even lower (more negative) than it would if the elastic forces existed alone. Of this additional decrease in intrapleural pressure from nonelastic resistances, 80% is due to pressure needed to overcome airway resistance; tissue viscous resistance accounts for only 20% of the nonelastic resistance.

At the end of inspiration, flow stops as intra-alveolar pressure equilibrates with atmospheric pressure. At this volume (FRC + TV), functional residual capacity (FRC) plus the tidal volume (TV), the intrapleural pressure reflects the elastic strength of the lungs tending to collapse. Since the lungs are stretched more during inspiration, the intrapleural pressure is lower (more negative) following inspiration than before. The functional residual capacity is the (tidal volume–anatomical dead space) × frequency of breathing. During normal breathing, the volume of air inspired (expired) is called the tidal volume.

During expiration, the elastic recoil strength of the lungs progressively decreases as the lungs deflate, and the intrapleural pressure rises (becomes less negative) accordingly. In addition, the elevated intra-alveolar pressure and the tissue viscous resistance oppose deflation and act outward against the intrapleural space. Therefore, the intrapleural pressure during expiration is higher (less negative) than it would be if the elastic forces were unopposed.

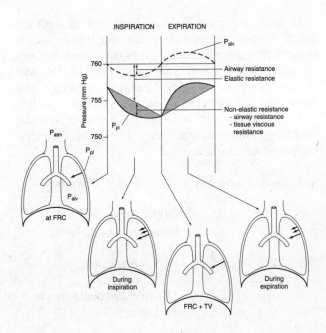

With a tidal volume of 500 ml, only 350 ml goes to the respiratory unit and 150 ml goes no further than the anatomic dead space. Most of the 350 ml that reaches the alveoli is involved in gas exchange, but some is a *"wasted volume"*—meaning it is a volume in excess of that needed to equilibrate with the blood passing through the capillaries of that area. A wasted volume occurs to some extent even in a healthy individual and will be produced when there is an elevated ventilation-perfusion ratio. An elevated ventilation-perfusion ratio occurs when either the blood flow is reduced or ventilation is in excess of that needed to equilibrate the volume of blood perfusing the area. Alveolar gas in an area with a high ventilation-perfusion ratio will exhibit increased oxygen and decreased carbon dioxide concentrations because of the excess oxygen delivery and carbon dioxide removal. The wasted volume plus the anatomic dead space equals the *physiologic dead space*. Even in a healthy individual the physiologic dead space is slightly larger than the anatomic dead space.

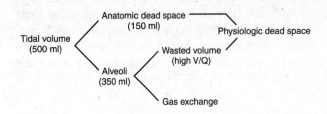

Alveolar ventilation refers to the volume of fresh air, which reaches the respiratory unit per minute and is equal to the rate of breathing times the volume of fresh air reaching the respiratory unit per breath (i.e., the tidal volume minus the anatomic dead space). *Dead space ventilation* is the volume of fresh air, which goes no further than the anatomic dead space per minute. Alveolar ventilation plus dead space ventilation equals the respiratory minute ventilation.

$$\text{Alveolar ventilation} = (TV - ADS) \times \text{Frequency}$$

$$= (500 - 150) \text{ ml} \times 12$$
$$\text{breaths/min} = 4.2 \text{ L/min}$$

$$\text{Dead space ventilation} = ADS \times \text{Frequency}$$

$$= 150 \text{ ml} \times 12 \text{ breaths/min} =$$
$$1.8 \text{ L/min}$$

The composition of alveolar air, reflecting the oxygen uptake by blood and carbon dioxide release from blood, has a lower PO_2 (100 mm Hg) and a higher PCO_2 (40 mm Hg) than that of atmospheric or moist tracheal air. Both alveolar air and atmospheric air have the same total pressures, since these compartments are connected by open tubes of the anatomic dead space.

Alveolar air is typically represented as having a constant composition. This is justified because the fluctuations which occur in PO_2 and PCO_2 with each breathing cycle are very slight. Because the volume of fresh air entering the alveoli (350 ml) is very small compared with the "pool" of alveolar air already in the lungs (FRC = 2,200 ml), the inspired fresh air is so diluted that the PO_2 will increase and the PCO_2 will decrease by only 1 or 2 mm Hg.

Assuming a constant oxygen uptake and carbon dioxide release by the body, the content of alveolar air will reflect the ventilatory rate of the lungs. Hyperventilation makes alveolar air more like fresh air, raising alveolar PO_2 and lowering PCO_2. Hypoventilation, in contrast, produces a lower PO_2 and an elevated PCO_2 in the alveoli. Similarly, not all areas of the lung have the same PO_2 and PCO_2. While some areas are relatively hyperventilated and have a high PO_2 and low PCO_2, other areas are simultaneously hypoventilated and have a low PO_2 and high PCO_2.

120. The driving pressure (ΔP) in breathing which causes air to flow into the lungs is:

(A) atmospheric pressure (P_{atm}).
(B) the intra-alveolar (intrapulmonary) pressure (P_{alv}).
(C) atmospheric pressure minus the intra-alveolar pressure.
(D) the intrapleural pressure (P_{pl}).

121. During inspiration, intra-alveolar pressure (P_{alv}):

(A) transiently goes below atmospheric pressure (P_{atm}).
(B) transiently goes above atmospheric pressure.
(C) equals atmospheric pressure.
(D) equals intrapleural pressure.

122. The alveolar ventilation per minute refers to the amount of fresh air that reaches the alveoli of the lungs per minute. Alveolar ventilation per minute equals the:

(A) functional residual capacity × frequency of breathing.
(B) physiologic dead space × frequency of breathing.
(C) anatomic dead space × frequency of breathing.
(D) (tidal volume − anatomic dead space) × frequency of breathing.

123. Hypoventilation produces which of the following changes in alveolar gas composition?

(A) The partial pressure of oxygen increases and the partial pressure of carbon dioxide decreases.
(B) The partial pressures of both oxygen and carbon dioxide increase.
(C) The partial pressure of oxygen decreases and the partial pressure of carbon dioxide increases.
(D) The partial pressures of both oxygen and carbon dioxide decrease.

Questions 124–126 are NOT based on a descriptive passage.

124. In an inducible operon such as the lac operon in *E. coli*, the repressor protein coded by the regulator gene binds to the _____ to inactivate the operon.

    (A) regulator gene
    (B) first structural gene in the operon
    (C) promoter
    (D) operator sequence

125. Ectoderm, mesoderm, and endoderm form as distinct layers during _____ in most animal embryos.

    (A) fertilization
    (B) organogenesis
    (C) cleavage
    (D) gastrulation

126. In humans, antibodies are synthesized by:

    (A) B lymphocytes and plasma cells.
    (B) granulocytes (neutrophils and eosinophils).
    (C) platelets.
    (D) the liver.

Passage V (Questions 127–131)

Toluene or methylbenzene is an important starting material for the synthesis of many aromatic compounds. The methyl group activates all unsubstituted carbons of the benzene ring for attack by electrophilic reagents, leading to substitution at one or more additional carbons. The *ortho, meta,* and *para* positions are substituted at different rates, depending on the capacity of the electron-donating methyl group to stabilize positively charged intermediates generated by the electrophilic attack. Unlike larger alkyl groups, the methyl group is too small to have a significant steric effect on the rate of substitution at the *ortho* position. Under appropriate conditions, the methyl group itself is often modified or derivatized, in which case, subsequent substitutions in the ring will be directed by the character of the modified group. Many different substituted products and positional isomers can be produced by manipulating reagents, reaction conditions, and the order of the various reactions. The *ortho, meta,* and *para* isomers usually differ sufficiently in properties to permit separation by standard physical methods. In any of the reactions of toluene, assume that ortho and para isomers can be separated.

127. The reaction of toluene with Br_2 in the presence of $FeBr_3$ would be expected to produce primarily:

    (A) benzyl bromide, $C_6H_5CH_2Br$.
    (B) *m*-bromotoluene.
    (C) *o* and *p*-bromotoluene.
    (D) an equimolar mixture of *m, o,* and *p*-bromotoluene.

128. The compound that undergoes electrophilic aromatic substitution more readily than toluene is:

    (A) chlorobenzene.
    (B) nitrobenzene.
    (C) acetophenone.
    (D) phenol.

129. The best sequence of reagents for conversion of toluene to *m*-nitrobenzoic acid is:

    (A) HNO_3-H_2SO_4, then oxidation with hot $KMnO_4$ or $K_2Cr_2O_7$.
    (B) Oxidation with hot $KMnO_4$ or $K_2Cr_2O_7$, followed by HNO_3-H_2SO_4.
    (C) Bromination of toluene with Br_2-$FeBr_3$, followed by displacement with $NaNO_2$.
    (D) Reaction of toluene with Br_2-$FeBr_3$, followed by oxidation with $KMnO_4$, or $K_2Cr_2O_7$, and then displacement of Br by $NaNO_2$.

130. The major product of the reaction of *p*-nitrotoluene with Br_2-$FeBr_3$ is:

    (A) 2-bromo-4-nitrotoluene.
    (B) 3-bromo-4-nitrotoluene.
    (C) *p*-nitrobenzyl bromide, *p*-$NO_2C_6H_4CH_2Br$.
    (D) 2, 6-dibromo-4-nitrotoluene.

131. Which of the following resonance structures is a contributor to the intermediate formed in the nitration of toluene to form *p*-nitrotoluene?

    (A)

    (B)

    (C)

    (D)

Passage VI (Questions 132–139)

The categories of necessary dietary nutrients include the essential amino acids, essential fatty acids, essential elements, and the vitamins. The nine essential amino acids for humans are found in all dietary proteins. They are called: phenylalanine, valine, threonine, tryptophan, isoleucine, methionine, histidine, leucine, and lysine. All other amino acids that are found in proteins are nonessential and can be synthesized in the body from other dietary sources. The one true essential fatty acid is linoleic. However, linoleic and arachidonic acids can help meet the nutritional requirement for this category of nutrients. Because generally all of these essential fatty acids are found in combinations of oils and fats, all three can be viewed as "essential" in a practical sense. Along with carbohydrates, we obtain both essential amino acid and fatty acids from the macronutrients (i.e., large quantities) of protein and fat respectively in our diet.

The essential elements are subcategorized as the electrolytes sodium, potassium, and chloride; the bulk essential minerals—calcium, phosphorus, and magnesium and the trace essential minerals—iron, zinc, selenium, iodine, cobalt, molybdenum, manganese, copper, chromium, and fluoride. All of these are needed, but the amount we need each day varies from micrograms to hundreds of milligrams. Vitamins are found in foods in water-soluble or fat soluble forms. The former includes vitamin C, thiamine, riboflavin, niacin, vitamin B_6, folacin, vitamin B_{12}, biotin, and pantothenic acid. The fat-soluble vitamins are vitamins A, D, E, and K. These are all required in the diet in trace amounts (i.e., micrograms to milligrams).

Choose the *one best* answer for each of the following:

132. Which of the following is *not* an essential nutrient?

    (A) valine
    (B) linoleic acid
    (C) glucose
    (D) vitamin E

133. Which of the following is *not* a vitamin?

    (A) thiamine
    (B) biotin
    (C) niacin
    (D) arachidonic acid

134. Which of the following is *not* a fat-soluble vitamin?

    (A) vitamin A
    (B) vitamin B_{12}
    (C) vitamin D
    (D) vitamin E

135. Which of the following is a bulk essential element?

    (A) selenium
    (B) copper
    (C) iron
    (D) calcium

136. A macronutrient is:

    I.   a carbohydrate.
    II. a protein.
    III a fat.
    IV. a vitamin.

    (A) I only
    (B) II only
    (C) I, II, and III
    (D) I, II, III, and IV

137. Regulation of the resorption of calcium from bone is controlled by the:

    (A) thyroid gland.
    (B) parathyroid glands.
    (C) thymus.
    (D) adrenal glands.

138. Undigested food is eliminated from the body by the process of:

    (A) exocytosis.
    (B) excretion.
    (C) egestion.
    (D) catabolism.

139. The energy released from the anaerobic respiration of a glucose molecule is less than that released from the aerobic respiration of a glucose molecule because:

    (A) aerobic respiration forms many more new, strong bonds than anaerobic respiration.
    (B) more enzymes are required for anaerobic respiration than for aerobic respiration.
    (C) anaerobic respiration occurs 24 hours a day, while aerobic respiration can occur only at night.
    (D) anaerobic respiration requires oxygen but aerobic respiration does not require oxygen.

Passage VI (Questions 140–142)

Blood samples from two groups of rats were assayed for luteinizing hormone (LH) in two separate radioimmunoassays. Half the rats were intact and half were orchidectomized. Some samples in each group were collected in the morning and some were collected in the afternoon. The data are summarized in the following table:

Assay I

	Intact or Orchid X	Sampled AM or PM	LH ng/ml
1	I	AM	5.0
2	O	AM	50
3	I	PM	4.8
4	O	PM	480
5	I	AM	5.2
6	O	AM	52
7	I	PM	5.1
8	O	PM	350
9	I	AM	4.9
10	O	AM	100

Assay 2

11	I	PM	7.5
12	O	PM	75
13	I	AM	7.7
14	O	AM	770
15	I	PM	7.3
16	O	PM	250
17	I	AM	7.4
18	O	AM	100
19	I	PM	7.6
20	O	PM	640

140. Based on the above table, which of the following statements is *not supported by* the information given?

    (A) Orchidectomy is followed by increased levels of LH in the blood.
    (B) Blood LH levels are higher in the afternoon than in the morning.
    (C) The differences between LH values in these two assays are probably explained by interassay variations because the ratios between intact and orchidectomized levels are similar.
    (D) LH release in the orchidectomized rats may be occurring episodically.

141. Which of the following conclusions is supported by the data?

    (A) The presence of the gonad inhibits LH secretion.
    (B) LH levels are higher in the morning than in the afternoon.
    (C) LH stimulates one or more functions in the gonad.
    (D) LH stimulates gamete production in the gonad.

142. The relationship between assay 1 and assay 2 is best explained by which of the following?

    (A) Values in assay 1 are higher than in assay 2.
    (B) Values in assay 2 are higher than in assay 1.
    (C) A systematic error occurred in assay 2.
    (D) A systematic error occurred in assay 1.

Questions 143–146 are NOT based on a descriptive passage.

143. Which hydrocarbon is a member of the series with the general formula C_nH_{2n-2}?

    (A) butane
    (B) ethene
    (C) benzene
    (D) ethyne

144. Which class of compounds has the general formula R–O–R′?

    (A) esters
    (B) alcohols
    (C) ethers
    (D) aldehydes

145. Of the functional groups listed below, which is incorrectly identified?

    (A) $-NH_2$ amino group

    (B) $-\overset{\text{O}}{\underset{\|}{C}}-CH_3$ acetyl group

    (C) $-\overset{\text{O}}{\underset{\|}{C}}-NH_2$ amide group

    (D) $-\overset{\text{O}}{\underset{\|}{C}}-OH$ hydroxyl group

146. An individual has at his disposal benzyl chloride, benzene, aluminum chloride, and sodium, and he wishes to synthesize diphenylmethane. He should react:

    (A) all four compounds.
    (B) benzyl chloride and sodium.
    (C) benzyl chloride, benzene, and aluminum chloride.
    (D) benzyl chloride, benzene, and sodium.

STOP

END OF TEST

Answer Key

MODEL EXAMINATION A

PHYSICAL SCIENCES

1. B	9. C	17. D	25. A	33. C	41. C	49. B
2. D	10. B	18. C	26. C	34. D	42. A	50. B
3. D	11. C	19. C	27. B	35. A	43. B	51. C
4. A	12. D	20. D	28. D	36. A	44. A	52. B
5. A	13. C	21. B	29. C	37. A	45. C	
6. B	14. A	22. A	30. C	38. D	46. D	
7. C	15. D	23. C	31. B	39. A	47. D	
8. B	16. B	24. A	32. B	40. B	48. C	

VERBAL REASONING

53. C	59. C	65. D	71. B	77. B	83. D	89. A
54. D	60. B	66. D	72. D	78. D	84. B	90. D
55. A	61. C	67. B	73. C	79. D	85. D	91. B
56. D	62. B	68. D	74. D	80. A	86. C	92. A
57. D	63. B	69. D	75. D	81. D	87. D	
58. B	64. A	70. B	76. D	82. D	88. B	

WRITING SAMPLE

93. See page 416 for a sample essay.

94. See page 417 for a sample essay.

BIOLOGICAL SCIENCES

95. B	103. B	111. C	119. D	127. C	135. D	143. D
96. C	104. D	112. A	120. C	128. D	136. C	144. C
97. C	105. D	113. C	121. A	129. B	137. B	145. D
98. D	106. C	114. C	122. D	130. A	138. C	146. C
99. D	107. B	115. C	123. C	131. B	139. A	
100. D	108. B	116. A	124. D	132. C	140. B	
101. D	109. C	117. B	125. D	133. D	141. A	
102. B	110. B	118. C	126. A	134. B	142. B	

ANSWERS EXPLAINED FOR MODEL EXAMINATION A

Physical Sciences

1. **(B)** The shortest wavelength corresponds to the highest photon energy, according to E = hc/λ. The maximum energy available occurs when the incident high-speed electron gives up all its energy at one time (in a bremsstrahlung process). If 80,000 volts is used to accelerate the electrons, the most energetic x-ray photon can have 80,000 eV of energy (but only a very small number of 80 keV photons will occur).

2. **(D)** The K_β transition is more energetic. This is shown by the shorter wavelength. The photon energy is $E = hf = hc/\lambda$. The K_α transitions are more probable. This is shown by the higher peak, which corresponds to a greater intensity due to a higher number of emitted photons.

3. **(D)** The minimum wavelength depends only on the accelerating voltage. The electrical work done in accelerating the electrons is equal to the maximum photon energy:

    $$eV_0 = hc/\lambda_{min}$$

4. **(A)** The peaks are characteristic of the *target* material. The photon energy emitted (say for an $n = 3$ to $n = 1$ transition) never changes. If V_0 is increased, the height of the peaks (intensity) will increase. (If the voltage is decreased to a very *low* value the peaks may not be seen because the incident electrons do not have enough energy to eject an inner shelf electron on the target. Thus a continuous spectrum can occur without the peaks.)

5. **(A)** The photon energy formula, $E = hc/\lambda$, shows that the photons of shortest (minimum) wavelength are the most energetic. Only a few of the incident electrons give up *all* their 35,000 eV of energy to create the photons of minimum wavelength (and maximum energy).

6. **(B)** The frictional work uses up all the kinetic energy. Frictional force is μmg, and frictional work is μmgs. Thus:

    $$W_f = KE_i - o = KE_i \quad \text{or} \quad \mu mgs = 1/2 \, mv^2$$

thus solving for skid length, s: $s = v^2/(2 \mu g)$, and the skid length is proportional to the *square of the speed*. The mass drops out of the equation.

7. **(C)** Because the skid length depends on speed squared, a car with twice the speed of another will slide *four* times as far.

8. **(B)** The forces during the collision *are* equal and opposite according to Newton's third law of motion. Each of the other responses is incorrect for the following reasons: **A.** The more massive van has *greater* momentum at the same speed. **C.** The forces are actually *equal* and opposite. **D.** It would require *more* mechanical work to stop the van because it has larger mass. In this case, the vehicles do not stop. The large van would actually reverse the velocity of the small car and "drive" the car backwards.

9. **(C)** As in the explanation for question 8, the forces during collision are equal and opposite. The other responses are incorrect because: **A.** The forces are always equal and opposite according to Newton's Third Law. **B.** Untrue, since the forces are actually equal and opposite. **D.** This is a true statement but it has nothing to do with the question asked, and does not explain why the car would suffer more damage in a head-on collision.

10. **(B)** In this particular experiment, the paint marks are three times farther apart when the speed (60 mph) is three times greater. Thus the times to travel between paint marks, which is the reaction time, remain the same. (The reaction times could vary from one test to another. Here the two times happened to be identical.)

11. **(C)** The reaction of calcium carbonate to form calcium bicarbonate requires water and carbon dioxide. Pure carbon dioxide gas is used. Therefore, no water enters the system and no reaction occurs.

12. **(D)** The passage states that calcium oxide is used to neutralize acidic soils. Therefore, the solution must be basic (pH > 7.0). Also, oxides of the alkaline earth metals are basic.

13. **(C)** Calcium chloride dissociates completely in water to form Ca^{2+} and $2Cl^-$. The resulting solution conducts electricity and is a strong electrolyte.

14. **(A)** Dissolved particles, calcium bicarbonate in this case, lower the freezing point of a solution.

15. **(D)** Calcium is a Group 2 element and forms ions with +2 charge.

16. **(B)** 56.1 g CaO corresponds to 1 mole of CaO (56.1 g CaO/56.1 g CaO = 1 mole CaO). According to the reaction stoichiometry in the passage, 1 mole of carbon dioxide is produced for each mole of CaO. One mole of gas at STP always occupies 22.4 L.

17. **(D)** The Archimedes Principle states that the buoyant force exerted on an object by a fluid is equal to the weight of the fluid displaced by the object. When an object floats, it displaces a volume of water the weight of which equals the weight of the floating object.

18. **(C)** A submerged object displaces a fluid volume equal to the volume of the submerged object.

19. **(C)** The buoyant force on the submerged block equals the weight of water displaced. This latter is greater than the weight of the block because the water density is greater than that of the wooden block.

20. **(D)** The speeds are the same because there is the same "pressure head," ρgy, to force the water out of the stopcocks where y is the 2 m depth, the same in both tanks. One can formally show this and find the actual speed by using Bernoulli's equation.

21. **(B)** Use conservation of mechanical energy. Let the initial gravitational potential energy equal the final kinetic energy at the bottom:

$$\frac{1}{2}mv^2 = mgh$$

where $h = 0.8$ meters.
The mass, m, cancels and:

$$v = \sqrt{2gh} = \sqrt{2(10 \text{ m/s}^2)(0.8 \text{ m})}$$

$$= 4.0 \text{ m/s}$$

22. **(A)** The period for any small angle of swing is given by the formula:

$$T = 2\pi\sqrt{L/g} = 2\pi\sqrt{0.8/10}$$

$$= 1.8 \text{ s}$$

23. **(C)** The period does not depend on the angle of swing (as long as the angle is small enough, less than about 10°).

24. **(A)** L can be found by squaring the equation for the period:

$$T^2 = 4\pi^2(L/g) = 4\pi^2(L/10) = 4 \text{ s}^2$$

Then:

$$L = 1.0 \text{ m.}$$

25. **(A)** T increases. The moon's force of gravity is $\frac{1}{6}$ that of Earth, so $g_{\text{moon}} = 1.6$ m/s^2. When used in the formula, the period will be longer by $\sqrt{6}$. ($T_{\text{moon}} = 4.9$ s). Video of the astronauts on the moon clearly showed the weaker force of gravity. They appeared to be moving in slow motion if they leaped upward.

26. **(C)** The equation of continuity for fluid flow is:

$$Av = \text{a constant value}$$

$$A_1v_1 = A_2v_2 = A_3v_3$$

Thus: $v_3 = A_1v_1/A_3$

$$v_3 = (3 \text{ m}^2)(2 \text{ m/s})/2 \text{ m}^2 = 3.0 \text{ m/s}$$

27. **(B)** Conservation of charge and mass requires the sum of the subscript (charge) numbers to be equal on both sides of the reaction as well as the sum of the superscript (mass) numbers to be equal. We must have then: $2 + 7 = 8 + 1$ and $4 + 14 = 17 + 1$. The missing subscript is 1, as is the missing superscript. The object is actually a proton initially, but we write the symbol for neutral hydrogen, since the proton will "grab" an electron to become hydrogen.

28. **(D)** The Coulomb force between two charged particles is given by: $F = kq_1q_2/r^2$. In this case, the ratio of the new force to the old force is:

$$\frac{k(3q_A q_B)/(3r)^2}{kq_A q_B/r^2} = 1/3$$

29. **(C)** The current through the 2-ohm resistor must split up with the larger portion going through the smaller resistor in the parallel branch. The 3-ohm and 6-ohm resistors are in the ratio of 1 to 2, so the 3-ampere current will split into the ratio of 2 to 1—that is, 2 amperes through the 3-ohm resistor and 1 ampere through the 6-ohm resistor.

30. **(C)** Since air friction is present, the ball will reach a "terminal velocity" shown as the value of *v* corresponding to the horizontal dotted line.

31. **(B)** Using Conservation of Mechanical Energy, $PE_A = PE_C + KE_C$. Then: $mgh_A = mgh_C + 1/2mv^2$ where *v* is the speed at point C. Cancel the mass *m* and solve for *v*. Note that we need not solve for the energies at B because the total mechanical energy is always constant.

32. **(B)** A real image is formed, so the focal length is positive. The lens is midway between the object and the screen, so the object and image distance are both equal to 30 cm and are positive. The thin lens equation gives the focal length:

$$1/f = 1/d_o + 1/d_i$$
$$= 1/30 + 1/30$$
$$1/f = 2/30$$
$$f = +15 \text{ cm.}$$

33. **(C)** The transmittance is the fraction of incident light that passes through the sample. This fraction is 72/81 = 0.889.

34. **(D)** The absorbance is defined as the negative logarithm of transmittance. $-\log 0.889 = 0.051$.

35. **(A)** The Beer-Lambert Law states that $A = -\log T = EMl$ where

A = absorbance
T = transmittance
E = a constant for the particular solute and wavelength of light
M = molarity of solution
l = path length of light

Thus absorbance varies directly with path length and with molar concentration; and decreasing the concentration by half will also halve the absorbance.

36. **(A)** In the above statement of the Beer-Lambert Law it is seen that absorbance varies directly with path length. Thus, halving the path length will halve the absorbance.

37. **(A)** The absorbance was 0.051. Doubling the concentration will double the absorbance to 0.102. Since absorbance = –log transmittance, and

$$\text{transmittance} = \frac{\text{reading with transmitted light}}{\text{reading with incident light}}$$

antilog (0.102) = 0.791
(0.791)(81) = 64

38. **(D)** The reading, the transmittance, and the absorbance will be affected by the wavelength of light, but the direction and magnitude cannot be readily predicted.

39. **(A)** HCl in water is expected to be virtually 100% ionized into H^+ (or H_3O^+) and Cl^-. $pH = -\log [H^+] = -\log (1 \times 10^{-2}) = 2$

40. **(B)** Because the volume has doubled, [HCl] = 0.005 molar = 5×10^{-3}.

Because HCl is virtually completely ionized,

$$[H^+] = 5 \times 10^{-3} \text{ molar}$$
$$pH = -\log (5 \times 10^{-3})$$
$$\log 10^{-3} = -3$$
$$\log 5 = \underline{0.6990}$$
$$\text{sum} = -2.3010$$
$$-(-2.3010) = 2.3010$$

You should recognize that the answer must be between 2 and 3 because log (5) is a positive number between zero and one.

41. **(C)** The Henderson-Hasselbalch equation states

$$pH = pK_a + \log \frac{[\text{salt}]}{[\text{acid}]}$$

The strongly ionized HCl will react with sodium propionate to yield propionic acid. Thus 0.01 moles of HCl will react with 0.01 moles of sodium propionate to yield 0.01 moles of propionic acid (HPr). An additional 0.01 moles of NaPr will remain unreacted.

$$pH = pK_a + \log \frac{[\text{salt}]}{[\text{acid}]} = 4.89 + \log \frac{(0.01)}{(0.01)} = 4.89$$

When the concentrations of weak acid and salt are equal,

$$\frac{[\text{Salt}]}{[\text{Acid}]} = 1 \text{ and } \log 1 = 0$$

At these concentrations, pH = pK_a. (The concentrations should be expressed in molarities rather than simply total moles. Reflection allows us to recognize that the end result will be the same as long as we are consistent in a single set of computations.)

42. **(A)** Hydrochloric acid is a strong acid; the other acids are weak acids.

43. **(B)** Look again at the Henderson-Hasselbalch equation. We have diluted [salt] and [acid] equally. Thus the pH remains at the pK_a.

44. **(A)** The stronger the acid, the lower its pK_a. Thus, pyruvic acid is the strongest acid among the three.

45. **(C)** Percent ionization = 100 (degree of ionization)

$$100 \times 0.12 = 12$$

46. **(D)** Remember Graham's Law:

$$\frac{V_1}{V_2} = \sqrt{\frac{m_2}{m_1}}$$

$$\frac{1}{0.5} = \sqrt{\frac{m_2}{m_1}}$$

Squaring $\dfrac{1}{0.25} = \dfrac{m_2}{20} = 4$

$$m_2 = 80$$

47. **(D)** $V_1 \times N_1 = V_2 \times N_2$
$$(20.0)(0.200) = (40.0)(0.100) = 4$$

This tells us nothing about the structure of the acid. Remember that the normality deals only with the available protons in solution rather than the molarity. The acid could be monoprotic, diprotic, or tripotic, but we have been given no information to allow us to decide.

48. **(C)** pK_w = pH + pOH = 14
4.5 + pOH = 14
pOH = 14 − 4.5 = 9.5

49. **(B)** pH = pK_a + log $\dfrac{[salt]}{[acid]}$
When the salt (dissociated anion) and acid concentrations are equal, log 1 = 0. Thus, pH = pK_a or 4.2 in this case.

50. **(B)** Buffering is always best at the pK_a.

51. **(C)** $\dfrac{P_1V_1}{T_1} = \dfrac{P_2V_2}{T_2}$

Since $T_1 = T_2$, they will cancel out.

$$(1)(1) = 2V \text{ and } V = \frac{1}{2} \text{ or } 0.50$$

52. **(B)** The step involved is a precipitation step. Increasing the Cl^- concentration will reduce the concentration of Ag^+ in solution. Remember K_{sp} = [Ag^+][Cl^-] and the source of the Cl^- is irrelevant. Thus increased concentration of Cl^- must result in decreased concentration of Ag^+ in order to maintain the solubility product constant. Addition of Ag_2SO_4 would probably be counterproductive, since additional Ag^+ is being added, and probably all will not be recovered.

Verbal Reasoning

53. **(C)** The central theme of the passage deals with the monumental amounts of research that have been done in the field of public education over the past 20 years. Mention of the vast research effort is made in paragraphs three, four, and five, whereas paragraph six makes it clear that research will continue.

54. **(D)** Paragraph two states that the outcry was created in part by declining economic conditions, as well as the publication of exhaustive studies of school resources and their impact.

55. **(A)** Paragraph one makes it clear that the reform in question for this passage deals with the nation's public school systems.

56. **(D)** All three statements are included in the answer. In education "the field" is considered the classroom (I). "Researchers" going into the field indicates that they are observing teachers and students in action (II). The fact that researchers have gone into the field in great numbers indicates that there is much interest in educational reform research (III).

57. **(D)** The combination of **B** and **C** encompasses educators who are researchers as well as those who are practicing in the field at all levels, and names three specific sets of practitioners who are closest to school settings. The question asks, what groups, and a choice is provided to include all the combinations.

58. **(B)** Paragraphs four and five discuss researchers in the field and some progress that has been made as a result of their efforts. The "tone" that the author sets in these paragraphs allows one to assume that she feels hands-on research is beneficial.

59. **(C)** Paragraph two traces the story back to seventh century China and goes on to state that the plot is universal. The central thesis of the passage is that all versions of the story share many ingredients, and the first paragraph asserts that one of these chronicles the transformation into womanhood. Paragraph three notes the evil stepmother as a feature common to various versions of the story.

60. **(B)** A main point of the passage is that a consistent aspect of Cinderella's character is her loving and forgiving spirit.

61. **(C)** No mention is made of Cinderella's need for warmth (**A** is incorrect). The skins clearly are important in a ritual sense (**B** is incorrect). Cinderella always returns to a clean, well-dressed state; and because it symbolically is essential that she give up the skins and there is no mention that she keeps them, **D** is incorrect.

62. **(B)** Cinderella, as the author notes in the final paragraph, is moving toward a condition of wholeness. There is nothing to suggest that she is less complex than she had thought (**A** is incorrect), that she exploits the prince (**C** is incorrect), or that her wholeness weakens her (**D** is incorrect).

63. **(B)** A central purpose of the essay is to show how various versions of this tale make concrete various aspects of Horney's theories. Nowhere is there a suggestion that Horney had in mind the Cinderella story or that Horney altered the story in any way, thus **A** and **D** are incorrect. And, though one might find that the parallel between Horney's theories and the fairy tale provide one illustration of how the theories appear to be supported by their presence in a given story like *Cinderella*, nowhere is there a suggestion that the validity of a theory could be based on a single story application such as this one. Thus **C** is incorrect.

64. **(A)** Although the first part of the title is a clever play on words, it also prepares the reader for the "fit" between Horney's theories and the Cinderella tale. The three other titles are not descriptive of the pattern of argument in the essay, and in the cases of **B** and **C**, contradict information in the text.

65. **(D)** The best and most encompassing title would be The Development of the Physician. The passage does not deal with professional growth and the development and training of the medical student exclusively. Although it is mentioned that the first two years of the study of medicine focus on the scientific aspects and thereafter the clinical practice predominates the life of the students, it is not examined specifically.

66. **(D)** The passage makes it clear that most students enter this profession because they care for their fellow man and want to serve him; in fact the passage ends on the note that "the secret of the care of the patient is in caring for the patient." Achieving public esteem is a part of becoming a physician and certainly although intelligence and a good background help, they are not enough in the making of a physician. Marriage among classmates is not discussed.

67. **(B)** Moral, clinical, and legal perspectives affect decision making and are in the order used upon first entrance into school. Socialization, however, elevates the clinical perspective to resolve the myriad of clinical situations. The issue of the influence of hospital administrators is not debated in the passage. The author quotes from Konner in respect to arrogance, but no conclusion is reached in respect to the statement that their extensive training gives anyone that right.

68. **(D)** Good health, although essential, is not enough for medical practice; the article stresses continuously that the overall, the broad, the human, the appreciation of life, love, and mankind must be considered and held in focus in order to serve appropriately.

69. **(D)** All the statements presented in this question are definitely contradicted by the information in the passage.

70. **(B)** The passage makes it clear that at the end of the reductional division the chromosomes are reduced to one-half their original number. Meiosis results in four gametes that possess one-half the chromosomal number of an adult. The production of gametes, or sex cells—egg and sperm—is known as gametogenesis. Because an individual possesses an equal amount of genetic

material from both parents and the same number of chromosomes as either parent, a reduction to one-half that number must be accomplished in the development of the egg and sperm.

71.	**(B)** During the process of meiosis, a recombination of genetic material is possible; this is effected through crossing-over, as noted in paragraph three. In crossing-over, comparable portions of chromatids are exchanged; crossing-over is more the rule than the exception. Replication results during the first part of meiosis in four chromatids and two of them may exchange materials. This exchange occurs before the tetrads separate.

72.	**(D)** The third paragraph indicates that replication of DNA occurs during interphase before meiosis starts. Interphase is the time during which the cell grows and prepares itself for meiosis.

73.	**(C)** See the explanation for previous questions dealing with this passage.

74.	**(D)** Eggs and sperm are haploid; a fertilized egg (zygote) possesses the diploid number of the parent again. Also see explanations for previous questions.

75.	**(D)** The first sentence of paragraph two mentions ten stages. Paragraph one states that sexual reproduction plays an important role in the expression of different phenotypes, and paragraph three indicates that replication of DNA occurs during interphase before meiosis begins.

76.	**(D)** The fact that ordinal position remains a little understood personality variable is stated in the opening paragraph and sets the tone for the passage.

77.	**(B)** Although much research has been done on birth order, it is not possible to make *absolute* statements about any of the ordinal positions. It has not been proven, for example, that the oldest is *always* the most mature. The opening paragraph implies that more studies need to be conducted.

78.	**(D)** The author states that primogeniture is "a perfect illustration of the importance of being first born." Because the custom began in feudal times, it is reasonable for the reader to conclude that the paragraph was inserted to provide a sense that the subject of ordinal birth has been the subject of study for some time.

79.	**(D)** All statements made in the question are correct. Parents attach to their firstborn such characteristics as a solid head on his/her shoulders, a mature behavior, and the ability to associate with adults, to be able to lead, to care for siblings, and to grow up as a pillar of the community. The youngest child is freer to develop into an exuberant and free-spirited individual because mothers do not expect the youngest to function in an adultlike manner. Many actions that were frowned upon previously are now considered cute in nature.

80.	**(A)** Although a comparison of the middle child to the older child is made, no direct comment or evidence is presented that this helps him/her reach higher levels of achievement; in fact because of the comparison and the desire of the child to establish his own identity, he may even become a problem student. The passage makes it clear that the firstborn usually performs better, and that the youngest feels the least need to excel. It is also stated in the passage that communication with adults is typically a problem of the second born.

81.	**(D)** All the statements are supported by the information in the passage.

82.	**(D)** The author of the passage neither supports nor contradicts the statements presented in the question.

83.	**(D)** All three statements are clearly contradicted by the information presented in the passage.

84.	**(B)** The charisma of the instructor is a factor in the evaluation of teaching effectiveness. There are objective methods available and grades do play a role in student ratings. Time of day is not discussed in the passage.

85.	**(D)** The difficulty of subject matter material and its effect on student ratings is not discussed in the passage.

86.	**(C)** Students are usually most interested in evaluations by students, believing that they are the "consumers" who are most directly affected by the quality of the "product" called teaching.

87.	**(D)** Paragraph five visualizes students as purchasers. Paragraph two points out that employers and employees benefit from evaluations, and paragraph four states that the end result is increased productivity.

88. **(B)** In paragraph one, the author plainly asserts that Tillich believes contemporary society is characterized by an absence of spirituality, whereas, ironically, there is a growing interest in religion.

89. **(A)** Tillich, according to the author, sees true religion as moving vertically, and thus being characterized by "depth." Tillich's main thesis deals with the ways in which (1) present-day religion runs counter to true religion and (2) present-day society discourages people from asking weighty eschatological questions.

90. **(D)** Although the author agrees with Tillich's assertions that modern man lacks true religion and is more materialistic now than in the past, he questions in his final paragraph the strictly "rational" ways that Tillich implies are the only ways of knowing spiritual truth. Nowhere in the essay does the author quarrel with Tillich's definition of spirituality.

91. **(B)** In paragraph three, the author states plainly that Tillich's ideas are perhaps even more insightful or relevant than they were 30 years ago.

92. **(A)** Though the author clarifies and qualifies Tillich's positions, he asserts that Tillich is still as relevant as he was "30 years ago."

Writing Sample

93. **Essay**

Herodotus's viewpoint here is clearly a fatalistic one. It is easy to see the logic behind it. Because mankind does not exist separately from either the rest of existence or the past, then every time that a person acts, she is in some ways also reacting to that surrounding existence and to the history that preceded that act. It is a frustrating point of view; and, in spite of its strange truth, it is probably a viewpoint best left without too much rumination. It is the given in life and the unchangeable. A resignation to this point of view would in some ways also be a voluntary denial of one's autonomy, of one's existence.

I say "voluntary" because I believe that the opposite viewpoint is, paradoxically, just as true. If I turn my head while driving in order to check my radio dial and in doing so also slightly turn my steering wheel causing an accident with an oncoming school bus, did not my act of turning my head create a circumstance whereby that accident occurred? Of course, it did. If I had not turned

my head, then I would have not turned the wheel; and if I had not turned the wheel then the bus would not have hit my car. However, from Herodotus's viewpoint, my act did not exist by itself. Had the radio not been in the car, had a different song even been on the station, then I would perhaps not have turned my head to adjust the dial. Had the bus driver waited longer at her last stop or had she not stopped for a cup of coffee on her way to work, then perhaps she would not have been at that place at that specific time. The issue is as puzzling as the issue of whether the chicken appeared first or the egg. It is the question of the identification of an original cause in a long line of causes.

What a thinking person is most likely to conclude is that individuals and their circumstances are mutually interdependent rather than mutually exclusive and that therefore a statement like that of Herodotus is, in a sense, meaningless. His is only a statement of perspective and, further, a rather negative one. But to say the opposite, that circumstances are dependent on individuals and not vice versa, would be naive and ignorant. A rational person would have to accept interdependence of individuals and circumstances in order to live realistically and effectively in the world. She would then act carefully, remaining aware both that there are circumstances over which she has no control and that her act will be part of the circumstances to come.

93. **Explanation of Response: 6**

The paper focuses sharply on the statement and addresses each of the three writing tasks. Paragraph one explains what the statement means, paragraph two gives a specific situation in which individuals do, in fact, determine circumstances (a reversal of the assertion that "men are dependent on circumstances, not circumstances on men"), and paragraph three reconciles the statement and the situation that illustrates that the opposite of the statement may also be true.

The paper provides an analysis of the potential dangers of all-or-none statements like the one in question. It does so by examining the logical extension of the idea that individuals are dependent on circumstances and by characterizing the implications of this assertion as "fatalistic." The logic of the paper's argument is sophisticated, on the one hand agreeing with the "strange truth" of Herodotus's point in paragraph one, but in paragraph two illustrating with a series of circumstances "dependent on individuals" that the reverse is also true. The final paragraph presents a balanced consideration of the interdependent relationship between individuals and the circumstances that they create and by which they are shaped.

The writing is clear and nicely controlled. The sentences are varied, containing simple (e.g., sentence one), compound (e.g., sentence four), and complex structures (e.g., sentence three). The first sentence of each paragraph serves as a topic sentence and gives unity to the paragraph that follows. Transitions, such as "however" in sentence five of paragraph two, provide coherence within the paragraph.

94.   **Essay**

Haeckel's quotation is an enigma because its meaning depends upon the interpretation of ambiguous words, "voluntary death," "intolerable suffering," and of course, "redemption." It is not clear whether the "voluntary death" is a suicide or a murder or any of the possibilities between these two extremes. So, even at the outset, the reader steps onto a shaky platform on which rests the remainder of Haeckel's statement. This "voluntary death" would specifically be the one that would put "an end to intolerable suffering." Because to "suffer" something is, in a sense, to "tolerate" it, then "intolerable suffering" would be an impossibility by definition. Finally, this enigmatic but "voluntary death," voluntary perhaps only because it is caused by a human act, is "an act of redemption." Naturally, one's thoughts might turn to the religious connotations of the word. In this case, it would mean a sort of act of deliverance from evil by sacrifice. If, however, you strip the mystery of religious aura from the word, it means simply a payback. Perhaps the redemption is the cashing in of the mortal life for freedom from human suffering. Keeping all of this in mind, Haeckel's statement, though, still a puzzle of sorts, must mean that for a person to cause or to allow death in order to discontinue the suffering of pain (of one sort or another) is an exchange of the body, which is only loaned for the duration of mortality, in exchange for the freedom of the human spirit.

Now, one could argue (and people certainly have argued) endlessly about the moral right and/or wrong of this idea because it is at the core of the controversies over euthanasia, abortion, and the execution of criminals. The argument is over, the "right" or "wrong" of this "redemption." Because "right" and "wrong" cannot really be defined but only agreed upon tentatively (as with laws), perhaps the literal meaning of the quote might be a better target for thought. The problem here is that it is not clear whose "intolerable suffering" is being

referred to in the statement. For example, if I refuse to tolerate or to suffer the presence of my annoying little brother, is my killing him or allowing him to die an act of redemption? The thought is appalling, of course, but, according to Haeckel, it would, in fact, be a redemptive act (even if the sacrifice entailed is only that of my own innocence). The way that Haeckel's quotation is worded, there are no real exceptions.

Haeckel's quotation could be used to try to justify morally the act of taking a human life. But the statement does not morally justify anything; it merely defines a type of "voluntary death" as a sort of exchange. The end of a human's life is always an exchange of one state for another. So the moral question, the "choice" perhaps, is a personal one (or a legal one). Morality is not defined by absolute natural laws; it is rather defined personally (or, in a social situation, legally). What governs the choice maker or the potential actor consists of nothing more absolute and nothing less vague than his or her conscience and personal beliefs. Haeckel's quote could be used loosely to justify an act that results in death. But "used" is the key word here. Moral decision, decisions about right and wrong, are not that easy. Ultimately, the choice of a *"voluntary* death" in "the face of intolerable suffering" is determined only by the judgment and conscience of the individual, the mysterious "volunteer."

94.   **Explanation of Response: 4**

The paper focuses on the topic defined by the statement and addresses the three writing tasks. The first paragraph responds to the task of explaining the statement, in this case a task complicated by the need to clarify definitions of words that have multiple meanings. In the second paragraph, the paper provides what is clearly one of the most extreme examples imaginable to demonstrate that, given the phrasing of the quotation, there are no specific situations in which "voluntary death" would not be an act of redemption. Paragraph three explores the factors that determine the choice of voluntary death in the face of intolerable suffering.

There is no question that Haeckel's statement raises difficult problems, and it is clear that this essay constructs a sophisticated argument that explores the complexity of these problems. The strategy of defining ambiguous terms in paragraph one is a good one; the choice to explore the connotations of these words also is effective, though anyone who chooses to spend this much time on definition in the first paragraph should be aware of the danger of overdoing it. This essay stops just short of this. The reason that this essay received a 4 rather than a 5 or 6 is that the second task ("Describe a specific situation in which the voluntary death by which a person puts an end to intolerable suffering would not be an act of redemption") is not confronted as directly as it might be. The paper maintains that "there are no real exceptions," virtually by definition. The writer might have used his or her skill with definition clearly demonstrated in paragraph one to construct at least one hypothetical situation that would provide a conceivable exception to Haeckel's statement. In addition to the need for a specific "exceptional" situation in paragraph two, the paper could be strengthened by the use of other examples to illustrate the major points in paragraphs one and three. This paper in general, however, is tightly reasoned, and it moves logically toward the conclusion that the choice of voluntary death in the face of intolerable suffering is ultimately a moral decision, one based on conscience.

Biological Sciences

95. **(B)** The thyroid hormones affect the rate of metabolism of all the tissues of the body; they control the growth, maturation, and differentiation of the organism. A goiter is any enlargement of the gland due to neoplasm or inflammatory disease. Endemic goiters are due to lack of iodine intake; this results in the increased production of TSH, compensatory hypertrophy and eventual exhaustion of the gland. Thyroxin deficiency leads to goiter; if the deficiency is not corrected, cretinism in the young and myxedema in the adult may be a consequence.

96. **(C)** Hypothyroidism would result in a patient who is fairly heavy, phlegmatic, is devoid of expression, and has rough and dry skin and laboratory tests would show a low basal metabolic rate, low protein bound iodine, and a high serum cholesterol level.

97. **(C)** The hypothyroid patient would have shown weight gain since less food is converted into energy and more food is stored as fat.

98. **(D)** See explanations for questions 95–97.

99. **(D)** A hyperthyroid patient would exhibit weight loss, nervousness, irritability, increased metabolic rate, rapid heart rate, sweating, and a protrusion of the eyeballs.

100. **(D)** This woman is not the mother. She can contribute only the O gene, and this child must receive an A gene from one parent and a B gene from the other parent. The man cannot be ruled out as the father with the limited information given, since he can contribute a B gene to a child.

101. **(D)** If the man previously fathered a child with blood type O, then the man must have a genotype of BO. The woman can contribute only the O gene. Since the man has an equal chance of contributing the B or the O gene, there is a 50% chance of the child being type O (genotype OO) or type B (genotype BO).

102. **(B)** The chance of any child of this couple being type B is 50% (see explanation for question 99). The chance that any child will be a girl is 50%. Since the blood type and the sex are independent of each other, multiply their individual chances (50% × 50% = 25%).

103. **(B)** Phenotypic and genotypic characteristics may be expressed as follows:

Phenotype	Genotype
A	A/O
B	B/O
O	O/O
AB	A/B

104. **(D)** Genotype refers to the genetic makeup of the organism. The genotype is expressed via phenotypic characteristics that are visible and observable under normal circumstances.

105. **(D)** An allele is one of a pair of genes that occupies the same locus on homologous chromosomes.

106. **(C)** Rhesus (Rh) agglutinogen is present in humans and is represented by a dominant gene R. The agglutinogen of an Rh positive fetus passes across the placenta, enters the maternal blood stream, and elicits the production of an agglutinin (antibody) by the mother. The agglutinin passes into the circulation of the fetus and if present in sufficient concentration can produce agglutination, at times fatal to the developing fetus.

107. **(B)** Hemophilia, a frequent disease of the royal houses of Europe, is a bleeding disorder transmitted through a sex-linked recessive gene. It results in abnormal coagulation; hemophilia A is the classical true hemophilia resulting from a

deficiency of factor VIII. Both sexes carry a complete complement of sex-linked genes. A female, with the XX arrangement, will only exhibit a recessive gene if she has received it from both parents (a rare event with an uncommon gene), whereas in the XY male the recessive gene cannot be masked because there is no partner X and so a larger number of recessive genes are expressed. A man receives his X from his mother and passes it on to his daughters. His daughters are the carriers of sex-linked traits and their sons may be affected.

108. **(B)** Synthesis of mRNA is catalyzed by RNA polymerase II.

109. **(C)** Proteins for secretion are made by ribosomes on rough endoplasmic reticulum and then modified in Golgi bodies.

110. **(B)** Skeletal muscle cells are striated due to the highly organized thick (myosin) and thin (actin) myofilaments and contain numerous nuclei.

111. **(C)** Reabsorption of useful solutes is the primary function of the proximal convoluted tubule.

112. **(A)** The corpus callosum connects the cerebral hemispheres.

113. **(C)** Pleiotropism is defined as multiple phenotypic effects of a gene (allele).

114. **(C)** 1-2, who manifests prolonged Q-T interval, has 14 descendants who are also affected and six who are not. Each of the 14 affected descendants has an affected parent; both parents (II-3&10) of four are affected. The trait thus shows unbroken lineal descent and is, therefore, *dominant*.

115. **(C)** *Deafness is not a pleiotropic affect of the gene producing prolonged Q-T*, for these abnormalities are observed *assorting* among the progeny of a male (II-1), who is doubly homozygous normal, and his wife (II-2), who is heterozygous for both abnormalities, that is, doubly heterozygous. Alleles segregate (Mendel's first law) from each other; non-alleles may assort. In the absence of linkage, *independent assortment* (Mendel's second law) of nonalleles occurs. Although the sample is not large enough to rule out weak linkage, it does rule out allelism.

116. **(A)** Every affected descendant of the affected progenitor (I-3) of the F. family has at least one parent affected, except III-21, a son of II-11, who marks the only break in lineal descent of the trait. If the trait were recessive, the three normal mothers (I-4, II-9, and II-12) of affected children would have to be carriers. Because of the rarity of the defect and the lack of biological kinship between these women and their spouses, it is highly unlikely that they are carriers. It is probable that the trait is dominant and that the allele has slightly reduced penetrance and failed to manifest itself phenotypically in II-11.

117. **(B)** If one were limited to the data on the W. family, it would be impossible to distinguish whether the defect is autosomal or X-linked. That is because we could not then rule out male-to-male transmission among the progeny of couple II-3&10, who have three arrhythmic sons. Nonetheless, prolonged Q-T and the arrhythmias are clinically indistinguishable and almost certainly determined by the same *autosomal dominant* allele as in the F. family, where male-to-male transmission shows that this dominant trait is autosomal. X-linked traits cannot be transmitted from father to son (male-to-male) because sons can receive their X chromosome (in which X-linked traits are transmitted) from only their mother, *not* from their father.

118. **(C)** All of the daughters of affected males would be affected if the trait were X-linked because they received their father's X chromosome which would have contained the (dominant) mutant allele had it been X-linked. None of the daughters of the affected fathers (II-3 and II-5) are affected, thus the mutant allele is *not* in the X chromosome; the trait is autosomal.

119. **(D)** Many autosomal dominant genes that produce rather mild phenotypic effects in the heterozygote produce much more extreme effects—in some cases, even lethality—in homozygotes. It is likely that *the propista* (III-10) *is homozygous* for the prolonged Q-T allele and demonstrates the more extreme phenotype frequently manifested by homozygotes for rare autosomal dominant traits.

120. **(C)** The driving force (ΔP) causing air to flow into or out of the lungs is the pressure difference between the atmospheric pressure (P_{atm}) and the intra-alveolar pressure (P_{alv}). The absolute atmospheric or intra-alveolar pressures do not dictate air flow, it is the pressure difference that is important. Intrapleural pressure reflects lung

elastic forces as well plus any smaller pressure difference between P_{atm} and P_{alv} while breathing. Thus, the absolute value of the intrapleural pressure has no bearing on inspiration.

121. **(A)** During inspiration the chest wall enlarges, expanding the lungs and the intra-alveolar air. Thus, the intra-alveolar pressure transiently drops below atmospheric pressure, pulling air into the lungs. During expiration the chest wall collapses causing the intra-alveolar pressure to transiently go above atmospheric pressure and air flows out of the lungs. When intra-alveolar pressure equals atmospheric pressure, no air will flow into or out of the lungs. The intrapleural pressure will always be lower than the intra-alveolar pressure by an amount equal to the elastic forces of the lungs. Thus, intra-alveolar pressure never goes below intrapleural pressure.

122. **(D)** As defined, the alveolar ventilation equals the amount of fresh air which reaches the alveoli per minute. Thus, alveolar ventilation is the amount of fresh air reaching the alveoli per breath times the number of breaths per minute. Because part of the fresh air inspired gets no farther than the anatomic dead space (i.e. it doesn't reach the alveoli), the fresh air actually reaching the alveoli equals the tidal volume minus the volume of the anatomic dead space. The frequency of breathing times any other lung volume equals something other than the alveolar ventilation.

123. **(C)** With hypoventilation, oxygen delivery to the alveolar gas is less than normal and the partial pressure of oxygen will decrease. Concurrently, the removal of carbon dioxide from the alveolar compartment is less than normal and the partial pressure of carbon dioxide will increase.

124. **(D)** The repressor protein binds to the operator sequence to block access to the promoter.

125. **(D)** The three germ layers become apparent during gastrulation.

126. **(A)** B lymphocytes and plasma cells are the only cells in humans that can form antibodies.

127. **(C)** The methyl group of toluene is an *o, p*-directing group.

128. **(D)** The hydroxyl group is a highly activating group, whereas the chloro, nitro, and acetyl groups deactivate the ring towards electrophilic aromatic substitutions.

129. **(B)** Oxidation of toluene yields benzoic acid. Nitration would yield the meta isomer because the carboxyl group is meta directing.

130. **(A)** The methyl group activates the *o, p*-positions and directs the Br to the ortho position. The nitro group is a meta directing deactivating group.

131. **(B)** The nitration of benzene involves the attack of a nitronium ion, NO^+_2, on toluene to form a cyclohexadienyl cation as the intermediate.

132. **(C)** Valine is one of the nine essential amino acids, whereas linoleic acid is the only true essential fatty acid. Vitamin E is fat soluble and found in foods. Glucose is essential, but is obtained in other forms, such as polysaccharides. Polysaccharides contain many monosaccharide units joined in long chains and among the most important are starch and cellulose. Starch is the reserve carbohydrate in plants and on complete hydrolysis it yields glucose.

133. **(D)** Linoleic, linolenic, and arachidonic acids (polyunsaturated) are listed as essential fatty acids, because they cannot be synthesized by the animal and must therefore be provided in the diet. Among the water soluble vitamins are thiamine, biotin, and niacin.

134. **(B)** The fat-soluble vitamins are vitamins A, D, E, and K. The water-soluble vitamins are vitamin C, thiamine, riboflavin, niacin, vitamin B_6, folacin, vitamin B_{12}, biotin, and pantothenic acid.

135. **(D)** The bulk essential minerals are calcium, phosphorus, and magnesium, whereas the trace essential minerals are iron, zinc, selenium, iodine, cobalt, molybdenum, manganese, copper, chromium, and fluoride.

136. **(C)** Amino acids are derived from proteins; carbohydrates that are polyhydroxy aldehydes and the simplest carbohydrate units are known as monosaccharides. The most important monosaccharide is glucose; it is obtained by the hydrolysis of starch. Fat and oil constitute one of the three main classes of food. Fats and oils are esters of glycerol with carboxylic acids.

137. **(B)** Parathyroid hormone acts upon bone, eliciting changes in calcium and phosphorus. Osteoclasts are the cells stimulated by parathyroid hormone to facilitate the resorption of calcium and phosphorus from bone. Administration of parathyroid hormone to animals without parathyroids results in an increase of phosphorus excretion in the urine, a fall in serum inorgamic phosphorus levels, an increase in serum calcium, and an increase of calcium excretion in the urine.

138. **(C)** Excretion concerns itself with the elimination of water (fluid) and metabolic wastes, whereas egestion is the process of eliminating undigested food materials. Catabolism is the chemical breakdown of molecules.

139. **(A)** In anaerobic respiration glucose is converted to two molecules of the 3-carbon compound pyruvic acid. In aerobic respiration, glucose is converted to six molecules each of carbon dioxide and water. Anaerobic respiration is only about 3% as efficient as aerobic respiration. The anaerobic pathway is the same as the aerobic to the pyruvic acid stage.

140. **(B)** LH (luteinizing hormone) is secreted by the pituitary gland. In the male, it is also called ICSH (interstitial, cell stimulating, hormone) from its effects on the testes. In our case, half of each group had its testes removed. This eliminates the feedback from testes to pituitary. Comparison of AM and PM readings for intact rats shows no significant differences in LH levels. For orchidectomized rats, levels vary widely, with no consistent AM-PM relationship.

141. **(A)** The strongest pattern in the data is higher LH values in orchidectomized rats. Choice B is not true. Choices C and D, although true, are not directly supported by the data given.

142. **(B)** Values are higher on average in each category in assay 2. This may be due to a systematic error in either assay, but that cannot be determined from the data given.

143. **(D)** The general formula C_nH_{2n-2} applies to all members of the alkyne series. The suffix for names in this series is "yne." Ethyne is the only choice that has the correct ending.

144. **(C)** Ethers have the general formula R–O–R′. The other compounds have the following general formulas:

$$\text{esters} \qquad R-\overset{\displaystyle O}{\underset{\displaystyle O-R'}{\overset{\|}{\underset{\backslash}{C}}}}$$

$$\text{aldehydes} \qquad R-\overset{\displaystyle O}{\underset{\displaystyle H}{\overset{\|}{\underset{\backslash}{C}}}}$$

$$\text{alcohols} \qquad R-OH$$

145. **(D)** This configuration:
$$-\overset{\displaystyle }{\underset{\displaystyle O}{C}}-OH$$

is characteristic of carboxyl groups. A hydroxyl group is identified by –OH.

146. **(C)** $\varnothing CH_2Cl + \varnothing \xrightarrow{AlCl_3} \varnothing-CH_2-\varnothing$

Friedel-Crafts Reaction

$\varnothing CH_2Cl + Na \longrightarrow \varnothing-CH_2CH_2-\varnothing$

Wurtz Reaction

Answer Sheet
MODEL EXAMINATION B

Directions: After locating the number of the question to which you are responding, fill in the circle containing the letter of the answer you have selected. Use pencil (not a ballpoint pen) to completely blacken the circle.

PHYSICAL SCIENCES

1 Ⓐ Ⓑ Ⓒ Ⓓ	27 Ⓐ Ⓑ Ⓒ Ⓓ	
2 Ⓐ Ⓑ Ⓒ Ⓓ	28 Ⓐ Ⓑ Ⓒ Ⓓ	
3 Ⓐ Ⓑ Ⓒ Ⓓ	29 Ⓐ Ⓑ Ⓒ Ⓓ	
4 Ⓐ Ⓑ Ⓒ Ⓓ	30 Ⓐ Ⓑ Ⓒ Ⓓ	
5 Ⓐ Ⓑ Ⓒ Ⓓ	31 Ⓐ Ⓑ Ⓒ Ⓓ	
6 Ⓐ Ⓑ Ⓒ Ⓓ	32 Ⓐ Ⓑ Ⓒ Ⓓ	
7 Ⓐ Ⓑ Ⓒ Ⓓ	33 Ⓐ Ⓑ Ⓒ Ⓓ	
8 Ⓐ Ⓑ Ⓒ Ⓓ	34 Ⓐ Ⓑ Ⓒ Ⓓ	
9 Ⓐ Ⓑ Ⓒ Ⓓ	35 Ⓐ Ⓑ Ⓒ Ⓓ	
10 Ⓐ Ⓑ Ⓒ Ⓓ	36 Ⓐ Ⓑ Ⓒ Ⓓ	
11 Ⓐ Ⓑ Ⓒ Ⓓ	37 Ⓐ Ⓑ Ⓒ Ⓓ	
12 Ⓐ Ⓑ Ⓒ Ⓓ	38 Ⓐ Ⓑ Ⓒ Ⓓ	
13 Ⓐ Ⓑ Ⓒ Ⓓ	39 Ⓐ Ⓑ Ⓒ Ⓓ	
14 Ⓐ Ⓑ Ⓒ Ⓓ	40 Ⓐ Ⓑ Ⓒ Ⓓ	
15 Ⓐ Ⓑ Ⓒ Ⓓ	41 Ⓐ Ⓑ Ⓒ Ⓓ	
16 Ⓐ Ⓑ Ⓒ Ⓓ	42 Ⓐ Ⓑ Ⓒ Ⓓ	
17 Ⓐ Ⓑ Ⓒ Ⓓ	43 Ⓐ Ⓑ Ⓒ Ⓓ	
18 Ⓐ Ⓑ Ⓒ Ⓓ	44 Ⓐ Ⓑ Ⓒ Ⓓ	
19 Ⓐ Ⓑ Ⓒ Ⓓ	45 Ⓐ Ⓑ Ⓒ Ⓓ	
20 Ⓐ Ⓑ Ⓒ Ⓓ	46 Ⓐ Ⓑ Ⓒ Ⓓ	
21 Ⓐ Ⓑ Ⓒ Ⓓ	47 Ⓐ Ⓑ Ⓒ Ⓓ	
22 Ⓐ Ⓑ Ⓒ Ⓓ	48 Ⓐ Ⓑ Ⓒ Ⓓ	
23 Ⓐ Ⓑ Ⓒ Ⓓ	49 Ⓐ Ⓑ Ⓒ Ⓓ	
24 Ⓐ Ⓑ Ⓒ Ⓓ	50 Ⓐ Ⓑ Ⓒ Ⓓ	
25 Ⓐ Ⓑ Ⓒ Ⓓ	51 Ⓐ Ⓑ Ⓒ Ⓓ	
26 Ⓐ Ⓑ Ⓒ Ⓓ	52 Ⓐ Ⓑ Ⓒ Ⓓ	

VERBAL REASONING

53 Ⓐ Ⓑ Ⓒ Ⓓ	73 Ⓐ Ⓑ Ⓒ Ⓓ
54 Ⓐ Ⓑ Ⓒ Ⓓ	74 Ⓐ Ⓑ Ⓒ Ⓓ
55 Ⓐ Ⓑ Ⓒ Ⓓ	75 Ⓐ Ⓑ Ⓒ Ⓓ
56 Ⓐ Ⓑ Ⓒ Ⓓ	76 Ⓐ Ⓑ Ⓒ Ⓓ
57 Ⓐ Ⓑ Ⓒ Ⓓ	77 Ⓐ Ⓑ Ⓒ Ⓓ
58 Ⓐ Ⓑ Ⓒ Ⓓ	78 Ⓐ Ⓑ Ⓒ Ⓓ
59 Ⓐ Ⓑ Ⓒ Ⓓ	79 Ⓐ Ⓑ Ⓒ Ⓓ
60 Ⓐ Ⓑ Ⓒ Ⓓ	80 Ⓐ Ⓑ Ⓒ Ⓓ
61 Ⓐ Ⓑ Ⓒ Ⓓ	81 Ⓐ Ⓑ Ⓒ Ⓓ
62 Ⓐ Ⓑ Ⓒ Ⓓ	82 Ⓐ Ⓑ Ⓒ Ⓓ
63 Ⓐ Ⓑ Ⓒ Ⓓ	83 Ⓐ Ⓑ Ⓒ Ⓓ
64 Ⓐ Ⓑ Ⓒ Ⓓ	84 Ⓐ Ⓑ Ⓒ Ⓓ
65 Ⓐ Ⓑ Ⓒ Ⓓ	85 Ⓐ Ⓑ Ⓒ Ⓓ
66 Ⓐ Ⓑ Ⓒ Ⓓ	86 Ⓐ Ⓑ Ⓒ Ⓓ
67 Ⓐ Ⓑ Ⓒ Ⓓ	87 Ⓐ Ⓑ Ⓒ Ⓓ
68 Ⓐ Ⓑ Ⓒ Ⓓ	88 Ⓐ Ⓑ Ⓒ Ⓓ
69 Ⓐ Ⓑ Ⓒ Ⓓ	89 Ⓐ Ⓑ Ⓒ Ⓓ
70 Ⓐ Ⓑ Ⓒ Ⓓ	90 Ⓐ Ⓑ Ⓒ Ⓓ
71 Ⓐ Ⓑ Ⓒ Ⓓ	91 Ⓐ Ⓑ Ⓒ Ⓓ
72 Ⓐ Ⓑ Ⓒ Ⓓ	92 Ⓐ Ⓑ Ⓒ Ⓓ

Answer Sheet
MODEL EXAMINATION B

WRITING SAMPLE

Use separate ruled
sheets of paper.

93

94

BIOLOGICAL SCIENCES

95	Ⓐ Ⓑ Ⓒ Ⓓ	121 Ⓐ Ⓑ Ⓒ Ⓓ
96	Ⓐ Ⓑ Ⓒ Ⓓ	122 Ⓐ Ⓑ Ⓒ Ⓓ
97	Ⓐ Ⓑ Ⓒ Ⓓ	123 Ⓐ Ⓑ Ⓒ Ⓓ
98	Ⓐ Ⓑ Ⓒ Ⓓ	124 Ⓐ Ⓑ Ⓒ Ⓓ
99	Ⓐ Ⓑ Ⓒ Ⓓ	125 Ⓐ Ⓑ Ⓒ Ⓓ
100	Ⓐ Ⓑ Ⓒ Ⓓ	126 Ⓐ Ⓑ Ⓒ Ⓓ
101	Ⓐ Ⓑ Ⓒ Ⓓ	127 Ⓐ Ⓑ Ⓒ Ⓓ
102	Ⓐ Ⓑ Ⓒ Ⓓ	128 Ⓐ Ⓑ Ⓒ Ⓓ
103	Ⓐ Ⓑ Ⓒ Ⓓ	129 Ⓐ Ⓑ Ⓒ Ⓓ
104	Ⓐ Ⓑ Ⓒ Ⓓ	130 Ⓐ Ⓑ Ⓒ Ⓓ
105	Ⓐ Ⓑ Ⓒ Ⓓ	131 Ⓐ Ⓑ Ⓒ Ⓓ
106	Ⓐ Ⓑ Ⓒ Ⓓ	132 Ⓐ Ⓑ Ⓒ Ⓓ
107	Ⓐ Ⓑ Ⓒ Ⓓ	133 Ⓐ Ⓑ Ⓒ Ⓓ
108	Ⓐ Ⓑ Ⓒ Ⓓ	134 Ⓐ Ⓑ Ⓒ Ⓓ
109	Ⓐ Ⓑ Ⓒ Ⓓ	135 Ⓐ Ⓑ Ⓒ Ⓓ
110	Ⓐ Ⓑ Ⓒ Ⓓ	136 Ⓐ Ⓑ Ⓒ Ⓓ
111	Ⓐ Ⓑ Ⓒ Ⓓ	137 Ⓐ Ⓑ Ⓒ Ⓓ
112	Ⓐ Ⓑ Ⓒ Ⓓ	138 Ⓐ Ⓑ Ⓒ Ⓓ
113	Ⓐ Ⓑ Ⓒ Ⓓ	139 Ⓐ Ⓑ Ⓒ Ⓓ
114	Ⓐ Ⓑ Ⓒ Ⓓ	140 Ⓐ Ⓑ Ⓒ Ⓓ
115	Ⓐ Ⓑ Ⓒ Ⓓ	141 Ⓐ Ⓑ Ⓒ Ⓓ
116	Ⓐ Ⓑ Ⓒ Ⓓ	142 Ⓐ Ⓑ Ⓒ Ⓓ
117	Ⓐ Ⓑ Ⓒ Ⓓ	143 Ⓐ Ⓑ Ⓒ Ⓓ
118	Ⓐ Ⓑ Ⓒ Ⓓ	144 Ⓐ Ⓑ Ⓒ Ⓓ
119	Ⓐ Ⓑ Ⓒ Ⓓ	145 Ⓐ Ⓑ Ⓒ Ⓓ
120	Ⓐ Ⓑ Ⓒ Ⓓ	146 Ⓐ Ⓑ Ⓒ Ⓓ

The MCAT
Model Examination B

PHYSICAL SCIENCES

TIME—70 MINUTES FOR 52 QUESTIONS

Directions: The following questions or incomplete statements are in groups. Preceding each series of questions or statements is a paragraph or a short explanatory statement, a formula or set of formulas, or a definition. Read the written material and then answer the questions or complete the statements. Select the ONE BEST ANSWER for each question and indicate your selection by marking the corresponding letter of your choice on the Answer Form. Eliminate those alternatives you know to be incorrect and then select an answer from among the remaining alternatives. A periodic table is provided (see p. 563). You may consult it whenever you wish to do so.

Passage I (Questions 1–6)

The law of definite proportion holds that when two elements react to form a compound, the compound formed will always contain the same ratio of elements by mass. The law of multiple proportions states that when two elements react to form several different compounds, the ratio by mass of the elements can be reduced to whole numbers.

A chemist chooses three gaseous compounds containing only nitrogen and oxygen and then analyzes each compound. Compound A is formed by reacting 7.0 g of nitrogen with 16.0 g of oxygen. Compound B is generated by reacting 7.0 g of nitrogen with 8.0 g of oxygen. Compound C is synthesized by reacting 7.0 g of nitrogen with 4.0 g of oxygen.

After conducting the analysis, the chemist compares the data obtained with the molecular weights of each gas. Compound A has a molecular weight of 46 g/mole. Compound B has a molecular weight of 30 g/mole. Compound C has a molecular weight of 44 g/mole.

1. Which gas effuses at the fastest rate?

   (A) compound A
   (B) compound B
   (C) compound C
   (D) SF_6

2. What is the empirical formula of compound C?

   (A) NO
   (B) N_2O
   (C) NO_2
   (D) NO_3

3. What volume is occupied by 15.0 g of compound B at 0°C and 1.0 atm?

   (A) 2.4 L
   (B) 10.2 L
   (C) 11.2 L
   (D) 22.4 L

4. What is the molecular formula of compound A?

  (A) NO
  (B) N_2O
  (C) NO_2
  (D) NO_3

5. The chemist characterizes another compound, N_2O_4. This has the same empirical formula as:

  (A) compound A.
  (B) compound B.
  (C) compound C.
  (D) NO_3.

6. What is the oxidation state of nitrogen in N_2O?

  (A) –1
  (B) 0
  (C) +1
  (D) +2

Passage II (Questions 7–11)

Wave motion is a fundamental topic in basic physics classes. Understanding how waves travel and interact with other waves and the media through which the waves travel is important. Assume a lab can produce most kinds of wave and measure their properties. These will include transverse waves on cords and longitudinal sound waves of many frequencies in different materials. Light sources with pure single wavelengths, lenses, and so on are available. The velocities, wavelengths, and frequencies are measured accurately.

7. Some properties of transverse and longitudinal waves are similar, and some differ. Fluids (gases and liquids) cannot transmit transverse waves. The speeds of both types generally do not depend on frequency. What experimental fact then most clearly distinguishes transverse and longitudinal waves?

  (A) Transverse waves will not travel through rock.
  (B) Transverse waves can be polarized.
  (C) Longitudinal waves have shorter wavelengths than transverse waves of the same frequency.
  (D) Longitudinal waves have longer wavelengths in liquids than in solids.

8. The energy of a photon of light is proportional to the frequency $E = hf$, where h is Planck's constant. When students measure the shortest and longest wavelengths of light that are visible they find the wavelengths range from about 400 nm to 750 nm (1 nm = 10^{-9} m) One wavelength is red, and the other is violet in color. Which color is the 750 nm wavelength, and which wavelength has the higher-energy photon?

  (A) red, 400 nm
  (B) red, 750 nm
  (C) violet, 400 nm
  (D) violet, 750 nm

9. A lighted object is 40 cm in front of an optical device that projects a clear image onto a screen 40 cm behind the device. Describe the device.

  (A) It is a converging lens of focal length 20 cm.
  (B) It is a converging lens of focal length 40 cm.
  (C) It is a diverging lens of focal length 15 cm.
  (D) It is a concave mirror of focal length 20 cm.

10. The professor cannot hear sounds higher in frequency than 14,000 Hz, while a student can hear a frequency of 19,000 Hz. What is the ratio of the speed of sound for the 19,000 Hz wave to the speed of the 14,000 Hz wave?

  (A) 1.36
  (B) 1.22
  (C) 1.00
  (D) 0.74

11. The professor holds a 2.0 m long thin aluminum rod at its center and strokes the rod with the rosin-covered fingers of his other hand. This causes a resonant longitudinal vibration. If the frequency of the sound heard is 1275 Hz, what is the speed of the sound wave in the aluminum rod?

  (A) 638 m/s
  (B) 2550 m/s
  (C) 1275 m/s
  (D) 5100 m/s

Passage III (Questions 12–16)

A number of apparatus are devised for the study of simple harmonic motion. Several masses can be attached to different springs and set into oscillation. The periods of these mass-spring systems are given by $T = 2\pi \sqrt{m/k}$, where k is the spring constant (N/m). A pendulum system has a bob of mass 1 kg on the end of a string 50 cm long. Bobs and strings of various masses and lengths are available. If the pendulum bob is displaced through an angle of less than about 10°, it behaves as a simple pendulum of length L with a period $T = 2\pi \sqrt{L/g}$. The speed of the pendulum bob and of the mass on the end of the spring can be measured by photogate timers.

12. The pendulum with the 1-kg bob and string length of 50 cm is starting to swing through an angle of about 9°. What is its period?

    (A) 3.2 sec
    (B) 6.1 sec
    (C) 1.4 sec
    (D) 5.5 sec

13. The bob is replaced with a 2-kg bob and the angle of swing is reduced to 5°. What is the period of this new pendulum?

    (A) 3.2 sec
    (B) 6.1 sec
    (C) 1.4 sec
    (D) 5.5 sec

14. A 500-gram mass is hung from a spring carefully so that it is at rest and the stretch of the spring is measured to be 49 cm. What is the spring constant of this spring?

    (A) 100 N/m
    (B) 40 N/m
    (C) 10 N/m
    (D) 80 N/m

15. The 500-gram mass is pulled down 5 cm from its rest position and released so that the mass executes simple harmonic motion. What is the period of this simple harmonic motion?

    (A) 4.4 sec
    (B) 1.4 sec
    (C) 2.8 sec
    (D) 5.6 sec

16. The 500 g mass is replaced with a 2 kg mass that is pulled down 5 cm from its rest position and released again. What happens to the period of this simple harmonic motion?

    (A) The period is only half as long.
    (B) The period increases by 4 times.
    (C) The period doubles.
    (D) The period triples.

Questions 17–19 are independent of any passage and each other.

17. What is the oxidizing agent in the following reaction?

    $$2Fe^{2+} + Cl_2 \rightarrow 2Fe^{3+} + Cl^-$$

    (A) Fe^{2+} (C) Cl^-
    (B) Fe^{3+} (D) Cl_2

18. Which molecule is nonpolar and contains a nonpolar covalent bond?

    (A) F_2 (C) HF
    (B) $CHCl_3$ (D) H_2O

19. Which compound reacts with an acid to form a salt and water?

    (A) CH_3Cl (C) KCl
    (B) CH_3COOH (D) KOH

Passage IV (Questions 20–24)

The Le Chatelier principle states roughly that when stress is placed upon an equilibrium system, the system will react in a direction to relieve the stress.

20. In the equilibrium reaction

$$CO(g) + Cl_2 (g) \leftrightharpoons COCl_2 (g),$$

the imposition of higher pressure will result in increased percentage(s) of:

(A) CO.
(B) Cl_2.
(C) $COCl_2$.
(D) A and B.

21. In the equilibrium reaction

$$2H_2S (g) \leftrightharpoons 2H_2 (g) + S_2 (g),$$

an increase in the applied pressure will result in higher percentage(s) of:

(A) H_2S.
(B) H_2.
(C) S_2.
(D) B and C.

22. In the equilibrium reaction

$$H_2 (g) + Cl_2 (g) \leftrightharpoons 2 HCl (g),$$

imposition of increased pressure would result in a higher percentage of:

(A) H_2.
(B) Cl_2.
(C) HCl.
(D) none of the above.

23. To an equilibrium mixture of H_2, Cl_2, and HCl in the equation in question 22, is added additional Cl_2. The result will be a (an):

(A) increase in the amount of HCl.
(B) decrease in the amount of H_2.
(C) increase in the amount of H_2.
(D) more than one of the above.

24. $X (g) + Y (g) \leftrightharpoons 2Z (g)$

If the above hypothetical reaction is at equilibrium, addition of more Z (without changing pressure or temperature) will result in:

(A) presence of more X.
(B) presence of less X.
(C) a change in K_{eq}.
(D) more than one of the above.

Passage V (Questions 25–29)

A physics instructor devises a simple electrical circuit setup in which one can easily insert various resistors and capacitors in series and parallel combinations. One can have only resistor combinations, only capacitor combinations, or capacitor-resistor combinations. The circuit is usually used for DC (direct current) studies but can also be used for AC (alternating current) studies. The DC battery voltage is 6 volts. The AC rms voltage is 120 volts (at 60 Hz). The student inserts the resistors and/or capacitors as instructed and has available suitable ammeters and voltmeters for both the DC and AC experiments. (There are three resistors, each of 2 ohms resistance. There are also three capacitors, each of 1 microfarad capacitance.)

25. All three resistors are connected in series and the combination is connected to the 6-volt DC battery. What voltage drop occurs across each individual resistor as measured by the voltmeter?

(A) 0.33 V
(B) 1.0 V
(C) 2.0 V
(D) 6.0 V

26. Two capacitors are connected in parallel. The ends of this combination are then connected to the 6-V DC battery. What are the final current and voltage, respectively, across the two capacitors?

(A) 0 A, 6 V
(B) 0.33 A, 3 V
(C) 0.33 A, 6 V
(D) 6 A, 6 V

27. Two of the 2-ohm resistors are connected in series, and the 6-volt battery is connected across the ends of the series combination. The current is measured. The same resistors are then connected in parallel, and the 6-volt battery is connected across the parallel pair. Which circuit, series or parallel, draws the most current from the battery?

   (A) Series
   (B) Parallel
   (C) Both draw about the same current
   (D) Cannot answer without knowing the current carrying values for the resistors

28. What are the highest and lowest resistance values that one can construct using all three of the 2-ohm resistors?

   (A) 3 ohms and 0.67 ohm
   (B) 6 ohms and 0.33 ohm
   (C) 6 ohms and 0.67 ohm
   (D) 6 ohms and 2 ohms.

29. Two of the 2-ohm resistors are connected in parallel. The other 2-ohm resistor is connected to the end (in series) with the parallel combination. The 120-volt AC source is applied to the ends of the group of three resistors. What current flows through the single 2-ohm resistor?

   (A) 3 A
   (B) 20 A
   (C) 40 A
   (D) 60 A

Passage VI (Questions 30–34)

An air track with carts is used as an (almost) frictionless system to study both elastic and inelastic collisions. The purpose is to understand the principle of conservation of linear momentum as well as the conservation of energy principle. It is assumed that total kinetic energy is conserved for the collision of air track carts with spring steel bumpers. The velocities of the carts are determined by the use of photogate timers, both before and after collisions. Carts with masses of 150 and 750 g are available. Some carts have "sticky" bumpers so that they stick together after colliding (in "completely inelastic" collisions). The total kinetic energy is not conserved (constant) in these latter collisions. Two of the different mass carts have a spring that can be compressed between them. A taut string tied between the carts keeps the spring compressed. The string is burned with a match and the two carts fly apart in opposite directions.

30. When the string is burned, the 150 g cart is observed to have a velocity of 3 m/sec. What is the magnitude of the opposite velocity of the 750 g cart?

   (A) 0.33 m/sec
   (B) 1 m/sec
   (C) 0.6 m/sec
   (D) 9 m/sec

31. One 50 g mass is added to a 150 g cart and another 50 g mass is added to a 750 g cart. With the carts initially at rest, forces of 2 N act for 2 seconds on each of the carts on the air track. Compare their final momenta after the 2 seconds.

   (A) They have equal momenta.
   (B) The heavier cart has the greater momentum.
   (C) The lighter cart has the greater momentum.
   (D) They are too fast to measure their momenta.

32. A 750 g cart passes through two photogates that are 2 m apart. It has a speed of 4.0 m/sec through the first photogate and a speed of 3.0 m/sec through the second photogate. About how much energy was lost to air friction during the passage between the gates?

    (A) 1.1 joules
    (B) 2.6 joules
    (C) 2.3 joules
    (D) 8.8 joules

33. One end of the air track is now elevated. A 450 g cart is given a push and then passes through a photogate. It ascends the track and comes to rest at a point that is measured to be a vertical height of 0.5 m above the photogate. Ignoring air friction, what was the speed of the cart through the photogate?

    (A) 1.24 m/sec
    (B) 3.13 m/sec
    (C) 4.55 m/sec
    (D) 6.26 m/sec

34. A cart of mass 750 g moving at a speed of 6 m/s collides with a cart of mass 150 g that is at rest. The carts stick together after the inelastic collision. What is the velocity of the combined carts after colliding?

    (A) 5 m/s
    (B) 6 m/s
    (C) 9 m/s
    (D) 1.5 m/s

Questions 35–40 are independent of any passage and of each other.

35. A ray of light is incident at an angle of 30° from air onto a glass surface with an index of refraction of 1.65. The angle of refraction in the glass is found to be 17.6°. Suppose the light ray were again incident at 30° but this time the incident angle is in the glass. The refracted angle in air as the ray leaves the glass will be:

    (A) larger than 30°.
    (B) smaller than 30°.
    (C) between 17.6° and 30°.
    (D) equal to 17.6°.

36. A steel ball is thrown straight up vertically and rises to its highest point, then falls back down. Which graph correctly shows the ball's velocity as a function of time during the time the ball is in free flight?

    (A)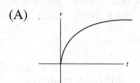

    (B)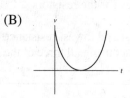

    (C)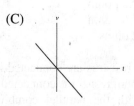

    (D)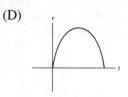

37. Radioactive Cobalt-60 decays, giving off very energetic gamma rays that have been used for many years to treat cancerous tumors. The half-life for decay is about 5.3 years. If a strong source of 5000 curies was originally furnished to the hospital, about how many curies would be left after 16 years? (The sources are actually changed more often to avoid lengthy treatment times for patients.)

    (A) 1667 curies
    (B) 3333 curies
    (C) 245 curies
    (D) 625 curies

38. A diffraction grating with grating constant $d = 1.67$ microns (1.67×10^{-6} meters) is used to produce an m-th order image of a spectral line of wavelength 417 nm (1 nm = 10^{-9} meters), which is seen at a diffracted angle of 30°. What is the value of the order m?

    (A) 1
    (B) 2
    (C) 3
    (D) 4

39. A 12 cm long board is on a fulcrum at its center and has masses of 30 grams and 15 grams on each end as shown. Where must a 20 gram mass be placed so that the system is balanced on the fulcrum?

    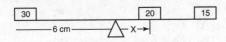

    (A) X = 5.5 cm
    (B) X = 3.0 cm
    (C) X = 4.5 cm
    (D) X = 2.5 cm

40. Neutron-induced fission of uranium-235 produces many possible reactions and decay products. One reaction is:

    $${}^{1}_{0}n + {}^{235}_{92}U \rightarrow {}^{A}_{Z}X + {}^{143}_{56}Ba + 3{}^{1}_{0}n$$

    The 3 neutrons may induce other fissions. What are the atomic number, Z, and mass number, A, and chemical symbol of the unknown isotope X?

    (A) ${}^{90}_{37}Rb$
    (B) ${}^{91}_{36}Rb$
    (C) ${}^{90}_{36}Kr$
    (D) ${}^{92}_{38}Sr$

Passage VII (Questions 41–47)

Ionization constants for weak bases may be dealt with in the same way as the ionization constants for weak acids.

$$B + H_2O \rightleftharpoons BH^+ + OH^-$$

$$K_b = \frac{[BH^+][OH^-]}{[B]} \quad \text{and} \quad pK_b = -\log \frac{[BH^+][OH^-]}{[B]}$$

41. Ammonia has a K_b of 1.8×10^{-5}. Its pK_b would be:

    (A) between 2 and 3.
    (B) between 3 and 4.
    (C) between 4 and 5.
    (D) greater than 5.5.

42. A 0.01 molar solution of ammonia in water would have a pOH of:

    (A) between 2 and 3.
    (B) between 3 and 4.
    (C) between 4 and 5.
    (D) greater than 5.5.

43. Hydrazine has a K_b of 1.7×10^{-6}. Its pK_b would be:

    (A) between 3 and 4.
    (B) between 4 and 5.
    (C) between 5 and 6.
    (D) between 6 and 7.

44. Assuming equal concentration (and solubility) the highest pH will be observed with an aqueous solution of a base having a pK_b of:

    (A) 3.5.
    (B) 4.8.
    (C) 6.2.
    (D) 6.8.

45. A theory of acids and bases that does NOT necessarily involve hydrogen or hydroxyl ions was developed by:

    (A) Arrhenius.
    (B) Brønsted and Lowry.
    (C) Gordon.
    (D) Lewis.

46. The base NaOH would be expected to have a pK$_b$ of:

(A) 2 ± 1.
(B) 5 ± 1.
(C) 9 ± 1.
(D) none of the above.

47. The pH of a 0.001 molar aqueous solution of NaOH would be:

(A) 3
(B) 5
(C) 9
(D) 11

Questions 48–52 are independent of any passage and each other.

48. What is the electron configuration of Ca^{2+}?

(A) $1s^2 2s^2 2p^6 3s^2 3p^4$
(B) $1s^2 2s^2 2p^6 3s^2 3p^6$
(C) $1s^2 2s^2 2p^6 3s^2 3p^6 4s^1$
(D) $1s^2 2s^2 2p^6 3s^2 3p^6 4s^2$

49. Which bond is formed by the transfer of an electron from one atom to another?

(A) ionic bond
(B) covalent bond
(C) peptide bond
(D) hydrogen bond

50. The maximum number of electrons that a single orbital of the 3d sublevel may contain is:

(A) 1
(B) 2
(C) 3
(D) 4

51. Given the following K_{sp} values, which compound will be the least soluble in water?

(A) AgBr = 5.0×10^{-13}
(B) AgCl = 1.8×10^{-10}
(C) AgIO$_3$ = 3.17×10^{-8}
(D) AgI = 8.3×10^{-17}

52. Which could act either as an oxidizing agent or a reducing agent?

(A) Fe^0
(B) Fe^{2+}
(C) Fe^{3+}
(D) Cu^0

VERBAL REASONING

TIME—60 MINUTES FOR 40 QUESTIONS

Directions: The questions are based on the accompanying seven passages. Read each passage carefully, then answer the following questions. Consider only the material within the passage. For each question, select the ONE BEST ANSWER and indicate your selection by marking the corresponding letter on the Answer Form.

Passage I (Questions 53–57)

What is the essence of graphic design? How do graphic designers solve problems, organize space, and imbue their work with those visual and symbolic qualities that enable it to convey visual and verbal information with expression and clarity? The extraordinary flowering of graphic design in our time—as a potent means of communication and a major component of our visual culture—increases the need for designers, clients, and students to comprehend its essence.

Traditionally, graphic designers looked to architecture or painting for their model. Certainly, a universal language of form is common to all visual disciplines, and in some historical periods the various design arts have shared styles. Too much dependence upon other arts—or even on the universal language of form—is unsatisfactory, however, because graphic design has unique purposes and visual properties.

Graphic design is a hybrid discipline. Diverse elements including signs, symbols, words, and pictures are collected and assembled into a total message. The dual nature of these graphic elements as both communicative sign and visual form provides endless fascination and potential for invention and combination. Although all the visual arts share properties of either two- or three-dimensional space, graphic space has a special character born from its communicative function.

Perhaps the most important thing that graphic design does is give communications resonance, a richness of tone that heightens the expressive power of the page. It transcends the dry conveyance of information, intensifies the message, and enriches the audience's experience. Resonance helps the designer realize clear public goals: to instruct, to delight, and to motivate.

Most designers speak of their activities as a problem-solving process because designers seek solutions to public communications problems. Approaches to problem solving vary, based on the problem at hand and the working methods of the designer. At a time when Western nations are evolving from industrial to information cultures, a comprehensive understanding of our communicative forms and graphic design becomes increasingly critical.

The general public does not understand graphic design and art direction. Designers tell the story of a graphic designer trying to explain this job to Grandmother. The designer shows Grandmother a recent project and says, "You were asking me about what I do, Grandmother. I'm a graphic designer, and I designed this."

Pointing to the photograph in the design, the grandmother asks, "Did you draw that picture?"

"No, Grandmother, it's a photograph. I didn't draw it, but I planned it, chose the photographer, helped select the models, assisted in setting it up, art-directed the shooting session, chose which shot to use, and cropped the picture."

"Did you write what it says, then?"

"Well, no," the designer replies, "But I did brainstorm with the copywriter to develop the concept."

"Oh, I see. Then you did letter these big words?" asks the grandmother, pointing to the headline.

"Uh, no, a typesetter set the copywriter's words in type, but I specified the typefaces and sizes to be used," responds the designer.

"Well, did you draw this little picture down in the corner?"

"No, but I selected the illustrator, told her what needed to be drawn, and decided where to put it and how big to make it."

"Oh. Well, did you draw this little, what do you call it, a trademark?"

"Uh, no. A design firm that specializes in visual identification programs designed it for the client."

The grandmother is somewhat confused about just what it is that her grandchild does and why credit is claimed for all these other people's work.

Used with permission of Philip B. Meggs and John T. Bryan, *Type and Image*, 1989.

53. The object of this passage is to:

    (A) convince the reader that graphic designers are artists.
    (B) illustrate the fact that the general public does not comprehend what graphic designers actually do.
    (C) underscore the fact that understanding graphic design is essential in an information culture.
    (D) provide the reader with a glimpse of the importance of graphic design in today's culture, as well as of its diverse nature.

54. According to this passage, graphic design today:

    (A) is an important communication tool, as well as a major component of our visual culture.
    (B) provides employment for people such as artists, directors, photographers, and writers.
    (C) depends too much on other art forms.
    (D) is a traditional discipline based on architectural design.

55. The author believes that the most important function of graphic design is to:

    (A) provide attractive visual displays for the public.
    (B) help Western culture make the transition from a technical to a communication-oriented society.
    (C) give communications resonance, thus helping the designer realize clear public goals: to instruct, to delight, and to motivate.
    (D) bring diversity to the art field.

56. Based on the information in the passage, what do graphic designers actually do?

    I. seek solutions to public communication problems
    II. organize space
    III. imbue their work with visual and symbolic qualities

    (A) I only
    (B) II only
    (C) I and II only
    (D) I, II, and III

57. Which of the following statements best supports the notion that graphic design is a *hybrid* discipline?

    (A) The extraordinary flowering of graphic design in our time increases the need for designers who have the ability to problem solve.
    (B) In graphic arts, diverse elements—including signs, symbols, words, and pictures—are collected and assembled into a total message.
    (C) Graphic design transcends the dry conveyance of information.
    (D) Graphic design has unique purposes and a special character.

Passage II (Questions 58–64)

Until recently, scientific data were a convenient tool in the scientific process, with the following steps: (1) formulating a question; (2) ascertaining what is known; (3) formulating a testable hypothesis; (4) conducting observations and collecting data; (5) analyzing the data and relating them to existing information; (6) formulating a new or modified hypothesis; and (7) initiating a new round of studies until the question is answered, abandoned or restated. At various periods in the age of enlightenment, different components of the scientific method have been emphasized. Early on, propositions were formulated and debated with minimum organized observation or collection of data. The age of philosophers gave way to the age of observers, such as the astronomers who gazed at the sky and mapped the thousands of points of light, the naturalists who described and collected plants and animals, and the explorers who mapped rivers and oceans, coasts and mountains. Observers of nature gave way to the industrial age, during which inventors focused on solutions, oftentimes without well-formulated questions, theory, or review of prior work. Naturalists and inventors recorded their observations in journals or log books as personalized memory aids. Inventors carried record keeping a step forward as a means of economy, to prevent repetition of failed trials. In all of these circumstances, however, the records were a convenient tool of and for the individual. Data records of concepts and observations took on a new meaning during the age of inventions. Inventors sought to profit from their creations, not only by building and selling a better "mousetrap" but also by seeking legal protection under constitutionally guaranteed rights to patent intellectual property. Records of data became a part of the documentation for priority, due diligence and breadth of a claim. Record keeping for

---

Adapted from *Basic Science*, S. Gaylen Bradley, 1990.

commercialization of intellectual property now has become formalized, standardized, and required.

During the past few decades, records of data have become essential components of the documentation for regulatory agencies approving utility, efficacy, or safety of new products or appliances. Progressively, regulatory agencies have extended the scope of their oversight, specifying some aspects of experimental design, data collection, and analysis. Most recently, regulatory agencies have insisted that all data collected be retained and made available for inspection, even data from aborted or defective studies. Data keeping and storage have become ends unto themselves, initially to ensure that work paid for was actually done and subsequently to ensure that unwanted results (e.g., toxicity of a drug) were not suppressed. It is perhaps a logical extension that managers of public funds have focused upon records of data as documentation that work paid for was actually done, much as an auditor of public accounts matches purchase orders, invoices, and disbursements. The managers of public funds, lacking the technical expertise to judge the quality and value of scientific investigations, have turned to process rather than product to demonstrate their diligence in protecting the taxpayers' money. The increased reliance on process rather than output measures reflects, in part, a loss of confidence by the public in the scientific community to have the ability and the will to judge and police itself. Regrettably, there are some bases for this loss of confidence in scientific peer review, and this loss of confidence permeates the scientific community itself as well as the managers of public funds.

Regardless of the cause, an increasing emphasis is now placed on data keeping and data storage. Any discussion on scientific data presupposes that there is general agreement on the definition of *data*. Unfortunately, there is no universally accepted definition of *data*. Perhaps the best we can do is conclude that, like pornography, we know *data* when we see them, or that data are defined by some unspecified *community standard*. Are data the holographic notes entered personally and immediately by the observer? Are data the printouts from apparatus? Are data the printouts of computers that accept input from the observer or directly from apparatus? Are data the embedded pieces of tissue from a treated animal, or the stained sections made from the tissue, or the notes of the observer examining the tissue, or all of these, or none of these? What are "materials and methods" as distinguished from "data" and from interpretation? How do we meet the demand that scientists must properly keep and store data, when we do not know what data are and whether or not they can be kept and stored other than by written notes of the observer or photographs of an event? Finally, who is responsible for keeping and storing data?

58. The passage could be entitled:

(A) Scientific Experimentation.
(B) Scientific Method.
(C) Scientific Responsibility.
(D) Scientific Data.

59. Throughout the history of experimentation and development of new knowledge:

(A) the scientific method has been painstakingly applied and followed.
(B) formulating a hypothesis has been a critical element in progress.
(C) emphasis within the application of the scientific method has varied.
(D) scientific data has been compared, analyzed, and scrutinized.

60. Using information provided in the passage, one would NOT be justified in concluding that:

I.   all scientific experimentation and observation throughout history was based on strict recording and analysis of data.
II. philosophy about matter eventually turned to the scientific approach.
III. with industrialization came a method of solving questions utilizing the scientific approach.
IV. industrialization was interested and emphasized practical solutions.

(A) I, II, and III
(B) I and III
(C) II and IV
(D) IV only

61. The passage contradicts which of the following?

I.   Inventors sought constitutional protection.
II. At the present, record keeping is an essential element of society.
III. Regulatory agencies can require complete documentation of data.
IV. Failed or aborted experiments do not need to be scrutinized because they are of little benefit.

(A) I, II, and III
(B) I and III
(C) II and IV
(D) IV only

62. Which of the following statement(s) is/are *supported by* the passage?

    I. The criteria for a definition of data are fairly well established.

    II. Data are verified by a computer printout.

    III. Data must be recorded and stored.

    IV. Responsibility for data storage rests upon the investigator.

    (A) I, II, and III
    (B) I and III
    (C) II and IV
    (D) none of the above

63. Which of the conclusions listed below follow(s) from the information contained in the passage?

    I. There has been an evolution in the methodology of recording data.

    II. After a foiled experiment, a modified hypothesis is part of the scientific approach.

    III. Data storage has been utilized as an end unto itself in order to ensure completion of a project.

    IV. Managers of public funds are usually well qualified to judge scientific work.

    (A) I, II, and III
    (B) I and III
    (C) II and IV
    (D) IV only

64. The passage argues that:

    (A) the public's money is well protected.
    (B) the public has trust in the scientific community.
    (C) the scientific community polices itself appropriately.
    (D) data collection and storage are increasingly stressed.

Passage III (Questions 65–69)

It has become obvious in recent years that the decision-making power in many school districts is shifting, and is becoming more liberalized as both teachers and parents realize that they are an important facet in the total school operation. They know that without their support and cooperation the system cannot continue to function smoothly.

Consequently, today's educator is no longer content to sit in the background and let decisions be made and programs formulated. New teachers want a voice, they demand a piece of the action, and they are daring enough to question the judgments of the system in their desire to achieve a better educational experience for their students as well as a more economically realistic position for themselves.

Not too many years ago, perhaps as little as a decade in some areas, the decision-making power in a school system could have been observed by quickly glancing at an organizational chart that would most probably have looked like this:

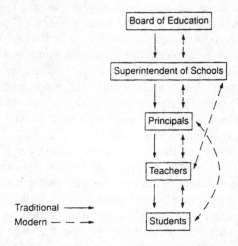

Although much simplified, the chart indicates a flow of power from the school board to the superintendent of schools down to the individual school principals and from there to the teachers and, finally, a minimal involvement of the students themselves.

The board of education was naturally found at the top, for it was assumed that this body represented the taxpaying community. Next in importance was the superintendent, whose word was considered to be law and who would, if so disposed, allow the principal some freedom to make decisions.

By the same token, those principals who prided themselves in being of a democratic nature would then allow

From Hugo R. Seibel and Kenneth E. Guyer, *How to Prepare for the Medical College Admission Test*, 6th ed. Hauppauge, New York: Barron's Educational Series, Inc., 1990.

teachers to have a voice in selected matters and would even possibly afford students the opportunity of making minute decisions in appropriate areas.

Within the confines of the individual school, the principal was looked upon as the one person who knew more about educational matters than any other member of the staff. Therefore, he or she was spotlighted not only as the chief administrator, but as the supreme educational leader of the complex. Teachers occupied the place of facilitators, whose main job it was to take the programs that were handed down to them and see that they were carried out satisfactorily. The students were viewed as receptacles for receiving and digesting information. Their major contribution rested in being accepted to an institution of higher learning, thus making the system look good and giving the taxpayers the feeling that the money they spent was, after all, worthwhile.

The entire pattern of decision making, as presented, was based on the very real fact that the board of education controlled the purse strings of a school system. Because money has always been of supreme importance, it was considered the most logical path to follow. Few people thought to question its wisdom or bothered to seek alternatives.

The modern public has slowly come to realize that even though money is still the most crucial factor in operating an efficient school system, there are also other vital and important elements that contribute to its success.

For example, parents are demanding a voice in the operation of local schools. They favor an open door policy that affords them the opportunity to see what is going on in the classrooms and allows many of them to get involved on a parent-volunteer basis. Parents speak out in many cases by manipulating a very vital school input, over which they have strict control, namely their children. Thus we read of such things as parents keeping their offspring out of school to protest situations that they find unsuitable and intolerable. Even though these actions may not in themselves solve the problems, they do cause those in authority to sit up, take notice, and search for possible solutions at a speedy rate.

Every bit as important as the public's realization of its powers is the teachers' realization that they too have a commodity that is of supreme importance to the system, and that is themselves. When teachers join forces and remove this vital input, school systems are forced to close and the educational machine comes to a halt. Teachers' strikes are now occurring more and more frequently in all areas of the country, and the threat of the entire profession becoming unionized is no longer a laughing matter.

Today's wise school systems have made note of these developments and are attempting to deal with them reasonably. Sharing the decision-making power by allowing more realistic and meaningful input from both parents and teachers has become a reality in many dis-

tricts. Although a revised look at the power flow chart today would probably show the players in the same basic positions, it would certainly have the arrows of decision coming not only down in a direct line, but also pointing up and out, allowing for a much more liberalized flow of communication and ideas.

65. The central theme of this passage deals with:

(A) the position of absolute power that is held by school boards in this country.
(B) the militant attitude that is displayed by many modern teachers.
(C) the shifting of decision-making power in today's school systems from that of a top down, authoritarian model to one that is more decentralized in nature.
(D) increased parent interest in the public schools and the establishment of strong parent-volunteer programs.

66. The role of the teacher is presented by the author as changing from that of mere program facilitator to one of a vital voice in educational planning. This change has come about partially because:

(A) the National Education Association represents modern educators throughout the United States.
(B) teachers are more willing than ever to speak out concerning the development of new programs and policies.
(C) teachers often go on strike if their demands for new programs are not met.
(D) according to the modern side of the flow chart, teachers now discuss their ideas directly with the board of education.

67. Which one of the following statements *contradicts* the central theme of this passage?

(A) Today's students are radical and demand a share in the decision-making process of local school boards.
(B) Principals are the instructional leaders in their schools.
(C) Students who get accepted to college make teachers look good.
(D) Because it has control over the purse strings, the board of education should have absolute power over all other facets of the educational machine within a school district.

68. Which of the following statements seems reasonable in light of the information presented in this passage?

   I. Parent-volunteer programs are one avenue of public involvement in local schools.
   II. Parents want to be placed above the board of education on the organizational chart.
   III. Parents are becoming a more powerful force in the operation of local schools.

   (A) I and II
   (B) II only
   (C) I and III
   (D) I, II, and III

69. Of the following statements, which one is NOT *supported nor contradicted by* the information presented in this passage?

   (A) Parents sometimes use their children as tools for getting what they want in a school system.
   (B) Teachers' strikes are taking place on a more frequent basis throughout the nation.
   (C) School systems of the future probably will see an equal division of power among the board of education, principals, and parents.
   (D) The board of education represents the tax-paying community in any given school district.

Passage IV (Questions 70–75)

Generally, state statutes grant school administrators the legal duty to establish, maintain, and protect the school's learning environment. It is a basic tenet of school law that school authorities may exclude from school any student whose conduct interferes with or in any way disrupts the operation of the school, or who openly defies school rules, or whose conduct is willfully insubordinate, or who poses a threat of harm to himself, to other persons, or to school property.

The terms used to characterize exclusion of students from school are suspension and expulsion. Generally, suspension denotes a temporary exclusion from school with a presumption that return to school is possible. Typically, by state code provision, school authorities possess the legal prerogative to suspend students from classes and from school. Expulsion denotes a longer term of exclusion from school with a presumption of

finality regarding the termination of one's status as a student. Considered the most severe student punishment available to school authorities, state statutes and local policies usually provide that only a local school board has the prerogative to expel a student.

In recent years, litigation has involved both the right of school authorities to suspend or expel, and the minimal procedural due process rights of students prior to suspension or expulsion. Following the landmark decision in *Gault,* in which the Supreme Court held that minor juvenile offenders in juvenile court were entitled to certain procedural due process protections, several lower courts began to clarify the procedural due process rights of students facing exclusion from school. The matter was ultimately treated by the United States Supreme Court in *Goss v. Lopez.*

Observing that a student possesses a property right to a public education, protected by the guarantees of the fourteenth amendment, the Supreme Court overturned an Ohio statute that allowed summary suspensions for up to ten days. In the Court's opinion, minimum procedures must be followed prior to exclusion from school. The Court held that in suspensions of ten days or less, notice of the charges and the right to be heard are required. And, if the student denies the charges, he or she must be informed of the evidence against him or her and be given the opportunity to present his or her side of the story. However, this requirement can be done informally and immediately after the incident. In *Goss,* the Supreme Court did not require that a public school system allow students to be represented by counsel, to present witnesses, or to confront and cross-examine witnesses. Nor did the Court rule on the elements of due process for suspensions of longer than ten days. The Court did observe that more procedural due process may be needed for longer suspensions.

Of major importance to the daily practice of school administrators is the Court's attitudes toward due process and school discipline, often missed by those who analyze this landmark case. First, the Court reemphasized the notion that procedural due process is a flexible legal standard, determined by the nature of the misconduct and the severity of the penalty. Second, the Court held that school officials are free to remove a student from school prior to a suspension if his or her presence is a danger to persons or property and/or is disruptive to teaching and learning.

Beyond the guidelines of the Supreme Court, a local school administrator is also bound by state statutory mandates and state court decisions, and these requirements vary. However, the following guidelines are generally accepted nationally and serve as excellent guidelines for school administrators: students must know in advance what standards of behavior are proscribed in their school and what modes of behavior are

---

Adapted from H. G. Hudgins and Richard S. Vacca, *Law and Education: Contemporary Issues and Correct Decisions,* 2nd ed. Charlottesville, Virginia: The Michie Company, 1985.

expected; they must know what specific disciplinary actions and punishments attach to violations of the rules; they must receive immediate and informed notice when they are accused of an infraction, and an opportunity to present his or her side of the story; and students must have an opportunity to appeal the decision to another administrative level within the school system. The administrator is reminded that these general elements become more formalized and technical when an expulsion is in process.

Two other student exclusion decisions from the United States Supreme Court should be briefly mentioned at this point because of their bearing on student procedural due process entitlements. The cases are *Wood v. Strickland,* and *Carey v. Piphus. Wood* involved the issue of students being allowed to sue local school board members for damages under Section 1983 for a denial of procedural due process in an expulsion hearing. In upholding the school board's actions, the Supreme Court held that individual board members could be sued if they knew or reasonably should have known that they denied students their constitutional rights or if board members acted with malicious intent.

Carey was a consolidation of two cases, both involving the suspension of a student from school. One student had violated a rule prohibiting the use of drugs at school, whereas the other student violated a rule against males wearing earrings at school. In rendering its decision in *Carey,* the Supreme Court held that students suspended from school without procedural due process are entitled to recover nominal damages of $1.00 and possibly extensive lawyers' fees. However, before any compensatory damages are awarded, a student must first submit proof of actual injury caused by the denial of due process. Punitive damages may be possible where a student can establish that school officials acted with the malicious intent to deprive him of his rights.

70. The main topic of this passage deals with:

   (A) the duty that school administrators have to establish, maintain, and protect the school's learning environment.
   (B) Fourteenth Amendment rights.
   (C) due process rights.
   (D) the exclusion of students from school by means of suspension and/or expulsion.

71. According to the information presented in this passage, exclusion from school refers to:

   I.   any time-out procedure directed at a student as a result of a disciplinary infraction.
   II. a temporary removal from the educational setting by means of suspension.
   III. a longer term and possibly permanent removal from the educational setting by means of expulsion.

   (A) I and II
   (B) I and III
   (C) II and III
   (D) all of the above

72. According to the information given in this passage, most state statutes and local policies give the prerogative of expelling a student from school to:

   (A) the classroom teacher.
   (B) the building administrator.
   (C) the school superintendent.
   (D) the school board.

73. The issue of student expulsion has produced numerous court cases. Litigation in this area generally involves:

   (A) the right of school authorities to suspend or expel, as well as the student's minimal due process rights prior to suspension or expulsion.
   (B) the flexible standard of the due process right as well as the length of time of the expulsion.
   (C) the past disciplinary record of a student as well as the type of punitive action that was taken previously.
   (D) all of the above.

74. In which of the following cases did the United States Supreme Court first treat the issue of procedural due process rights for students?

   (A) *Wood v. Strickland*
   (B) *Brown v. Board of Education*
   (C) *Goss v. Lopez*
   (D) *Carey v. Piphus*

75. Which of the following statements concerning the right to a public education is the *most* significant in *Goss v. Lopez*?

    (A) Every student has the right to a public education.
    (B) Public education is an inalienable right.
    (C) The right to a public education is a property right.
    (D) The right to a public education is protected by the Fourteenth Amendment.

Passage V (Questions 76–80)

Students in institutions of higher education hold diverse interests and backgrounds. There are average students as well as bright ones. Are the needs of average students different from those headed toward graduate school? Both need qualified and enthusiastic teachers.

When students evaluate teaching ability, they may or may not know a faculty member's academic qualifications or tenure status. Some nontenure-eligible faculty members have credentials comparable to tenure-track faculty members. The fact that a faculty member has a master's degree and teaches only lower level courses does not reflect on his or her teaching ability. Yet criteria used to evaluate full-time faculty members are similar to those applied to part-time faculty members. In addition, there is often an abuse of nontenure-eligible faculty members who may be requested to teach five courses a semester while receiving only 20 percent of the pay of the full-time faculty member.

Some faculty members contend that tenure is the freedom to teach, speak and write. Both tenured and nontenure-eligible faculty members, in fact, enjoy these freedoms. Academic freedom is not necessarily contingent upon tenure because the university protects the constitutional right of freedom of speech for all faculty members.

Tenure means job security, and bonds an individual to the institution. Nontenure-eligible faculty members are expected to bond with the institution; yet how can this be accomplished when they often experience employment uncertainty? The response is that tenure is not the only way to achieve bonding. Long-term contracts or "rolling contracts" are alternatives. There are some faculty members who may not want or need job security.

These are individuals in business or technical and professional fields who want to bond with a scholarly community in order to teach. They may have a primary career elsewhere or they may be pausing between career moves.

Tenure affects attitude and morale. What makes so many nontenure-eligible faculty members feel they are second-class citizens? Often they do not have offices or have not been accorded recognition for their teaching excellence. Faculty attitudes are inhibitive of change as are economic considerations. Why do nontenure-eligible faculty have to teach only lower level courses? Many nontenure-eligible faculty members may, in fact, be better equipped to teach some upper level courses. In addition, as the pool of faculty members in certain disciplines, English, for example, diminishes, the salaries needed to hire nontenure-eligible faculty members will increase. This competitive situation will encourage nontenure-eligible faculty members to voice their complaints about the lack of diverse teaching assignments or the failure to be treated as professional equals.

Pay differential between tenure track and nontenure-eligible faculty members will vary, but issues of bonding will remain on the table.

There is a need to determine the role and purpose of research in the university. Although the tripartite foundation of teaching, public service, and research is espoused, the institution's reward system leans toward research. At the same time, legislators, students, and parents cry out for excellence in teaching in order to raise the standards of quality. This conundrum must be addressed.

Nontenure-eligible research faculty experience other concerns that are not necessarily bound to tenure. They want job security during the transitional periods, i.e., from receipt of one grant to another. They lose even their second-class citizenship when job security is jeopardized. Long-term contracts are suggested in lieu of tenure.

Nontenure-eligible clinical faculty members practice usually in the medical and human services professions (dentistry, medicine, nursing, veterinary medicine, social work, clinical psychology, and counseling). In medicine and social work, much of the clinical teaching of patient care is delivered by nontenure-eligible faculty members who serve on a short-term basis. They represent the "off-site" faculty and serve as preceptors for clinical training of students. Their appointments cement the relationship between the practice and school. The clinical activities of nontenure-eligible faculty are not linked solely with the generation of income.

Tenure, for individuals in these disciplines, is usually accorded to individuals who have the M.D., Ph.D., or D.Ed. degrees. Lacking of tenure fosters the two-class system in which the vast majority of clinical care providers/teachers are, once again, made to feel they are relegated to the second class. Incentives and recognition of clinical performances are very important to clinical faculty members. Is it realistic to expect and demand

Adapted from A. Nancy Avakian. "Some Reflections on Nontenure-Eligible Faculty Members." In *Role of Nontenure-Eligible Faculty in the Academy*, 1990.

excellence in all endeavors (teaching, research, public service) by the nontenure-track clinical faculty?

Usually complexity of clinical teaching and practice dictates the need for a large number of nontenure-eligible faculty members whose financial compensations vastly exceed the number of tenure positions and available resources. Does tenure have a place in clinical departments which have the potential to generate substantial income for the private practitioner?

76. Which of the following types of faculty is NOT discussed by the passage?

   (A) research faculty
   (B) clinical faculty
   (C) part-time faculty
   (D) administrative faculty

77. Addressing as it does issues related to job security of various categories of faculty, the passage supports all but which of the following conclusions?

   (A) Institutions should promote opportunities by which individuals may feel a bonding.
   (B) Multiyear contracts would be beneficial to elicit identity with the institution.
   (C) There is a need to clarify the roles and differences of tenure and nontenure-eligible faculty.
   (D) Tenure is probably the only way to achieve bonding.

78. Issues of concern regarding nontenure-eligible faculty are:

   I.   job security.
   II. compensation.
   III. evaluation.
   IV. academic freedom.

   (A) I, II, and III
   (B) I and IV
   (C) II and IV
   (D) I, II, III, and IV

79. One could conclude from the information provided in the passage that:

   (A) responsibilities and qualifications of tenure and nontenure-eligible faculty are quite similar in many instances.
   (B) there is a difference between undergraduate and graduate bond students and the instructors they need.
   (C) tenure-track faculty are apt to initiate changes.
   (D) students are knowledgeable about instructor's status.

80. Which of the following statement(s) is/are NOT *supported nor contradicted by* the passage?

   I.   Pensions should be reviewed as separate from issues of intellectual and academic freedom.
   II   State legislatures must be educated or reeducated about the role of faculty.
   III. Institutions should provide support for nontenure-eligible research faculty between receipt of grants.
   IV. Nontenure-eligible faculty members should have access to the institution's grievance procedures.

   (A) I, II, and III
   (B) I and III
   (C) II and IV
   (D) I, II, III, and IV

Passage VI (Questions 81–86)

Herbert Hoover's initial reputation in public life arose from his legendary success in feeding the victims of World War I. Already established as a successful consulting engineer, he had responded to overwhelming human need at the outbreak of the war and had set up the Commission for Relief in Belgium to facilitate humanitarian responses to the dislocations of German occupation. From 1914 until the American declaration of war in April 1917, Hoover administered a complex organization to raise funds, obtain food, and transport it to the needy. Along the way, he negotiated and renegotiated with the warring governments, persuading them to permit his rescue operations. At the conclusion of the war, Hoover resumed international feeding with the American Relief Administration. And, during the 1920s, when he perceived need, he responded in the same fashion—in Russia from 1921 to 1923, for example, and again during the Mississippi floods of 1927.

The feeding, relief, and rescue operations made him one of the most beloved and admired men in the world. But that personal prestige was of small importance to Hoover, compared with the sense of satisfaction at having "saved the lives of 1,400,000,000 human beings, mostly women and children, who otherwise would have perished."

In all of his rescue efforts, children represented Hoover's first concern. Orphaned himself by age ten, he showed a lifetime commitment to children—to making sure that all children should have the opportunity to grow up with adequately nourished bodies and minds. In public life, his efforts may be seen in the White House Conference on Child Health and Protection; in private life, he and Mrs. Hoover engaged in countless hidden charities, providing for destitute families and educating needy youngsters. Each of Hoover's relief operations also began with the concern for suffering children, and then expanded to include mothers, other women, the aged, and finally able-bodied men.

But Hoover's purpose stretched beyond mere feeding. He understood that the Four Horsemen of the Apocalypse rode together, and that Famine's grim companions could warp minds as well as bodies. Not often poetic, Hoover nevertheless printed this verse at the beginning of his great documentary study of his relief activities:

I am the stalking aftermath of all wars.
Pestilence is my companion.
Tumult and Revolution rise round my feet
We kill more than all of the guns.
I breed fears and hates that bring to man more wars.
From me comes no peace to mankind.
My legacy is to Children of Famine—
Stunted bodies and twisted minds.

The battle against starvation had critical long-term political and ideological aspects. The hungry could not long defend themselves—or defend Freedom.

The outbreak of World War II in Europe in September 1939 immediately raised the relief question again. Within less than two weeks, in conversations with representatives of the Franklin Roosevelt Administration, Hoover suggested centralizing all relief activities under a single agency, preferably the Red Cross. When invited to join the executive committee of the Red Cross, Hoover declared himself willing to accept only if the Red Cross would "take on the whole job," dealing with food, clothing, medicine, and other aspects of relief. Norman Davis, head of the Red Cross, defined its role more narrowly, arguing that there was a fundamental difference between emergency relief that had been the normal function of the Red Cross and that could be

financed by private contributions, and the mass feeding and relief over an extended period that would require government financing. Hoover and Roosevelt's emissaries had reached an impasse.

81. In this passage the Red Cross:

(A) pictured itself as a broad-based, capable relief organization.
(B) viewed its role as supplying emergency relief.
(C) wanted Hoover to lead the organization.
(D) depended on government to finance its operation.

82. It is quite clear from the passage that Hoover's passion was:

(A) the hungry.
(B) the homeless.
(C) the children.
(D) the indigent.

83. Hoover was trained as:

(A) a politician.
(B) a businessman.
(C) a relief specialist.
(D) an engineer.

84. Which of the following is *contradicted by* the passage?

(A) Roosevelt supported Hoover's efforts.
(B) Hoover was active in negotiating between warring governments.
(C) Hoover's efforts were broad based.
(D) Hoover helped natural disaster victims.

85. Which of the following is/are *supported by* the passage?

   I. Hoover believed that a centrally coordinated effort would serve best.
  II. Deprived people will rise to the occasion and defend their liberties.
 III. Hoover was quick to act.
 IV. Hoover did not have his family's support.

(A) I, II, and III
(B) I and III
(C) II and IV
(D) none of the above

We gratefully acknowledge the help of Dr. Susan Esterbrook Kennedy, Professor of History and Geography, Virginia Commonwealth University, 1990.

86. Which of the following would describe/fit Herbert Hoover best?

    (A) He was a socialist.
    (B) He was a republican.
    (C) He was a globalist.
    (D) He was a humanitarian.

Passage VII (Questions 87–92)

Aristotle believed that "right reasoning" or ethical thinking could best be taught by tragedies. He particularly liked *Antigone* in this regard. He pointed out that tragedies first capture the heart of the reader by having a hero (or someone with whom we can associate) and then showing that this likable person committed an "error in judgment" *(hamartia)*. Aristotle believed in training the *heart* as well as the *mind* and that pity and fear *(pathos)* can best be aroused by a hero's downfall that is actually his fault. The "error in judgment" is all the more terrifying when we realize that it could have happened to us just as easily. Tragedies show our worst fear: good and logical people can fail!

Tragedies can test the limits of a culture to function; they can depict institutional and national failures. Tragedies can also show a particular culture to be the source of error. For instance, in the historical examples, unchecked scientific research and religious proselytizing resulting from a cultural misjudgment. Modern cultural misjudgments are the Catholic persecution in Ireland, black slavery in America, and the Jewish holocaust in Germany. Yet, in these three modern cases, it is important to realize the role of *pathos,* or empathy, in teaching wisdom. The reader must *identify with those who made the error in judgment* to be motivated toward determining that reasoning. For instance white Americans can feel guilt, humility (the "beginning of wisdom"), and uncertainty by studying slavery, whereas black Americans will feel mostly anger and resentment. Black Americans, for instance, should be introduced to the persecutions of other groups in other settings to obtain "true" or underlying wisdom about man's capacity for logical errors. Similarly, the holocaust is not a Jewish tragedy nor is the Irish persecution a Catholic tragedy in the classical sense of motivating the reader toward wanting to make good judgments. For such motivation, a person must "see" himself making the logical error, not just being a victim.

Tragedies can also show conflicts in values within one group or even within one person. Samuel Johnson criticized Shakespeare for a lack of morality in his plays; the hero often was a liar or an adulterer. What Shakespeare was actually so good at was showing the complexity of judgments in clear ways.

If tragedies are potentially effective for developing ethics and even wisdom, how can they be used in the educational arena? In his 1908 book, *Ethics,* John Dewey pointed out the "danger of either dogmatism or a sense of unreality when students are introduced abruptly to theoretical ideas." Dewey went on to propose an efficiency: ". . . he is encouraged to try them on simple problems before attempting the problems of the present." Following his lead, I propose to first introduce students to simple cases and then proceed to the more complex. Across the grades, this means beginning with picture books and one-page examples and eventually progressing to case studies in college. Of course, care must be taken to have the necessary elements of an empathetic character, moral dilemma, and mistake in judgment at all of these levels.

Sources for ethical tragedies are the Bible, classical literature, history, newspapers, books, and actual experiences. Shorter versions and profiles must be developed to make an ethical lesson in a reasonable amount of time. Uses or formats are Xerox pages, pamphlets, published articles, workbooks, and computer "what if" simulations with or without video accompaniments.

The main idea is that all these tragedies, regardless of format, must be short but not too short. For instance, John F. Kennedy wrote a book called *Profiles in Courage,* which contained about a dozen stories of U.S. senators faced with ethical dilemmas. The stories are short in length, but long enough in description to capture the heart of the reader to wish the hero well. In this way, we can take the need for such virtues as wisdom and courage "to heart."

The renewal of ethical *skills* to each generation can be helped by understanding capitalistic and market mechanisms. (Notice I did not say ethical *knowledge* because we are not trying to transmit facts but to develop right reasoning.) For instance, if teachers at a certain grade level or in a certain subject area have a case study or pamphlet "fair" where their works are displayed, the better works will become known and used increasingly. A school district, university, or state education department could encourage development, publication, and "survival of the fittest" of ethical tragedies by similar display mechanisms, sales shows, or annotated bibliographies. Eventually, a *general* curriculum could be prescribed by the state education department.

Ethical pamphlets or booklets are being proposed instead of textbooks because of the modular or "mix and match" possibilities that they allow. For instance, a high school teacher can use a pamphlet to supplement a history course at a strategic point, whereas a business

Adapted from material by Dr. James J. McGovern, Virginia Commonwealth University. Presented at the Conference on Educating the Gifted for the 21st Century (1990).

teacher in college can allow students to choose among some case studies and compare one of them to a recent event. The combination of student feedback and teacher rewriting should produce better case studies for the future. In this way, we can develop a naturally self-improving mechanism or *Tao* in this important area.

Encouraging teachers in various fields to write, desktop publish, and trade ethical cases has another advantage. It not only keeps the cases current, but it encourages teachers in the present generation to put the "key ideas" together to allow wise leadership to be "unlocked" in individuals in the next generation. In many ways, our teachers determine and give birth to the future.

It is primarily through education that the process of heredity, which from the beginning has caused the world to rise to higher zones of consciousness, is furthered in a reflective form and in its social dimensions. The educator, as an instrument of Creation, should derive respect and ardor for his efforts from a profound, communicative sense of the development already achieved or awaited. . . .

Pierre Teilhard de Chardin
The Future of Man

87. The material in this passage is an excerpt from a longer selection. Based on the tone of the content, which of the following statements describes the probable communication vehicle of the original piece?

(A) The material comes from a methods textbook on education.
B   The material is part of a talk presented at a conference on educating gifted students.
(C) The material comes from a theatrical article.
(D) The material is taken from a speech given to college graduates.

88. The main theme of this passage is that:

(A) studying plays or stories that have a tragic ending tends to make the reader view the lead character as a hero despite any judgment errors that he may be responsible for.
(B) tragedies, such as those created by Shakespeare, lack moral character because the hero generally is a liar or an adulterer.
(C) the skills needed to develop ethical thinking in new generations can be fostered by studying tragedies.
(D) an understanding of market mechanisms is needed to understand ethics.

89. The author's sense of the Greek word *hamartia* is:

(A) unavoidable mistakes.
(B) faulty logic.
(C) major injustices.
(D) personal grief.

90. In his book *Ethics,* John Dewey cautioned teachers to:

(A) avoid dogmatism.
(B) begin with theoretical overviews.
(C) start with simple cases.
(D) limit discussions to current situations.

91. Having teachers write their own ethical case studies:

(A) allows a standard curriculum to be developed.
(B) provides a free market mechanism.
(C) keeps the cases current.
(D) allows the writer to identify with the victim.

92. Passing on a sense of ethics from one generation to another can be accomplished by:

(A) teaching a basic body of knowledge.
(B) inspiring students to live good lives.
(C) teachers formulating good and humane reasoning, and this skill being picked up by students.
(D) reading about tragedies and other cases where evil doers suffer.

WRITING SAMPLE

TIME—2 ESSAYS
    60 MINUTES (30 MINUTES/TOPIC)

Directions: This is a test of your writing skills. The test consists of two parts. You will have 30 minutes to complete each part. Use your time efficiently. Before you begin writing each of your responses, read the assignment carefully to understand exactly what you are being asked to do. Because this is a test of your writing skills, your response to each part should be as well organized and clearly written as you can make it in the time allotted.

93. Consider this statement:

It is no wise man that will quit a certainty for an uncertainty.

Samuel Johnson

Write a unified essay in which you perform the following tasks. Explain what you think the above statement means. Describe a specific situation in which a wise person would quit a certainty for an uncertainty. Discuss the circumstances that you think determine whether or not one should or should not give up certainty for uncertainty.

94. Consider this statement:

Destruction is, after all, a form of creation.
Graham Greene

Write a unified essay in which you perform the following tasks. Explain what you think the above statement means. Describe a specific situation in which an act of destruction is not a form of creation. Discuss what you consider to be the circumstances that determine the relationship between destruction and creation.

BIOLOGICAL SCIENCES

TIME—70 MINUTES FOR 52 QUESTIONS

> **Directions:** The following questions or incomplete statements are in groups. Preceding each series of questions or statements is a paragraph or a short explanatory statement, a formula or set of formulas, or a definition. Read the written material and then answer the questions or complete the statements. Select the ONE BEST ANSWER for each question and indicate your selection by marking the corresponding letter of your choice on the Answer Form. Eliminate those alternatives you know to be incorrect and then select an answer from among the remaining alternatives.

Passage I (Questions 95–99)

The diagram below represents three generations of a human family, some of whose members have a non-lethal birth defect. Individuals 1, 3, and 4 are distantly related and come from a family in which the defect has occurred for many generations. Information on the occurrence of the defect among the ancestors of individual 2 is unavailable. The preceding four generations of the family and the siblings of individual 19 included no individuals who expressed the defect. The defect is caused by a single gene for which new mutations are very rare. The individuals with birth defects are represented by solid black symbols and the individuals who have a normal phenotype are represented by open symbols. Males are represented by squares and females are represented by circles.

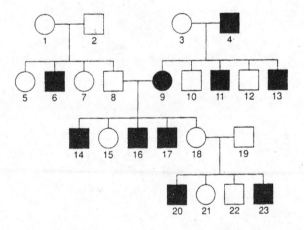

95. The defect is most likely caused by:

   (A) an autosomal gene for which the defective allele is recessive to the normal allele.
   (B) an X-linked gene for which the defective allele is recessive to the normal allele.
   (C) an autosomal gene for which the defective allele is dominant to the normal allele.
   (D) an X-linked gene for which the defective allele is dominant to the normal allele.

96. The genotype of individual number 1 in the family:

   (A) is most likely to contain only normal alleles.
   (B) is most likely to contain only defective alleles.
   (C) is most likely to contain both normal and defective alleles.
   (D) cannot be determined from the pedigree.

97. The genotype of individual number 6 in the family:

   (A) is most likely to contain only normal alleles.
   (B) is most likely to contain only defective alleles.
   (C) is most likely to contain both normal and defective alleles.
   (D) cannot be determined from the pedigree.

98. The genotype of individual number 8 in the family:

    (A) is most likely to contain only normal alleles.
    (B) is most likely to contain only defective alleles
    (C) is most likely to contain both normal and defective alleles.
    (D) cannot be determined from the pedigree.

99. The genotype of individual number 9 in the family:

    (A) is most likely to contain only normal alleles.
    (B) is most likely to contain only defective alleles.
    (C) is most likely to contain both normal and defective alleles.
    (D) cannot be determined from the pedigree.

Passage II (Questions 100–103)

Many scientists think of the pituitary gland as the master gland responsible for the secretion of many different hormones. A reciprocal relationship operates between the hormones secreted by the pituitary and the hormones produced by the target organs; this delicate control of balance of production of secretory product between the pituitary and the target organs is known as "negative feedback." Among the many hormones produced by the adenohypophysis of the pituitary gland are ACTH, FSH, LH, TSH, and STH. The following experiments were set up to demonstrate the actions of some of the above factors. Twenty-five, day-old immature male and female rats were subjected to the following treatment for 10 days: Group I was given a 0.5 cc saline injection; Group 2 was given a 0.5 cc FSH injection; and Group 3 was given a 0.5 cc crude pituitary extract injection. The results were recorded in table form.

MALE RATS

Group	Body Weight grams	Testes mg	Seminal Vesicles mg	Prostate mg	Thyroid mg	Adrenals mg
1	86	3750	18	71	6.0	20
2	82	5310	57	176	6.1	21
3	83	4830	24	163	7.5	27

FEMALE RATS

Group	Body Weight grams	Ovaries mg	Uterus mg	Thyroid mg	Adrenals mg
1	83	20	25	5.9	22
2	82	43	83	5.7	21
3	84	33	61	7.1	37

100. Based on the information provided, which of the following statements is/are *supported* by the data?

    (A) From the table it seems as if the crude pituitary extract had a lesser effect on the sex organs than did FSH.
    (B) Pituitary extract affected every organ under investigation.
    (C) Hypophysectomy probably would have resulted in a decreased weight of the organs under investigation.
    (D) All of the above.

101. Based on the information provided, which of the following statement(s) is/are *supported* by the data?

    (A) The administration of FSH alone to an immature rat will produce follicular growth, but uterine and vaginal configurations will remain infantile since LH is also needed. The experimental data indicate uterine growth, casting doubt on the purity of the FSH preparation.
    (B) Both FSH and LH are necessary for the production of estrogen.
    (C) FSH has as its target organs the organs of reproduction.
    (D) A and C of the above.

102. Based on the information provided, which of the following, statement(s) is/are *contradicted* by the data?

(A) FSH in the male had the greatest effect on the weight of the prostate gland; the tissue is therefore most reactive to it.

(B) The adrenal weight probably would drop if the animals were deprived of ACTH.

(C) In these experiments, none of the hormones in the pituitary extract probably were as effective as a purified fraction of them might have been.

(D) Body weights were not a significant experimental parameter.

103. Each of the following is under control of the adenohypophysis EXCEPT the:

(A) thyroid
(B) adrenal medulla
(C) testis.
(D) adrenal cortex.

Questions 104–108 are NOT based on a descriptive passage.

104. Characteristics of phylum Chordata include:

(A) a dorsally located nervous system.
(B) a vertebral column.
(C) mammary glands.
(D) epidermally derived scales.

105. A typical protein-coding gene in a eukaryote requires _____ between the time the gene is transcribed and the time that the mRNA is translated.

(A) chemical modification of the 5′ cap
(B) removal of introns
(C) addition of a poly-A tail to the 3′ end
(D) all of these

106. Sustained muscle activity leads to fatigue, which is accompanied by accumulation of:

(A) ATP.
(B) ADP.
(C) troponin.
(D) lactic acid.

107. A eukaryotic cilium or flagellum contains _____ microtubules.

(A) 7 outer doublets and 2 inner
(B) 9 outer doublets and 2 inner
(C) 7 outer doublets and 3 inner
(D) 9 outer doublets and 3 inner

108. Transfer RNA carries _____ to the site of _____ synthesis.

(A) nucleotides, DNA
(B) nucleotides, RNA
(C) amino acids, protein
(D) amino acids, DNA

Passage III (Questions 109–116)

In order for a thoracic surgeon to visualize the heart, he or she must open up the pericardium, which is a sac that covers the heart. A human heart is four-chambered and is composed of right and left atria, which are separated by an interatrial septum that is frequently marred by defects. In the fetus the foramen ovale is an opening in this septum and blood passes from the right atrium to the left atrium so that the pulmonary circulation may be bypassed. A patent foramen ovale may contribute to the condition known as "blue baby." Two ventricles are also present; specifically we can speak of a right ventricle that pumps deoxygenated blood to the lungs and a left ventricle that pumps oxygenated blood to the tissues of the body. Between the ventricles is located the interventricular septum.

The superior and inferior vena cava and the coronary sinus empty into the right atrium. From here blood passes into the right ventricle to be pumped into the lungs via the pulmonary arteries. Blood from the lungs is returned to the left atrium by the pulmonary veins; it then passes into the left ventricle to leave upon its contraction via the aorta to supply the arterial system of the body. The heart alternately contracts and relaxes, and this cardiac cycle is repeated about 75 times per minute; the duration of one cycle is about 0.8 second. Atrial systole (contraction), which takes about 0.1 second, is followed by ventricular systole lasting about 0.3 second, and absolute diastole (relaxation) follows, lasting about 0.4 second.

The heart has an automatic rhythmic beat, but it is also under the influence of nerves that, however, serve only to change the force or frequency of the contractions of the muscle in accordance with the physiologic needs of the organism. The modification of the intrinsic rhythmicity is by way of the two parts of the autonomic nervous system; stimulation occurs through the sympathetic portion, whereas homeostatic maintenance is mainly a function of the parasympathetic portion. Stimulation through the sympathetic nerves increases the rate and force of the heart beat; slowing and reduction in force are the result of parasympathetic stimulation. Vasodilation of the coronary arteries is brought about by sympathetic stimulation, whereas vasoconstriction is elicited by parasympathetic stimulation.

109. When a physician informs a patient that his blood pressure reading is 160/90, she refers respectively to:

   (A) systolic blood pressure of the left ventricle.
   (B) blood pressure in the veins of the arm.
   (C) systolic and diastolic pressures of the brachial artery.
   (D) systolic pressure of the aorta and diastolic pressure in the superior vena cava.

110. The vital centers for control of heart rate, respiratory rate, and blood pressure are located in the:

   (A) pons.
   (B) medulla
   (C) cerebellum.
   (D) hypothalamus.

111. Blood in the pulmonary veins is rich in:

   (A) oxyhemoglobin.
   (B) carbaminohemoglobin.
   (C) hemoglobin.
   (D) uric acid.

112. Running to catch the bus to go to work has produced a rapid heart rate, an increase in the respiratory rate, and an increase in blood pressure in an individual. We can attribute these changes to:

   (A) the peripheral nervous system.
   (B) the central nervous system.
   (C) the parasympathetic component of the autonomic nervous system.
   (D) the sympathetic component of the autonomic nervous system.

113. Which of the following muscle types is NOT under the control of the autonomic (involuntary) nervous system?

   (A) heart (cardiac)
   (B) smooth
   (C) skeletal (striated)
   (D) arrector pili

114. The functional unit of a striated muscle is known as the sarcomere. A sarcomere on an electron micrograph is the region between:

   (A) two A bands.
   (B) two I bands.
   (C) two H bands.
   (D) two Z bands.

115. If we examine the three types of muscles in respect to their characteristics, which of the series below is false?

	Characteristic	Cardiac	Skeletal	Smooth
(A)	No. of Nuclei	One-Several	Many	One
(B)	Position of Nuclei	Central	Central	Central
(C)	Striations	Present	Present	Absent
(D)	Control	Autonomic	Voluntary	Autonomic

116. Heartbeat is initiated by the:

   (A) vagus nerve.
   (B) sympathetic nervous system.
   (C) A-V (atrio-ventricular) node.
   (D) S-A (sino-atrial) node.

Passage IV (Questions 117–121)

The A B O blood grouping system is explained on the basis of a single triallelic system with genes A, B, and O operating at a single genetic locus. Phenotypic and genotypic characteristics may be expressed as follows:

Phenotype	Genotype
A	A/A; A/O
B	B/B; B/O
O	O/O
AB	A/B

The A and B genes appear to be codominant; they are dominant over O, which is recessive.

117. Utilizing this system, transfusions have become relatively safe. The universal recipient is considered to be type:

    (A) A.
    (B) B.
    (C) O.
    (D) AB.

118. Which of the following agglutinogens do these individuals carry on their red blood cells?

    (A) A.
    (B) B.
    (C) O.
    (D) A, B.

119. A person of blood type A can receive blood of type(s):

    (A) A.
    (B) B; A.
    (C) O.
    (D) A; O.

120. Two people are planning to have a family. The woman has blood type A/A and the man B/B. Their children might have the following:

    (A) A and B.
    (B) B only.
    (C) A/B only.
    (D) A and B and A/B.

121. A man with blood cell genotype B/O marries a woman with type A/B. Their offspring could have any of the following:

    (A) A/B, B/B, A/O, B/O
    (B) A/B and B/O only.
    (C) A/O and B/B only.
    (D) none of the combinations above.

Questions 122–129 are NOT based on a descriptive passage.

122. Social stress will most severely affect the:

    (A) pancreas.
    (B) pineal.
    (C) adrenal.
    (D) parathyroid.

123. The codons that specify the sequence of amino acids in a protein occur in:

    (A) rRNA.
    (B) mRNA.
    (C) tRNA.
    (D) ribosomes.

124. The template (information course) for DNA synthesis is:

    (A) DNA.
    (B) mRNA.
    (C) tRNA.
    (D) rRNA.

125. Follicle-stimulating hormone is to estrogen as luteinizing hormone is to:

    (A) progesterone.
    (B) testosterone.
    (C) vasopressin.
    (D) luteotrophic hormone.

126. Energy is routinely released from ATP in cells by:

    (A) converting the entire molecule to CO_2 and water.
    (B) hydrolyzing the adenine from the ribose.
    (C) hydrolyzing one or two phosphates from the ATP.
    (D) converting ATP into NADH.

127. Simple squamous epithelium is found in all of the following EXCEPT:

   (A) alveoli of the lung.
   (B) glomerulus of the kidney.
   (C) epidermis of the skin.
   (D) endothelium of blood vessels.

128. Most carbon dioxide is transported in blood as:

   (A) carboxyhemoglobin.
   (B) carbaminohemoglobin.
   (C) dissolved carbon dioxide in blood plasma.
   (D) bicarbonate ions.

129. The function of DNA ligase in DNA replication in prokaryotes is to:

   (A) fill in gaps created by primer removal on the lagging strand.
   (B) synthesize RNA primers on the lagging strand.
   (C) add deoxynucleotides to the new leading strand.
   (D) join adjacent Okazaki fragments on the lagging strand.

Passage V (Questions 130–134)

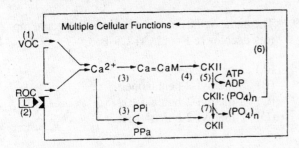

Many of the physiological functions of neurons are mediated by signal transduction systems. By way of intermediate messengers, transduction systems relay extracellular signals to intracellular effector elements which produce a physiologic response. Depending on their position in the relay chain, the intermediate relay elements are known as second messengers, tertiary messengers, and so on.

In the stylized neuron above, the extracellular signal (a neurotransmitter) is signified by the letter "L" (ligand). When "L" binds to its receptor, it opens the associated channel which admits extracellular calcium into the neuron. This constitutes a Receptor Operated Channel (ROC). Admission of calcium via the ROC serves to depolarize the neuron. With depolarization, the Voltage Operated Channel (VOC) can also open to admit calcium. When the cell is sufficiently depolarized, both channels close and no more calcium is admitted.

An elevation of calcium within the cell serves to activate the calcium binding protein Calmodulin (CaM). Activated CaM, in turn, activates a Calcium/Calmodulin-dependent Kinase (CKII). A kinase is a specialized enzyme that can transfer a phosphoryl group from a high energy donor such as ATP to an appropriate substrate phosphoprotein. CKII can transfer phosphoryl groups to itself in a process known as autophosphorylation. The autophosphorylated form of CKII is active and is able to carry out multiple cellular functions including increasing neurotransmitter synthesis and release.

CKII is inactivated by dephosphorylation. The initial calcium influx also serves to activate inactive Protein Phosphatases (PP), the enzymes that remove phosphoryl groups from phosphoproteins. The activity of these phosphatases is, however, somewhat slower than the other components in the system. Thus, the complete system contains all of the elements necessary for transducing an initial extracellular signal into a physiologic response. It also contains an internal mechanism for terminating the response.

130. Increasing the activity of CKII could be best achieved by blocking step(s):

   (A) 3.
   (B) 5.
   (C) 7.
   (D) 3 and 7.

131. Decreasing the activity of CKII could be achieved by blocking step(s):

   (A) 2 only.
   (B) 5 only.
   (C) 2 or 4 or 5.
   (D) 7.

132. An electrode is used to depolarize the neuron to the same extent as activation of the ROC. No neurotransmitter ligand (L) is present to bind to its receptor. Calcium, present in normal extracellular concentrations, would enter the cell through:

   (A) the ROC.
   (B) the VOC.
   (C) ROC and the VOC.
   (D) none of the above.

133. The enzyme responsible for transfer of a phosphoryl group from a high energy donor to a suitable substrate is known as a:

    (A) phosphatase.
    (B) catalase.
    (C) transferase.
    (D) kinase.

134. CKII can perform its multiple cellular functions because:

    (A) there is more kinase than phosphatase.
    (B) there is more phosphatase than kinase.
    (C) the inactivation pathway is slower than the activation pathway.
    (D) the activation pathway is slower than the inactivation pathway,

Passage VI (Questions 135–139)

A student is given four unknown clear colorless liquids, each having the molecular formula $C_5H_{10}O$. Assume that the compounds shown below are in bottles labeled I-IV. The contents of these bottles are to be associated with their chemical or physical properties.

$$\underset{\text{I}}{\underset{\overset{|}{CH_3}}{\overset{\overset{O}{\|}}{CH_3CCHCH_3}}} \qquad \underset{\text{II}}{\underset{\overset{|}{CH_3}}{CH_3CHCH_2CH=O}}$$

$$\underset{\text{III}}{\underset{\overset{|}{CH_3}}{CH_3CH=CHCH_2OH}} \qquad \underset{\text{IV}}{\overset{\overset{O}{\|}}{CH_3CH_2CCH_2CH_3}}$$

135. The compound above that has the highest boiling point would be:

    (A) I.
    (B) II.
    (C) III.
    (D) IV.

136. The compound above that would react with 2,4-dinitrophenyl hydrazine to form a hydrazone and gives a positive Tollen's test with $Ag(NH_3)_2OH$ is:

    (A) I.
    (B) II.
    (C) III.
    (D) IV.

137. The compound above that on hydrogenation with H_2 in the presence of a catalyst, such as Pt or Ni, forms a chiral center, and that can be resolved into R and S enantiomers is:

    (A) I.
    (B) II.
    (C) III.
    (D) IV.

138. The reaction of acetaldehyde (ethanal) with isopropyl Grignard reagent, $\underset{\overset{|}{CH_3}}{CH_3CHMgBr}$, followed by hydrolysis and then oxidation with $K_2Cr_2O_7$ would be expected to produce:

    (A) I.
    (B) II.
    (C) III.
    (D) IV.

139. The name of the compound above that would rapidly decolorize Br_2 in CH_2Cl_2 is:

    (A) 3-pentanone.
    (B) 2-methyl-2-pentanone.
    (C) 3-methyl-2-buten-1-ol.
    (D) 2-methyl-2-buten-4-ol.

Passage VII (Questions 140–142)

Ten milliliters of blood were removed from a patient, and centrifugation was utilized to separate 5 ml of plasma from the blood cells. A 3-ml sample of the plasma was extracted with 100 ml of an appropriate lipid solvent. The lipid solvent was then evaporated to 10 ml, and a 0.1-ml sample was analyzed for cholesterol. The color produced in the calorimetric analysis at 560 millimicrons was exactly equal to a standard in which 0.5 mg of cholesterol was known to be present.

140. The cholesterol concentration of the patient's plasma was:

   (A) 200 mg cholesterol/100 ml plasma.
   (B) 295 mg cholesterol/100 ml plasma.
   (C) 867 mg cholesterol/100 ml plasma.
   (D) 1667 mg cholesterol/100 ml plasma.

141. In order to make the above calculations it was *not* necessary to know:

   (A) the volume of plasma separated from the blood.
   (B) the volume of plasma subjected to extraction.
   (C) the solvent volume after evaporation.
   (D) the volume of sample that was subjected to colorimetric analysis.

142. If the addition of twice the volume of standard produces more than twice the absorbance at 560 millimicrons, this is probably best explained by:

   (A) exceeding the linear range of the method.
   (B) error in pipetting.
   (C) error in weighing to prepare the standard solution.
   (D) any or all of the above.

Questions 143–146 are NOT based on a descriptive passage.

143. Cholesterol is an intermediate in the biosynthesis of:

   (A) essential fatty acids.
   (B) steroid hormones.
   (C) essential amino acids.
   (D) prostaglandins.

144. The essential fatty acids are required in the human body in the biosynthesis of:

   (A) ascorbic acid
   (B) bile acids.
   (C) estrogen.
   (D) prostaglandins.

145. $$A + B + C \xrightarrow{\text{E(enzyme)}} ABCD \rightarrow D + F + E$$
$$\quad\;(1) \qquad\qquad (2) \qquad (3) \qquad\qquad (4)$$

In the above reaction, the enzyme-substrate complex is represented by:

   (A) 1.
   (B) 2.
   (C) 3.
   (D) 4.

146. Phenylamine is cooled to 0°C and treated with HCl and $NaNO_2$. After a few minutes of reaction time cuprous bromide is added, and the solution is heated.

What percent nitrogen is contained in the final aromatic product?

   (A) 20
   (B) 15
   (C) 8
   (D) 0

Model Examination B

STOP

END OF TEST

Answer Key
MODEL EXAMINATION B

PHYSICAL SCIENCES

1. B	9. A	17. D	25. C	33. B	41. C	49. A
2. B	10. C	18. A	26. A	34. A	42. B	50. B
3. C	11. D	19. D	27. B	35. A	43. C	51. D
4. C	12. C	20. C	28. C	36. C	44. A	52. B
5. A	13. C	21. A	29. C	37. D	45. D	
6. C	14. C	22. D	30. C	38. B	46. D	
7. B	15. B	23. D	31. A	39. C	47. D	
8. A	16. C	24. A	32. B	40. C	48. B	

VERBAL REASONING

53. D	59. C	65. C	71. C	77. D	83. D	89. B
54. A	60. B	66. B	72. D	78. A	84. A	90. C
55. C	61. D	67. D	73. A	79. A	85. B	91. C
56. D	62. D	68. C	74. C	80. D	86. D	92. C
57. B	63. B	69. C	75. C	81. B	87. B	
58. D	64. D	70. D	76. D	82. C	88. C	

WRITING SAMPLE

93. See page 461 for a sample essay.
94. See page 462 for a sample essay.

BIOLOGICAL SCIENCES

95. B	103. B	111. A	119. D	127. C	135. A	143. A
96. C	104. A	112. D	120. C	128. D	136. B	144. D
97. B	105. D	113. C	121. A	129. D	137. B	145. C
98. A	106. D	114. D	122. C	130. C	138. D	146. D
99. B	107. B	115. B	123. B	131. C	139. C	
100. D	108. C	116. D	124. A	132. B	140. B	
101. D	109. C	117. D	125. A	133. D	141. C	
102. A	110. B	118. D	126. C	134. C	142. B	

ANSWERS EXPLAINED FOR MODEL EXAMINATION B

Physical Sciences

1. **(B)** Graham's law of effusion gives the formula for calculating the relative rates of effusion for two gases. The important thing to recognize is that the lighter the gas (lower molecular weight), the faster it effuses.

2. **(B)** Compound C forms from 7.0 g (7.0 g/28.0 g = 0.25 mole) of nitrogen gas and 4.0 g (4.0 g/32.0 g = 0.125 mole) of oxygen gas. The ratio of these elements in compound C is 2:1.

3. **(C)** According to the passage, the molecular weight of compound B is 30 g/mole. Thus, 15.0 g of compound B is equal to 0.50 mole of compound B (15.0 g/30.0 g = 0.50 mole). A mole of any gas at STP (0°C and 1 atm) occupies 22.4 L; half that amount occupies half the volume.

4. **(C)** The molecular formula is found by dividing the empirical formula mass by the molecular mass. Compound A forms from 7.0 g (7.0 g/28.0 g = 0.25 mole) of nitrogen gas and 16.0 g (16.0 g/32.0 g = 0.5 mole) of oxygen gas. Compound A has empirical formula NO_2; the empirical formula mass is 46 g/mole. Dividing by the molecular mass (46 g/mole) gives a ratio of 1:1. So the empirical formula and the molecular formula are the same.

5. **(A)** Compound A forms from 7.0 g (7.0 g/28.0 g = 0.25 mole) of nitrogen gas and 16.0 g (16.0 g/32.0 g = 0.5 mole) of oxygen gas. Compound A has empirical formula NO_2, as does N_2O_4.

6. **(C)** The oxidation state of oxygen is –2. To balance this and make a neutral molecule, each nitrogen must be +1.

7. **(B)** Only transverse waves can be polarized. Choices A, C, and D are untrue. Light (electromagnetic) waves can be polarized and are therefore transverse. However, longitudinal sound waves cannot be polarized.

8. **(A)** The long-wavelength end (750 nm) of the visible spectrum is red in color, but waves with the shorter wavelengths are the most energetic.

$E = hf = hc/\lambda$, where c is the speed of light. For example, the energies of diagnostic X-ray photons are often hundreds of thousands of times more energetic than visible light photons.

9. **(A)** Only a converging lens can form a real image, behind the lens, of an object in front. The focal length cannot be 40 cm because an object 40 cm in front would not form any image (the image distance would be infinite). A diverging lens cannot form a real image by itself. A concave mirror can form a real image but not behind itself.

10. **(C)** Sound waves of all frequencies travel with the same speed. This is fortunate for communicating since we voice several different frequencies with each sound we utter. If the frequencies had differing speeds, we could not understand anyone who was some distance away.

11. **(D)** The speed of any type of wave is always given by:

$$v = f\lambda.$$

The rod vibrates in a standing wave with antinodes at each end where the rod vibrates freely and a node at the center where it is held. This produces the lowest natural frequency, the fundamental. The antinodes at the end are one-half wavelength apart

$$\lambda/2 = 2 \text{ m}$$
$$\lambda = 4 \text{ m}$$
$$v = 1275 \text{ Hz} \times 4.0 \text{ m} = 5100 \text{ m/s}$$

12. **(C)** The given formula allows calculation of the period. The string length must be in meters. $L = 0.5$ m.
$$T = 2\pi \sqrt{L/g} = 6.28 \sqrt{0.5/9.8} = 1.41 \text{ sec}$$

13. **(C)** The formula for the pendulum is independent of the mass and the angle of swing (so long as the angle is *small*; 10° or less). Thus the period is unchanged, since the length of the string is still 0.5 m.

14. **(C)** Hooke's Law for the elastic spring states that the stretch or elongation, x, of a spring is proportional to the stretching force, $F = kx$, where k is the "spring constant." Here, $F = mg = kx$, so that $F = 0.5 \text{ kg} \times 9.8 \text{ m/sec}^2 = k \times 0.49$ m. Thus $k = 10$ N/m.

15. **(B)** We use the formula given for a mass on the end of a spring. $T = 2\pi \sqrt{m/k}$ (The 5-cm amplitude does not appear in the expression for T. It is characteristic of simple harmonic oscillators that their periods do not depend on the starting amplitudes. For the pendulum above, the amplitude was the initial angle.)

$$T = 2\pi \sqrt{m/k} = 6.28 \sqrt{0.5\text{kg}/10\text{N}/m} = 1.4 \text{ sec}$$

16. **(C)** The mass is increased by a factor of 4 over the previous question. Since the mass appears under the square root sign and the root of 4 is 2, the period will double.

17. **(D)** The half-reactions for the given reaction are as follows:

    oxidation: $2Fe^{2+} \rightarrow 2Fe^{3+} + 2e^-$
    reduction: $Cl_2 + 2e^- \rightarrow 2Cl^-$

    An oxidizing agent is defined as the substance being reduced. In this redox equation, Cl_2 is being reduced and is the oxidizing agent.

18. **(A)** Nonpolar covalent bonds are formed between atoms of the same element or atoms with the same electronegativity. The F_2 molecule has one nonpolar covalent bond only and is therefore a nonpolar molecule.

19. **(D)** An acid reacts with a base to form a salt and water. KOH is a base.

20. **(C)** It is noted that there are two moles of gas on the left side of the equation and one mole on the right side. Considering the fact that one mole of gas occupies a volume of 22.4 liters at standard temperature and pressure, imposition of greater pressure should favor the shift of equilibrium to the right, thus reducing the total number of moles of gas.

21. **(A)** Two moles of gas are noted on the left side of the equation and three moles on the right. Thus, greater pressure should shift the equation to the left, favoring H_2S.

22. **(D)** Because two moles of gas are noted on each side, a pressure change should not affect the equilibrium of the reaction.

23. **(D)** A and B are both correct, Without a change in K_{eq}, the addition of either reactant on the left side will result in more of the product on the right side, which uses up some of the H_2.

24. **(A)** Without a change in temperature or pressure, addition of material on one side of an equilibrium equation will result in more of a product or products on the other side. This will occur without a change in K_{eq}.

25. **(C)** The equivalent resistance for series connections of resistors is equal to the sum of the individual resistances.

    $R_s + R_1 + R_2 + R_3$, and so on. Then $I = V/R_s$ from Ohm's law; so $I = 1$ A.

    The individual voltage drops are also found using Ohm's law,

    $$V = 1 \text{ A} \times 2 \text{ ohm} = 2 \text{ volts.}$$

26. **(A)** No DC current can flow through the parallel capacitors. The 6 volts does appear across the ends of the capacitors when they are fully charged.

27. **(B)** The parallel combination has the lower equivalent resistance. The series resistance equals 4 ohms (2 ohms + 2 ohms). The parallel resistance is found by the reciprocal formula:

    $$1/R_p = 1/R_1 + 1R_2 = 1/2 + 1/2$$
    $$= 1 \text{ ohm}$$

    The current from Ohm's law is:

    $$I = V/R_p = 6 \text{ amperes}$$

28. **(C)** Three resistors in series yield an equivalent 6-ohm resistance:

    $$R_s = 2 + 2 + 2 = 6 \text{ ohms}$$

    In parallel:

    $$1/R_p = 1/2 + 1/2 + 1/2 = 3/2$$
    $$R_p = 2/3 = 0.67 \text{ ohm}$$

29. **(C)** We need to find the equivalent resistance. The two resistors in parallel have a resistance of 1 ohm:

    $$1/R_p = 1/2 + 1/2 = 1$$
    $$R_p = 1 \text{ ohm}$$

    The other 2-ohm resistor is in series with this equivalent 1-ohm resistor:

    $$R_s = 2 + 1 = 3 \text{ ohms.}$$

Since these are pure resistances, the current can be found by:

$$I = V/R_s = 120 \text{ V}/(3 \text{ ohm})$$
$$= 40 \text{ A}$$

30. **(C)** The energy for the motion comes from the expanding compressed spring so that energy is not "conserved" here. However, the total momentum of the two cart system is constant. Because the initial total momentum was zero, the final momentum of the system is also zero, i.e.,

$$P_i = P_f, \text{ or}$$
$$0 = m_1 v_1 + m_2 v_2$$
and $\quad v_2 = - m_1 v_1 / m_2 = -0.6 \text{ m/sec.}$

31. **(A)** The different carts experience the same impulse and therefore undergo the same change in momentum.

impulse = force × time = Ft
Ft = change in momentum = Δp

Since both carts start from rest we have:

Impulse = final momentum – zero = $p_f - 0$

Their <u>final momenta</u> are equal. (Of course the lighter cart has the greater velocity.)

32. **(B)** In this question the energy dissipated due to air friction is apparent because of the decrease in the kinetic energy of the cart.

$$E_{lost} = 1/2 \, m v_i^2 - 1/2 \, m v_f^2 = 2.6 \text{ joules}$$

(m = 0.75 kg, v_f = 3.0 m/sec, and v_i = 4.0 m/sec).

33. **(B)** This question deals with the interchange of energy between the forms of kinetic energy and gravitational potential energy. The total energy is conserved but does change form.

$$KE_i = PE_f$$

$1/2 \, m v^2 - 0 = mgh$. Solving this for $v = \sqrt{2gh}$ we find that $v = 3.13$ m/sec.

34. **(A)** All interactions conserve total momentum of the objects involved. Some of the initial kinetic energy is dissipated, but the total momentum of the two carts will not change. The initial momentum (0.75 kg × 6 m/s) is equal to the final momentum of the "stuck together" carts.

$$(0.75 \text{ kg})(6 \text{ m/s}) = (0.75 \text{ kg} + 0.15 \text{ kg})v$$

$$v = + 5.0 \text{ m/sec}$$

35. **(A)** Snell's Law of Refraction, $n_1 \sin\theta_1 = n_2 \sin\theta_2$, applies to this problem. Solving for $\sin\theta_2$:

$$\sin\theta_2 = (n_1/n_2) \sin\theta_1$$

θ_2 will be larger than θ_1 if n_1 is greater than n_2 (and vice versa). In this case, when the ray of light is incident from inside the glass n_1 = 1.65 is indeed larger than n_2 = 1.0 for air. θ_2 will be larger than 30°.

36. **(C)** The ball's constant downward vertical acceleration is a = g. For constant acceleration the velocity is given by v = v_o + at. The formula shows that the velocity is linearly proportional to the time, t, and the graph of velocity versus time will be a straight line. The initial velocity is positive upward and decreases linearly with time until the ball reaches its high point, where its velocity is zero momentarily. The velocity then increases linearly in the negative direction.

37. **(D)** The number of half-lives is 16/5.3 or about 3 half-lives. The activity in curies is reduced by half (0.5) for each half-life, so the activity remaining is approximately 5000 curies × 0.5 × 0.5 × 0.5 = 625 curies. The exact exponential decay formula should be used if the time is not some integer number of half-lives:

$A = A_0 e^{-0.693t/T}$
T = half-life
t = actual time
A_0 = initial activity

38. **(B)** The diffraction grating equation $m\lambda = d\sin\theta$ can be solved for the value of m. λ is the wavelength and θ is the angle of diffraction.

$$m = (d/\lambda) \sin\theta = 1.67 \times 10^{-6} \, m \sin 30°)/$$
$$417 \times 10^{-9} \, m = 1.99 = 2$$

39. **(C)** The torques about the fulcrum must add to zero for balance. The counterclockwise torques are positive and the clockwise torques are negative. (The 30 gram mass on the left causes a positive torque.) We find that:

$$(30)(6 \text{ cm}) - (15)(6 \text{ cm}) - (20)(X \text{ cm}) = 0$$

So that: X = 4.5 cm

40. **(C)** The total mass numbers and atomic numbers must match on both sides of the reaction. The mass numbers on the left add to 236. Subtract the mass numbers of Ba and the 3 neutrons.

$$236 - 143 - 3 = 90 = A$$

We do the same with the atomic numbers:

$$92 - 56 = 36 = Z$$

$Z = 36$ shows the element is Krypton.

41. **(C)** $pK_b = -\log K_b$ = between 4 and 5 (by inspection).

42. **(B)** $$K_b = \frac{[NH_4^+][OH^-]}{[NH_3]} = \frac{[OH^-]^2}{0.01}$$
$$= 1.8 \times 10^{-5}$$
$$[OH^-]^2 = (0.01)(1.8 \times 10^{-5})$$
$$= 1.8 \times 10^{-7}$$
$$[OH^-] = 4 \times 10^{-4}$$
$$pOH = -\log [OH^-] = \text{between 3 and 4}$$
$$\text{(by inspection).}$$

43. **(C)** $pK_b = -\log K_b$ = between 5 and 6 (by inspection).

44. **(A)** As the smallest pK_a will give the lowest pH, the smallest pK_b will give the lowest pOH and the highest pH.

45. **(D)** The Lewis theory or concept does not deal specifically with hydrogen ions or hydroxyl ions.

46. **(D)** NaOH is a strong base and is assumed to be virtually completely ionized.

47. **(D)** $pOH = -\log [OH^-] = -\log (1 \times 10^{-3}) = 3$
$pH = 14 - pOH = 11$.

48. **(B)** The electron configuration is determined by filling orbitals from lowest to highest energy, starting with the $1s$ orbital. The calcium ion contains two fewer electrons than calcium.

49. **(A)** This is a definition of an ionic bond. It results in two ions of opposite charge.

50. **(B)** Although different sublevels have different maximum numbers of orbitals, any one orbital can hold a maximum of two electrons.

51. **(D)** The smaller the K_{sp}, the less soluble the salt. Of the four choices, AgI has the smallest K_{sp} (the largest negative exponent).

52. **(B)** A substance can act as both an oxidizing agent and a reducing agent only if the oxidation state of the element can become higher and lower than it is. There are no lower oxidation states for Fe^0 and Cu^0; there are no higher oxidation states for Fe^{3+}.

Verbal Reasoning

53. **(D)** At the end of the first paragraph, the author states the need for designers, clients, and students to understand the essence of graphic design. The remainder of the passage provides examples of the many objectives that this discipline accomplishes.

54. **(A)** In sentence number two, the author speaks about the extraordinary flowering of this art form and describes it as a potent means of communication as well as a major component of our visual culture.

55. **(C)** Paragraph four describes resonance as being the most important thing that graphic design provides. Resonance is viewed as a richness of tone that heightens the expressive power of a page.

56. **(D)** Graphic design is a diverse field. The first five paragraphs include mention of each of the tasks given above. Problem solving can be found in paragraphs one and five; organization of space in paragraphs one and three; visual and symbolic qualities in paragraphs one, two, and three.

57. **(B)** In paragraph three the author states that graphic design is a hybrid discipline in which, "Diverse elements, including signs, symbols, words, and pictures are collected and assembled into a total message."

58. **(D)** The passage clearly discusses all four answers to the question. The scientific method is detailed at the onset, scientific experimentation and responsibility are discussed, but definitely the author has written this text to debate and clarify the issues that surround the gathering, recording, and storing of scientific data.

59. **(C)** The author makes the point that at various periods, different components of the scientific method have been emphasized. It is also emphasized that early on propositions were formulated and debated with minimum organized observation or collection of data. The above statement would eliminate the several critical elements of the strict application of the scientific method as mentioned in **A, B,** and **D** of the question.

60. **(B)** The passage makes it clear that throughout history a great deal of haphazard observing, recording, and analysis have occurred. It is stated in the article that with the coming of the indus-

trial age, inventors focused on solutions, but that oftentimes they did not start with well formulated questions. The scientific method requires the above. Philosophers did give way to the age of the observers and observers gave way to the industrial age. There is no support in the passage for the claim that, as industrialization progressed, a clear scientific approach became standard for solving problems.

61. **(D)** The passage does point out that inventors sought legal protection under constitutionally guaranteed rights to patent intellectual property. It is clearly stated at the end of paragraph one that record keeping now has become formalized, standardized, and required. Regulatory agencies not only can, but do require (according to the passage) that they be allowed to inspect complete records of product development. Statement IV is contradicted in paragraphs one and two; failed experiments should be recorded to eliminate repetition, and also unwanted results (e.g., toxicity of drug) should not be suppressed because harm might result.

62. **(D)** None of the statements is supported by the passage. In paragraph three, the author makes the point that there is no universally accepted definition of data. The question asked in paragraph three is "are data the printouts of computers?" But no answer is provided, and this question is raised because we don't know what data are. Can we require scientists to record and store it? The paragraph ends asking who is responsible for keeping and storing data.

63. **(B)** It is quite clear from the passage that an evolutionary process has been involved in the data collection process and that data keeping and storage have become ends unto themselves in order to ensure that work paid for was actually done. No mention is made regarding the must of a modified hypothesis, and the fact that managers of public funds are clearly inadequate to judge scientific work is inescapable.

64. **(D)** The passage focuses on data collection and storage and makes it quite clear that the public's money is not well protected, that the public truly has no great trust in science, and that above all, scientific peer review and policing are flawed.

65. **(C)** The main theme of the passage deals with the shifting of decision-making power in school districts, from one where the board of education is the most important player to one where power is shared. Paragraph one states this in the opening sentence. The remainder of the passage goes on to name the parties that are becoming more powerful, especially teachers and parents. The flow chart, which represents both traditional and modern decision-making power, graphically supports the information presented in the passage.

66. **(B)** Paragraph two discusses the fact that today's teachers want to have a voice in program development as well as in determining salary scales. Later in the passage teachers are presented in an even more forceful light as their power to bring an educational system to a halt by means of strikes is noted.

67. **(D)** Because the central theme of the passage discusses the fact that the board of education no longer holds absolute power in most school districts, **D** is a direct contradiction to the theme since it proposes that the power remain with the board.

68. **(C)** Statement I, which talks about the emergence of parent volunteer programs in schools, and statement III, which claims that parents are becoming more powerful in schools, are both true according to the passage.

69. **(C)** The *degree* of decision-making power desired by the parties described in this passage is not mentioned and therefore **C**, which calls for *equality* of power, is not supported. The statement is not contradicted because a specific degree of power is not a topic of the passage.

70. **(D)** Although the Fourteenth Amendment is the vehicle that guarantees and protects a student's right to a public education, the main focus of this passage concerns expulsion from school, which would be a denial of that right.

71. **(C)** Time-out procedures are not mentioned in this passage. Exclusion from school is the actual removal of a student from the educational setting. The difference between suspension and expulsion is described in paragraph two.

72. **(D)** Expulsion from school generally is considered to be the most severe student punishment available to school administrators. In paragraph two of the passage, the author writes that state statutes and local policies usually provide that only a local school board has the prerogative to expel a student.

73. **(A)** Paragraph three notes that in recent years litigation has involved both the right of school officials to exclude students as well as the rights that students have to due process prior to suspension and/or expulsions,

74. **(C)** Although the matter had been treated in lower courts, *Goss v. Lopez* brought the exclusion question to the United States Supreme Court. The case is explained in paragraphs three through five.

75. **(C)** Paragraph four points out that the right to a public education is a property right. Because the Fourteenth Amendment protects an individual's right to his/her property, the removal of a student from school would constitute an affront to his/her property.

76. **(D)** Paragraph two discussed the fact that criteria used in evaluations are similar for full-time and part-time faculty. Paragraphs seven and eight deal with research faculty, whereas the remaining paragraphs discuss clinical faculty. The issue of administrative faculty is not addressed specifically by the passage.

77. **(D)** Paragraph four addresses the issues of bonding and identifying with an institution and also points out that long-term contracts would be one solution in the job security issue. The whole passage deals with the roles of several categories of faculty and the diverse issues posed and the need to find appropriate solutions. It is clearly stated in paragraph four that tenure is *not* the only way to achieve bonding.

78. **(A)** Job security is discussed in paragraph four. The inequity of compensation and the evaluation criteria are addressed in paragraph two. Academic freedom is discussed in paragraph three and is a nonissue according to the author.

79. **(A)** Paragraph two indicated that qualifications do not necessarily distinguish faculties and the level of the course taught does not reflect teaching ability. The argument that all students need qualified and enthusiastic instructors is made at the onset of paragraph one. Paragraph three indicates that academic freedom protects all faculty and introduction of changes is not limited. Paragraph two makes it quite clear that when students evaluate teaching, they may or may not know a faculty member's academic qualifications or tenure status.

80. **(D)** None of the statements made is discussed in the passage.

81. **(B)** Paragraph five makes it clear that the Red Cross believed that it should serve as an emergency relief organization and obtain its funds from private contributions. Hoover was invited to join the executive committee; Norman Davis was the head of the Red Cross.

82. **(C)** Paragraph three points out that in all of Hoover's rescue efforts, children represented his first concern.

83. **(D)** Paragraph one states that Hoover was a successful consulting engineer before he undertook his relief activities.

84. **(A)** The last line of the passage leaves no doubt that Hoover's and Roosevelt's camps did not agree with each other. Paragraph one mentions that Hoover took an active part in negotiating between the warring factions and that his efforts were not limited to war victims. He readily helped the victims of the Mississippi floods of 1927.

85. **(B)** Hoover (paragraph five), within less than two weeks of outbreak of hostilities, raised the relief question and suggested that one organization should provide a focal point. Paragraph four ends with the line that hungry people cannot defend themselves nor defend freedom. Paragraph three makes it clear that Mrs. Hoover supported her husband's efforts.

86. **(D)** There can be no doubt in the reader's mind that Hoover was a humanitarian with an interest in helping victims.

87. **(B)** This question truly should awaken the reader to the fact that the whole passage, including the references and credits, should be read. In the credit it is pointed out that the material was presented at a conference on education of the gifted for the twenty-first century.

88. **(C)** Paragraph four states that tragedies are potentially effective for developing ethics and even wisdom. The last paragraph emphasizes that teachers can put key ideas together for wise leadership in individuals of the next generation. It is proposed that teachers determine and give birth to the future. **D** tries to mislead you drastically, but careful reading of paragraph seven points out that the author distinguishes between

ethical skills and ethical knowledge, which is the development of right reasoning.

89. **(B)** The author in paragraph one does not speak of unavoidable mistakes major injustices, or personal grief. However, faulty logic is presented and associated with the word *hamartia*.

90. **(C)** In paragraph four it is pointed out that Dewey feared a danger of either dogmatism or a sense of unreality when students are abruptly introduced to theoretical ideas. He proposes to first introduce students to simple cases and then proceed to the more complex.

91. **(C)** Paragraph nine reasons that teacher preparation of material keeps the cases current, and in this way the cases help future generations.

92. **(C)** Paragraphs seven through nine emphasize the combination of student feedback and teacher production of material (formulating good and humane reasoning) to be an essential skill in the passing on of a sense of ethics from one generation to another.

Writing Sample

93. **Essay**

A wise person, according to Johnson, is one who knows that dreams and hopes are no substitute for reality. Though it may not always be pleasant or exciting to know what the next day will bring, there is no wisdom in reaching out for something exciting or pleasant when one cannot be sure that it is there. A realist has more hope to find happiness if he takes his reality and alters it than one who casts about in the dark hoping to find a pot of gold. A person may take his last dollar and buy a lottery ticket, hoping to win a jackpot, but the wise individual will take his last dollar and use it to buy food. Though the foolish person may think that because he is desperate, good, and deserving and that God or fate will intervene on his behalf, the wise one knows that fate and God will do little to even the odds. The wise person knows he needs food more than he needs a one-in-seven-million chance of becoming rich.

But what courage does it take to face each day that is the same as the last? Is it wise to keep one's feet firmly planted on the ground, taking no risks? To stay with what is certain out of fear of the unknown is certainly safe, but it may be unwise. Imagine a shoe retailer is approached by a partner who has developed a new last and leather that will make women's shoes more comfortable to wear, but they will appear just as stylish. The partner asks the store owner to place the new shoes in his front window, and for this favor the two will share whatever profits come from the venture in half. The shoe salesperson refuses, knowing that the shoes he has shown in his window for the last five years have brought in a steady stream of customers. Though he is not getting rich, at least he is certain that his current display works. The partner sets off to find another store owner, discovering one only three doors down from the first shop he visited. The second owner takes the risk, for he knows that nothing great is achieved without some peril. For days the first shoe salesperson sees streams of people walking by his store, and wondering where they are going, peeks outside to see them entering his competitor's shop. Word has spread, and even the first shopkeeper's regular male customers desert him for the shop down the street. Though women buy the new shoes for themselves, men pick them up for their wives; and while they are in the shop, they find it convenient to buy their own shoes there, too. The first shopkeeper goes out of business, blaming himself for not having the wisdom to have faith in a good, albeit unproved, idea.

Had the shopkeeper been wiser, perhaps what he would have seen was that this was not a matter of uncertainty. It is possible that had he been thinking, he would have recognized that it was a certainty that women would want to wear a more comfortable shoe, and that though it seemed new and risky to stock the new shoes, there was no risk involved at all. The wisdom is not in an unwillingness to make a change, it is in the unwillingness to make a change without considering the realistic possibilities of it. The chances involved in buying a lottery ticket make it such an impossible odd that the wise individual will reject the notion of spending his last dollar on it. The chances that women will prefer comfortable and stylish shoes over uncomfortable and stylish shoes, however, is not a chance at all. It is reasonable to assume that given the choice between discomfort and comfort the customer will choose comfort. A wise person knows a certainty when he sees it, and he knows that sometimes what appears to be a risk is not a risk at all. By the same token, a wise person knows when a safe offer is really a risk, and no matter how often he says, "I need this money, surely fate will let me have it. It is only fair that one who is as deserving as I should win" will not change the odds in a lottery.

So the wise individual is indeed one who will not quit certainty for uncertainty, but it is the same wise individual who knows the difference.

93.   **Explanation of Response: 6**

This essay focuses clearly on Johnson's statement and addresses each of the three writing tasks. Paragraph one explains what the statement means, paragraph two gives a specific situation in which one would not be wise to give up a certainty for an uncertainty, and paragraph three explores circumstances that determine whether it is wise or unwise to give up a certainty for an uncertainty.

The paper provides an explanation of the quotation by introducing "reality" as a qualifier for "certainty" and "dreams and hopes" for "uncertainty." This allows the author to cite concrete examples like the one that refers to the lottery to complete the explanation by referring to realistic and unrealistic acts. Through an effective example in paragraph two, the paper illustrates that safety, contrary to the implication of the quotation, may sometimes be unwise, as the first owner discovers. Finally the passage provides a balanced analysis of the things that determine whether quitting certainty for uncertainty is wise or unwise.

The writing in this essay is clear and controlled. The writer's use of concrete examples is one of the strongest features of the passage. They grow logically out of the main ideas of each paragraph and illustrate the ideas very effectively. The lottery ticket example is easy to relate to as an example of the uncertainty of taking a long shot, whereas the shoe shop example provides a clear example of a time when acting on at least mild uncertainty can be wise indeed. There is variety in the sentence structure, and the paper flows smoothly from one sentence to the next.

94.   **Essay**

Graham Greene's definition of destruction is really only an argument of semantics. Because "create" only means to bring into being, to cause to exist, then any act of change is also an act of creation. The idea is not a new one and appears in even as ancient a myth as that of the phoenix, who rises again out of the ashes of its own funeral pile. What Greene is suggesting is an alternative perspective by which one could view or interpret destruction. The connotations of "destruction" are generally negative ones. Greene is offering another option and a more optimistic one, a view of destruction as a new beginning or a sort of rebirth.

Taken only at literal face value, Greene's statement could be a dangerous one. It could be taken as an argument for anarchy, chaos, or, even more specifically, violence and murder. Of course, this would all depend on whether or not the interpreter sees "creation" as always a positive end. Further, it would depend on whether or not creation is viewed as an end or a means. For example, murder, for most people, is certainly not a positive thing. It is, however, undeniably an act of destruction. It is also undeniably an "end" of sorts, as an unalterable change. Murder is an act of destruction that separates the corporeal existence from the spiritual one. Because there is nothing really *new* that exists as a result, because it is not a means of propagating other possibilities, one could argue that murder is an act of destruction that is not, in fact, also an act of creation.

To destroy is to disintegrate or to demolish, to cause a cessation of one form of existence. What would follow would inevitably be another form of existence. For example, if I demolish my house, then I, by default, create a pile of rubble. I could even say that I have created that pile of rubble, because it did not exist before I demolished my house. To create is to bring into being. Because (granted that we are not dealing with the loss of matter) destruction is the ceasing of one thing to exist in its present state, then one is always creating a new state of being with every destruction. The taking of a life would be one possible exception because the dead body has not been cremated and there is no accounting for the spirit that has been "lost." In general, however, the relationship between destruction and creation is inevitable, as one necessitates the other.

94.   **Explanation of Response: 4**

This essay does a nice job with tasks one and three. Paragraph one explains the statement by giving a traditional definition of "create," commenting then on connotations of destruction, and finally suggesting how Greene offers another option for seeing acts of creation. Paragraph two expands the explanation and moves toward a general example, murder, which might not, because it is not "positive," be considered an act of creation. The final paragraph examines the circumstances that determine the relationship between creation and destruction.

The paper has many strengths. The essay is thoughtful, and it flows smoothly from sentence to sentence, paragraph to paragraph. The use of transitions, such as "however" in the final sentence, provides coherence. The paper shows sensitivity to language, particularly in its examination of the denotation and connotation of creation and destruction. The paper would have received a rating of 5 or 6 if it had dealt more directly with the second task: that of providing a specific situation in which destruction is not a form of creation. The example of murder as such remains too general. The example of the demolition of the house in the final paragraph is effective in making the paper more concrete. Other such examples in the rest of the paper would be helpful.

Biological Sciences

95. **(B)** Individuals 6, 20, and 23 could be produced by dominant defective alleles (either autosomal or sex-linked) only if all three cases resulted from new mutations since the parents in all three cases have only normal phenotypes. Because mutations are specified as rare, this is unlikely. A recessive autosomal defective allele could explain all observations down through individual 18, but the presence of a defective allele in individual 19 is unlikely due to no occurrences of the defect in that individual's ancestors and the low incidence of new mutations. The sex ratio of defective individuals (all male except for one female, and she had a defective father) is highly unlikely for an autosomal recessive defective allele. The expected probability of males among defective offspring is 1/2 for a recessive autosomal allele (i.e., normal chance of male offspring), so the probability of the observed sex ratio among defective offspring is very unlikely. For these reasons, a defective autosomal recessive allele is not a likely explanation. An X-linked recessive defective allele easily explains all observations. Defective male offspring received an X chromosome containing a recessive defective allele from their mothers (most of whom are normal due to a dominant normal allele on their other X chromosome) and the recessive allele determined their phenotype since the Y chromosome contained no allele for the characteristic. Most females were normal due to a normal allele on the X chromosome received from their fathers. The defective female (9) received a defective X from both parents.

96. **(C)** Female 1 must contain one normal allele (because she has a normal phenotype and she produced normal male 8) and one defective allele (because she produced defective male 6).

97. **(B)** Male 6 would contain only one allele to the characteristic since he (like all normal human males) has only one X chromosome. The Y chromosome from his father lacks an allele for the characteristic. His defective phenotype must be produced by a defective allele on his X, so he contains only defective alleles.

98. **(A)** Male 8 would have one allele for the characteristics (on his single X chromosome—see explanation for question 3), Because his phenotype is normal, the allele must be normal and he would contain only normal alleles.

99. **(B)** Female 9 must have two X chromosomes (like all normal human females). Because her phenotype is defective, both X chromosome must contain defective alleles. Female 9 would therefore contain only defective alleles.

100. **(D)** All of the statements of the question were supported by the data. Although it would have been a good assumption that crude pituitary extract would have a lesser effect than pure FSH, one must examine the data. In our case the extract did affect every organ; however, the weight increase was less than when FSH was administered. With the data available concerning the effect of pituitary extract, it is safe to assume that hypophysectomy would have resulted in decreased organ weights. Remember, FSH in the female stimulates the growth of the ovarian follicle, whereas in the male it stimulates the testes to produce sperm.

101. **(D)** FSH in the female stimulates the development of the ovarian follicle and the production of estrogen; LH and prolactin are responsible for the corpus luteum, which secretes progesterone and prepares the uterus for implantation of the fertilized egg. Because uterine growth was observed in our case, it is safe to assume that FSH was not of the highest purity. Our data neither supports nor contradicts the statement that FSH and LH are necessary for estrogen secretion. Because our data shows that FSH did not affect the thyroid and adrenal glands, the statement that FSH primarily affects the reproductive organs is supported.

102.   **(A)** The data shows that FSH in the male had its greatest effect on the seminal vesicles and not the prostate gland. Statements (B) and (C) are not supported nor contradicted, whereas statement (D) is a truism supported by the data; body weights did not vary significantly.

103.   **(B)** The pituitary secretes ACTH, FSH, LH, TSH, and STH. ACTH acts on the adrenal cortex; FSH and LH on the gonads; TSH on the thyroid, and STH on the general system. The adrenal medulla can be considered to house the post ganglionic neurons for part of the sympathetic portion of the autonomic nervous system and is responsible for epi- and norepinephrine production.

104.   **(A)** All chordates have a dorsally located nerve cord. A vertebral column occurs in vertebrates, mammary glands occur in mammals, and epidermal scales occur in reptiles, all of which are groups within the chordates. These features, though, are not shared by all chordates.

105.   **(D)** All of these modifications typically occur between transcription and translation in eukaryotes.

106.   **(D)** Sustained muscle activity leading to fatigue results in anaerobic glycolysis, which causes accumulation of lactic acid.

107.   **(B)** A eukaryotic cilium or flagellum has 9 outer doublets and a central pair of microtubules.

108.   **(C)** Transfer RNA carries amino acids (as aminoacyl groups) to the ribosomes and inserts them into the growing polypeptide.

109.   **(C)** Blood pressure is usually measured by placing the sphygmomanometer cuff around the arm compressing the brachial artery and vein. Maximum blood pressure is obtained during ventricular contraction (systole); in our case 160. Minimum blood pressure indicates ventricular rest (diastole); in our case 90.

110.   **(B)** The medulla is a part of the brain stem and connects to the spinal cord at the foramen magnum. The following cranial nerves are associated with the medulla: a, XII—hypoglossal nerve; b, XI—spinal accessory nerve; c, X—vagus nerve; d, IX—glossopharyngeal nerve; e, VIII—stato-acoustic nerve; and f, portions of the facial nerve (VII). The vagus nerve (X) is the most important parasympathetic nerve. Stimulation of vagal fibers slows the heart rate; constricts the smooth muscles of the bronchial tree; stimulates secretion by the bronchial mucosa; and promotes peristalsis, gastric, and pancreatic secretions. Blood pressure control also involves aortic body, carotid sinus, and carotid body receptor modulation by the glossopharyngeal (IX) and vagus (X) nerves.

111.   **(A)** From the right ventricle blood is sent the lungs via the pulmonary arteries; this blood is rich in carbaminohemoglobin and the CO_2 will be exchanged for O_2. Blood returns from the lungs to the left auricle via the pulmonary veins; this blood has been oxygenated and is rich in oxyhemoglobin. Blood then passes to the left ventricle and then out via the aorta to supply the tissues of the body.

112.   **(D)** The sympathetic component of the autonomic nervous system mobilizes the body reserves in case of emergencies.

113.   **(C)** Skeletal (striated) muscle is under voluntary control. The autonomic nervous system innervates cardiac muscle, smooth muscle and glands. Arrector pili musculature is associated with skin and is smooth musculature.

114.   **(D)** A sarcomere is the region between two bands. In simple terms we are dealing with this unit: ZIAHAIZ. Contraction of the sarcomere is due to the fine filaments (actin) sliding between the thick filaments (myosin) pulling the Z bands to which they are attached. This pulls the Z bands closer together, and so the sarcomeres are shortened.

115.   **(B)** In skeletal muscle, the nuclei are found peripherally. To complete the chart, the speed of contraction should also be mentioned. Skeletal muscle is the fastest working, smooth muscle the slowest, and cardiac muscle occupies an intermediate position.

116.   **(D)** Heartbeat is initiated by the S-A (sino-atrial) node, which is also known as the pacemaker.

117–119. **(117-D) (118-D) (119-D).** As can be seen from the table, there are four major blood types, and the explanation as to universal donor and recipient is based on the following:

Type	Agglutinogens on Cells	Agglutinogens in Serum and Plasma
AB—can receive A, B, AB, or O (universal recipient)	A, B	none
A—can receive A, O	A	anti b
B—can receive B, O	B	anti a
O—can receive only O, but can give to all; therefore, O is the universal donor	O	anti ab

120. **(C)** The ABO blood grouping system is explained on the basis of a single triallelic system with genes A, B, and O operating at a single genetic locus. Phenotypic and genotypic characteristics may be expressed as follows:

Phenotype	Genotype
A	A/A; A/O
B	B/B; B/O
O	O/O
AB	A/B

The A and B genes appear to be codominant; they are dominant over O, which is recessive.

121. **(A)** See explanations for questions 117–120. One gene from each parent can produce any of the four combinations named.

122. **(C)** Social stress causes adrenal enlargement.

123. **(B)** mRNA contains codons specifying amino acids. tRNA contains anticodons.

124. **(A)** DNA is the template for both DNA and RNA symthesis.

125. **(A)** FSH stimulates estrogen synthesis as LH stimulates progesterone synthesis.

126. **(C)** Routine energy release from ATP is by hydrolysis of phosphates.

127. **(C)** The epidermis is stratified squamous, not simple squamous epithelium.

128. **(D)** All of these occur, but the majority of carbon dioxide is carried as bicarbonate.

129. **(D)** DNA ligase joins DNA fragments, including the Okazaki fragments on the lagging strand.

130. **(C)** Although blocking the activation of the phosphatases by blocking the effect of calcium (step 3), the CKII activation pathway would also be blocked. For this reason, (A) and (D) are incorrect. The autophosphorylation of CKII at step 5 is the final step in the activation of CKII. A block here, as suggested by **B**, would not increase but inhibit CKII activity; hence **B** is also a poor choice.

131. **(C)** CKII activity could be decreased by blocking calcium influx, calmodulin activation of CKII, or autophosphorylation. There are more than the single sites suggested in (A) and (B). Blocking dephosphorylation by the phosphatase, step 7, **D**, would serve to *increase,* not decrease, CKII activity.

132. **(B)** Only a Voltage Operated Channel (VOC) is opened by depolarization alone. As stated in the passage, a Receptor Operated Channel (ROC) is opened by the binding of an appropriate ligand. The question states that depolarization is produced and no neurotransmitter ligand is present, so **A** and **C** are incorrect.

133. **(D)** This comes straight out of the reading: A kinase is an enzyme that transfers phosphoryl groups from a high energy donor to a suitable substrate. **A** is incorrect, because a phosphatase antagonizes the actions of a kinase by *removing phosphoryls* from phosphoproteins. Catalases and transferase, **B** and **C**, are enzymes, but their specific functions are not phosphorylating phosphorproteins. If you chose one of these answers you attempted to address more than the question asked. Stick with the simple approach and do not read anything extraneous into the question.

134. **(C)** The question requires that you synthesize two pieces of given information. First, that both the CKII activation and inactivation (phosphatase) pathways are activated by calcium and, second, that the phosphatase response to calcium is slower than other components of the system. **D** suggests the reverse of this situation and is there-

fore wrong. It is plausible that is less phosphatase than kinase **B**; however, this is not addressed in the reading and you would have no basis for arriving at this interpretation. **A**, also not addressed in the reading, would not constitute a plausible mechanism for CKII to function. It would suggest a mechanism that would render CKII permanently nonfunctional.

135. **(C)** All have the same molecular formula, and only III is capable of intermolecular hydrogen bonding.

136. **(B)** II is the only aldehyde of the four. I and IV form hydrazones but do not give a positive Tollen's test.

137. **(A)** On hydrogenation I is converted to:

$$
\begin{array}{c}
\text{OH} \\
| \\
CH_3{-}C{-}CHCH_3 \\
| \quad | \\
\text{H} \ \ CH_3
\end{array}
$$

in which the carbon with the hydroxyl group is chiral.

138. **(A)** The reaction sequence is:

$$CH_3CH{=}O + CH_3CHMgBr \xrightarrow[\ ]{then} \underset{\substack{| \\ CH_3}}{CH_3CHCHCH_3}^{\overset{OH}{|}} \xrightarrow[H_2O^+]{K_2Cr_2O_7}$$

139. **(C)** Compound III has a double hand to react with Br_2. The hydroxyl group is given priority in numbering.

140. **(D)** $\dfrac{0.5 \text{ mg}}{0.1 \text{ ml}} = \dfrac{X}{10 \text{ ml}}$

$$X = \frac{(0.5)(1)}{0.1} = 50 \text{ mg}$$

This 50 mg represents the total amount in the entire 3 ml of plasma that was extracted.

$$\frac{50 \text{ mg}}{3 \text{ ml}} = \frac{X}{100 \text{ ml}}$$

$$X = \frac{(50)(100)}{3} = 1667 \text{ mg/100 ml}$$

141. **(A)** See the explanation to answer 140. The calculation is based on 100 ml plasma, not on the total amount of plasma.

142. **(B)** Exceeding the linear range would ordinarily lead to a lower absorbance than expected. An error in weighing to prepare the standard solution would introduce a constant error. The remaining possibility, a pipetting error, is most likely. Pipetting errors may be positive or negative.

143. **(B)** Cholesterol is an intermediate in the biosynthesis of steroid hormones, bile acids, and vitamin D. Essential fatty acids and essential amino acids must be consumed by the organism in the diet.

144. **(D)** Prostaglandins are potent compounds; they are structurally unique in the respect that they contain 20 carbon atoms and are formed from essential fatty acids. They affect the nervous system, circulation, reproductive organs, and metabolism.

145. **(C)** Substrate(s) or reactants) react(s) with the enzyme to form an enzyme-substrate complex. This complex breaks down into product(s) and frees enzymes ready for formation of a new enzyme-substrate complex.

146. **(D)** We have described conditions for the formation of a diazonium salt and then replacement of the diazonium salt by Br to produce monobromobenzene. (The replacement is known as the Sandmeyer reaction.) The intermediate diazonium salt is often unstable at room temperature, so a lower temperature is used.

Answer Sheet

MODEL EXAMINATION C

Directions: After locating the number of the question to which you are responding, fill in the circle containing the letter of the answer you have selected. Use pencil (not a ballpoint pen) to completely blacken the circle.

PHYSICAL SCIENCES

1 Ⓐ Ⓑ Ⓒ Ⓓ
2 Ⓐ Ⓑ Ⓒ Ⓓ
3 Ⓐ Ⓑ Ⓒ Ⓓ
4 Ⓐ Ⓑ Ⓒ Ⓓ
5 Ⓐ Ⓑ Ⓒ Ⓓ
6 Ⓐ Ⓑ Ⓒ Ⓓ
7 Ⓐ Ⓑ Ⓒ Ⓓ
8 Ⓐ Ⓑ Ⓒ Ⓓ
9 Ⓐ Ⓑ Ⓒ Ⓓ
10 Ⓐ Ⓑ Ⓒ Ⓓ
11 Ⓐ Ⓑ Ⓒ Ⓓ
12 Ⓐ Ⓑ Ⓒ Ⓓ
13 Ⓐ Ⓑ Ⓒ Ⓓ
14 Ⓐ Ⓑ Ⓒ Ⓓ
15 Ⓐ Ⓑ Ⓒ Ⓓ
16 Ⓐ Ⓑ Ⓒ Ⓓ
17 Ⓐ Ⓑ Ⓒ Ⓓ
18 Ⓐ Ⓑ Ⓒ Ⓓ
19 Ⓐ Ⓑ Ⓒ Ⓓ
20 Ⓐ Ⓑ Ⓒ Ⓓ
21 Ⓐ Ⓑ Ⓒ Ⓓ
22 Ⓐ Ⓑ Ⓒ Ⓓ
23 Ⓐ Ⓑ Ⓒ Ⓓ
24 Ⓐ Ⓑ Ⓒ Ⓓ
25 Ⓐ Ⓑ Ⓒ Ⓓ
26 Ⓐ Ⓑ Ⓒ Ⓓ

27 Ⓐ Ⓑ Ⓒ Ⓓ
28 Ⓐ Ⓑ Ⓒ Ⓓ
29 Ⓐ Ⓑ Ⓒ Ⓓ
30 Ⓐ Ⓑ Ⓒ Ⓓ
31 Ⓐ Ⓑ Ⓒ Ⓓ
32 Ⓐ Ⓑ Ⓒ Ⓓ
33 Ⓐ Ⓑ Ⓒ Ⓓ
34 Ⓐ Ⓑ Ⓒ Ⓓ
35 Ⓐ Ⓑ Ⓒ Ⓓ
36 Ⓐ Ⓑ Ⓒ Ⓓ
37 Ⓐ Ⓑ Ⓒ Ⓓ
38 Ⓐ Ⓑ Ⓒ Ⓓ
39 Ⓐ Ⓑ Ⓒ Ⓓ
40 Ⓐ Ⓑ Ⓒ Ⓓ
41 Ⓐ Ⓑ Ⓒ Ⓓ
42 Ⓐ Ⓑ Ⓒ Ⓓ
43 Ⓐ Ⓑ Ⓒ Ⓓ
44 Ⓐ Ⓑ Ⓒ Ⓓ
45 Ⓐ Ⓑ Ⓒ Ⓓ
46 Ⓐ Ⓑ Ⓒ Ⓓ
47 Ⓐ Ⓑ Ⓒ Ⓓ
48 Ⓐ Ⓑ Ⓒ Ⓓ
49 Ⓐ Ⓑ Ⓒ Ⓓ
50 Ⓐ Ⓑ Ⓒ Ⓓ
51 Ⓐ Ⓑ Ⓒ Ⓓ
52 Ⓐ Ⓑ Ⓒ Ⓓ

VERBAL REASONING

53 Ⓐ Ⓑ Ⓒ Ⓓ
54 Ⓐ Ⓑ Ⓒ Ⓓ
55 Ⓐ Ⓑ Ⓒ Ⓓ
56 Ⓐ Ⓑ Ⓒ Ⓓ
57 Ⓐ Ⓑ Ⓒ Ⓓ
58 Ⓐ Ⓑ Ⓒ Ⓓ
59 Ⓐ Ⓑ Ⓒ Ⓓ
60 Ⓐ Ⓑ Ⓒ Ⓓ
61 Ⓐ Ⓑ Ⓒ Ⓓ
62 Ⓐ Ⓑ Ⓒ Ⓓ
63 Ⓐ Ⓑ Ⓒ Ⓓ
64 Ⓐ Ⓑ Ⓒ Ⓓ
65 Ⓐ Ⓑ Ⓒ Ⓓ
66 Ⓐ Ⓑ Ⓒ Ⓓ
67 Ⓐ Ⓑ Ⓒ Ⓓ
68 Ⓐ Ⓑ Ⓒ Ⓓ
69 Ⓐ Ⓑ Ⓒ Ⓓ
70 Ⓐ Ⓑ Ⓒ Ⓓ
71 Ⓐ Ⓑ Ⓒ Ⓓ
72 Ⓐ Ⓑ Ⓒ Ⓓ

73 Ⓐ Ⓑ Ⓒ Ⓓ
74 Ⓐ Ⓑ Ⓒ Ⓓ
75 Ⓐ Ⓑ Ⓒ Ⓓ
76 Ⓐ Ⓑ Ⓒ Ⓓ
77 Ⓐ Ⓑ Ⓒ Ⓓ
78 Ⓐ Ⓑ Ⓒ Ⓓ
79 Ⓐ Ⓑ Ⓒ Ⓓ
80 Ⓐ Ⓑ Ⓒ Ⓓ
81 Ⓐ Ⓑ Ⓒ Ⓓ
82 Ⓐ Ⓑ Ⓒ Ⓓ
83 Ⓐ Ⓑ Ⓒ Ⓓ
84 Ⓐ Ⓑ Ⓒ Ⓓ
85 Ⓐ Ⓑ Ⓒ Ⓓ
86 Ⓐ Ⓑ Ⓒ Ⓓ
87 Ⓐ Ⓑ Ⓒ Ⓓ
88 Ⓐ Ⓑ Ⓒ Ⓓ
89 Ⓐ Ⓑ Ⓒ Ⓓ
90 Ⓐ Ⓑ Ⓒ Ⓓ
91 Ⓐ Ⓑ Ⓒ Ⓓ
92 Ⓐ Ⓑ Ⓒ Ⓓ

Answer Sheet
MODEL EXAMINATION C

WRITING SAMPLE

Use separate ruled
sheets of paper.

93

94

BIOLOGICAL SCIENCES

95 Ⓐ Ⓑ Ⓒ Ⓓ	121 Ⓐ Ⓑ Ⓒ Ⓓ
96 Ⓐ Ⓑ Ⓒ Ⓓ	122 Ⓐ Ⓑ Ⓒ Ⓓ
97 Ⓐ Ⓑ Ⓒ Ⓓ	123 Ⓐ Ⓑ Ⓒ Ⓓ
98 Ⓐ Ⓑ Ⓒ Ⓓ	124 Ⓐ Ⓑ Ⓒ Ⓓ
99 Ⓐ Ⓑ Ⓒ Ⓓ	125 Ⓐ Ⓑ Ⓒ Ⓓ
100 Ⓐ Ⓑ Ⓒ Ⓓ	126 Ⓐ Ⓑ Ⓒ Ⓓ
101 Ⓐ Ⓑ Ⓒ Ⓓ	127 Ⓐ Ⓑ Ⓒ Ⓓ
102 Ⓐ Ⓑ Ⓒ Ⓓ	128 Ⓐ Ⓑ Ⓒ Ⓓ
103 Ⓐ Ⓑ Ⓒ Ⓓ	129 Ⓐ Ⓑ Ⓒ Ⓓ
104 Ⓐ Ⓑ Ⓒ Ⓓ	130 Ⓐ Ⓑ Ⓒ Ⓓ
105 Ⓐ Ⓑ Ⓒ Ⓓ	131 Ⓐ Ⓑ Ⓒ Ⓓ
106 Ⓐ Ⓑ Ⓒ Ⓓ	132 Ⓐ Ⓑ Ⓒ Ⓓ
107 Ⓐ Ⓑ Ⓒ Ⓓ	133 Ⓐ Ⓑ Ⓒ Ⓓ
108 Ⓐ Ⓑ Ⓒ Ⓓ	134 Ⓐ Ⓑ Ⓒ Ⓓ
109 Ⓐ Ⓑ Ⓒ Ⓓ	135 Ⓐ Ⓑ Ⓒ Ⓓ
110 Ⓐ Ⓑ Ⓒ Ⓓ	136 Ⓐ Ⓑ Ⓒ Ⓓ
111 Ⓐ Ⓑ Ⓒ Ⓓ	137 Ⓐ Ⓑ Ⓒ Ⓓ
112 Ⓐ Ⓑ Ⓒ Ⓓ	138 Ⓐ Ⓑ Ⓒ Ⓓ
113 Ⓐ Ⓑ Ⓒ Ⓓ	139 Ⓐ Ⓑ Ⓒ Ⓓ
114 Ⓐ Ⓑ Ⓒ Ⓓ	140 Ⓐ Ⓑ Ⓒ Ⓓ
115 Ⓐ Ⓑ Ⓒ Ⓓ	141 Ⓐ Ⓑ Ⓒ Ⓓ
116 Ⓐ Ⓑ Ⓒ Ⓓ	142 Ⓐ Ⓑ Ⓒ Ⓓ
117 Ⓐ Ⓑ Ⓒ Ⓓ	143 Ⓐ Ⓑ Ⓒ Ⓓ
118 Ⓐ Ⓑ Ⓒ Ⓓ	144 Ⓐ Ⓑ Ⓒ Ⓓ
119 Ⓐ Ⓑ Ⓒ Ⓓ	145 Ⓐ Ⓑ Ⓒ Ⓓ
120 Ⓐ Ⓑ Ⓒ Ⓓ	146 Ⓐ Ⓑ Ⓒ Ⓓ

The MCAT
Model Examination C

PHYSICAL SCIENCES

TIME—70 MINUTES FOR 52 QUESTIONS

Directions: The following questions or incomplete statements are in groups. Preceding each series of questions or statements is a paragraph or a short explanatory statement, a formula or set of formulas, or a definition. Read the written material and then answer the questions or complete the statements. Select the ONE BEST ANSWER for each question and indicate your selection by marking the corresponding letter of your choice on the Answer Form. Eliminate those alternatives you know to be incorrect and then select an answer from among the remaining alternatives. A periodic table is provided (see p. 563). You may consult it whenever you wish to do so.

Passage I (Questions 1–6)

A human centrifuge is used to test and train pilots and astronauts to withstand the large "g-forces" experienced during flight. The centrifuge arm length is such that the subject moves in a large circle of radius 9 m. The maximum angular velocity is 4 radians/sec. The subject normally faces inward toward the center of the circular path. ("eyeballs in").

During a test, the subject's respiratory and metabolic rate rise. The energy released per liter of oxygen consumed in human metabolism averages about 20,000 J/L.

1. What is the maximum linear (tangential) speed of the subject along the circular path at the maximum angular velocity of 4 radians/s?

   (A) 18 m/sec
   (B) 25 m/sec
   (C) 36 m/sec
   (D) 226 m/sec

2. A pilot of mass 82 kg (180 lbs) experiences 8 "g's" during one test for a period of 2 minutes. What is centripetal force, in newtons, acting on the pilot?

   (A) 16 N
   (B) 660 N
   (C) 960 N
   (D) 6400 N

3. In the earth frame of reference, what centrifugal force acts *on the pilot* during the test?

   (A) The centrifugal force *on the pilot* is equal and opposite the centripetal force on the pilot.
   (B) The centrifugal force *on the pilot* is 1 "g" larger than the centripetal force on the pilot.
   (C) The centrifugal force *on the pilot* is 1 "g" smaller than the centripetal force on the pilot.
   (D) There is *no* centrifugal force *on the pilot*.

4. The pilot's metabolic rate rises to 450 W and remains at that level during the 2 minute test period. What is the approximate number of liters of oxygen consumed by the pilot during the test period?

(A) 3 L
(B) 4 L
(C) 6 L
(D) 10 L

5. What force acts on the back of the pilot's seat?

(A) 0 N
(B) 88 N
(C) 960 N
(D) 6400 N

6. The pilot now faces outward ("eyeballs out"). What effect does this have on the centripetal force acting on the pilot?

(A) The centripetal force now points outward.
(B) The seat back now exerts an outward force.
(C) The centripetal force is replaced by the centrifugal force (now supplied by the pilot's seat harness).
(D) The centripetal force is unchanged (now supplied by the pilot's seat harness).

Passage II (Questions 7–13)

The most common method of preparing hydroiodic acid is passing a stream of hydrogen iodide gas through water:

$$HI(g) + H_2O(l) \rightarrow H_3O^+(aq) + I^-(aq)$$

The hydrogen iodide can be prepared using several different reactions. Iodine reacts with hydrazine in water as follows:

$$2I_2(aq) + N_2H_4(aq) \rightarrow 4HI(aq) + N_2(g)$$

The iodine used in the preparation of hydrogen iodide can be purified by sublimation. Hydrogen iodide can be distilled from a solution of concentrated acid and potassium iodide. Additionally, gaseous iodide and hydrogen can be used according to the reaction:

$$H_2(g) + I_2(g) \rightarrow 2HI(g)$$

A chemist uses this procedure to produce a pure sample of hydroiodic acid. The chemist combines 0.010 g H_2 gas with 1.26 g iodine and collects the gas produced in 1.00 L of water.

7. Compared with fluorine, iodine is:

(A) more electronegative.
(B) less electronegative.
(C) oxidized.
(D) reduced.

8. The intermolecular forces involved in solid iodine are:

(A) ionic forces.
(B) hydrogen bonds.
(C) dipole forces.
(D) London dispersion forces

9. What is the pH of the hydroiodic acid prepared by the chemist?

(A) 1.0
(B) 2.0
(C) 4.5
(D) 6.0

10. In the reaction of hydrogen and iodine:

(A) hydrogen is oxidized and iodine is reduced.
(B) hydrogen is oxidized and iodine is oxidized.
(C) hydrogen is reduced and iodine is reduced.
(D) hydrogen is reduced and iodine is oxidized.

11. The chemist finds that the hydroiodic acid solution prepared conducts electricity. This is because:

(A) HI is nonpolar.
(B) HI is polar.
(C) HI is a weak electrolyte.
(D) HI is a strong electrolyte.

12. What phase change occurs during sublimation?
(A) gas → liquid
(B) liquid → solid
(C) solid → gas
(D) solid → liquid

13. The bond between atoms in I_2 can best be described as:

(A) nonpolar covalent.
(B) polar covalent.
(C) ionic.
(D) electrostatic.

Passage III (Questions 14–19)

A periscope viewing system is to be used to observe the behavior of primates in a large environmentally controlled room on the upper floor of a large research facility. The periscope, like those used on submarines, is essentially a large, folded-path, low-power telescope (using prisms to fold the light path). A sketch of the preliminary design appears below. Like all Newtonian telescopes, it uses a relatively long focal length objective lens to form a real image in front of the eyepiece lens (of shorter focal length). The observer looks through the eyepiece lens to see the final image, in the same manner that one would use a magnifying glass. The distance between the lenses is approximately equal to the sum of their focal lengths. The eyepiece, in this design, can be moved forward or back in order to focus on the primates as they move closer to or further away from the objective lens.

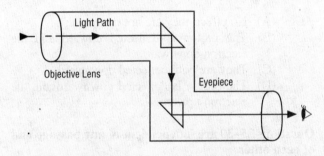

14. The total tube length of the three sections is to be 4 m. The objective lens available has a focal length of 3 m. What should the focal length of the eyepiece lens be?

    (A) 0.75 m
    (B) 1 m
    (C) 1.33 m
    (D) 7 m

15. A visitor seeing the sketch points out an important flaw that will require a design change. What is the flaw?

    (A) The focal length of the eyepiece lens is too short.
    (B) The images of the primates will be inverted.
    (C) The objective lens should be a diverging lens.
    (D) The prisms cannot be used in this way.

16. What will be the approximate magnification of this periscope?

    (A) 0.67 ×
    (B) 1 ×
    (C) 3 ×
    (D) 300 ×

17. The prisms (45-45-90° prisms) turn the light path through 90° by "total internal reflection" from the inside hypotenuse faces of the prisms when the incident angle is 45° as in the sketch. Can one use crown glass with an index of refraction of 1.52 for the prism?

    (A) Yes, because the critical angle for crown glass is 47°.
    (B) Yes, because the critical angle for crown glass is 41°.
    (C) No, because the critical angle for crown glass is exactly 47°.
    (D) No, because the critical angle for crown glass is 41°.

18. Describe the properties of the image that one sees with this preliminary design.

    (A) real, inverted, magnified
    (B) real, upright, magnified
    (C) virtual, upright, same size as object
    (D) virtual, inverted, magnified

19. The telescope is focused on a primate rather far away on the far side of the large habitat. As the primate moves rather closer to the telescope, what must the observer do to see the primate clearly?

    (A) No change, the image remains clear.
    (B) Move the eyepiece away from the objective.
    (C) Move the eyepiece closer to the objective.
    (D) Use an inverting eyepiece because the image flips.

Passage IV (Questions 20–24)

A glass tube has a set of parallel metal plates and is evacuated of air. The plates are attached to a battery of 100 volts. An electron, starting from rest at the negative plate, accelerates uniformly toward the positive plate. At the same instant, a proton (which is 1835 times more massive than the electron) starts from rest at the positive plate and accelerates toward the negative plate. One can also apply a magnetic field across the region between the plates by the use of externally mounted current-carrying coils of wire.

20. Compare the kinetic energies in electron-volts of the proton and electron at the instant each reaches its opposite plate.

    (A) proton: 183,500 eV and electron: 0.05 eV
    (B) proton: 1 eV and electron: 183,500 eV
    (C) proton: 100 eV and electron: 100 eV
    (D) proton: 0.05 eV and electron: 100 eV

21. Assume that the original accelerating electric field points horizontally north. A horizontal magnetic field pointing west is now applied using the external coils. What are the paths of the electron and proton now?

    (A) They both travel in a straight line without deflecting.
    (B) They are both deflected vertically upward.
    (C) The proton is deflected vertically upward and the electron downward.
    (D) The proton is deflected to the west and the electron to the east.

22. How does the magnetic field affect the speed of the electron and proton?

    (A) The speeds of both are not affected.
    (B) The proton speeds up and the electron slows down.
    (C) Both speed up due to the magnetic force.
    (D) The electron speeds up and the proton slows down.

23. The magnetic coils are rotated so that the magnetic field is now parallel to the electric field (north). What are the paths of the electron and proton now?

    (A) They are both deflected upward.
    (B) The proton deflects downward and the electron upward.
    (C) Neither is deflected upward or downward.
    (D) The proton is deflected to east and the electron to west.

24. The magnetic coils are turned off and an additional small set of parallel plates is mounted horizontally to produce a vertically upward electric field. The proton and electron, which were traveling horizontally, enter the region where the upward **E** field exists. What effect does this field have on the paths of the proton and electron?

    (A) No effect; they are not deflected.
    (B) The proton is deflected upward and the electron downward.
    (C) They are both deflected downward.
    (D) The proton is deflected downward and the electron upward.

Questions 25–30 are independent of any passage and of each other.

25. Following bombardment of the Hg-198 isotope with neutrons, the resulting compound nucleus emits a deuteron, $^2_1$H. What is the isotope, X, that results?

    $$^1_0n + {}^{198}_{80}Hg \rightarrow {}^A_ZX + {}^2_1H$$

    (A) $^{197}_{80}$Hg
    (B) $^{98}_{81}$Tl1
    (C) $^{197}_{79}$Au
    (D) $^{197}_{78}$Pt

26. A centrifuge starts from rest and reaches a final angular speed of 57,300 rev/min in 2 minutes. (Recall that 1 rev = 2π radians.) What is the angular acceleration of the centrifuge?

    (A) 50 rad/sec^2
    (B) 32 rad/sec^2
    (C) 3000 rad/sec^2
    (D) 12 rad/sec^2

27. A student makes a simple refracting telescope using both a long focal length converging lens and a shorter-length converging lens. Will it be possible for the student to make a telescope using the same long focal length lens and a diverging lens?

    (A) No, the diverging lens can form only a virtual image.
    (B) Yes, the student must use the diverging lens as the eyepiece.
    (C) No, the diverging lens has too long a focal length.
    (D) Yes, the student must use the diverging lens as the objective.

28. A woman can see clearly only those objects that are no more than 50 cm from her eyes. (Her "far point" is at 0.5 m.) She needs glasses with a focal length of –0.5 m. State the power of this lens in Diopters and whether it is a converging lens or a diverging lens.

    (A) –2.0 D, converging
    (B) –2.0 D, diverging
    (C) –0.5 D, converging
    (D) –0.5 D, diverging

29. One of the naturally occurring radioactive decay series is that of $^{238}_{92}$U, which decays by a succession of alpha and beta decays to a stable, non-radioactive isotope. The series is α, β, β, α, α, α, α, α, β, β, α, β, β, α.

    What is the final, stable isotope?

    (A) $^{206}_{82}$Pb

    (B) $^{210}_{83}$Bi

    (C) $^{214}_{82}$Pb

    (D) $^{210}_{84}$Po

30. The index of refraction of water is $n_w = 1.33$. The speed of light in a certain substance is 83% of its value in water. What is the index of refraction, n_u, of this substance?

    (A) 1.6
    (B) 1.8
    (C) 1.1
    (D) 2.1

Passage V (Questions 31–36)

In a neutral atom, the number of orbital electrons is equal to the number of protons in the nucleus (atomic number). Orbital electron configurations may be shown in shorthand form and may be used to predict reactivity and valence. Krypton, for example, may be shown as $1s^22s^22p^63s^23p^63d^{10}4s^24p^6$. Neon is $1s^22s^22p^6$.

31. A neutral atom of the element $1s^22s^22p^63s^1$ would be expected to:

    (A) readily lose an electron to become an ion with a charge of +1.
    (B) readily lose two electrons to become an ion with a charge of +2.
    (C) readily gain three electrons to become an ion with a charge of –3.
    (D) be an unreactive (noble) element.

32. A neutral atom of the element $1s^22s^22p^63s^1$ has an atomic number of:

    (A) 8.
    (B) 11.
    (C) 18.
    (D) 19.

33. A neutral atom of the element $1s^22s^22p^63s^23p^63d^{10}4s^24p^5$ would be expected to react by:

    (A) losing one electron.
    (B) losing two electrons.
    (C) gaining one electron.
    (D) gaining three electrons.

34. An atom of atomic number 9, having an electron configuration of $1s^2 2s^2 2p^6$, would be:

    (A) a neutral atom.
    (B) an ion with a charge of +1.
    (C) a noble element.
    (D) an ion with a charge of –1.

35. Noble elements include all of the following EXCEPT:

    (A) helium.
    (B) argon.
    (C) neon.
    (D) scandium.

36. In a particular atom, the number of electrons that possess all four quantum numbers identical to those of another electron is:

    (A) zero.
    (B) one.
    (C) two.
    (D) three.

Passage VI (Questions 37–41)

The production of carbon disulfide proceeds via the following reaction:

$$CH_4(g) + S(s) \rightarrow CS_2(l) + H_2S(g)$$

The hydrogen sulfide gas produced can be captured and bubbled through water to produce a slightly acidic aqueous solution:

$$H_2S(aq) + H_2O(l) \rightarrow HS^-(aq) + H_3O^+(aq)$$
$$pK_a = 6.89$$

Carbon disulfide reacts with chlorine gas to produce liquid carbon tetrachloride and sulfur dioxide gas. Sulfur dioxide is a component of acid rain and so must be captured to avoid polluting the atmosphere. A common method for capturing sulfur dioxide is to react it with hydrogen peroxide:

$$H_2O_2(aq) + SO_2(g) \rightarrow H_2SO_4(aq)$$

The pH of the resulting solution can be used to assess the amount of sulfur dioxide present in a sample of a gas.

37. What volume does 32.0 g of methane gas occupy at STP?

    (A) 11.1 L
    (B) 22.4 L
    (C) 33.5 L
    (D) 44.8 L

38. In solution, hydrogen sulfide is:

    (A) a weak acid.
    (B) a strong acid.
    (C) a weak base.
    (D) a strong base.

39. What is the pH of a solution containing equal molar amounts of $H_2S(aq)$ and $HS^-(aq)$?

    (A) 3.40
    (B) 4.40
    (C) 6.89
    (D) 7.57

40. The intermolecular forces between molecules of CH_4 are:

    (A) covalent bonds.
    (B) ionic bonds.
    (C) hydrogen bonds.
    (D) London dispersion forces.

41. When H_2O_2 in 100.0 mL of water is reacted with SO_2, the pH of the resulting solution is 2.0. How much SO_2 was involved in the reaction?

    (A) 0.001 mole
    (B) 0.01 mole
    (C) 0.05 mole
    (D) 0.10 mole

Passage VII (Questions 42–47)

A set of laboratory experiments designed to physically involve the students is planned for a high school physics course. They are to verify Newton's laws of motion and the conservation laws for linear and angular momentum. A pair of low carts on which the student sits are fitted with two complete skateboard wheel sets each. A laser beam and photogate can measure the velocities of such large objects using a commercial computer timing system. The forces required are measured with calibrated spring scales. The experiments are performed in the gymnasium to make use of its large smooth floor area. The instructor has devised a pulley and falling mass system to provide the constant forces to accelerate the cart student systems, but most of the time she has the student provide the accelerating forces by walking backward while keeping the force reading constant on a spring scale. The experience of providing a constant force while accelerating gives the pulling student a "feel" for the real meaning of acceleration.

42. A student practices until he can pull a classmate at constant speed to just overcome friction. This requires a force of 9 N when the mass of cart-student is 90 kg. The student then accelerates the cart-student by pulling with a constant force of 18 N. What is the measured acceleration?

 (A) 0.1 m/sec^2
 (B) 0.8 m/sec^2
 (C) 1.2 m/sec^2
 (D) 4.2 m/sec^2

43. Two students of different masses sit on carts close together. They push off from each other and their velocities are measured just after they separate. The 60 kg student-cart has a speed of 1.2 m/sec. The other student-cart has an opposite speed of 0.8 m/sec. What is the mass of the second student-cart?

 (A) 40 kg
 (B) 90 kg
 (C) 110 kg
 (D) 120 kg

44. A student stands on a rotating frictionless stand with two large weights in his hands. While holding his arms in close to his sides, another student starts him spinning with a rotational angular velocity of 0.3 rev/sec. He then sticks his arms out straight at shoulder height and his angular velocity slows to 0.2 rev/sec. What is the ratio of his moment of inertia about his vertical spin axis when his arms are extended to his moment of inertia when his arms are at his sides?

 (A) 0.6
 (B) 0.8
 (C) 1.5
 (D) 2.5

45. Two students whose cart-student masses are 120 kg and 80 kg sit on the essentially frictionless carts. They hold the ends of a light rope and pull until the carts bump together. They meet at their common center-of-mass. If they start 2 m apart, how far from the starting point of the heavier 120 kg mass is the meeting point?

 (A) 0.4 m
 (B) 0.8 m
 (C) 1.2 m
 (D) 1.4 m

46. One student-cart of mass 80 kg has an initial speed of 4 m/sec and collides with another 80 kg student-cart that is at rest. The two carts lock together (due to a coupling mechanism) and move off together. What is their common velocity?

 (A) 0.5 m/sec
 (B) 1 m/se
 (C) 2 m/sec
 (D) 2.5 m/sec

47. In another trial, an 80 kg student-cart is to be accelerated from rest over a 10 m distance. The students calculate that the net force (including the tension in the cord and the opposing friction force) accelerating the cart is 100 N. What is the speed of the 80 kg student-cart at the end of the 10 m distance?

 (A) 2 m/sec
 (B) 4.5 m/sec
 (C) 5 m/sec
 (D) 10 m/sec

Questions 48–52 are independent of any passage and of each other.

48. Which of the following aqueous solutions will have the lowest freezing point?

    (A) 1 *M* NaCl.
    (B) 0.3 *M* Na$_2$SO$_4$.
    (C) 1.5 *M* glucose.
    (D) H$_2$O.

49. Consider this reaction: Fe^{2+} $\rightleftharpoons$ Fe^{3+} + e$^-$. Which of the following is correct?

    (A) The reaction toward the right is an oxidation.
    (B) The reaction toward the right is a reduction.
    (C) The reaction toward the left is a reduction.
    (D) A and C are correct.

50. The hydronium ion is:

    (A) a protonated water molecule.
    (B) formed by removal of H$^-$ from a water molecule.
    (C) an ion with the formula of H$_2$O$^+$.
    (D) an uranium byproduct.

51. How many milliliters of 0.5*N* NaOH are required to neutralize 50 ml of 0.25*N* HCl?

    (A) 25
    (B) 50
    (C) 0.25
    (D) 2.5

52. A zwitterion is a molecule containing:

    (A) both cationic and anionic functional groups.
    (B) more than one cationic or anionic functional groups.
    (C) polar and nonpolar groups.
    (D) a Z$^+$ charge.

VERBAL REASONING

TIME—60 MINUTES FOR 40 QUESTIONS

Directions: The questions are based on the accompanying seven passages. Read each passage carefully, then answer the following questions. Consider only the material within the passage. For each question, select the ONE BEST ANSWER and indicate your selection by marking the corresponding letter on the Answer Form.

Passage I (Questions 53–58)

In the early 1920s, dozens of F. Scott Fitzgerald's short stories such as "The Offshore Pirate," "Head and Shoulders," "Rags Martin-Jones and the Prince of Wales" as well as his first two novels, *This Side of Paradise* and *The Beautiful and Damned* contained strong, free spirited female characters; and early in his professional career he realized that he had created a type, the Fitzgerald Flapper, for which there came to be increasing public demand. "I know that the magazines want only flapper stories from me," he told his agent Harold Ober in 1922. In the years leading up to the composition of *The Great Gatsby* (1920–1924) he struggled with the difficulty of beginning his fictional work, both the popular stories for magazines like the *Saturday Evening Post*, the more serious ones for magazines like *The Smart Set* and *Scribner's Magazine*, and his novels with independent women, whose very independence fitted them in advance into the broad cultural stereotype of the American Flapper. It was inevitable, however, that Fitzgerald, who would go on to create complex female characters, among many others, like Nicole Diver in *Tender Is the Night* and Kathleen in the unfinished *The Last Tycoon*, characters who defy easy stereotyping, would have to sacrifice the flapper he had created or else *begin* over and over again with a type solidly constructed by the public whose appetite he had, for some time, satisfied. The process by which Fitzgerald created the flapper with a gallery of memorable characters allowed her to ride the wave of popular opinion into a permanent place in the American psyche, and then laid her to rest in the service of his own artistic development is a classic study of the central dilemma of professional authorship: how one who earns his living through his writing can, at the same time, move beyond the dictates of popular culture and create enduring art.

Fitzgerald proclaimed in 1922 that "There always were flappers." And while this is, of course, true in the sense that there have always been women who openly and proudly defied the social conventions of their time, the term "flapper" as Fitzgerald is broadly using it originated in Britain in the years just before 1918, where the term characterized a young girl who had not yet been introduced into society. John O'Hara, in calling attention to the misuse of the term "flapper" in America, offers a slight variation of this usage describing "flapper" as British slang referring to "a society girl who had made her debut and hadn't found a husband." The word "flapper" came into wide currency in the postwar decade in America to describe "a girl or young woman whose conduct and dress [were] characterized by somewhat daring freedom and boldness"—particularly one who wore rouge, flapping galoshes, dresses whose hemlines were more than 9 inches above ground, and bobbed hair. The American Flapper historically is a product of what Frederick Lewis Allen in *Only Yesterday* characterizes as the revolution in manners and morals brought about by an interaction of forces related to World War I and its aftermath. Among these Allen cites the "eat-drink-and-be-merry-for-tomorrow-we-die spirit that accompanied the departure of the soldiers to the training camps and the fighting front"; the war neurosis, which led individuals to find solace in unconventional diversions like drinking, smoking, and dancing; the winning of women's suffrage in 1920; the "growing independence of the drudgeries of housekeeping," brought about by the introduction of household appliances; an increasing tendency of women to join the work force and gain a measure of financial independence. Additional forces, according to Allen, included prohibition (with its invitation to rebel against restrictions), the automobile, the confession and sex magazines, and the movies.

The American flapper, who came into existence during the revolution of manners and morals described by Allen and who owes her name, in part, to the British flapper, came to be associated in the 1920s with the illustrations of John Held, Jr., America's leading cartoonist of the Jazz Age. In film the first flapper was Colleen Moore, who appeared in the movie *Flapperdom* in 1922, and was shortly joined by Clara Bow, the "It" girl, who came to be considered as the quintessence of the flapper. But it is

Adapted from "The Fitzgerald Flapper," VCU, 1995 and used with permission of Dr. Bryant Mangum.

Fitzgerald who is, over and over in the popular magazines of his time, credited with inventing or discovering the flapper, as the following samples demonstrate. A 1921 article in *Shadowland*, entitled "Fitzgerald, Flappers and Fame," acknowledges Fitzgerald as "the recognized spokesman of the younger generation . . . since the publication of his now famous flapper tale 'This Side of Paradise.'" In a newspaper clipping from 1922 pasted in the Fitzgeralds' scrapbooks, Fitzgerald is called "The Flapper Laureate." Another from the same period is headlined "F. Scott Fitzgerald Tells How He Discovered the Flapper." Even into the 1930s editors and reviewers continued to associate Fitzgerald with his tales of the Jazz Age and to echo the call for the flapper stories. Magazine editors continued into the mid-1930s to ask for the old Fitzgerald stories on flappers and "flask gin," but by the mid-1920s he had given up his creation for which he is now perhaps most often remembered in favor of fictional individuals that he hoped would defy stereotyping. The popular magazines of the Jazz Age, now in the bound periodicals section of most libraries, remain the most accessible shrine, though now perhaps a dusty one, to the Fitzgerald Flapper.

53. The best title for this passage would be:

(A) Social Customs of the 1920s.
(B) The Novels of F. Scott Fitzgerald.
(C) F. Scott Fitzgerald: Creator of the American Flapper.
(D) America in the Post–World War I Decade.

54. Which of the following statements best describes the origin of the term "flapper" as it is explained in the passage?

(A) It refers to a young bird, colloquially known as a "flapper."
(B) It originated in Britain and at one time referred to a young girl who had not made her entrance into society.
(C) It was originally an American term that was associated with the flapping arm movements of women who where dancing.
(D) No one is certain where the word "flapper" came from.

55. According to John O'Hara:

(A) a particular quality of the British flapper was that she had not yet found a husband.
(B) Fitzgerald did not invent the flapper.
(C) flappers had been associated in Britain with prostitution.
(D) the movies are primarily responsible for popularizing the flapper.

56. Frederick Lewis Allen attributes the development of the flapper to:

(A) the war neurosis.
(B) women's growing independence from the drudgeries of housekeeping.
(C) the postwar revolution in manners and morals.
(D) all of the above.

57. Which of the following statements is/are *supported* by the passage?

(A) Fitzgerald is the creator of the flapper in fiction.
(B) Fitzgerald was writing about flappers in the mid-1930s.
(C) Clara Bow was the first flapper in film.
(D) Fitzgerald wanted to continue writing about flappers but the public had tired of his stereotype.

58. Which of the following is/are *neither supported nor contradicted* by the passage?

I.   Fitzgerald will be remembered as a better short story writer than a novelist.
II. Fitzgerald will be remembered for creating the flapper in fiction.
III. John Held, Jr. was a better cartoonist than writer.
IV. Fitzgerald gave up writing about the flapper because he wanted to create less stereotyped characters.

(A) I, II, and III
(B) I and III
(C) II and IV
(D) IV only

Passage II (Questions 59–64)

The dependence process begins with an initial exposure to a psychoactive drug. The drug experience allows an individual to perceive two contrasting altered states of consciousness, the normal state versus the drug-induced state. If the drug state is perceived by an individual as more pleasurable (or producing a less painful state) than the nondrug state, then such an individual may make a choice of maintaining the drug state. The word "pleasurable," however, has many meanings, and may not be related to "feeling good." Thus, someone may initiate smoking tobacco, for example, not because it makes him/her feel good (most times it doesn't) but because his/her specific peer group dictates tobacco use as a means of acceptance. Belonging to the group is pleasurable, not the use of tobacco; any drug can serve such a purpose. Many examples of this drug–human interaction can be noted, and the lesson learned, is that humans take drugs for many reasons that essentially meet their own individual needs, whether it be feeling good, peer pressure, or whatever.

Therefore, drugs may not always serve primarily as reinforcers of behavior but may have important secondary reinforcing qualities as well. Regardless of the reasons for using a specific chemical agent, however, it should be understood that most drugs produce their effects via an alteration of brain neurochemistry, which can lead to other more long-term problems, especially if the drug is consumed on a chronic basis.

Once an individual takes on the responsibility of using a given chemical agent chronically, then he/she is beginning to allow other variables to take over his/her own drug-taking behavior, and to some degree will lose his/her ability to control this behavior. Taking drugs repeatedly means that one swallows, injects, sniffs, or smokes a given agent at certain times, in certain places and possibly with certain people. Each time a drug is taken all these events become cumulatively conditioned with the drug, forming a conditioned-stimulus (cs) complex (learned associations). If repeated enough times, the drug takes on stimulus properties initiating certain effects psychologically. Thus, if one associates smoking behavior with feeling good with friends (peer control), then one may need to smoke when those friends are not present to feel good. Conversely, the presence of friends may also act as a stimulus to smoking. What occurs is that the use of the drug can come under environmental (stimulus) control and behavior comes under drug-induced stimulus control. Over time these events can merge to a point where drug taking becomes more and more contingent upon environ-

mental events. The example of this stimulus-complex may be too simplistic, but one may be able to significantly reduce his/her pain by going through the drug taking ritual without administering the drug. Thus, the pharmacological effects of morphine, for example, may be elicited by going through the ritual including an injection of water. Counselors feel that some heroin addicts may be addicted to the needle, and thus the term "needle freaks." Much of these effects are difficult to detect but have been verified in controlled human experiments. We should not take these effects lightly and should suspect that similar CS complex can occur with most drugs we take.

Acute behaviorally effective doses of psychoactive drugs generally disrupt most learned behaviors. Thus, alcohol acutely disrupts the ability of any individual to drive an automobile. However, if the individual continues to drive under the influence of alcohol, then two things can occur. First, the individual will develop behavioral tolerance to the alcohol. That is, such a person will learn to adapt to the drug state and will learn how to manage his/her automobile in spite of the pharmacological effects of alcohol. As this process continues, the learning of how to drive the car and how to get to certain places (to the ABC store) can also become contingent upon the alcohol state. Thus, an individual may have difficulties finding the ABC store when sober. This phenomena is called *drug-induced state dependent learning*. Its premise is that the retention of information learned under the drug state is contingent upon the reinstitution of the drug state. There are many examples of this with most psychoactive drugs. In fact, one might consider this a form of dependence. Thus, a person may need to continue using a specific drug in order to perform specific tasks learned under the drug state.

Drugs that are abused by man appear to have very subtle but profound effects on specific neurotransmitter systems in the brain. In the normal state these chemicals, which are the means by which nerves communicate with each other, are in a very delicate balance, allowing one to perceive his/her environment and make adjustments to act in accordance with his/her own needs. Psychoactive drugs tend to disrupt this balance, which in effect alters an individual's ability to respond in his/her environment.

At this point there is one theoretical model that suggests that the drug-dependent person's neurochemical system is out of balance and that the individual uses a given drug to allow his/her neurochemical systems to function in a more normal fashion. This theory has been promoted as a mental health model in order to explain the success of chemotherapy in the control of several psychotic states. However, this has yet to be substantiated in the substance abuse area.

Adapted from John A. Rosecrans, "Psychological and Neurochemical Mechanisms Involved in the Maintenance of Chemical Dependencies" *Drug Dependence Outline*, MCV/VCU, 1990.

59. This passage deals with:

    I. the acute pharmacolgical experience.
    II. the habitual drug use: the condition of drug effects as a prelude to dependency.
    III. learning aspects.
    IV. neurochemical aspects.

    (A) I, II, and III
    (B) I and III
    (C) II and IV
    (D) I, II, III, and IV

60. Which of the following statements is *supported by* the passage?

    (A) A drink here and there really does not hurt.
    (B) Your first drink starts you on your way to drug abuse.
    (C) A pleasurable state is associated with euphoria.
    (D) Drug use follows certain patterns.

61. Human beings partake in drugs because of:

    (A) peer pressure.
    (B) psychological need.
    (C) depression due to marital pressure.
    (D) all of the above.

62. Chemical agents consumed chronically:

    (A) alter the mind.
    (B) seem to act in a predictable fashion.
    (C) modulate neurochemical mechanisms.
    (D) have relatively short-term effects.

63. Once an individual is addicted:

    (A) ritual becomes the order of the day.
    (B) environmental conditions may play a dominant role.
    (C) injection of a placebo replaces the chemical.
    (D) the side effects decrease and use becomes less harmful.

64. According to the author:

    (A) certain tasks can be better learned while under the effects of drugs.
    (B) certain tasks can be better performed while under the effects of drugs.
    (C) certain tasks may be difficult to perform if not under the influence of drugs.
    (D) behavioral tolerance will lessen the influence of drug affliction.

Passage III (Questions 65–69)

For almost a thousand years Alexandria was the world's center of higher learning. The library eventually contained a half million scrolls, and the museum contained a zoo, botanical garden, astronomical observatory, anatomical exhibit, and treasures from around the world. Teaching was limited only to what was necessary to train researchers for the next generation. The main focus was on improving understanding so that each generation could inherit a more advanced civilization. Teaching was not an end or good in itself.

The school of Alexandria was modeled after the Lyceum of Aristotle. What Aristotle received from Plato and was passed to the school at Alexandria was a sense of optimism and dedication in seeking the truth. We know that Plato marveled at the underlying principles of mathematics, such as the Pythagorean theorem, and that he tried to find underlying principles or "truths" in other fields of study. Aristotle's improvement was to take this idea of generalization apart and show that when deduction and induction were used alternately, we had a *method* of finding underlying principles.

The first librarian was Herodotus of Ephesus, who with these new methods of logic dared to edit Homer's *Iliad* and *Odyssey*. The second librarian was Eratosthenes of Cyrene, who, to mention one specific item, measured the size of the earth. First, he measured the angle of the sun (six degrees) at midday on midsummer's day at Alexandria because he knew from previous trips to Cyrene (near today's Aswan Dam) that the sun shone to the bottom of its wells (zero degrees) on that very day and time each year. Then, he only had to measure the distance between these two places to calculate the circumference of the earth (60/360 = distance/circumference).

The third librarian, Aristophanes of Byzantium, commissioned 70 scholars to translate the Bible into Greek; and this translation, used by Jesus Christ, became known as the *Septuagint*. (There is other evidence to suggest that the "flight into Egypt" took place in Alexandria.) The fourth librarian was Aristarchus of Samosthrace, who developed the eight parts of speech and wrote commentaries on the works of Homer, Pindar, and Aristophanes of Athens.

Returning to the faculty, we should not fail to aknowledge what we owe to Euclid beyond geometry. Euclid, who was commissioned to start a school of mathematics around 300 B.C., established a mode of accumulating understanding by starting with a few axioms and theories, stacking conclusions into workable structures of knowledge. Examples today would be the Periodic Chart of Elements, the Myers-Briggs Personality Types,

Adapted from Dr. James McGovern, "Alexandria: The First Research University," MCV/VCU, 1990.

and the concept of management schools, to name a few structures or inferential models in different disciplines.

Apollonius and Archimedes were in the next generation of scholars. Whereas Apollonius gave us the conic sections, Archimedes gave us number systems (myriads) capable of counting the sands of the earth. That same generation included Aristarchus of Samos, who taught that the earth moved around the sun and whose name appeared in the margin of a book used by Copernicus while studying at Bologna in the seventeenth century.

During the following century, Hipparchus of Nicea calculated the length of the year to within minutes and the length of the month to a few seconds. Around 150 A.D. Claudius Ptolemy wrote 13 books on astronomy, called the *Almagest*. This set also explained that finding a descriptive model for understanding was more important than accounting for every fact or observation. In his books on astrology, he summarized the beliefs of the Greeks, Egyptians, and Persians and gave us the horoscopes and Zodiac signs used today. Also around 150 A.D. Galen came to Alexandria to study. He was the authority on medicine for more than a thousand years; when physicians found parts of the body to differ from his descriptions, they concluded that the person was abnormal.

During the early days of Alexandria, prisoners were dissected alive. However, evil was not limited to "pagans" but discrimination and killing occurred between Jews and Greeks, Christians and Egyptians, and so on. Around 400 A.D., a Christian mob under Cyril ripped the flesh off the mathematician Hypatia because her beliefs were not like theirs.

Whereas understanding could be accumulated in libraries and transmitted by books from generation to generation, wisdom (seeing the importance of doing good for others, i.e., human truths) has to be reinspired again and again by individuals in each generation.

Through the centuries, religion and classical humanism have contended to underwrite the meaning of wisdom. Sometimes, religion (morality) provided the rationale for justice, at other times, humanism (ethics). Whatever, the lesson from Alexandria's past is that whenever a true sense of the underlying principles of morality *or* ethics was not present, minorities and individuals suffered. Thus, during periods of ebbing or pluralistic religious beliefs (like today), ethics becomes necessary to form a behavorial consensus, to "hold these truths." Accordingly, the university's first mission is not to acquire new understandings nor to teach many students, but to reinspire wisdom at an effective level in each new generation.

65. Which statement best summarizes the attitude at the ancient library-museum at Alexandria?

(A) It was bascially a teacher-training school.
(B) It was an academy of philosophers.
(C) It was a natural history museum.
(D) It was mostly a scholarly research institute.

66. Plato's sense of "truth" was:

(A) what was revealed by God.
(B) limited to mathematical proofs.
(C) underlying principles in any field.
(D) what was agreed to by consensus.

67. Eratosthenes was able to measure the angle of the sun at two distant places on the earth's surface *simultaneously* by:

(A) measuring at one place at midday on midsummer's day a year after measuring at the other place at the same time and date.
(B) having two teams measure angles at the same time and date.
(C) calculating the transit of the sun between measurements.
(D) calculating the movement (turning) of the earth between measurements.

68. One argument given that the "flight into Egypt" of Jesus Christ took place in Alexandria was:

(A) Jesus Christ spoke Greek.
(B) Jesus Christ knew the Greek version of the Bible.
(C) Jesus Christ used the accentuation and punctuation of Alexandria.
(D) Jesus Christ was against plagiarism.

69. What statement best fits Claudius Ptolemy?

(A) He was an ancient astronomer.
(B) He was an ancient astrologer.
(C) He was both an astronomer and astrologer.
(D) He was a historian.

Passage IV (Questions 70–75)

Charles James Correll (February 2, 1890–September 26, 1972), radio comedian and co-creator with Freeman Gosden of *Amos 'n Andy*, was the son of Joseph Boland Correll and (though there are some inconsistencies about his mother's first name) Julia A. Fiss Correll. He was born in Peoria, Illinois, where he grew up in a stable, working class family. While still in school, he worked as an usher in a local vaudeville house and developed an interest in show business. After graduating from Peoria's public high school, he began to follow his father's trade as a bricklayer. In his spare time, however, he played piano in Peoria's silent movie houses and sang, danced, and took small parts in local shows.

In 1918, after being noticed by the director of a local show, Correll was offered a job with the Joe Bren Company of Chicago. Bren specialized in producing minstrel shows as fund-raisers for charitable groups in small cities. For the next 6 years Correll traveled the country, directing productions for Bren. In 1919, doing a show in Durham, North Carolina, he first met Freeman Gosden, who had just been hired by Bren and was to be trained by Correll. The two became friends, often sharing an apartment during summers when both men were in Chicago, preparing for the next season. In 1924 both men were brought to Bren's Chicago home office, Gosden to manage Bren's new circus division, Correll to manage the shows division.

Sharing an apartment, Correll and Gosden began to write musical reviews together, and they worked up a "song and chatter" act. In March 1925, they began an 8-month series of weekly appearances on Chicago's radio station WEGH. Soon they were doing occasional appearances in shows and on radio programs in St. Louis, in Columbus, Ohio, and other places in the Midwest. During the summer of 1925 they both resigned from the Bren Company and began concentrating on a career in vaudeville. However, the Chicago *Tribune*'s radio station offered them $200 a week, and in November 1925, they began a series of nightly broadcasts on WGN.

At the suggestion of the station's management, Correll and Gosden used their experiences with minstrel shows to work up a "radio comic strip" about two African American boys, and on January 12, 1926, *Sam 'n Henry* began a series of nightly 10-minute broadcasts on WGN. The show was an immediate hit. In 1928, however, a rival Chicago newspaper lured Correll and Cosden away from WGN, though the *Tribune* retained all rights to *Sam 'n Henry* and continued broadcasting the show with two new men.

At the Chicago *Daily News*'s radio station WMAQ, on March 19, 1928, Correll and Gosden began broadcasting six nights a week with a 15-minute show about two African American men living in Harlem. *Amos 'n Andy* focused on the misadventures of Amos Jones, played by Freeman Gosden as energetic, enterprising, and honest, and Andrew H. Brown, played by Correll as indolent but good-hearted. Gradually, the team added characters, but until the 1940s all the writing and voices were done by Correll and Gosden.

The show was a huge success, and with the help of the *Tribune*'s publicity staff, in 1929 Correll and Gosden even put out a book (*All About Amos 'n Andy and Their Creators Correll and Gosden*) to satisfy Chicago listeners' curiosity. Within a short time NBC was offering Correll and Gosden $100,000 a year, and on August 19, 1929, Pepsodent toothpaste began sponsoring *Amos 'n Andy* on NBC's Red network.

Amos 'n Andy became network radio's first huge success. Within a few years, Correll and Gosden had moved to California, where they appeared in movies, published books of *Amos 'n Andy* dialogue, and lived the life of Hollywood stars. Despite protests about the racial stereotyping of *Amos 'n Andy*, especially from the African American press, Correll and Gosden's show remained popular throughout the Great Depression and into the 1940s. Short, stocky, and dark haired (later gray), Correll became the relaxed, gregarious half of the partnership, balancing Freeman Gosden's more tempermental, difficult, and creative personality.

Correll enjoyed his success. He bought a large, lavish home in Beverly Hills; he indulged in expensively stylish clothes and became an enthusiastic golfer. After a divorce from his first wife, Marie Janes (whom he married in 1927), he married the dancer Alyce Mercedes McLaughlin in 1937. They eventually had four children.

With World War II, listenership began to drop. In February 1943, after changing networks and sponsors several times, *Amos 'n Andy* left the air. In October it returned as a half-hour weekly variety program featuring guest stars, an orchestra, outside writers, and a studio audience. This show continued with NBC until 1948, when Correll and Gosden, along with Jack Benny and other stars, left NBC. For $2.5 million Correll and Gosden sold CBS the rights to *Amos 'n Andy* for the next 20 years, and they also received star salaries to play the chief parts.

Within a few years, television ended the success of their variety show, but from 1954 into the 1960s, Correll and Gosden stayed on CBS radio with a new show, The Amos and Andy Music Hall, mixing skits with popular records. On November 25, 1960, they left the air permanently.

Adapted from "Charles James Correll," VCU, 1995 and used with permission of Dr. Nicholas Sharp.

In the mid-1950s, CBS developed a situation comedy based on *Amos 'n Andy* characters. Correll and Gosden were creative consultants, but the cast was entirely African American. The show had modest success with audiences, but it was embroiled in constant racial controversy. The NAACP protested the show vehemently, and the cast had frequent problems with the scripts. Neither Correll nor Gosden was prepared for the kind of bitterness that the TV show had engendered, and both men, especially Gosden, felt deeply wounded by some accusations.

After the TV series ended and their last radio show was over, Correll and Gosden remained friends, living near each other in quiet retirement in their Beverly Hills homes. Correll continued throughout his life to maintain warm and friendly connections with his mid-western roots, and returning to Chicago, he died there at the age of 82.

70. Which of the following is supported by the passage?

(A) Correll's interest in vaudeville came through his mother and father, both of whom were performers.
(B) Correll was independently wealthy and took up vaudeville because he could find nothing else that interested him.
(C) Correll's interest in vaudeville began when he was an usher in a vaudeville house.
(D) Correll preferred his father's profession of bricklaying to show business, but he was better at entertainment than at bricklaying.

71. According to the passage, which quality more characterizes Gosden than it does Correll?

(A) He was more even-tempered.
(B) He was more temperamental.
(C) He was a better pianist.
(D) He was the funniest.

72. What event marked the beginning of the first decline of popularity of the *Amos 'n Andy Show*?

(A) The Great Depression
(B) The arrival of Correll's first child.
(C) Gosden's hospitalization.
(D) World War II.

73. What does the passage indicate happened to the *Sam 'n Henry Show* after Correll and Gosden left radio station WGN?

(A) They carried their show with them to rival station WMAQ.
(B) WGN retained rights to the show and continued it without Correll and Gosden.
(C) Correll and Gosden retained rights to the show but changed its name to the *Amos 'n Andy Show.*
(D) The show was canceled.

74. From the Great Depression onward, the *Amos 'n Andy Show* was criticized for its racial stereotyping. According to the passage, which of the words below best describes Correll's response to this criticism?

(A) Angry
(B) Vindictive
(C) Wounded
(D) Indifferent

75. In retirement, both Correll and Gosden were financially secure. What was the state of their friendship in the later years of their lives?

(A) Their friendship was weakened by the turmoil and controversy caused by the show, and they drifted apart.
(B) They remained friends and lived near each other in Beverly Hills.
(C) They quarreled bitterly over money and parted enemies.
(D) They occupied adjoining suites in the Beverly Hilton until Correll returned to Peoria.

Passage V (Questions 76–80)

The process involved in the recovery from either chronic alcohol or substance abuse is a long one, mainly a lifetime pursuit. AA teaches that an alcoholic can never drink again, and it is generally held that relapse occurs more often when someone stops going to "meetings." Although empirical observations such as these have caused a considerable amount of doubt in the past, a measure of light is now being shed on the situation.

For example, some of the answers to the puzzle of the recovery process are suggested in two articles published in the first issue of the *Informer* by O'Brien and Rosecrans. They focus primarily on the environmental contingencies that cause drug-dependent individuals problems when trying to stop using a specific chemical. Thus, the drug-dependent individual is faced with many problems outside of his or her own internal need to feel good. For example, drug effects such as their self-administration, and the withdrawal syndrome following chronic use, can be elicited by external stimuli previously associated with previous drug use. A heroin-dependent individual in recovery may experience severe withdrawal symptoms if he or she enters a bar or restaurant previously associated with heroin withdrawal. Furthermore, an alcoholic when not under the influence of alcohol may have difficulty finding his or her car when parked during an alcoholic bout, but can remember where it is when drinking is resumed. This latter phenomena is better known as drug-induced state dependent learning, a pharmacological effect well documented in the human literature.

Thus, when one considers what a drug can do to an individual internally, and in conjunction with his or her environment, one wonders how anyone could become drug-free under the burden of such effects. However, it does happen many times over, regardless of the odds. Thus, is recovery a magical phenomena, or is it scientifically based? The answer is not simple. One experiment conducted in rats may help us appreciate what might be going on during the recovery process. In this study, Esposito *et al.* (*Science 224*: 306–309 (1984) at the National Institute of Mental Health were evaluating how electrical stimulation (like ECS) affects energy metabolism in rat brains. Two groups of rats were studied; one group was allowed to stimulate itself by pressing a lever (self-stimulation); the other group was stimulated within the same parameters, but the stimulation was elicited by the experimenter. The second group, thus, had no part in the electrostimulation of their brains. Interestingly, even though both groups of rats received the same level of stimulation, the brain area distribution pattern of increases in energy metabolism were quite different and contingent upon whether rat or experimenter turned on the stimulator.

This experiment is important, not because it provided a specific set of data, but because it demonstrated that a specific change in brain energy metabolism was controlled by each individual rat. The effect on energy metabolism was quite different when elicited by the experimenter. This simple experiment suggests that each individual, to recover from drug dependency, must operate on him or herself. This concept may have importance for two other reasons. First, treatment works only when the individual decides to take on recovery. Although this may appear to be a logical statement, many good professionals, including some in the areas of medical and mental health, do not appear to appreciate the difference between treatment and recovery. Second, during the recovery process, the individual is basically altering his or her behavioral conditioning and neurochemistry, which will allow the process to go forward. This can be done by extinguishing or altering the stimulus properties of the drugs that the individual is dependent on. "Don't drink and go to meetings." In scientific terms, the reinforcing effects of drugs are extinguished by not using them, and the stimulus properties are altered by joining forces with people who have also changed their environments. In addition, the social reinforcement and support in AA is also important to recovery because one is substituting alcohol or drugs with people, a much finer euphoriant. Therefore, success in recovery may not be as magical as was once thought, and may have a very precise and orderly basis. The awareness and knowledge of this scientific base can be helpful to both client and therapist.

76. An appropriate title for this passage could be:

    (A) Withdrawal Syndrome.
    (B) Behavioral Conditioning and Withdrawal.
    (C) The Recovery Process.
    (D) Environmental Contingencies and Drug Use.

77. Recovery from drug addiction:

    (A) involves a lifelong process.
    (B) is modulated by environmental factors.
    (C) can be associated with withdrawal symptoms.
    (D) includes all of the above.

Adapted from John A. Rosecrans, *Drug Dependence Outline*, MCV/ VCU, 1990.

78. According to the author:

    (A) certain tasks can be better learned while under the influence of psychoactive drugs.
    (B) certain tasks are easily performed while under the influence of drugs.
    (C) certain tasks may be difficult if not under the influence.
    (D) learning and performing of tasks are not drastically affected by drug use.

79. Which statement(s) is/are *supported by* the passage?

    (A) Neurochemical mechanisms play a role in drug addiction and recovery.
    (B) Environmental conditions may have drastic effects on an individual.
    (C) The individual is a key determinator.
    (D) All of the above.

80. According to the passage:

    (A) the addiction process is well understood.
    (B) the recovery process is well understood.
    (C) recovery is the reverse of addiction and depends solely on substitution of compounds.
    (D) none of the above statements is supported.

Passage VI (Questions 81–87)

Physicians like Hippocrates, Thomas Browne, and John Gregory emphasized that physicians must do the "right thing" for their patients, and most physicians take this to mean curing illness and preventing death. Gregory refreshingly reminds us that physicians are not always perfect. "I may reckon among the moral duties incumbent on a physician, that candor, which makes him open to conviction, and ready to acknowledge and rectify his mistakes. An obstinate adherence to an unsuccessful method of treating a disease, is based on a high degree of self-conceit, and a belief of the infallibility of a system." Erik Erikson takes the Golden Rule as his "baseline . . . for wise and proper conduct" and points out that even though systematic ethicists may believe the concept too simple, the rule has "marked a mysterious meeting ground between ancient peoples surrounded by oceans and eras and is a theme hidden in the most memorable sayings of many thinkers." The Talmudic version of the Golden

Rule, "What is hateful to yourself, do not to your fellow man," is similar to the Christian "Love thy neighbor as thyself." The Golden Rule is not a sufficient ethical principle, however, because it conceptualizes the idea that what is good for the physician is good for the patient. It expresses *beneficence,* which means that the physician, because of specialized knowledge and motivation, knows what is best for each patient.

The principle of beneficence, however, must be tempered by the countervailing idea of *autonomy*. The idea of human rights is a relatively recent development in social evolution. When physicians and priests were one and the same, the principle of beneficence was taken for granted. Patients were expected to do what they were told and "doctors orders" became an everyday expression. The ethical principle of autonomy echoes Rousseau, Washington, and Jefferson in emphasizing the patient's primacy in making moral judgments about himself. The courts have generally held that constitutional rights permit an individual to determine what happens to himself and his property; many of these rights have been codified in what has been called a "Patient's Bill of Rights."

Rousseau pointed out that a social contract was necessary because of the inherent inequality among human beings. Some are wise, whereas others are dull, some are strong, whereas others are weak. This inequality is particularly striking in the patient-physician relationship. Physicians have wide knowledge and experience, whereas the patient may understand his own needs and value but has little information about his clinical state. Only detailed conversations with patients and their families can narrow this gap in such a way that people can make truly autonomous judgments about their own care.

Physicians frequently appear to ignore the required balance between the principles of beneficence and autonomy. A physician recommends radical mastectomy for breast cancer. No options are provided because the physician believes he knows best. The patient asks for a second opinion and the physician refuses, saying, "I cannot take care of you unless I can make all important decisions." Here is presumed beneficence gone amok. A moment later the patient refuses all surgery and the physician says kindly, "It's your life and you are free to do anything you like." Here the physician is ignoring the obvious worried state of the patient and threatening abandonment if the patient does not obey.

Aside from the physician's obvious arrogance and insensitivity, the key question must be: Is the patient completely autonomous when she refuses all treatment and walks out of the doctor's office? She has been told that she has cancer and must have what she believes to be a destructive surgical procedure. Fear of disfigurement and death have produced uncontrollable anxiety that causes her to attempt escape from the situation.

Adapted from Dr. Stephen M. Ayres, "Moral Reasoning and Medical Decision Making," MCV/VCU, 1990.

True beneficence in this situation demands that the physician seek out the patient, and her family, and make certain that repeated efforts are made to present the true gravity of the situation. Beneficence does not mean the quick delivery of a series of commands, but implies shared responsibility, patient education, and understanding, and gentle persuasion where necessary. *Indeed, correctly interpreting the proper balance between these two moral principles in any given situation could be considered one of the key responsibilities of the practice of medicine.*

The beneficence/autonomy concept must be related to the burden/benefit relationship of any proposed action. The balance between the risks or burden of continued treatment relative to any anticipated benefits must be carefully considered. Sometimes life itself, or the treatment proposed to sustain life, is so burdensome that the patient claims the right to allow the dying process to proceed. Granting seriously ill patients, or their families, the right to refuse life-lengthening treatment is an important human issue that is central to professional practice. In many respects, the judicial system is ahead of most physicians in understanding the issues under discussion. Artificial feeding, for example, a technique that many would consider to be part of the basic humane care required for all patients may also become burdensome in certain situations where any benefits from such intervention is minimal.

Obviously, the accuracy of a group of physicians to predict that meaningful life is no longer possible for the individual is central to any such decision. Such a need raises the issue of who can determine what is "meaningful life" and how physicians can best learn how to decide when the burden outweighs the benefit of any course of action.

81. Which of the following statement(s) is/are *supported by* the passage?

(A) The Golden Rule is not a sufficient ethical statement.
(B) Most physicians emphasize curing illness and preventing death.
(C) The Golden Rule views the physician as knowing what is best for the patient.
(D) All of the above.

82. Which of the following would probably have been chosen by the author as a title for this passage?

(A) The Development of the Medical Decision Making Process
(B) Physician Reasoning and Autonomy
(C) The Practice of the Golden Rule
(D) Moral Reasoning and Medical Decision Making

83. Regarding human rights, which statement(s) is/are NOT *supported by* the passage?

(A) Hippocrates lived before that principle was established.
(B) Physicians must attempt to defeat the disease first and then explain their protocol.
(C) The courts generally have backed the physician as to knowing what is best for the patient.
(D) All of the above.

84. From information provided in the passage, one would be justified in concluding that:

I. patients are perfectly capable of making autonomous judgments.
II. beneficence implies understanding.
III. Rousseau believed that people are quite similar.
IV. beneficence and autonomy go hand in hand to achieve good medical practice.

(A) I, II, and III
(B) I and III
(C) II and IV only
(D) IV only

85. Hippocrates is cited as one of several who believed that physicians should do the "right thing" for their patients. Which other specific beliefs, thoughts, or perceptions are directly attributed to Hippocrates in the passage?

    I. He perceived medicine as a tripartite relationship between patient, disease, and doctor.
    II. He believed that disease was determined to a great extent by the patient's environment and way of life.
    III. He believed that there was nothing sacred about sickness and that each malady followed a distinct pattern (three stages).
    IV. He thought of the physician as nature's helper who should reinforce the body's own defenses.

    (A) I, II, and III
    (B) I and III
    (C) II and IV
    (D) I, II, III, and IV

86. According to the passage, which of the following is/are correct?

    I. Life itself at times can be burdensome.
    II. Patient education is an essential element in true beneficence.
    III. The courts have a better grasp of the right to die concept than the physician.
    IV. Basic humane treatment must always be provided no matter what the benefit is.

    (A) I, II, and III
    (B) I and III
    (C) II and IV
    (D) I, II, III, and IV

87. The author of the passages argues for:

    I. education.
    II. balance.
    III. consultation.
    IV. patient rights.

    (A) I, II, and III
    (B) I and III
    (C) II and IV
    (D) I, II, III, and IV

Passage VII (Questions 88–92)

Another kind of editorial begins in the April 1942 issue. It was the first to acknowledge America's entry into World War II. This informed youth how they could contribute to the war effort and attempted to inspire them to make such contributions. In an editorial "Little Things Can Help Win the War," the points were simple—stay healthy so you can work hard; assume minor responsibilities so adults can take major roles; save your pennies and dimes to buy Defense Stamps; and "most important of all," be confident. Confidence would provide "vision to see beyond today and its efforts and worries to the glorious day when we can all say, 'We, too, have fought a good fight and, all pulling together for the right cause, . . . we have won!' "

War effort editorials emphasized the need for collecting scrap metal and rubber, for maintaining fitness, and for growing "victory gardens."

To stress the need for staying fit, Hecht published the first guest editorial in *True Comics*. Colonel Theodore P. Bank, chief of the Athletic and Recreation Branch, Special Services Division of the War Department, wrote "The Importance of Physical Fitness Today." Bank mentioned time and effort being wasted because army recruits were unfit and work days were being lost in factories "because of sickness or injuries which are traceable directly to (young people's) lack of physical fitness."

On youth's involvement in food production, Hecht invited another guest writer, Wayne H. Darrow, director, U.S. Agricultural Labor Administration. His piece "You Can Help the Farmer Win the War," was carried on the first page of the August 1943 issue rather than on the inside front cover. Darrow wrote:

> When the harvest is in this fall, everyone who has toughened his hands at farm work will be able to say that he has helped to win the war. Out on our farms this year there is a man's and a woman's job waiting for many thousand boys and girls. Our soldiers, sailors, and marines are counting on the farmers. Can the farmers count on you?

It could be thought that Hecht used editorials merely to sell magazines and to advance patriotism. He was indeed a skillful promoter, and he wanted the United States to win the war, but these aspects were less important than his major goal—a world of democracy, unity, and concord. He was an avid internationalist, a globalist.

In February 1943, in the midst of his war effort editorials, he wrote "It's Your World." The arguments were unusual, perhaps even risky for his own well-being,

From Dr. William E. Blake, Jr., "True Comics," VCU, 1990.

made as they were when the battle was at last shifting in favor of the Allies. This would not seem an appropriate moment to hint to children that the United States must bear some responsibility for the war. However, he attacked the retreat of the United States into isolationism following World War I. "So we celebrated our victory, crawled into our national shell and left the young democracies set up by the Versailles peace treaty to get along the best they could," he wrote. He continued the argument, "We hope and believe that never again will we be guilty of such failure to stand by. For one thing, we know now that withdrawing from our responsibilities after the last war was in a great measure responsible for World War II." He urged young people "to make this battle-scarred planet a safe and sane place to live in."

A similar article in January 1944 pointed out the rapid development of transportation and communication making the world smaller. "Learn to write, read, and speak another langauge—or two or three, if you can," he wrote. According to Hecht, advantages would be easier travel and more friendships in foreign countries. But also the linguist would be able to explain the principles of democracy.

In the following issue Hecht wrote another daring piece, which aroused hostility among some Americans. There was nothing subtle in the title, "An International Police Force." He maintained nations should not be free to act as they pleased. Nations should take their grievances to an international court and let judges decide. He advocated an international police force to enforce court decisions. "We can't have it both ways," he concluded. "We can't have lasting peace and at the same time insist upon all those national 'rights' which make the waging of wars inevitable."

March 1944 was the last issue of *True Comics* to carry an editorial. Paper had become scarce, and all comic magazines were forced to cut the number of pages. Features had to be discontinued and editorials seemed the most dispensable item.

Circulation figures for *True Comics* are available for each year of its publication, but it is impossible to know how widely young people were reading the editorials or what sort of impact they made.

The idea of a comic book with true stories was unique. Other publishers responded, turning our similar products, but *True Comics* stood alone in carrying editorials. These essays were clear witness to the broad, humanistic, and internationalist values and goals held by George J. Hecht; his determination to spread those ideals; and his confidence in the ability and willingness of American youth to read, to learn, and to do.

88. Which statement(s) is/are *supported by* the passage?

    I.   The passage essentially is a history lesson.
    II.   America's war effort is described.
    III. Youth and fitness are the main themes.
    IV. The fate of a comic book is described.

    (A) I, II, and III
    (B) I and III
    (C) II and IV
    (D) IV only

89. The publication was unique because it incorporated:

    (A) true stories.
    (B) color photographs.
    (C) editorials.
    (D) war stories.

90. The editorials stressed:

    (A) recycling.
    (B) patriotism.
    (C) fitness.
    (D) all of the above.

91. The publisher of this series could be considered a(an):

    (A) communist.
    (B) idealist.
    (C) internationalist.
    (D) socialist.

92. In providing information related to the editorials contained in *True Comics* during the World War II period, the author of this passage asserts that:

    (A) the publisher was the first to portray America's entry into World War II in comic form.
    (B) the publisher hoped to reach the young.
    (C) the publisher himself wrote the editorial on fitness.
    (D) isolationism was proposed.

WRITING SAMPLE

TIME—2 ESSAYS
     60 MINUTES (30 MINUTES/TOPIC)

Directions: This is a test of your writing skills. The test consists of two parts. You will have 30 minutes to complete each part. Use your time efficiently. Before you begin writing each of your responses, read the assignment carefully to understand exactly what you are being asked to do. Because this is a test of your writing skills, your response to each part should be as well organized and clearly written as you can make it in the time allotted.

93. Consider this statement:

> **Probably all laws are useless; for good men do not want laws at all, and bad men are made no better by them.**
>
>   **Demonax**

Write a unified essay in which you perform these tasks. Explain the meaning of the above quote. Give specific examples of a time when good people would want laws and when bad ones would be made better by them. Discuss the purpose of a set of imposed laws, what makes them useful or useless in serving this purpose.

94. Consider this statement:

> **And thus your freedom when it loses its fetters becomes itself the fetter of a greater freedom.**
>
>   **Kahlil Gibran**

Write a unified essay in which you complete the following tasks. Explain what you think the above statement means. Describe a specific situation in which freedom that has lost its fetter does not become the fetter of a greater freedom. Discuss the manner in which one type of freedom might put a restraint or a confinement on another type of freedom.

BIOLOGICAL SCIENCES

TIME—70 MINUTES FOR 52 QUESTIONS

Directions: The following questions or incomplete statements are in groups. Preceding each series of questions or statements is a paragraph or a short explanatory statement, a formula or set of formulas, or a definition. Read the written material and then answer the questions or complete the statements. Select the ONE BEST ANSWER for each question and indicate your selection by marking the corresponding letter of your choice on the Answer Form. Eliminate those alternatives you know to be incorrect and then select an answer from among the remaining alternatives.

Passage I (Questions 95–99)

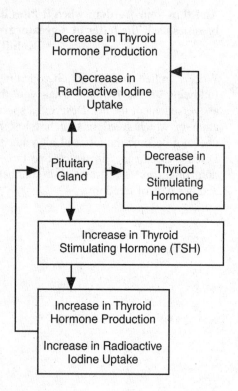

The pituitary gland is responsible for the secretion of thyroid stimulating hormone (TSH), which elicits an increased production of thyroid hormone from the gland; this thyroid hormone then may inhibit the pituitary via a negative feedback. Under hyperthyroid conditions, the following tests would give elevated values:

1. Basal metabolic rate (BMR)
2. Protein bound iodine (PBI)
3. Radioactive iodine uptake (RAI)

95. When TSH secretion falls, the secretion by the thyroid of thyroid hormone:

(A) stays the same.
(B) increases.
(C) decreases.
(D) will feed back upon the pituitary.

96. According to the schema given, if a normal individual is given an injection of TSH, his/her thyroid hormone production will first

(A) show no noticeable change.
(B) increase.
(C) decrease.
(D) lead to a decrease in pituitary TSH output.

Use the information in the flow chart and paragraph above, and in the following charts, to answer questions 97–99.

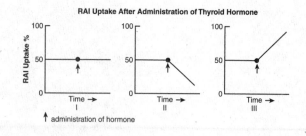

97. In which of the graphs is there evidence of thyroid malfunction?

(A) I
(B) I and II
(C) I and III
(D) III

98. Which graph(s) probably represent(s) the case of a typical hyperthyroid person?

    (A) II
    (B) I
    (C) I and III
    (D) II and III

99. Which of the graphs lead(s) you to believe that there is a breakdown in the normal thyroid-pituitary functional relationship?

    (A) I and III   (C) II
    (B) III   (D) II and III

Questions 100–103 are NOT based on a descriptive passage.

100. A lack of iodine in the diet usually is associated with which disorder?

    (A) acromegaly   (C) rickets
    (B) goiter   (D) skin rash

101. Thyroid stimulating hormone (TSH) is produced by which of the following?

    (A) acidophils (alpha cells)
    (B) basophils (beta cells)
    (C) delta cells
    (D) chromophobes

102. Which of the following statements concerning the thyroid are correct?

    (A) The gland is derived from the pharynx (foramen cecum of the tongue).
    (B) Colloid is located extracellularly.
    (C) T_3-triiodothyronine and T_4 thyroxine are the active principles.
    (D) All of the above.

103. Hypersecretion of which hormone will result in acromegaly (giantism)?

    (A) TSH—thyroid stimulating hormone
    (B) STH—somatotropin (growth hormone)
    (C) ACTH—adrenocorticotrophic hormone
    (D) thyroxin

Passage II (Questions 104–108)

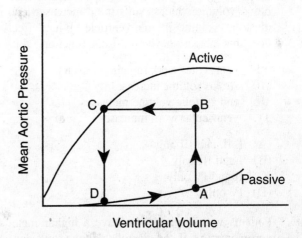

As the left ventricle of the heart contracts, it generates a pressure, which when more than that in the aorta causes the ejection of a volume of blood. The action of the ventricle can be represented as the relationship between the volume of blood in the ventricle and the intraventricular pressure. The relationship between ventricular pressure and volume is known as the Frank-Starling Law of the Heart and is shown above.

The lower curve represents the pressure volume relationship when the heart is being passively filled with blood during diastole (i.e., at rest). The upper curve represents the pressure-volume relationship as a result of contraction (i.e., systole). The volume at Point A is known as the end diastolic volume, which is the volume of blood in the ventricle immediately preceding contraction. During systole, the ventricle contracts, but no blood is ejected until the pressure in the ventricle exceeds the pressure in the aorta. This phase of the cardiac cycle is known as isovolumetric contraction and is represented by line segment AB. When the aortic valve opens (Point C), blood is ejected without further increase in the ventricular pressure (line segment BC). Therefore, this phase of contraction is isotonic and results in the ejection of a volume of blood known as the stroke volume.

When the pressure that the ventricle can generate exactly equals the aortic pressure, the ejection of blood ceases, and the ventricle undergoes isovolumetric relaxation as represented by the line segment CD. The blood from the atrium then fills the ventricle, and the pressure increase is the result of passive resistance of the ventricle (curve DA).

104. Assuming a constant mean aortic pressure, patients with renal failure may have an increased blood volume which results in an increased end diastolic volume in the ventricle. What effect does this increase have on cardiac function?

    I.   ventricular work remains constant
    II. stroke volume increases
    III. end systolic volume increases
    IV. ventricular work increases

    (A) I, II, and III only
    (B) I and III only
    (C) II and IV only
    (D) IV only

105. Patients with hypertension have a higher mean aortic pressure. If end diastolic volume stays constant:

    I.   stroke volume increases.
    II. ventricular work increases.
    III. end systolic volume decreases.
    IV. ventricular work may or may not increase.

    (A) I, II, and III only
    (B) I and III only
    (C) II and IV only
    (D) IV only

106. Patients with heart failure have an active pressure curve (i.e., upper curve), which is shifted downward and to the right as compared with that of normal. Assuming the end diastolic volume and the mean aortic pressure remain constant and the ventricle is capable of ejecting blood:

    I.   stroke volume decreases.
    II. end systolic volume increases.
    III. ventricular work decreases.
    IV. end systolic volume decreases.

    (A) I, II, and III only
    (B) I and III only
    (C) II and IV only
    (D) IV only

107. With time, the blood volume of patients with heart failure tends to increase resulting in an increased end diastolic volume with a continued downward shift in the active pressure curve (i.e., upper curve). The increase in the end diastolic volume, as compared with the case of a failing ventricle without compensation referred to in the preceding question, will result in:

    I.   a stroke volume that may or may not increase.
    II. an increase in cardiac work.
    III. a decrease in end systolic volume.
    IV. an increase in stroke volume.

    (A) I, II, and III only
    (B) I and III only
    (C) II and IV only
    (D) IV only

108. With a constant mean aortic pressure and as compared to normal, a compensated failure will show:

    I.   an increase in stroke volume.
    II. a stroke volume that may or may not decrease.
    III. a decrease in cardiac work.
    IV. an increase in end systolic volume.

    (A) I, II, and III only
    (B) I and III only
    (C) II and IV only
    (D) IV only

Passage III (Questions 109–113)

The diagram below represents three generations of a human family, some of whose members have a non-lethal birth defect. The defect is caused by a single gene for which new mutations are very rare. The individuals with birth defects are represented by solid black symbols, whereas the individuals who have a normal phenotype are represented by open symbols. Males are represented by squares and females are represented by circles.

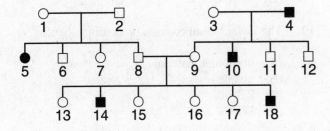

109. The defect is most likely caused by:

(A) an autosomal gene for which the defective allele is recessive to the normal allele.
(B) an X-linked gene for which the defective allele is recessive to the normal allele.
(C) an autosomal gene for which the defective allele is dominant to the normal allele.
(D) an X-linked gene for which the defective allele is dominant to the normal allele.

110. The genotype of individual number 1 in the family:

(A) is most likely to contain only normal alleles.
(B) is most likely to contain only defective alleles.
(C) is most likely to contain both normal and defective alleles.
(D) cannot be determined from the pedigree.

111. The genotype of individual number 4 in the family:

(A) is most likely to contain only normal alleles.
(B) is most likely to contain only defective alleles.
(C) is most likely to contain both normal and defective alleles.
(D) cannot be determined from the pedigree.

112. The genotype of individual number 7 in the family:

(A) is most likely to contain only normal alleles.
(B) is most likely to contain only defective alleles.
(C) is most likely to contain both normal and defective alleles.
(D) cannot be determined from the pedigree.

113. The genotype of individual number 8 in the family:

(A) is most likely to contain only normal alleles.
(B) is most likely to contain only defective alleles.
(C) is most likely to contain both normal and defective alleles.
(D) cannot be determined from the pedigree.

Questions 114–116 are NOT based on a descriptive passage.

114. Microvilli should be most abundant on the surface of a cell involved in:

(A) secretion.
(B) protection.
(C) motility.
(D) absorption.

115. Introns are found in:

(A) most prokaryotic protein genes.
(B) most eukaryotic protein genes.
(C) a few eukaryotic protein genes.
(D) most prokaryotic and eukaryotic genes.

116. The initial mechanism that acts to prevent infection by most types of bacteria in a normal human is:

(A) skin.
(B) blood clotting.
(C) inflammatory reactions.
(D) specific immune reactions.

Passage IV (Questions 117–126)

Blood is the fluid that circulates around in blood vessels to provide for gas exchange, waste removal, and nutrient procurement by the cells of the body. Blood is composed of various types of cells and cell fragments (referred to as formed elements) and a fluid called plasma. The formed elements include erythrocytes or RBCs (red blood corpuscles), various types of leucocytes or WBCs (white blood cells), and thrombocytes or platelets.

In a clinical setting a number of tests are conducted on blood. One of these is to determine the packed cells volume or *hematocrit* (which is defined as the volume of formed elements relative to the total volume of blood). In order to determine an individual's hematocrit, 10 milliliters of blood are collected and placed in a heparinized centrifuge tube. Heparin is used to prevent clotting. The tube is spun for 15–20 minutes at 2500 rpm to sediment all the formed elements. The tube is then examined to determine the volume (in milliliters) of the packed formed elements. On the average, blood consists of approximately 45% formed elements and approximately 55% plasma; in other words, each 10 ml of blood will contain 4.5 ml of formed elements. The average "normal" packed cell volume or hematocrit is therefore 45% (i.e., 4.5 ml is 45% of 10 ml). Most of the sedimented formed elements are RBCs. A small region of WBCs and platelets will be located at the top of the region of formed elements; this layer is often referred to as the "buffy" coat.

A patient was seen by a physician who ordered a hematocrit as part of the patient's lab workup. Ten millimeters of blood were collected and treated as previously described. The diagram below shows the hematocrit tube at the end of centrifugation.

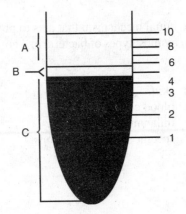

117. Region A consists of:

    (A) fibrin clot material.
    (B) plasma.
    (C) serum.
    (D) WBCs.

118. Region B consists predominantly of:

    (A) fibrin clot material.
    (B) plasma.
    (C) RBCs.
    (D) WBCs.

119. The lower 5.5 ml consists predominantly of:

    (A) fibrin clot material.
    (B) platelets.
    (C) RBCs.
    (D) WBCs.

120. The hematocrit of this patient is:

    (A) 45%.
    (B) 55%.
    (C) 4.5 ml.
    (D) 5.5 ml.

121. The hematocrit of this patient is:

    (A) normal.
    (B) above normal.
    (C) lower than normal.
    (D) cannot be determined from the information given.

122. The components of the blood responsible for binding and carrying oxygen would be located in:

    (A) region A
    (B) region B
    (C) region C.
    (D) regions A and C.

123. The cellular components of the blood responsible for fighting infections would be located in:

   (A) region A.
   (B) region B.
   (C) region C.
   (D) regions B and C.

124. The components of the blood responsible for initiating blood clotting would be located in:

   (A) region A.
   (B) region B.
   (C) region C.
   (D) regions B and C.

125. The major component found in region A would be:

   (A) water.
   (B) hemoglobin.
   (C) sodium chloride.
   (D) glucose.

126. The hematocrit of the patient, as compared to the normal value, suggests that the patient:

   (A) lives at a high altitude.
   (B) has sickle cell anemia.
   (C) has pernicious anemia.
   (D) has recently undergone excessive X ray treatment.

Passage V (Questions 127–131)

All of the possible ketopentose sugar isomers have been synthesized in a research project. The ketopentose isomers have been reduced with sodium borohydride, converting the ketone function to an alcohol.

127. The total number of 2-ketopentose isomers is:

   (A) two.
   (B) four.
   (C) six.
   (D) eight.

128. The total number of isomers of the sugar alcohols produced by sodium borohydride reaction is:

   (A) two.
   (B) three.
   (C) four.
   (D) five.

129. If all the sugar alcohols in the previous question were selectively oxidized so that the number 3 hydroxyl was converted to a ketone, there would be _____ chiral center(s) in each molecule.

   (A) one
   (B) two
   (C) three
   (D) four

130. The pentose(s) found in RNA usually consists of:

   (A) deoxyribose.
   (B) ribose.
   (C) various pentoses.
   (D) glucose.

131. If the sugar alcohols in question 128 were oxidized to convert carbon numbers 1 and 5 to carboxyls, the number of chiral centers would be:

   (A) none.
   (B) one.
   (C) two.
   (D) three.

Questions 132–136 are NOT based on a descriptive passage.

132. The primary source or repository of information concerning synthesis of nucleic acids and proteins is considered to be:

   (A) protein.
   (B) DNA.
   (C) RNA.
   (D) peptides.

133. In the polymer that directs protein biosynthesis, there is a requirement of _____ unit(s) (or monomers) to code for each amino acid.

    (A) one
    (B) two
    (C) three
    (D) four

134. In a chromosome of higher animals there is (are) _____ strand(s) of DNA.

    (A) one
    (B) two
    (C) three
    (D) four

135. If 100 somatic cells of higher animals are allowed to divide once in ^2H_2O (water containing only deuterium), _____ of the cells will have only DNA containing deuterium.

    (A) none
    (B) one fourth
    (C) one half
    (D) all

136. Ultimately, sythesis of protein requires:

    (A) DNA.
    (B) RNA.
    (C) protein.
    (D) all of the above.

Passage VI (Questions 137–139)

The graphs represent experimental results obtained when the pituitary gland was removed (A), the ovaries were removed (B), and lesions were placed in the hypothalamus (C), that part of the brain most closely related to the pituitary gland. The hormones LH and prolactin were measured in blood by radioimmunoassay.

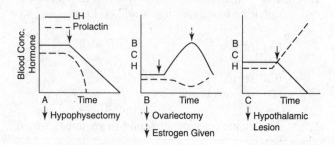

137. It can be concluded from these results that:

    (A) prolactin is produced by the ovaries.
    (B) LH release stimulates prolactin release.
    (C) ovarian hormones inhibit LH release, but not prolactin release.
    (D) presence of the ovaries inhibits removal of LH from the blood.

138. According to the data, LH secretion is inhibited by:

    (A) hypophysectomy.
    (B) estrogen.
    (C) hypothalamic lesion.
    (A) all three.

139. The results suggest that:

    (A) LH stimulates prolactin release.
    (B) LH inhibits prolactin release.
    (C) LH and prolactin are released by the same cells.
    (D) LH and prolactin are secreted independently.

Passage VII (Questions 140–142)

The following graph represents an experiment designed to measure the rate of collagen synthesis in developing chondrocytes. Chondrocytes were isolated from developing sterna of chick embryos and incubated in culture media containing proline–^{3}H, a precursor of collagen. Specimens were fixed after various time intervals and prepared for autoradiography. The graph represents number of silver grains counted (μm/square of organelle).

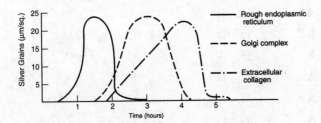

140. The following statements are related to the information presented. Select the statement *supported by* the information given.

    (A) The radioactive label found in the rough endoplasmic reticulum is transferred directly into the extracellular collagen without passing through the Golgi complex.
    (B) Radioactive isotope is incorporated into the extracellular collagen within 2 hours.
    (C) Collagen is a highly stable molecule and is not degraded.
    (D) The amount of rough endoplasmic reticulum in the cell increases during collagen synthesis.

141. The most likely path for the reactive label in the experiment is:

    (A) nucleus → rER → Golgi → extracellular.
    (B) nucleus → rER → extracellular.
    (C) rER → Golgi → extracellular.
    (D) rER → extracellular.

142. The pattern followed by the radioactive label in this experiment is:

    (A) typical of label in secreted proteins.
    (B) typical of label in mRNA.
    (C) probably unique to collagen.
    (D) typical of most proteins made in eukaryotic cells.

Questions 143–146 are NOT based on a descriptive passage.

143. Amino acids found in higher animals are usually:

    (A) optically inactive.
    (B) of the L-series.
    (C) of the D-series.
    (D) a racemic mixture.

144. Carbohydrates found in higher animals (such as glucose, fructose, and galactose) are usually:

    (A) optically inactive.
    (B) of the L-series.
    (C) of the D-series.
    (D) a racemic mixture.

145. D-glucose and L-galactose, both aldohexoses, could be said to be:

    (A) epimers.
    (B) diastereomers.
    (C) enantiomers.
    (D) A and B.

146. Foods with the highest number of kcal/g are the:

    (A) carbohydrates.
    (B) proteins.
    (C) fats.
    (D) nucleic acids.

STOP

END OF TEST

Answer Key

MODEL EXAMINATION C

PHYSICAL SCIENCES

1. C	9. A	17. B	25. C	33. C	41. A	49. D
2. D	10. A	18. D	26. A	34. D	42. A	50. A
3. D	11. D	19. B	27. B	35. D	43. B	51. A
4. A	12. C	20. C	28. B	36. A	44. C	52. A
5. D	13. A	21. C	29. A	37. D	45. B	
6. D	14. B	22. A	30. A	38. A	46. C	
7. B	15. B	23. C	31. A	39. C	47. C	
8. D	16. C	24. B	32. B	40. D	48. A	

VERBAL REASONING

53. C	59. D	65. D	71. B	77. D	83. D	89. C
54. B	60. B	66. C	72. D	78. C	84. C	90. D
55. A	61. D	67. A	73. B	79. D	85. D	91. C
56. D	62. C	68. B	74. C	80. D	86. A	92. B
57. A	63. B	69. C	75. B	81. D	87. D	
58. B	64. C	70. C	76. C	82. D	88. D	

WRITING SAMPLE

93. See page 505 for a sample essay.

94. See page 505 for a sample essay.

BIOLOGICAL SCIENCES

95. C	103. B	111. B	119. C	127. B	135. A	143. B
96. B	104. C	112. C	120. B	128. B	136. D	144. C
97. C	105. D	113. C	121. B	129. B	137. C	145. B
98. B	106. A	114. D	122. C	130. B	138. D	146. C
99. A	107. C	115. B	123. B	131. C	139. D	
100. B	108. C	116. A	124. B	132. B	140. B	
101. B	109. A	117. B	125. A	133. C	141. C	
102. D	110. C	118. D	126. A	134. B	142. A	

ANSWERS EXPLAINED FOR MODEL EXAMINATION C

Physical Sciences

1. **(C)** The tangential (linear) velocity of an object moving around a circular path (velocity tangent to the circle) is proportional to the angular velocity. $v = rw$, where r is the radius (9 m in this case) and w is the angular velocity (which must be in radians/sec for use in this formula).

2. **(D)** A "g" force is equal to the actual weight, mg, of a person or object, so:

   8 "g's" = 8(82 kg)(9.8 m/sec^2) = 6429 N.

3. **(D)** The centrifugal force is the "equal and opposite force" of Newton's third law and thus does NOT act *on* the *pilot*. It is the force that the pilot exerts *on the back of his seat*.

4. **(A)** Power in watts is the rate of energy use, thus the energy, $E = P \times t$ or $E = 450$ watts $\times$ 120 sec = 54,000 joules and liters of O_2 consumed = 54,000 J/(20,000 J/L) = 2.7 L.

5. **(D)** According to Newton's third law, the pilot exerts a force of 8 "g's" on his seat back. Notice that this *is* the centrifugal force and it *is* a real outward force on the seat back. (The pilot, in his rotating "frame of reference," feels as if a large outward force is pushing him into the seat back. This force is a "fictitous" force because the only real force acting on him is the inward centripetal force.)

6. **(D)** The necessary inward-pointing centripetal force is unchanged. Nothing has changed except the device that supplies the centripetal force.

7. **(B)** Electronegativity decreases going down a group.

8. **(D)** Iodine is nonpolar. The large iodine atoms are polarizable—meaning the molecule forms a temporary dipole. This is the main intermolecular force involved.

9. **(A)** The chemist combined 1.26 g I_2 (1.26 g I_2/253 g I_2 = 0.005 mole I_2) with 0.010 g H_2 (0.010 g H_2/2.01 g H_2 = 0.005 mole H_2) and produced 0.01 mole of HI. In 1.00 L of water, this produced a 0.01 M HI solution. The pH = $-\log[H^+]$ = $-\log[0.01]$ = 2.0

10. **(A)** The oxidation state of hydrogen goes from 0 to +1; it is oxidized. The oxidation state of iodine goes from 0 to –1; it is reduced.

11. **(D)** HI is a strong acid and dissociates completely in solution. Thus, it is a strong electrolyte and conducts electricity.

12. **(C)** Sublimation is the phase change going from a solid to a gas.

13. **(A)** The iodine atoms share electron density equally. The bonding is thus nonpolar covalent.

14. **(B)** It is given in the passage that the telescope length is approximately equal to the sum of the focal lengths. If the total length is 4 m, then the value of f_e is 4 m $- f_o$ = 1 m.

15. **(B)** The objective lens forms a real, inverted image. The eyepiece acts in the same way that a magnifying glass does. The observer looks through the eyepiece and sees a final, virtual image that has the same orientation as the first image (that is, the final image is still inverted). This can be corrected by inserting a third lens, known as an erecting lens, between the objective and eyepiece.

16. **(C)** The magnification of a simple Newtonian telescope is the ratio of the objective focal length to the eyepiece focal length:

    $M = f_o/f_e = 3/1 = 3 \times$.

17. **(B)** This question requires an understanding of total internal reflection. The critical angle is the incident angle for which Snell's law of refraction predicts a refracted angle of 90°, for light rays traveling from a medium of larger index of refraction toward a medium of lower index of refraction. Here the light ray is incident inside the glass prism toward air of index, $n_{air} = 1$. Using Snell's law:

    $n_{glass} \sin \varnothing_c = n_{air} \sin 90°$, and because n_{glass} = 1.52; $\sin \varnothing_c$ = 1/1.52 and $\varnothing_c$ = 41°.

18. **(D)** The objective lens is a projection lens, producing an inverted real image. The first image lies within the focal length of the eyepiece, which therefore acts as a magnifying glass, forming a virtual, enlarged image. The eyepiece does not invert the image.

19. **(B)** As the object (primate) moves closer to the objective, the real image formed by the objective

is further away from the objective, i.e., closer to the original position of the eyepiece. To see the image clearly, the eyepiece must be moved "back" away from the objective in order to focus the second (virtual) image clearly. (It is the eyepiece that is adjustable in telescopes and binoculars.) This is similar to holding this printed page too close to your eyes to see clearly. If you hold the page still and move your head away you will be able to see the print clearly.

20. **(C)** The work done on charged particles by electric fields depends on the charge of the particle and the voltage difference (not on the mass of the particle). The electric work, $W = qV$, increases the kinetic energy of the particles, in this case from zero to the final KE. Because the charges for electron and proton are equal, they have equal final kinetic energies (although the electron has a greater speed).

21. **(C)** We need to know the force ($F = qvB \sin\theta$) on a moving charge in a magnetic field and we need the "right-hand rule" for the vector direction of the force on a positively charged particle (knowing the vector velocity and vector magnetic field, B). For a positive charge moving horizontally north through a magnetic field pointing horizontally west, the magnetic force is vertically *upward*. The negative electron is equivalent to a positive charge moving in the *opposite* direction so the force on *both* electron and proton is upward.

22. **(A)** The magnetic force acts only at right angles to the velocity of a charged particle. It can change the direction of the velocity vector but not its magnitude (speed *is* the magnitude of velocity).

23. **(C)** The charged particles are now moving parallel to the magnetic field direction so that $\sin \theta$ is zero in the magnetic force equation ($F = qvB \sin \theta$). The magnetic force on each is zero, and their paths are not deflected.

24. **(B)** The electric force, $F = qE$, shows that the direction of the force is parallel to E for positive charges like protons, and opposite (antiparallel) for negative charges like electrons.

25. **(C)** The total charge (atomic number) must be conserved so that the total number of subscript numbers must be the same on both sides of the nuclear equation, $(0 + 80 = 79 + 1)$. Thus $Z = 79$.

The total of superscript numbers must also be the same since the total number of nucleons A (mass numbers) are also constant $(1 + 198 = 197 + 2)$. Thus $A = 197$.

26. **(A)** The angular acceleration is the change in angular velocity divided by the time taken, or $\alpha = (\varpi_f - \varpi_i)/t$. Converting ϖ to rad/sec:

$$\varpi_f = 57{,}300 \text{ rev/min} \times 2\pi \text{ rad/rev} \times 1 \text{ min/60sec} = 6000 \text{ rad/sec}$$

$$\alpha = (6000 \text{ rad/sec} - 0)/120 \text{ sec} = 50 \text{ rad/sec}^2$$

27. **(B)** The diverging lens can be used. This type of telescope is known as a Galilean telescope. It has the advantage of forming an upright, final image and the disadvantage of having rather low power.

28. **(B)** A lens with a negative focal length is a diverging lens. The power in Diopters is the reciprocal of the focal length in meters; thus

$$P = -1/0.5 = -2.0 \text{ D}.$$

29. **(A)** Each α-decay reduces the nuclear charge (the atomic number) by 2 units and reduces the mass number by 4 units. Each negative β-decay increases the charge by 1 unit without changing the mass number. Thus 8 α-decays decrease the charge by 16 and decrease the mass number by 32. The 6 β-decays increase the charge by 6 units, so the net change in charge is -10. The element with atomic number $92 - 10 = 82$ and mass number $238 - 32 = 206$ is lead, $^{206}_{82}$Pb.

30. **(A)** The index of refraction is $n = c/v$, where c is the speed of light in a vacuum (3×10^8 m/sec) and v is the speed of light in the material. Here, $v_s = 0.83 \, v_w$. Or $v_s = 0.83 \, c/n_w = c/n_s$. Cancel c and solve for $n_s = 1.6$.

31. **(A)** Loss of a single electron in the $3s$ orbital leaves the stable electronic configuration of the noble gas, neon.

32. **(B)** In a neutral atom, the number of electrons in orbitals equals the number of protons in the nucleus. The latter defines the atomic number.

33. **(C)** Gain of an additional electron would give the stable electronic configuration of the noble element, krypton.

34. **(D)** Note that the number of electrons exceeds the atomic number (and the number of protons) by one. Thus, this would be an ion with a charge of –1.

35. **(D)** Noble elements include helium, neon, argon, krypton, xenon, and radon.

36. **(A)** No two electrons in an atom possess all four identical quantum numbers.

37. **(D)** 32.0 g methane is the same as 2.0 moles of methane (32.0 g/16.0 g = 2.0 moles). At STP, 1 mole of gas occupies 22.4 L; 2 moles of gas occupy twice that amount, or 44.8 L.

38. **(A)** Hydrogen sulfide gives up a proton, making it an acid. It is not one of the six strong acids, and so it is a weak acid.

39. **(C)** Using the Henderson-Hasselbach equation:

$$pH = pK_a + \log \frac{[\text{conjugated base}]}{[\text{conjugated acid}]}$$

the logarithm term equals 0 since the $\log(1) = 0$. Thus, the $pH = pK_a = 6.89$.

40. **(D)** Methane is nonpolar. The intermolecular forces involved in nonpolar compounds are London dispersion forces.

41. **(A)** A pH of 2.0 means a 0.01 M concentration of H^+ ($pH = -\log[H^+]$; $[H^+] = 10^{-pH} = 10^{-2} = 0.01$ M). This corresponds to 0.001 mole/100 mL. For every 1 mole of acid produced, 1 mole of SO_2 is required; thus, 0.001 mole of SO_2 were involved in the reaction.

42. **(A)** Newton's second law states that the net force equals the product of mass and acceleration: $F_{net} = ma$. In this case the net force is the difference between the applied force (18 N) and the force of friction (9 N): $F_{net} = F_a - F_f = 18 - 9 = (90)a$.

43. **(B)** The total momentum of the two-cart system is zero before the students push off, and remains zero after they separate. Then: $0 = m_1v_1 + m_2v_2$. Thus, $v_2 = 60$ kg(1.2 m/sec)/(0.8 m/sec).

44. **(C)** We know that the total angular momentum of the student is conserved (constant). Because he is capable of changing his moment of inertia about the vertical axis of spin by extending his arms or pulling them in, we can find the ratio of the moments of inertia by using the conservation law in the form: $I_1 \Omega_1 = I_2 \Omega_2$. Then $I_2/I_1 = \Omega_1/\Omega_2 = 1.5$.

45. **(B)** The center-of-mass will not move because the forces exerted by pulling on the rope are internal forces to the two-cart system. It is nearer the larger mass, and is found by using the formula for the cm: $X_{cm} = (m_1x_1 + m_2x_2)/(m_1 + m_2)$. We are allowed to place the origin of the coordinate system anywhere we choose. Placing the origin at the original position of the larger mass, $x_1 = 0$ and $x_2 = 2$ m. $X_{cm} = (0 + (80)(2))/(200$ kg$) = 0.8$ m.

46. **(C)** Conservation of momentum applies to this completely inelastic collision as follows: $m_1v_1 = (m_1 + m_2)V$. Then $V = (80$ kg$)(4$ m/sec$)(80 + 80) = 2$ m/sec.

47. **(C)** The work done in accelerating the cart is equal to the gain in kinetic energy: $F_{net}x = 1/2\ mv^2$, or (100 N)(10 m) = (1/2) 80v^2 and then $v = 5$ m/sec.

48. **(A)** Freezing point depression in water depends only on the number of solute particles per unit volume

1 M NaCl = $2 \times 1 \times 6.02 \times 10^{23}$ particles per liter
0.3 M Na_2SO_4 = $3 \times .3 \times 6.02 \times 10^{23}$ particles per liter
1.5 M glucose = $1 \times 1.5 \times 6.02 \times 10^{23}$ particles per liter
0.5 M $BaSO_4$ = $2 \times 0.5 \times 6.02 \times 10^{23}$ particles per liter
Dividing by 6.02×10^{23} we can see that the comparative figures are NaCl, 2; Na_2SO_4, 0.9; glucose, 1.5; and $BaSO_4$, 1.0. Thus, the NaCl solution has the greatest number of particles per unit volume (considering the ionization of NaCl, Na_2SO_4, and $BaSO_4$), and it will have the lowest freezing point.

49. **(D)** A reaction in which electrons (e^-) are removed is termed an oxidation reaction; the adding of electrons to an atom or molecule is termed a reduction reaction.

50. **(A)** The hydronium ion, H_3O^+, is a protonated water molecule. $2H_2O \rightleftarrows H_3O^+ + OH^-$

51. **(A)** As long as the volume units are the same, $N_1V_1 = N_2V_2$

$$V_2 = \frac{N_1V_1}{N_2} = \frac{(50)(0.25)}{0.50} = 25 \text{ ml}$$

52. **(A)** This is a definition of the zwitterion; an example is the amino acid, glycine.

Verbal Reasoning

53. **(C)** The entire passage presents the thesis that Fitzgerald created the American flapper through his short stories and novels. It is true that the flapper is a part of the social history of America in the post-World War I decade and thus a vehicle of social customs in America during the time; but this is not a major point of the passage. The author mainly attempts to establish the claim that Fitzgerald, not John Held, Jr. and not various flappers in film, invented or created this character type. Though there are allusions to Fitzgerald's novels, the passage mentions them only in passing, and thus **B** would be incorrect.

54. **(B)** Paragraph two of the passage chronicles the origin and evolution of the term "flapper," clearly locating one of its early associations with women in Britain who had not yet been introduced into society, the answer supplied by **B**. It is actually also true, according to the *Oxford English Dictionary,* that the word may have originally come from the term that designated a young bird (**A**), a "flapper," but this information is not supplied by the passage and, therefore, would not be a correct answer for this question. Some have also suggested that the flapping arm movements of dancing flappers prompted the name. Again, however, the passage does not include this bit of information, and **C**, therefore, would be an incorrect response.

55. **(A)** John O'Hara notes that the term "flapper" had been misused and that it had designated a girl who had not yet found a husband. His comment suggesting this variation is found in paragraph two.

56. **(D)** The social historian Frederick Lewis Allen cited numerous conditions, summarized in paragraph two, that contributed to the development of the flapper. All of those cited, as well as others, are included in paragraph two.

57. **(A)** As outlined in the explanation to question one (above), the central thesis of the passage is that Fitzgerald was the creator, through his fiction, of the type known as the American Flapper.

58. **(B)** The passage does not deal with comparative studies of the worth of Fitzgerald's novels as opposed to his short stories, nor does it address the relative merits of John Held, Jr.'s cartoons versus his writing. Therefore, I and III are neither supported nor contradicted by the passage, which does, however, deal in detail with Fitzgerald's role in developing the flapper and with his ultimate decision to discontinue the stereotype because it limited him in the creation of complex characters. This information is presented in paragraph one.

59. **(D)** Paragraphs one and two could be entitled acute pharmacological experience, whereas paragraph three deals with drug effects as a prelude to dependency. Paragraph four discussed learning aspects, and paragraphs five and six deal with neurochemical aspects.

60. **(B)** Paragraph one makes it perfectly clear that the dependence process starts with the initial exposure. It is also emphasized that after taking a drug an individual may feel pleasure (or less pain), but that the word "pleasurable" has many meanings and may not be related to "feeling good."

61. **(D)** Paragraph one emphasizes that people take psychoactive drugs for many reasons that essentially meet their own individual needs, whether it be feeling good, peer pressure, or whatever.

62. **(C)** Paragraphs two and five make the statement that most drugs produce their effects via an alteration of brain neurochemistry, which can lead to other more long-term problems. Alteration of the mind is not specific, and drugs do not act in a very predictable way.

63. **(B)** Paragraph three discusses the phenomenon of conditioned stimulus and points out that the use of a drug can come under environmental control. Although the role of ritual is mentioned, it certainly is not the order of the day. Placebo does not routinely replace the chemical substance. No mention is made anywhere in the passage as to side effects.

64. **(C)** Paragraph four deals with learned behaviors. There is no implication that learning or performing of tasks is enhanced by the consumption of psychoactive drugs. The point is made that there is the development of behavioral tolerance and that people learn to adapt to the drug state to a degree. The example is given of an individual having difficulty finding the liquor store when sober. No credence is given in the passage to the statement that behavioral tolerance lessens the effects of drug affliction.

65. **(D)** Paragraph one indicates that at Alexandria teaching was limited to only what was necessary to train researchers for the next generation. The focus was on improving understanding so that each generation could inherit a more advanced civilization.

66. **(C)** Paragraph two makes it clear that Plato marveled at the underlying principles of mathematics and tried to find underlying principles or "truths" in other fields of study.

67. **(A)** Paragraph three deals with the second librarian Eratosthenes, who measured the size of the earth; he measured the angle of the sun (six degrees) at midday on mid-summer's day at Alexandria because he knew from previous trips to Cyrene (near today's Aswan Dam) that the sun shone to the bottom of its wells (zero degrees) on that very day and time each year. He only had to measure the distance between these two places to calculate the circumference of the earth.

68. **(B)** Paragraph four indicates that Aristophanes, the third librarian, commissioned 70 scholars to translate the Bible into Greek and that this translation, which became known as the *Septuagint,* was used by Jesus Christ. The point is also made that evidence suggests that the "flight into Egypt" took place in Alexandria.

69. **(C)** Paragraph seven tells us that Ptolemy wrote 13 books on astronomy, and that in his books on astrology he summarized the beliefs of the Greeks, Egyptians, and Persians and gave us the horoscope and Zodiac signs used today.

70. **(C)** Paragraph one tells of his boyhood in Peoria, and of his early job as usher in a vaudeville house through which he first became interested in show business. His father was a bricklayer, and there is no evidence in the passage that either his mother or father ever worked in show business.

71. **(B)** In paragraph seven we are told that Correll's relaxed, gregarious half of the partnership balanced Gosden's more temperamental and creative temperament.

72. **(D)** The first sentence in paragraph nine informs the reader that listenership began to drop following the beginning of World War II.

73. **(B)** Though the passage provides few details regarding the possible evolution of the *Sam 'n Henry Show* into the *Amos 'n Andy Show,* the author of the passage states explicitly in paragraph four that the *Tribune* retained the rights to *Sam 'n Henry* and ran it with two other men.

74. **(C)** Both Correll and Gosden were surprised by the controversy surrounding the show, and the passage indicates in the last sentence of paragraph 11 that Gosden, especially, was wounded by it.

75. **(B)** We learn in the final paragraph that Correll and Gosden maintained a close friendship into their later years, living close to each other in Beverly Hills until Correll returned to Illinois and, at the age of 82, died.

76. **(C)** A thorough reading of the passage will leave the reader with only one major theme. The writer has clearly focused on the recovery process and its many facets.

77. **(D)** Paragraph one indicates that a long-term proposition is encountered in the recovery from addiction. It is a lifetime pursuit and, as AA points out, relapse frequently occurs when people stop attending meetings. Drug use and recovery depend on many factors, and the environment plays a major role in both. As is common with many compounds taken for a long period (psychoactive drugs or steroids administered under supervision), stoppage usually results in withdrawal symptoms.

78. **(C)** Under no circumstances is the point made that drug use enhances learning or the performing of tasks. Psychoactive drugs are definitely detrimental to all aspects of an individual's functioning. The point is made that there is a drug-induced state dependent learning and the example is that a person sober might have a problem finding the car, but when under the influence the person "may" remember where it is.

79. **(D)** Every statement is substantiated by the passage. Drugs or electrical stimulation produce their effects via an alteration of the brain's neurochemistry. The environment, it is pointed out in paragraph two, plays a key role in the addiction and recovery process. Paragraph four emphasizes that the individual determines to a great extent his/her own fate.

80. **(D)** Neither addiction nor recovery is a simple or well-understood process. Recovery, as paragraph four indicates, involves commitment on the part of the user to stop using the drug and to reinforce his actions by changing and utilizing environmental and social phenomena to help him in the lifelong process.

81. **(D)** The passage in paragraph one emphasizes that the Golden Rule is not a sufficient ethical principle because it fosters the idea that what is good for the physician is good for the patient. Paragraph one also emphasizes that physicians must do the "right thing" and indicates that most feel that this means curing illness and postponing death. Gregory does point out that physicians are not perfect and should acknowledge and rectify their mistakes.

82. **(D)** Although the passage touches upon medical decision making, reasoning and autonomy of the patient, the application and interpretation of the Golden Rule, the central theme is philosophical and the best and most encompassing title would be "Moral Reasoning and Medical Decision Making."

83. **(D)** None of the statements posed are supported by the passage. The passage points out that Hippocrates preached the Golden Rule and that certainly is part of the principle of human rights. A very strong argument is made in paragraphs four and five in favor of the physician explaining in an appropriate, understanding, sensitive, compassionate, and thorough manner the disease process to the patient and reaching a mutual consensus in order to deliniate an appropriate course of action suitable for the individual, the family, and accepted medical practice. Paragraph two makes it quite clear that the courts generally have held that the constitutional rights permit an individual to decide what happens to himself, and these rights have been called the "Patient's Bill of Rights."

84. **(C)** Throughout the passage it is stressed that a give and take attitude must exist in the decision making process, and paragraph three points out that Rousseau advocated a social contract because human beings are different. Paragraph four leaves no doubt that beneficence and autonomy must be weighed and applied to reach a decision.

85. **(D)** Although every statement is correct and was espoused by Hippocrates, the passage does not deal with them, and so it neither contradicts nor supports the information presented in the question.

86. **(A)** Paragraph six emphasizes that burden/benefit aspects of treatment must be weighed. Sometimes life itself, or the treatment proposed to sustain life, is so problematical that patients opt for the right to die. It was previously pointed out that education of the patient is essential for proper medical practice. Paragraph six makes the point that the courts understand the concept of the right to die better than most physicians. The paragraph gives the example of artificial feeding, which may become so problematical in the respect that any benefit from the intervention is minimal.

87. **(D)** There should be no doubt in the reader's mind that the passage argues strongly for education, a balance in the decision-making process, consultation between physician and patient, and among physicians, and above all that patients' rights should never be negated.

88. **(D)** The last paragraph makes it perfectly clear that the history of a comic book (*True Comics*) is detailed.

89. **(C)** The last paragraph points out that the idea of a comic book with true stories was unique, but *True Comics* stood alone in the respect that it carried editorials.

90. **(D)** A thorough reading leads the reader to conclude that besides selling magazines, the publisher preached recycling, patriotism, and fitness.

91. **(C)** Paragraph three ends with the statement that the publisher was an avid internationalist, a globalist.

92. **(B)** Paragraph one clearly indicates that it was an editorial in the comic book that was the first acknowledgment of America's entry into World War II. The editor was interested in reaching the young and making them aware of how they could contribute to the national effort.

Writing Sample

93. Essay

One must point out that Demonax begins his assertion with "probably." The statement then takes on a more questioning or probing tone, as if he is asking for a contradiction. This tone colors an attitude that is already filled with a sort of shrugging resignation or apathy. Demonax clearly believes that laws do not serve their intended purpose. It seems that, to him, that purpose would be to change the nature of people who are not "good." He says, in effect, that good individuals do not need laws in order to be good and that bad ones will remain bad with or without laws.

This is probably true. However, it is not clear that Demonax explored the possibility that laws might serve another purpose. Among some probable other things, laws serve as guidelines by which individuals can operate in social groups. Even a very good person might want to know on which side of the street she should drive. Laws might also be a deterrent to bad behaviors as well. A bad person who might steal the purse of an elderly blind woman might be deterred by the knowledge that the law calls for a prison sentence for so doing. The individual is made no better by the law, but the life of the blind woman might be.

Laws are useful as a set of guidelines, rules, or agreements, accepted by a group of people who wish to live interdependently. They save time for people who otherwise would have to continuously be deciding upon the methods to use in everyday social interactions. More controversial, but also inevitable, is the fact that they also uphold a moral code that is agreed upon, ideally by the majority. Without any laws, we would, in fact, be less free to move about in more important endeavors because we would be constantly battling each other for time and space. Imagine an interstate highway with no traffic regulations, for example. Or imagine trying to maintain possession of one's home if there were no laws to say that it was your home between the time you left for work and the time you returned from work. As an effort to change the nature of a human being, laws are, indeed, probably useless. But, as an effort to change the nature of our social lives, they are clearly invaluable and mean the difference between living in civilization and living in chaos.

93. Explanation of Response: 5

The paper focuses on the statement and addresses each of the three writing tasks. In the first paragraph the writer begins the explanation of the statement by noting that it is qualified with the word "probably," an explanation that is completed with a paraphrase of the quotation. The second paragraph presents specific situations in which laws do, in fact, serve good purposes. The final paragraph balances the extremes, exploring those things about laws that make them useful for people living together in social situations, which is a pragmatic position, but arguing that laws probably do not change human beings.

This is a tightly reasoned essay that makes good use of concrete examples. The writing is clear, and the sentences are nicely paced. Paragraph two is potentially a strong one, with its example of the elderly woman's purse; but it would benefit from a bringing together of ideas at the end, a sentence to clinch the paragraph. With fuller development of this paragraph and a brief expansion of the idea in paragraph one that, to Demonax, laws do not serve their intended purpose, the essay would receive a 6 rather than a 5.

94. Essay

With the thought of the concept of freedom comes naturally the question, from what? Freedom does not exist without the possibility, really the latent presence of restraint. What Gibran says is that an increase in one freedom would necessarily imply a restraint on another. This is because an increase in a person's freedom always means also an increase in his domain of responsibility. For example, as an infant, a person could be seen as either totally free or totally without freedom. An infant is totally free from responsibility and obligation, yet totally dependent on and restrained by his caretakers. What Gibran understands is that, the greater one's realm of existence and the broader one's scope of knowledge, the greater also is one's realm and scope of responsibility. As you commit an act, the act becomes a part of you, a fetter perhaps, and certainly a history or past to which you are then forever confined and from which you never will be free.

From this point of view, there are certainly no possible examples of a freedom that implies no restraints, for existence itself implies a certain restraint. Even a freedom to die would imply a restraint from the opportunity to live. The point is that one thing or act at a point in the realm of time and space forbids the existence of another at that point. With every act and thought then, we redefine our own existence; with definition comes restraint, and with restraint comes the inhibition of some freedom.

What Gibran is apparently trying to do is to point beyond an immediate goal of freedom to the new existence beyond it. For example, once a person is free of the yoke of his parents and family, that freedom puts a new and greater yoke, that of responsibility on his shoulders throughout the remainder of his life. Gibran is not arguing against freedom, however, but is suggesting a more mature, wiser view of freedom than that of freedom as an end in itself. As one's vision expands, one will have greater and greater freedoms. But with that vision will also come knowledge and with knowledge will come responsibility. And so, as we seek to broaden our scope of existence, we also seek to make our burden a bit heavier. And this becomes a good thing.

94. **Explanation of Response: 4**

The paper addresses all three objectives, and it does an especially nice job with one and three. Paragraph one focuses sharply on the explanation of the quotation. This is perhaps the most difficult of the tasks for this quotation because of its seeming paradox. The paragraph also provides the example of the infant, who could be considered either totally free or totally without freedom. Paragraph two does not confront the second task as directly as does paragraph one. Though there is a clear attempt here to explore the possibility of a freedom that would not imply a burden or an obstacle to a greater freedom, the paragraph stops short of providing a specific situation that illustrates the point. If there were a more direct confrontation of the second task, this essay would receive a higher rating. Paragraph three reconciles the extremes and examines the implications of the statement.

The writing in this paper is clear and well controlled. Each of the paragraphs is organized around a topic that gives unity to the paper. Its sentences are varied and flow nicely from one to the next. The weakest aspect of the paper is that it lacks concrete details to illustrate its points from the beginning of paragraph two to the end. With the addition of such details and with a direct confrontation of the task in paragraph two, its rating would move to 5 or 6.

Biological Sciences

95. **(C)** Thyroid stimulating hormone (TSH) produced by the pituitary gland stimulates the thyroid gland to produce its hormones T_3 (triiodothyronine) and T_4 (tetraiodothyronine or thyroxine). TSH modulates the iodide trapping mechanisms; hypersecretion results in goiter and exophthalmos, whereas hyposecretion leads to diminished thyroid function and lethargy.

96. **(B)** See explanation for question 95.

97. **(C)** When thyroxin is administered, one would expect that the iodide uptake would decrease; in graph I it stayed level, whereas in graph III an increase of uptake is exhibited. Both experimental conditions indicate some evidence of thyroid malfunction.

98. **(B)** A hyperthyroid individual would not be expected to show additional uptake because the gland already is working at an elevated level. When thyroid hormone was administered as in our experiments, normally the uptake should have decreased; it stayed the same however.

99. **(A)** When thyroxin is administered, TSH production diminishes and RAI uptake should drop. This did not occur in graph I while graph II demonstrates the expected normal. Graph III shows an increase in uptake indicating that the pituitary is not responding to the negative inhibitory feedback that thyroxin elicits; TSH production should decrease at the time of thyroxine administration.

100. **(B)** Acromegaly is a result of pituitary oversecretion of growth hormone. Lack of iodine will result in goiter development of the thyroid gland. Rickets is due to vitamin D deficiency. A skin rash is not a specific lesion that can be associated with only one specific cause as the others listed.

101. **(B)** Acidophils produce somatotropic hormone (STH) and luteotropic hormone (LTH) or prolactin. Beta cells produce thyroid stimulating hormone (TSH), adrenocorticotropic hormone (ACTH), and melanocyte stimulating hormone (MSH). Delta cells produce luteinizing hormone (LH) (called interstitial cell stimulating hormone in the male), and follicle stimulating hormone (FSH). Chromophobes are considered resting cells.

102. **(D)** All statements are correct. The thyroid originates from the foramen cecum region of the tongue. Its structural unit is the follicle, a unit of epithelial cells that surround a colloid space. Colloid is located extracellularly and contains thyroglobulin. T_3 and T_4 are the active thyroid principles and are released into the bloodstream and carried on proteins to the tissues.

103. **(B)** Acromegaly and (or) giantism is due to overactivity of the alpha cells of the pituitary, which secrete growth hormone. If a person is affected before puberty, he or she will develop into a fairly well-proportioned giant. After maturity, an increase in the size of the hands and feet and massive development of the bones comprising the face are consequences. In the adult, strictly speaking, the term acromegaly must be applied to this condition.

104. **(C)**

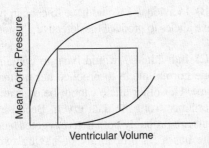

If aortic pressure is unchanged and end diastolic volume increases, the stroke volume or the difference between end diastolic volume and end systolic volume is larger. Ventricular work is equal to:

Work = Pressure · Stroke Volume = Force/Area · Volume = Force · Length

or the area under the curve. The kinetic energy of the ejected blood can be ignored because it represents $\approx 5\%$ of the total energy and stays constant under most conditions. The area subtended by the pressure-volume loop increases as does the work in this case. Because the contractility of the heart represented by the upper curve remains constant, the end systolic volume also remains constant.

105. **(D)**

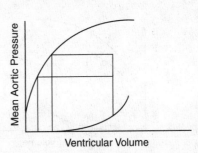

Whereas the pressure to eject blood must increase, the volume of blood the ventricle ejects is less. Therefore, the ventricular work depends on the exact nature of the two curves. Because the ventricle cannot maintain the required pressure at low volumes, the total volume of blood ejected is less and the end systolic volume is increased.

106. **(A)**

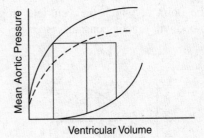

In this case, the ventricle is incapable of generating the same pressure at low volumes. Therefore, the volume of blood ejected is less (i.e., the stroke volume is smaller), and the end systolic volume is correspondingly larger. Note that this question is a play on words. If the stroke volume decreases with a constant end diastolic volume, the volume left in the ventricle after contraction will be more. The ventricular work is reduced because the pressure remains constant while the volume of blood ejected falls so that the product of the two decreases.

107.   **(C)**

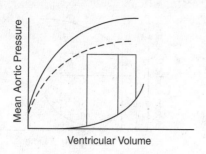

The key to this question is to remember which two cases are being compared. The increase in end diastolic volume allows the failing ventricle to increase the stroke volume as compared to the uncompensated case. With a constant pressure, an increase in stroke volume causes an increase in the work (i.e., pressure • stroke volume). Because the aortic pressure is constant and the active pressure curve is unchanged in the two cases, the volume remaining in the ventricle at the point at which the ventricle stops ejecting blood will remain constant.

108.   **(C)**

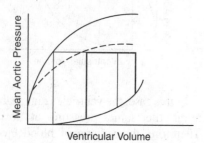

The key to this question, as in question 107, is that one must remember what conditions are being compared. Increasing the end diastolic volume sufficiently could theoretically allow a failing ventricle to eject a larger stroke volume than is the case in normals. However, the compensation for a failing ventricle usually is not sufficient for this to occur under physiological conditions. Because the stroke volume is indeterminate relative to the normal condition, the ventricular work is also indeterminate given a constant mean aortic pressure. Because by definition a failing ventricle cannot maintain the same pressure at low volumes, the end systolic volume must increase in comparison to that of normal.

109.   **(A)** The defect cannot be dominant because individual 5 was produced by two normal parents who would have no defective alleles if the defect is dominant (either autosomal or X-linked). The defect is unlikely to be X-linked recessive because unless a new mutation occurred, individual 5 should have received a normal allele for the gene on her X from her father (individual 2) and therefore could not express a recessive X-linked defect. Therefore the most likely possibility (using the assumptions of a single controlling gene and very rare mutations) would be an autosomal gene for which the defective allele is recessive to the normal allele.

110.   **(C)** Unless a new mutation occurred, individual 1 would have to have one normal allele (which produced the normal phenotype) and one defective allele (which was contributed to individual 5 along with a defective allele from individual 2) to produce individual 5's defective phenotype.

111.   **(B)** Individual 4 would have to contain two defective alleles to produce the defective phenotype.

112.   **(C)** Individual 7 would have to contain at least one normal allele to produce her normal phenotype. Her other allele cannot be determined with certainty from the data given. Because her parents are probably both heterozygotes (see above), she has a $1/3$ probability of having two normal alleles and a $2/3$ probability of having one normal and one abnormal allele.

i.e., $Nn \times Nn$

$1/4\ NN$: $2/4\ Nn$: $1/4\ nn$

defective phenotype

$2/3$ of normal phenotype

$1/3$ of normal phenotype

Therefore she is most likely to contain one normal and one defective allele.

113.   **(C)** Individual 8 would have to contain one normal allele (to produce his normal phenotype) and one abnormal allele (because he contributed one of the two defective alleles in each of offspring 14 and 18).

114.   **(D)** Microvilli are typically most numerous on cell surfaces involved in absorption, frequently by active transport.

115. **(B)** Introns occur in most eukaryotic protein genes but are absent in most prokaryotic genes.

116. **(A)** Skin is the initial defense against most bacteria. All of the other mechanisms are also protective but come into play when skin has been bypassed.

117. **(B)** The upper region consists of the fluid portion of the blood, the plasma.

118. **(D)** The thin "buffy" layer is the white blood cells and platelets.

119. **(C)** After centrifugation, the packed volume of formed elements was 5.5 ml. As stated previously, most of the formed elements are RBCs.

120. **(B)** After centrifugation, the volume of packed formed elements of the patient was 5.5 ml. Because hematocrit is defined as the relative volume of formed elements, the hematocrit of this patient is 55% (i.e., 5.5 ml out of 10 ml, or 55% of the total blood volume, was occupied by formed elements).

121. **(B)** The hematocrit of this patient, 55%, is higher than the normal average value of 45%.

122. **C.** Region C consists of RBCs. These cells contain hemoglobin, which binds and carries oxygen.

123. **(C)** Region B, the "buffy" coat, consists of WBCs and platelets. The WBCs consist of a number of cell types, some of which are responsible for fighting infections.

124. **(B)** Region B, the "buffy" coat, consists of WBC and platelets. The platelets are responsible for triggering the cascade of events that results in the formation of blood clots.

125. **(A)** The major component of blood plasma is water.

126. **(A)** Because the patient's hematocrit is higher than the normal value, the patient has more formed elements, largely RBCs, than a normal individual. Because RBCs are responsible for binding and carrying oxygen, a higher hematocrit might suggest that the individual has a higher physiological demand for oxygen. Such a condition is seen in individuals living at high altitudes where the oxygen concentration of the air is lower (compared to the oxygen concentration of air at sea level).

127. **(B)** The number of possible isomers is four. Note that positions 3 and 4 are chiral and thus may have the hydroxyl group on either side. Thus $2 \times 2 = 4$.

128. **(B)** Although there appear at first glance to be three chiral centers, this is not so; the number 3 carbon is *not* attached to four nonidentical groups. Thus only four isomers appear to be possible, but it can be seen that two of these are identical and thus there are two optically active isomers and one optically inactive isomer.

129. **(B)** There are two chiral centers.

130. **(B)** Ribose is found in RNA, contributing to the name, ribonucleic acid. Deoxyribose is found in DNA.

131. **(C)** As seen in the explanation for question 128, there are only two chiral centers (carbons 2 and 4).

132. **(B)** DNA is the primary source of information. It is usually considered that DNA directs the synthesis of RNA and that RNA directs the synthesis of protein. DNA also directs its own replication. In some cases (for example the retroviruses), RNA can direct the synthesis of DNA.

133. **(C)** RNA directs the synthesis of protein (see above) and three nucleotide bases are required to code for each amino acid.

134. **(B)** Paired strands of DNA are found in the chromosomes of higher animals.

135. **(A)** None of the cells will have only DNA containing deuterium. Each cell will have two strands of DNA for each chromosome, and one strand of each pair will contain deuterium.

136. **(D)** As stated above, DNA is required to code for RNA and RNA is required to code for protein. The enzymes that actually carry out the biosynthesis are protein. (It might be argued that DNA is not required, but *ultimately* DNA is required for RNA synthesis.)

137. **(C)** From the experimental data, one can conclude that prolactin and LH are both produced by the pituitary, and that the hypothalamus stimulates LH release, but inhibits prolactin release, and that ovarian hormones inhibit LH release, but not prolactin release. Lactogenic hormone or luteotrophic hormone (LTH) or prolactin is secreted by the aci-

dophils (alpha cells) of the pituitary. This hormone: (1) promotes growth of the breast, which has been stimulated already by estrogen and progesterone; (2) promotes and maintains lactation; (3) helps in maintenance of the corpus luteum; and (4) promotes maternal instinct.

138.   **(D)** The data clearly indicates inhibition of LH secretion by all three factors.

139.   **(D)** LH and prolactin appear to be secreted independently. Hypophysectomy inhibits secretion of both, but hypothalamic lesions have opposite effects on LH and prolactin. In addition, ovariectomy and estrogen alter LH secretion with little effect on prolactin.

140.   **(B)** The fiber components of connective tissue add strength and support. They are collagenous, elastic, and reticular in nature; collagen fibers are the most numerous fiber type. The graphs show that labeled proline starts to appear in the collagen in under 2 hours, so **B** was supported by the evidence. Statements **A** and **C** were contradicted by the information given, and **D** is neither supported nor contradicted.

141.   **(C)** The apparent sequence in the graph is rER to Golgi and then very quickly to the extracellular space.

142.   **(A)** The pattern follows the typical pattern for secreted proteins.

143.   **(B)** Glycine has no chiral center, but other amino acids in higher animals are ordinarily of the L-series.

144.   **(C)** Carbohydrate monosaccharides found in higher animals are generally of the D-series.

145.   **(B)** Epimers differ in configuration at only one carbon. Enantiomers are nonsuperimposable mirror images. Diastereomers are nonsuperimposable nonmirror images.

146.   **(C)** The number of kcal/g for the classes of food material are: carbohydrates, 4; proteins, 4; and fats, 9. The nucleic acids are not considered as a class of food.

Answer Sheet

MODEL EXAMINATION D

Directions: After locating the number of the question to which you are responding, fill in the circle containing the letter of the answer you have selected. Use pencil (not a ballpoint pen) to completely blacken the circle.

PHYSICAL SCIENCES

1 Ⓐ Ⓑ Ⓒ Ⓓ
2 Ⓐ Ⓑ Ⓒ Ⓓ
3 Ⓐ Ⓑ Ⓒ Ⓓ
4 Ⓐ Ⓑ Ⓒ Ⓓ
5 Ⓐ Ⓑ Ⓒ Ⓓ
6 Ⓐ Ⓑ Ⓒ Ⓓ
7 Ⓐ Ⓑ Ⓒ Ⓓ
8 Ⓐ Ⓑ Ⓒ Ⓓ
9 Ⓐ Ⓑ Ⓒ Ⓓ
10 Ⓐ Ⓑ Ⓒ Ⓓ
11 Ⓐ Ⓑ Ⓒ Ⓓ
12 Ⓐ Ⓑ Ⓒ Ⓓ
13 Ⓐ Ⓑ Ⓒ Ⓓ
14 Ⓐ Ⓑ Ⓒ Ⓓ
15 Ⓐ Ⓑ Ⓒ Ⓓ
16 Ⓐ Ⓑ Ⓒ Ⓓ
17 Ⓐ Ⓑ Ⓒ Ⓓ
18 Ⓐ Ⓑ Ⓒ Ⓓ
19 Ⓐ Ⓑ Ⓒ Ⓓ
20 Ⓐ Ⓑ Ⓒ Ⓓ
21 Ⓐ Ⓑ Ⓒ Ⓓ
22 Ⓐ Ⓑ Ⓒ Ⓓ
23 Ⓐ Ⓑ Ⓒ Ⓓ
24 Ⓐ Ⓑ Ⓒ Ⓓ
25 Ⓐ Ⓑ Ⓒ Ⓓ
26 Ⓐ Ⓑ Ⓒ Ⓓ

27 Ⓐ Ⓑ Ⓒ Ⓓ
28 Ⓐ Ⓑ Ⓒ Ⓓ
29 Ⓐ Ⓑ Ⓒ Ⓓ
30 Ⓐ Ⓑ Ⓒ Ⓓ
31 Ⓐ Ⓑ Ⓒ Ⓓ
32 Ⓐ Ⓑ Ⓒ Ⓓ
33 Ⓐ Ⓑ Ⓒ Ⓓ
34 Ⓐ Ⓑ Ⓒ Ⓓ
35 Ⓐ Ⓑ Ⓒ Ⓓ
36 Ⓐ Ⓑ Ⓒ Ⓓ
37 Ⓐ Ⓑ Ⓒ Ⓓ
38 Ⓐ Ⓑ Ⓒ Ⓓ
39 Ⓐ Ⓑ Ⓒ Ⓓ
40 Ⓐ Ⓑ Ⓒ Ⓓ
41 Ⓐ Ⓑ Ⓒ Ⓓ
42 Ⓐ Ⓑ Ⓒ Ⓓ
43 Ⓐ Ⓑ Ⓒ Ⓓ
44 Ⓐ Ⓑ Ⓒ Ⓓ
45 Ⓐ Ⓑ Ⓒ Ⓓ
46 Ⓐ Ⓑ Ⓒ Ⓓ
47 Ⓐ Ⓑ Ⓒ Ⓓ
48 Ⓐ Ⓑ Ⓒ Ⓓ
49 Ⓐ Ⓑ Ⓒ Ⓓ
50 Ⓐ Ⓑ Ⓒ Ⓓ
51 Ⓐ Ⓑ Ⓒ Ⓓ
52 Ⓐ Ⓑ Ⓒ Ⓓ

VERBAL REASONING

53 Ⓐ Ⓑ Ⓒ Ⓓ
54 Ⓐ Ⓑ Ⓒ Ⓓ
55 Ⓐ Ⓑ Ⓒ Ⓓ
56 Ⓐ Ⓑ Ⓒ Ⓓ
57 Ⓐ Ⓑ Ⓒ Ⓓ
58 Ⓐ Ⓑ Ⓒ Ⓓ
59 Ⓐ Ⓑ Ⓒ Ⓓ
60 Ⓐ Ⓑ Ⓒ Ⓓ
61 Ⓐ Ⓑ Ⓒ Ⓓ
62 Ⓐ Ⓑ Ⓒ Ⓓ
63 Ⓐ Ⓑ Ⓒ Ⓓ
64 Ⓐ Ⓑ Ⓒ Ⓓ
65 Ⓐ Ⓑ Ⓒ Ⓓ
66 Ⓐ Ⓑ Ⓒ Ⓓ
67 Ⓐ Ⓑ Ⓒ Ⓓ
68 Ⓐ Ⓑ Ⓒ Ⓓ
69 Ⓐ Ⓑ Ⓒ Ⓓ
70 Ⓐ Ⓑ Ⓒ Ⓓ
71 Ⓐ Ⓑ Ⓒ Ⓓ
72 Ⓐ Ⓑ Ⓒ Ⓓ

73 Ⓐ Ⓑ Ⓒ Ⓓ
74 Ⓐ Ⓑ Ⓒ Ⓓ
75 Ⓐ Ⓑ Ⓒ Ⓓ
76 Ⓐ Ⓑ Ⓒ Ⓓ
77 Ⓐ Ⓑ Ⓒ Ⓓ
78 Ⓐ Ⓑ Ⓒ Ⓓ
79 Ⓐ Ⓑ Ⓒ Ⓓ
80 Ⓐ Ⓑ Ⓒ Ⓓ
81 Ⓐ Ⓑ Ⓒ Ⓓ
82 Ⓐ Ⓑ Ⓒ Ⓓ
83 Ⓐ Ⓑ Ⓒ Ⓓ
84 Ⓐ Ⓑ Ⓒ Ⓓ
85 Ⓐ Ⓑ Ⓒ Ⓓ
86 Ⓐ Ⓑ Ⓒ Ⓓ
87 Ⓐ Ⓑ Ⓒ Ⓓ
88 Ⓐ Ⓑ Ⓒ Ⓓ
89 Ⓐ Ⓑ Ⓒ Ⓓ
90 Ⓐ Ⓑ Ⓒ Ⓓ
91 Ⓐ Ⓑ Ⓒ Ⓓ
92 Ⓐ Ⓑ Ⓒ Ⓓ

Answer Sheet

MODEL EXAMINATION D

WRITING SAMPLE

BIOLOGICAL SCIENCES

Use separate ruled
sheets of paper.

93

94

95	Ⓐ Ⓑ Ⓒ Ⓓ	121	Ⓐ Ⓑ Ⓒ Ⓓ
96	Ⓐ Ⓑ Ⓒ Ⓓ	122	Ⓐ Ⓑ Ⓒ Ⓓ
97	Ⓐ Ⓑ Ⓒ Ⓓ	123	Ⓐ Ⓑ Ⓒ Ⓓ
98	Ⓐ Ⓑ Ⓒ Ⓓ	124	Ⓐ Ⓑ Ⓒ Ⓓ
99	Ⓐ Ⓑ Ⓒ Ⓓ	125	Ⓐ Ⓑ Ⓒ Ⓓ
100	Ⓐ Ⓑ Ⓒ Ⓓ	126	Ⓐ Ⓑ Ⓒ Ⓓ
101	Ⓐ Ⓑ Ⓒ Ⓓ	127	Ⓐ Ⓑ Ⓒ Ⓓ
102	Ⓐ Ⓑ Ⓒ Ⓓ	128	Ⓐ Ⓑ Ⓒ Ⓓ
103	Ⓐ Ⓑ Ⓒ Ⓓ	129	Ⓐ Ⓑ Ⓒ Ⓓ
104	Ⓐ Ⓑ Ⓒ Ⓓ	130	Ⓐ Ⓑ Ⓒ Ⓓ
105	Ⓐ Ⓑ Ⓒ Ⓓ	131	Ⓐ Ⓑ Ⓒ Ⓓ
106	Ⓐ Ⓑ Ⓒ Ⓓ	132	Ⓐ Ⓑ Ⓒ Ⓓ
107	Ⓐ Ⓑ Ⓒ Ⓓ	133	Ⓐ Ⓑ Ⓒ Ⓓ
108	Ⓐ Ⓑ Ⓒ Ⓓ	134	Ⓐ Ⓑ Ⓒ Ⓓ
109	Ⓐ Ⓑ Ⓒ Ⓓ	135	Ⓐ Ⓑ Ⓒ Ⓓ
110	Ⓐ Ⓑ Ⓒ Ⓓ	136	Ⓐ Ⓑ Ⓒ Ⓓ
111	Ⓐ Ⓑ Ⓒ Ⓓ	137	Ⓐ Ⓑ Ⓒ Ⓓ
112	Ⓐ Ⓑ Ⓒ Ⓓ	138	Ⓐ Ⓑ Ⓒ Ⓓ
113	Ⓐ Ⓑ Ⓒ Ⓓ	139	Ⓐ Ⓑ Ⓒ Ⓓ
114	Ⓐ Ⓑ Ⓒ Ⓓ	140	Ⓐ Ⓑ Ⓒ Ⓓ
115	Ⓐ Ⓑ Ⓒ Ⓓ	141	Ⓐ Ⓑ Ⓒ Ⓓ
116	Ⓐ Ⓑ Ⓒ Ⓓ	142	Ⓐ Ⓑ Ⓒ Ⓓ
117	Ⓐ Ⓑ Ⓒ Ⓓ	143	Ⓐ Ⓑ Ⓒ Ⓓ
118	Ⓐ Ⓑ Ⓒ Ⓓ	144	Ⓐ Ⓑ Ⓒ Ⓓ
119	Ⓐ Ⓑ Ⓒ Ⓓ	145	Ⓐ Ⓑ Ⓒ Ⓓ
120	Ⓐ Ⓑ Ⓒ Ⓓ	146	Ⓐ Ⓑ Ⓒ Ⓓ

The MCAT
Model Examination D

PHYSICAL SCIENCES

TIME—70 MINUTES FOR 52 QUESTIONS

Directions: The following questions or incomplete statements are in groups. Preceding each series of questions or statements is a paragraph or a short explanatory statement, a formula or set of formulas, or a definition. Read the written material and then answer the questions or complete the statements. Select the ONE BEST ANSWER for each question and indicate your selection by marking the corresponding letter of your choice on the Answer Form. Eliminate those alternatives you know to be incorrect and then select an answer from among the remaining alternatives. A periodic table is provided (see p. 563). You may consult it whenever you wish to do so.

Passage I (Questions 1–7)

Sodium is a reactive alkali metal. It is most readily produced by electrolysis of molten sodium chloride as follows:

$$2NaCl(l) \rightarrow 2Na(l) + Cl_2(g)$$
$$E° = -4.07 \text{ V}$$

The sodium metal generated must be stored under an inert liquid to prevent oxidation. Electrolysis of aqueous sodium chloride is an important reaction used commercially to generate sodium hydroxide as follows:

$$2NaCl(aq) + 2H_2O(l) \rightarrow 2NaOH(aq) + Cl_2(g) + H_2(g)$$
$$E° = 0.53 \text{ V}$$

1. What is the electron configuration of sodium?

   (A) $1s^2 2s^2 2p^6$
   (B) $1s^2 2s^2 2p^6 3s^1$
   (C) $1s^2 2s^2 2p^6 3s^2$
   (D) $1s^2 2s^2 2p^6 3s^2 3p^6$

2. The standard reduction potential for the sodium half reaction is –2.71 V. What is the standard reduction potential for the reduction of chlorine?

   (A) 0.83 V
   (B) –0.83 V
   (C) 1.36 V
   (D) –1.36 V

3. In the second reaction, what occurs at the anode?

   (A) $2H_2O + 2e^- \rightarrow H_2 + 2OH^-$
   (B) $Cl_2 + 2e^- \rightarrow 2Cl^-$
   (C) $Na^+ + e^- \rightarrow Na$
   (D) $2Cl^- \rightarrow Cl_2 + 2e$

4. A chemist conducts an experiment involving the second reaction to produce hydrogen gas. What is the likely pH of the solution after electrolysis has occurred?

   (A) 1.0
   (B) 4.0
   (C) 7.0
   (D) 9.0

5. The enthalpy associated with the melting of solid sodium chloride to make liquid sodium chloride is the:

    (A) heat of sublimation.
    (B) heat of fusion.
    (C) heat of vaporization.
    (D) heat of deposition.

6. What describes the interaction between Na$^+$ and Cl$^-$ in NaCl(s)?

    (A) nonpolar covalent bonding
    (B) polar covalent bonding
    (C) ionic bonding
    (D) hydrogen bonding

7. Sodium chloride is:

    (A) a weak acid.
    (B) a strong acid.
    (C) a weak electrolyte
    (D) a strong electrolyte.

Passage II (Questions 8–13)

A newly discovered reaction is being studied. It is concluded that the reaction consists of

$$2A + 3B \rightleftharpoons 3C + 2D$$

(The letters A, B, C, and D represent hypothetical compounds.)

8. The equilibrium constant as written may be calculated as:

    (A) $\dfrac{[C]^3 [D]^2}{[A]^2[B]^3}$

    (B) $\dfrac{3[C]\, 2[D]}{2[A]\, 3[B]}$

    (C) $\dfrac{[A]^2[B]^3}{[C]^3[D]^2}$

    (D) $\dfrac{[C]\, [D]}{[A]\, [B]}$

9. If the equilibrium constant is 0.001:

    (A) reaction to the right will be favored.
    (B) reaction to the left will be favored.
    (C) the reaction rate is fast.
    (D) the reaction rate is slow.

10. If A, B, and D are gases and C is a solid, the reaction will:

    (A) be improved toward the right with increased pressure.
    (B) be improved toward the left with increased pressure.
    (C) be unaffected by increased pressure.
    (D) not proceed in either direction in the presence of increased pressure.

11. At standard temperature and pressure, the volume represented by 3 moles of C is about:

    (A) 22 liters.
    (B) 45 liters.
    (C) 67 liters.
    (D) more than 80 liters.

12. A small equilibrium constant is indicative of:

    (A) a fast reaction rate.
    (B) a slow reaction rate.
    (C) no reaction.
    (D) none of the above.

13. Adding a catalyst to the reaction will:

    (A) shift equilibrium toward the products.
    (B) shift equilibrium toward the reactants.
    (C) increase the rate of reaction.
    (D) decrease the rate of reaction.

Passage III (Questions 14–18)

In a physics class, an experimental motion experiment is devised to allow the study of the motion of a number of objects under a variety of conditions. One part involves projecting identical steel or wooden balls at a variety of initial angles and speeds, starting at various heights above the floor. Equipment, such as protractors and photogate timers, is available so the angles and speeds are known. Rectangular metal blocks of various masses can be slid across horizontal surfaces and also down inclined planes. The surfaces vary from essentially frictionless to quite rough surfaces. The balls can be rolled down the inclined planes also. The masses of each object are measured in advance and the velocities can be measured at any point of the motion with the photogate timers.

14. One of the identical steel balls is dropped from the edge of a lab table 1.0 m high, and at the same instant another one is projected horizontally with an initial velocity of 2 m/sec. If there is no air resistance, what are the times for the two balls to strike the floor?

    (A) 0.22 sec, 0.22 sec
    (B) 0.32 sec, 0.52 sec
    (C) 0.45 sec, 0.45 sec
    (D) 1.20 sec, 1.50 sec

15. One ball is projected horizontally with an initial horizontal velocity of 10 m/sec while the second is projected at an angle of 30° *above* the horizontal with the same initial speed. Both balls strike a vertical wall that is exactly 10 m away. How long does it take each ball, respectively, to hit the wall?

    (A) 0.87 sec, 1.5 sec
    (B) 1 sec, 0.87 sec
    (C) 1 sec, 1 sec
    (D) 1 sec, 1.15 sec

16. A rectangular block of mass 1 kg and one of mass 3 kg are projected across a rough surface with the same starting speed of 4 m/sec. The coefficient of friction is 0.4. How far do the blocks slide, respectively?

    (A) 2 m, 2 m
    (B) 3 m, 2 m
    (C) 4 m, 4 m
    (D) 6 m, 2 m

17. One of the balls is released from rest at the top of an inclined plane 0.5 m high and rolls down without slipping. At the same instant a rectangular block is released and slides down a frictionless plane which is also 0.5 m high. Which of the two objects has the greater speed at the bottom of the inclines?

    (A) The ball.
    (B) The block.
    (C) Both have the same speed.
    (D) The question cannot be answered because there is not enough information given.

18. A wooden ball of mass 0.6 kg is dropped down a circular stairwell in a tall building and reaches a terminal velocity of 39 m/sec, continuing to fall at that speed. What is the force of air friction acting on the ball?

    (A) 5.9 N
    (B) 8.7 N
    (C) 16 N
    (D) 31 N

Passage IV (Questions 19–23)

Most of the students in an introductory physics class are in premedicine, so the instructor devises a lab in which all the topics are related to the human body. Each student's blood pressure, temperature, weight, height, metabolic rate, pulmonary function, and so on can be measured with reasonable accuracy. A lab handout supplies the following information:

   1 kg is equivalent to 2.2 pounds
   1 kcal = 4186 joules
   Average aortic pressure = 100 mm Hg
   1×10^5 N/m^2 = 750 mm Hg
   Density of blood = 1050 kg/m^3
   Energy of oxidation of fats and oils = 9.5 kcal/gram = 39,700 joules/gram
   Oxygen consumption in humans releases about 20,000 joules/liter O^2 (consumed)
   1 watt = 1 joule/sec

19. A student with a basal metabolic rate of 100 W exercises vigorously for 10 minutes. During that 10-minute period his average metabolic rate is 730 W. What is the approximate number of liters of oxygen the student consumes during the exercise period?

   (A) 22 L
   (B) 30 L
   (C) 109 L
   (D) 210 L

20. The student is trying to lose 2.3 kg of fat by exercising. The average rate of energy expended *above* that required for ordinary metabolism is 630 W. For how many hours will the student have to exercise?

   (A) 3 hr
   (B) 4 hr
   (C) 9 hr
   (D) 40 hr

21. The metabolism for a woman in the class is about 2000 kcal/day. If she has a food intake of 3100 kcal/day for four weeks, what mass of fat, corresponding to the excess intake, might accumulate?

   (A) 880 grams
   (B) 3242 grams
   (C) 1280 grams
   (D) 6650 grams

22. What is the gauge pressure in the foot artery, which is 1.35 m below the aorta?

   (A) 120 mm Hg
   (B) 205 mm Hg
   (C) 405 mm Hg
   (D) 660 mm Hg

23. You consume only about 25% of the oxygen that you take into your lungs. If you work for 4 hours at a metabolic rate of 350 W, how many *total liters of oxygen* do you inhale? (The volume of air will be 5 times larger, since O$_2$ is 20% of the atmosphere.)

   (A) 216 L
   (B) 1000 L
   (C) 3200 L
   (D) 4300 L

Passage V (Questions 24–28)

Students in a physics laboratory use the circuit shown. An ammeter can measure the "conventional" current in the circuit, which flows anticlockwise. Circuit elements can be added or removed. A voltmeter is available to measure the voltage across any circuit component.

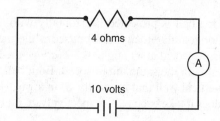

24. What is the current in the original circuit?

   (A) 7.5 A
   (B) 5.0 A
   (C) 2.5 A
   (D) 1.5 A

25. Another 4-ohm resistor is added in parallel with the first resistor. What happens to the total current in the circuit?

   (A) The current increases by a factor of 2.
   (B) The current decreases by a factor of 2.
   (C) The current remains the same.
   (D) The current decreases by a factor of 4.

26. A capacitor, *C*, of 2 microfarads is inserted into the circuit between the battery and the ammeter. Which graph shows how the charge on the capacitor changes with time?

(A)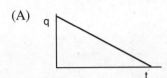

(B)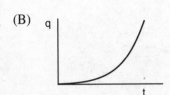

(C)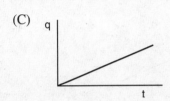

(D)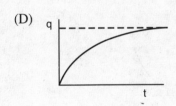

27. What is the value of the final charge on the capacitor?

(A) 0 C
(B) 5×10^{-6} C
(C) 2.0×10^{-5} C
(D) 20.0×10^{-6} C

28. With the capacitor in the circuit, the two resistors are reconnected in series. What happens to the value of the final charge on the capacitor?

(A) It will increase by a factor of 2.
(B) It will decrease by a factor of 2.
(C) It will decrease by a factor of 4.
(D) It will remain the same.

Passage VI (Questions 29–34)

A liquid is isolated, containing 5.9% hydrogen and 94.1% oxygen by mass. The elements are 50% hydrogen and 50% oxygen by volume. The molecular weight is determined to be 34.0. In a decomposition reaction this liquid produces water, oxygen, and no other products.

29. The empirical formula is:

(A) HO.
(B) H_2O_2.
(C) H_3O_3.
(D) H_3O_4.

30. The molecular formula is:

(A) HO.
(B) H_2O_2.
(C) H_3O_3.
(D) H_3O_4.

31. The balanced equation for the decomposition indicates that one mole of the liquid will produce _____ moles of oxygen.

(A) 0.25
(B) 0.50
(C) 1.0
(D) 2.0

32. The balanced equation for the decomposition of the liquid indicates the formation of _____ liters of oxygen at STP from one mole of the liquid.

(A) 1.12
(B) 2.24
(C) 11.2
(D) 22.4

33. For an equilibrium reaction at 25°C, the decomposition we have been considering would be _____ by an increase in pressure.

(A) favored
(B) unaffected
(C) adversely affected
(D) affected, but in an unpredictable direction

34. The order of the reaction, from information given above, will be definitely

    (A) zero.
    (B) first.
    (C) second.
    (D) unpredictable.

Questions 35–41 are independent of any passages and of each other.

35. The naturally occurring radioactive decay series known as the Actinium series begins with the long-lived isotope $_{92}U^{235}$. It decays by a series of alpha (α) and beta (β) decays as follows: α, β, α, α, β, α, α, β, α, α, β. What isotope is the final result of this series?

    (A) $_{88}Ra^{208}$
    (B) $_{82}Pb^{210}$
    (C) $_{88}Ra^{220}$
    (D) $_{82}Pb^{207}$

36. Radium-226 (Ra226) has a half-life of 1600 years. The activity of a radium needle used to treat skin cancers in the early 20th century was 1.0 curie. What is the approximate activity at the present time, 100 years later?

    (A) 0.44 curie
    (B) 0.26 curie
    (C) 0.96 curie
    (D) 0.62 curie

37. The absolute temperature of an ideal gas increases by 50% at constant volume. What happens to the absolute pressure of the gas?

    (A) The pressure doubles.
    (B) The pressure increases by 50%.
    (C) The pressure increases by 150%.
    (D) The pressure decreases by 50%.

38. A constant force F acts on a mass m which can move without friction. The mass is at rest at the origin of coordinates ($x = 0$) at time $t = 0$. Which graph correctly shows the velocity of the mass as a function of time?

(A)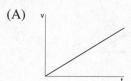

(B)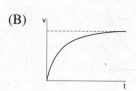

(C)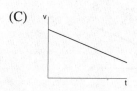

(D)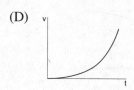

39. What are the highest and lowest values of resistance that one can construct using three 3-ohm resistors?

    (A) 12 ohms and 0.33 ohm
    (B) 9 ohms and 0.33 ohm
    (C) 9 ohms and 1 ohm
    (D) 12 ohms and 0.67 ohm

40. A net force of 6 N acts on a mass of 3 kg, accelerating it from rest. If the force acts over a distance of 4 m, what is the final speed of the mass?

    (A) 4.0 m/sec
    (B) 3.6 m/sec
    (C) 5.1 m/sec
    (D) 2.8 m/sec

41. A homeowner working in a crawl space touches a "hot" 120 V source. A current of 120 milliamperes passes through his heart and initiates a dangerous ventricular fibrillation. What is the body resistance in ohms?

    (A) 400 ohms
    (B) 1000 ohms
    (C) 1400 ohms
    (D) 800 ohms

Passage VII (Questions 42–45)

A set of experiments to study all aspects of sound waves is devised. Several identical audio oscillators with loudspeakers can be used for experiments in audible sound at any frequency between 25 Hz and 40,000 Hz. An old ultrasound (US) unit (an "A scan" unit) is available to study the propagation of ultrasound waves. The unit has a US transducer that transmits a pulse of US and then "rests" and acts as a receiver of the US echo. The transmitted signal and echo are observed on an oscilloscope. The time for the echo to return can be read from the horizontal scope face. Since the returned signals are quite weak, the US unit has the ability to highly amplify the echo. The student can study the conditions of waves in pipes closed on one end or open on both ends. The audio units can be mounted on carts to study the Doppler effect. The waves from the oscillator and US unit are sent through air, water, and aluminum. The speed of sound in these materials is measured by determining the time for the echo to return from a surface a known distance from the transducer. Some of the results are:

Apparatus	Material	Speed of sound	Frequencies
Audio oscillator	Air	340 m/sec	50 Hz, 1000 Hz
	Water	1440 m/sec	50 Hz, 1000 Hz
	Aluminum	5100 m/sec	50 Hz, 1000 Hz
US unit	Air	340 m/sec	2.5 MHz (megahertz)
	Water	1440	2.5 MHz
	Aluminum	5100	2.5 MHz

42. Which signal has the longest wavelength?

    (A) The 50 Hz signal in air
    (B) The 2.5 MHz signal in air
    (C) The 50 Hz signal in aluminum
    (D) The 2.5 MHz signal in aluminum

43. The audio system is used to send a sound wave from a small speaker into a 25-cm long cylindrical tube which is open on both ends. Both open ends must be antinodes for a standing wave. As the frequency is slowly increased, a louder resonant fundamental is heard. What is the frequency of this fundamental?

    (A) 340 Hz
    (B) 680 Hz
    (C) 170 Hz
    (D) 1020 Hz

44. The US transducer at 2.5 MHz is placed just below the surface in a water tank and pointed straight down at a horizontal wooden surface. A reflected echo from the surface is detected after 0.35 milliseconds. How far is the wooden surface from the transducer?

    (A) 0.82 m
    (B) 0.34 m
    (C) 1.1 m
    (D) 0.25 m

45. The audio system is mounted on a cart and pushed away from a student at 30 m/s while emitting a 2000 Hz signal. What will happen to the frequency that the student hears?

    (A) The frequency will increase.
    (B) The frequency will remain unchanged.
    (C) The frequency will decrease.
    (D) The frequency will increase and then decrease.

Questions 46–52 are independent of any passages and of each other.

46. Catalysts:

(A) are changed and consumed during a reaction.
(B) have virtually no effect on the overall rate of the reaction.
(C) are changed but not consumed during a reaction.
(D) speed up the rate of the reaction.

47. If solution A is less concentrated in dissolved particle content than solution B, then solution B is said to be:

(A) hypertonic.
(B) hypotonic.
(C) isoosmotic.
(D) isotonic.

48. Compared to one mole of oxygen, how many more molecules do two moles of carbon dioxide contain?

(A) 25×10^6
(B) 12.04×10^{46}
(C) 6.02×10^{23}
(D) 12.04×10^{23}

49. Which one of the following acids does not commonly form acid salts?

(A) $HC_2H_3O_2$
(B) H_2SO_4
(C) H_2CO_3
(D) H_3PO_4

50. Which of the statements listed below is false?

(A) An aqueous solution in which $[H^+] > 1 \times 10^{-7}$ is said to be acidic.
(B) Ions are atoms or groups of atoms that have lost or gained one or more electrons.
(C) HCl is a Brønsted acid because it furnishes H^+ ion in solution.
(D) NaOH is called a base because it furnishes Na^+ ions in solution.

51. In the decomposition of $KClO_3$ to generate oxygen gas, a small amount of MnO_2 is added in order to:

(A) increase the volume of oxygen obtained from the $KClO_3$.
(B) produce oxygen of higher purity.
(C) reduce the temperature at which decomposition of $KClO_3$ takes place.
(D) increase the temperature at which decomposition of $KClO_3$ takes place.

52. The name applied to a substance such as MnO_2 used in the reaction above is a (an):

(A) enzyme.
(B) catalyst.
(C) isotope.
(D) free radical scavenger.

VERBAL REASONING

TIME—60 MINUTES FOR 40 QUESTIONS

Directions: The questions are based on the accompanying seven passages. Read each passage carefully, then answer the following questions. Consider only the material within the passage. For each question, select the ONE BEST ANSWER and indicate your selection by marking the corresponding letter on the Answer Form.

Passage I (Questions 53–57)

In the fall of 1990, a vigorous debate broke out at the University of Texas at Austin, a debate that turned into a heated national conversation on the purpose of the writing classroom and, to some extent, the purpose of liberal education. Among composition specialists the debate delineated two separate ways of thinking about freshman composition and the field of composition studies.

The debate focused on a proposed curriculum for the freshman composition program at the University of Texas, English 306, a curriculum that required students to produce approximately 3,900 words of writing and taught students to conduct and sustain rhetorical inquiry into a single topic. Some of the goals of the curriculum were to introduce undergraduates to the intellectual demands of college through the teaching of skills such as analysis, research, and synthesis, to create an intimate, participatory classroom experience for the students whose freshman schedules are often otherwise confined to huge lecture halls, and to help the new graduate student teachers focus on the teaching of writing by creating a bridge between skills learned in the study of literature and the teaching of freshman composition. All seemingly laudable, standard goals for freshman composition. The problem, the reason for the violent debate, was the topic chosen for the class: difference, specifically difference related to legal opinions given in court cases involving issues such as race, gender, bilingualism, and sexual orientation. The debate that followed the submission and ultimate rejection of the program in many ways disregarded the course itself; the discussion became a forum for stating the purpose of composition and liberal education.

One group, that I will call the traditionalists, views the writing classroom as the place to focus on process, a place where students write, primarily, personal essays to engage in the writing process. The other group, the radical pedagogists, believe that the purpose of the writing classroom is to engage the student as critical thinker, often defined as one who rethinks cultural assumptions and becomes committed to social change. There are varying views among radical pedagogists of the ways and means of teaching critical thinking. . . .

. . . The traditionalist point of view is, relatively speaking, fairly new. It arose in the past 25 years or so, in tandem with the advent of composition studies as a legitimate academic discipline. The traditionalist approach focuses on process, and states that a primary way to engage the student is to have the student determine essay topics. As Richard Graves says, "the first lesson in teaching composition is that the writer must find his or her own subject." This student-centered approach assumes that the student will not only be more invested in the essay if the idea originates with her, but that the student learns that she has a wealth of information inside her, information that once organized not only reflects her knowledge base but proves interesting to others. This new knowledge engages the student in her own writing, making it a forum for her voice, thus giving her a sense of legitimacy to her own experiences and reflections. Although aware of the powerful effects of writing on the student as thinker, the primary concern for the traditionalists is the student as writer, as they seek to engage the students in the process and act of writing.

The radical pedagogists are more concerned with the student as thinker and want to use the mind power generated in the writing process to foster social change. Patricia Bizzell states that "we rhetoricians like to see ourselves as social reformers, if not revolutionaries." . . . This concern with social and political change is prevalent among the radial pedagogists. Sharon Crowley states that "freshman composition can be radicalized in the service of social justice" and commends writers who "would put literacy to work with the specific goal of effecting social change." There is little mention among these highly political pedagogists of the student as writer, or of developing writing skills in a student for the sake of individual education.

Donald Lazere, a committed leftist educator and radical pedagogist, offers an alternative to both schools of composition theory. He sees student empowerment and

---

Adapted from a paper by Abby Arnold, "Empowerment Pedagogy and the Writing Classroom," English 636, VCU, 1996 and used with permission of the author.

social change as coming through the student's learning to write, thus learning to access and manipulate the dialogue of mainstream culture. He criticizes both the "process" contention that skills are less important than the act of writing and the "radical" determination to focus on critical thinking at the expense of writing instruction. He states that "the lack of basic skills and factual knowledge is an obstacle to autonomous critical thinking" and that "a sophisticated level of literacy is virtually necessary, or at least highly advantageous, for effective opposition to the dominant culture in today's society."

Although committed to his view of social change, Lazere is also committed to the growth of the student. He recognizes the coercive nature of some radical pedagogy, the kind of belief in one's agenda that led Sharon Crowley to state that composition teachers "must give up our traditional subscription to liberal tolerance if we are to bring about social change through [our students]." Lazere believes that to force any ideology on students "is only to replace the coercion . . . in mainstream education with coercion into accord with an opposing ideology."

53. Which of the following was **not** a stated goal of the freshman curriculum at the University of Texas when the debate over English 306 broke out?

   (A) to create a smaller, more intimate classroom experience than freshmen typically have
   (B) to help new graduate student teachers focus on the teaching of writing
   (C) to teach freshmen how to bring about social change through their writing
   (D) to introduce freshmen to the intellectual demands of college by teaching various skills

54. Of the two main groups in opposition with each other in the University of Texas debate, which of the following groups have as a goal to use writing and the teaching of writing to bring about social change?

   (A) the traditionalists
   (B) the pragmatists
   (C) the radical pedagogists
   (D) the purists

55. According to the passage, Donald Lazere could best be characterized as:

   (A) a leftist educator.
   (B) a person who would disagree with the methods proposed by Sharon Crowley.
   (C) a radical pedagogist.
   (D) all of the above.

56. The proposed topic for English 306 was to include:

   (A) a study of world literature.
   (B) an examination of the relationship between writing for the mass media and writing for scholarly journals.
   (C) a study of legal opinions from court cases involving, among other things, sexual orientation.
   (D) an analysis of fiction and creative nonfiction.

57. Based on the quotations attributed to Sharon Crowley in the passage, we can deduce that she belongs to the group referred to as:

   (A) the traditionalists.
   (B) the radical pedgaogists.
   (C) the free thinkers.
   (D) the grammar advocates.

Passage II (Questions 58–64)

To establish a prima facie case of sex discrimination in compensation, an employee must present data that compare her salary with that of male coworkers doing the same job under the same circumstances. The standard or test that has emerged from case law is called the equal pay for equal work standard. Not to be confused with the idea that one must hold a job identical to that of someone else, that standard is built on a concept that evaluates jobs within a context of substantial equivalency. The issue to probe thus becomes: Is complainant's job equal in effort and responsibility to that of a male counterpart? A corollary question also is asked. Do the two incumbents in these jobs (the male and the female) possess comparable skills?

On March 11, 1974, the Secretary of Labor took action against Columbia University and its president, seeking to enjoin the university from discriminating

Adapted from Richard S. Vacca: "Sex Discrimination in Public School Employment." In S. B. Thomas, N. H. Cambron-McCabe, and M. M. McCarthy, Eds., *Education and the Law,* New York: Institute for School Law and Finance, 1983.

against its female custodial workers (classified as light cleaners). Alleging a violation of the Equal Pay Act on the basis of sex, the evidence showed that female light cleaners were paid a lower hourly rate than male heavy cleaners. At trial, the court came to the conclusion that the jobs of light cleaners and heavy cleaners were different. And, because the job of heavy cleaners involved greater effort than that of light cleaners, the plaintiff had failed to sustain the burden of establishing the idea of equal work within the meaning of the act.

On appeal, the Second Circuit Court of Appeals focused its attention on the "equal effort" criteria in connection with the workers' primary duties. The court stated:

> The concept of "effort" in the act is straightforward. It calls for a direct comparison of the amount of physical exertion required by the jobs; there is no factor added to compensate for physiological differences between men and women. Based on our careful review of the record before us we cannot say that the district court was clearly erroneous in making this direct comparison and the finding as a fact that heavy cleaning involves "greater effort."

The court also noted that the differences between the heavy cleaner and light cleaner jobs were known by the employees. Furthermore, no heavy cleaner job had ever been denied to a woman. In fact, in 1972, Columbia opened a heavy cleaner category to women, and seven light cleaners were accepted into on-the-job training for that position. However, after seven weeks, four of the seven workers transferred back to light cleaning.

In conclusion, the circuit court held that based on the evidence of the understanding and experience of the individuals most closely involved, together with the undisputed fact that heavy cleaning called for greater effort, there was no valid claim of unequal pay for substantial equivalent work within the meaning of the Equal Pay Act.

A new and more controversial standard in sex discrimination cases involves the notion of comparable worth. Under the theory of comparable worth, one must look beyond the equal pay for equal work criterion. In such cases, the female plaintiff argues the intrinsic worth, or the intrinsic difficulty of her job, as compared to other jobs in the same organization. Such an argument thus carries the complaint beyond the confines of an equal wage matter and places it under the broader umbrella protection of Title VII.

The judiciary has not yet endorsed the notion of comparable worth, but the Supreme Court has ruled that Title VII provides a remedy for sex discrimination in compensation beyond that covered by the Equal Pay Act. The matter arose in Washington County, Oregon, when four women guards in the female section of the county jail alleged that they were paid unequal wages for work substantially equal to that performed by male guards. In their complaint, the women guards charged that because of intentional discrimination, the county set the pay scale of female guards (but not male guards) "at a level lower than that warranted by its own survey of outside markets and the worth of the jobs."

After an adverse decision at trial, the female guards appealed to the Eighth Circuit Court of Appeals. The appellate court reversed the trial court and held that petitioners were not precluded from suing under Title VII, solely because their jobs were not substantially equal to higher-paying jobs held by male employees. The Supreme Court agreed and ruled in County of *Washington v. Gunther* that the wage differentials were based on intentional sex discrimination even though female guards did not actually perform work equal to that of male guards. Although not adopting the controversial concept of comparable worth, the Court left the door open for a comparable worth argument to be raised in future litigation.

It is significant to note that Justice Rehnquist for the four dissenters in *Gunther* strongly stated that this decision could spell the nullification of the Equal Pay Act if future plaintiffs are allowed to substitute the comparable worth standard for that of the equal pay for equal work standard. He asserted that the majority's opinion must be read narrowly ("the opinion does not endorse the so-called 'comparable worth' theory): though the Court does not indicate how a plaintiff might establish a prima facie case under Title VII, the Court does suggest that allegations of unequal pay for unequal, but comparable, work will not state a claim on which relief may be granted."

Others would argue that the Supreme Court's decision in *Gunther* establishes a possibility for plaintiffs in future cases to be given the opportunity to produce evidence showing a Title VII violation based on a comparable worth, rather than on an equal work basis. For example, female teachers might argue that over the years the historical pattern and practice in public school systems have inflated the value and salaries of certain jobs simply because they were held by men, while depressing the value and salaries of other jobs because they were held by women, even though each of the jobs is of comparable worth to the school system.

58. When one investigates an equal pay issue, attention must be given to:

    I. equal worth.
    II. equal effort.
    III. equal length of employment.
    IV. equal responsibility.

    (A) I, II, and III
    (B) I and III
    (C) II and IV
    (D) I, II, III, and IV

59. From information provided in the passage, which of the following conclusions is one justified in drawing?

    (A) Identical jobs should receive equal reimbursement.
    (B) Substantial equivalency is at the bottom of the issue.
    (C) The question also to be asked is whether the concerned possess equal levels of education.
    (D) Effort, attitude, drive, and determination are important considerations in equal pay for equal work cases.

60. In sex discrimination cases the courts:

    I. have considered the fact that women bear children.
    II. have decided that maternity leave is a constitutional right.
    III. have allowed the notion of physical and physiological differences.
    IV. view the Equal Pay Act and the Title VII laws as equal in impact.

    (A) I, II, and III
    (B) I and III
    (C) II and IV
    (D) neither I, II, III, nor IV

61. The Columbia University case illustrates:

    (A) that on-the-job training is essential in avoiding problems.
    (B) the haphazard approach used by the Department of Labor in filing suit.
    (C) that employees are not always aware of differences in their jobs.
    (D) the well-defined limits of the Equal Pay Act in regard to the equal effort interpretation.

62. Which of the following statement(s) is/are *supported by* the passage?

    I. Comparable worth is a complex issue.
    II. In comparable worth issues one must probe well beyond the equal pay for equal work issues.
    III. The Supreme Court considers Title VII as a remedy for sex discrimination.
    IV. The judiciary has endorsed Title VII.

    (A) I, II, and III
    (B) I and III
    (C) II and IV
    (D) I, II, III, and IV

63. In the Oregon case:

    I. the first trial ended with a ruling for the county.
    II. the first trial resulted in no definitive decision.
    III. the appellate court did not preclude a suit based on job unequality.
    IV. the Supreme Court adopted the concept of comparable worth.

    (A) I, II, and III
    (B) I and III
    (C) II and IV
    (D) I, II, III, and IV

64. The passage substantiates which of the following observations?

    I. There were four dissenters to the Supreme Court decision.
    II. Concern was voiced about the future effectiveness of the Equal Pay Act.
    III. It is anticipated that litigation might substitute the principle of comparable worth for the argument equal pay and equal work.
    IV. The majority opinion clearly defined the limits of the decision in the *County of Washington v. Gunther* case.

    (A) I, II, and III
    (B) I and III
    (C) IV only
    (D) I, II, III, and IV

Passage III (Questions 65–69)

There have been two controversies over Eoanthopus, and it is the first of them that has incongruous mandible for its theme. The question at issue was whether this specimen represents a single creature or two different ones. Scientist made reconstructions reconciling jaw and skull; however, one group described the jaw as an ape's separately from the skull that was assigned to Homo sapiens. The finder's argument ran as follows: All of the remains were found very close together. The lower jaw and brain case were both of a similar brown color and apparently in the same state of fossilization. The jaw, even though ape-like, did have human features, particularly in the teeth. The molar teeth had apparently been worn to a flatness never seen in apes, and only expected if the jaw had belonged to a type of human being. The roots of the teeth seen radiologically also resembled human teeth. The appearance of this ape-like man at the beginning of the Ice Age was just what many authorities expected to find. Shortly thereafter, a canine tooth, ape-like, but worn in a way never found in modern apes, was found. This was strong support for the missing link interpretation and man's ape-like ancestry. Questions remained concerning how anatomically the jaw could have worked as part of a human skull, and a wear of the teeth.

Three years later, about two miles away from the first site, pieces of a thick braincase and a molar tooth (both similar to the first find) were unearthed. The climate was ripe for the view that the human ancestor would show a combination of ape and man. However, as more human fossils were found in other parts of the world, this particular specimen differed from all in regard to skull characteristics. Their braincases were far more ape-like and their jaws less so, and a consistent line of evolution was found. Restorations of the cranium resulted in the revisions of brain volume, but in the end the controversial specimen had a brain of modern size to go with its modern skull.

If the remains were old, they would be accepted even though odd and isolated. When the fluorine method was applied, it was found that neither jawbone nor braincase contained more than small traces of fluorine meaning that the specimen did not date before the Ice Age. The specimen was now believed to be 50,000 and not 500,000 years old, making it an evolutionary absurdity with no known ancestor or descendants. An explanation was to suppose that a piece of modern ape jaw had been deliberately placed with an ancient braincase and both suitably stained. Another fluorine analysis placed the braincase as ancient, but the jaw and teeth in modern times. In fact, chemical analysis showed that the jaw and teeth contained the same amount of nitrogen and organic carbon as modern specimens, the calvarium, however, much less. Ruling out that the organic matter was not gelatin or glue with which the specimen had been impregnated as a means of hardening was accomplished with electron microscopy because the jaw showed preserved fibers of organic tissue and the calvarium laced this feature. Besides this, it was established that the jaw had been colored artificially with iron to match the calvarium.

The first specimen was apparently made up by placement of an artificially abraded molar tooth of an orangutan with a piece of thick frontal bone; the last fragment found duplicated the thinnest part of the first skull. Chromium detected in the jaw indicates that a dichromate solution was used in an attempt to assist the oxidation of iron salts used to stain these specimens.

65. The skull was classified to belong to:

   I. a vertebrate.
   II. a mammal.
   III. a man.
   IV. an ape.

(A) I, II, and III
(B) I and III
(C) II and IV
(D) I, II, III, and IV

66. This passage was probably written by:

(A) a historian.
(B) an anthropologist.
(C) a sociologist.
(D) an archeologist.

67. From the passage one could surmise that fluorine:

(A) was obtained from drinking water.
(B) was absorbed from the soil.
(C) becomes more concentrated.
(D) is a by-product of the decay process.

68. If the jawbone was modern, its fluorine content in relation to the braincase would have been:

(A) the same.
(B) more.
(C) less.
(D) not important in the solution.

From H. R. Seibel, "The Piltdown Hoax," *Bioscope*, 1962.

69. The analysis of iron was used to establish:

(A) a color comparison.
(B) the organic matrix pattern.
(C) the age of the specimens.
(D) none of the above.

Passage IV (Questions 70–75)

Many who have seen photographs of Zelda Sayre Fitzgerald note that no two images of her resemble each other. She had many different, unforgettable faces, among them the polished and strikingly beautiful one that appeared on the cover of *Hearst's International* magazine in the early 1920s and that she referred to as her Elizabeth Arden face. But the different faces of Zelda, as the Fitzgeralds' friend Sara Murphy observed shortly after Zelda's first mental breakdown, had much less to do with subtle changes in makeup or lighting than with inner complexity and mystery that no one, not even her husband, Scott, ever touched. There have been many constructions of Zelda Fitzgerald, all hinting at the complexity that Sara Murphy noted. But, not surprisingly, the various constructions like the various photographs of Zelda's face rarely resemble each other.

From the actual Zelda Sayre of Montgomery, Alabama, Scott Fitzgerald constructed a fairy princess, hidden away in a tower to be rescued from her provincial surroundings and taken by him into the more sophisticated world of Princeton and New York. She had been born July 24, 1900, the sixth child of Alabama Judge Anthony Sayre and his wife, Minnie, who named Zelda after a gypsy queen in a novel she had read and who spoiled her from the beginning, nursing her, some say, until she was 4 years old. By the time Fitzgerald arrived at Fort Sheridan, near Montgomery, in his tailored Brooks Brothers uniform Zelda was, at 18, thought of as an original, a daring local beauty who was known not only in Montgomery but in most college towns in Alabama. She became not only Scott's idealized version of the Southern Belle but also the incarnation of all that was desirable in woman. He went back to New York from Montgomery after the war was over, finished the novel that was to become *This Side of Paradise*, sent for Zelda, and married her in the rectory of St. Patrick's Cathedral.

The process of Scott's invention and reinvention of Zelda, which had already begun with his creation of the heroine of "The Ice Palace," set in a small southern town, would be repeated numerous times in the next two decades, among other places in Gloria in *The Beautiful and Damned* and in Daisy in *The Great Gatsby*. His two

---

Adapted from "Zelda," VCU, 1995 and used with permission of Dr. Bryant Mangum.

final fictional recreations of Zelda in fiction, as Nicole Diver in *Tender Is the Night* and as Ailie Calhoun in "The Last of the Belles," remain strong at the end, though the hero has lost the ability to sustain a romantic vision of her. Fitzgerald constructed and reconstructed Zelda for as long as he had the emotional vitality to do so. But after Zelda's mental collapse, precipitated in part by her obsessive pursuit of ballet—in effect her obsessive pursuit of an artistic identity of her own that she could have separate from Scott's imagined version of her—Scott began his descent into alcoholism. He left his capacity for hope, he said, on the road leading away from Zelda's sanitarium.

Nancy Milford, Zelda's first major biographer, constructs a Zelda shaped in large part by Scott's exploitation of her, by his appropriation of her image and even of the prose from her diaries for the purpose of enhancing his own literary reputation. There was no room for two artists in the Fitzgerald household, as Milford's description of the bitter conflict that surrounded the publication of Zelda's 1932 novel *Save Me the Waltz* demonstrates. She was, as Scott reminded her, a third-rate talent. But his assault on Zelda's self-esteem is only part of Milford's picture of a self divided by internal forces beyond her control. Her entrapment in a world with little understanding or appreciation of her predicament makes Milford's Zelda a symbol for our time, her death in 1948 by fire while locked away in the upper reaches of a mental institution dramatically underscoring the powerlessness of her plight. Sara Mayfield's competing portrait of Zelda, who was Mayfield's girlhood friend, depicts a southern belle whose major misfortune was her loss of the traditions of the genteel South at the hands of Scott, who took Zelda from her home and set in motion the tragedy of two "exiles from paradise." These are only two of many recreations of Zelda.

The actual Zelda Sayre Fitzgerald is fragmented in the many constructions of her life that we have. Once, in an attempt to establish the historical truth about Zelda's role in Scott's life and his role in hers, someone asked Scott for his analysis. He replied that if one asked Zelda's friends, they would say that his drinking drove her to insanity. His friends would say that her insanity drove him to drink. But the truth, he noted, is that "liquor on my mouth is sweet to her and I cherish her wildest hallucinations." And here we are back where we began. Historically, Scott did cherish, celebrate, and enshrine as art Zelda's wildest hallucinations, particularly during the decade of the Roaring Twenties, which marked the high point of their lives together. After the stock market crash of 1929 and Zelda's first mental collapse, which shortly followed it, Scott went through the motions of supporting her, among other things by paying her hospital bills, until his death in 1940.

But, in effect, Scott left Zelda in the mid-1930s to herself and to the biographers, poets, and playwrights who continue to create versions of her from the known facts of her life, from the gallery of her paintings, from her scrapbooks, from her published and unpublished novels, stories, essays, and letters—and from their own imaginations.

70. According to the passage, Zelda Fitzgerald rarely looked the same in any two of the many pictures taken of her. Sara Murphy attributed this to

   (A) Zelda's inner complexity.
   (B) the unpredictable quality of photographic equipment in the 1920s and 1930s, during which most of the photographs were taken.
   (C) Zelda's careful use of makeup.
   (D) Zelda's insistence that photographers take her picture from unusual angles.

71. Zelda Fitzgerald's first major biographer, according to the passage, was

   (A) Sara Mayfield.
   (B) Sara Murphy.
   (C) Arthur Mizener.
   (D) Nancy Milford.

72. One could deduce from the passage that Zelda Fitzgerald's husband, F. Scott Fitzgerald,

   (A) married Zelda on the rebound from his first love, Ginevra King.
   (B) had known Zelda all of his life and became romantically interested in her only after he had gone off to college.
   (C) met her when he was stationed near her home in Alabama during the war.
   (D) agreed to marry Zelda only if she would not pursue her career as a ballet dancer.

73. Minnie Sayre, Zelda's mother, the passage states, named her daughter after

   (A) a gypsy queen in a novel she was reading.
   (B) a distant relative who had agreed to remember Zelda in her will.
   (C) her maternal grandmother.
   (D) a character in a popular radio drama of the time.

74. The passage would support the following conclusion:

   (A) Insanity ran in Zelda's family, according to family medical records.
   (B) Zelda was exploited by Scott, but she also suffered from internal conflicts probably not attributable to her husband, according to a major biographer.
   (C) Zelda was unpopular in her hometown of Montgomery, Alabama, one of her high school friends maintained.
   (D) Zelda had always wanted to marry a popular author, she told her brother many years after her marriage to Scott.

75. According to the passage, when asked about his role in Zelda's life and her role in his, Scott made an observation that revealed his own belief about their relationship:

   (A) Their mutual friends were better qualified to comment on this than he was.
   (B) They were mutually destructive of each other.
   (C) Zelda was to blame for driving him to drink.
   (D) His drinking was responsible for driving her to insanity.

Passage V (Questions 76–80)

"In this way you shall set the fiftieth year apart and proclaim freedom to all the inhabitants of the land." In this way the ancient writer of Leviticus had God speak through Moses for the purpose of commemorating the entrance of the people of Israel into the "Promised Land." This is not the oldest reference to the celebration of an "anniversary," but it does show that celebrating anniversaries is a very old practice, and it also illustrates the role of round numbers in such celebrations.

Thus, the institution's celebration of its one hundred fiftieth year of existence adheres to a very old tradition. We celebrate birthdays and wedding anniversaries annually, whereas we usually commemorate the formation of institutions, businesses, churches, nations and schools on the round-numbered years. (Even with birthdays and weddings we call special attention to the "big" years—tenth, twenty-fifth, fiftieth, and so on.) That we do so may have something to do with the fact that our numbering is on the base ten system, and the round numbers are those that finish the pattern. Although that explains why we pick the round numbers for our large celebrations, it does not

From Dr. William E. Blake, Jr., VCU's Sesquicentennial Celebration, 1989.

explain why we think it important to celebrate such occasions. A brief discussion of why we *do* observe anniversaries is also an argument for why we *should* do so.

Perhaps the most obvious reason for celebrating the birth of an institution or the commemoration of some dramatic event is our belief that there was a good in it worth perpetuating. Thus, John Adams said of the 1776 Resolution of Independence:

> I am apt to believe that it will be celebrated by succeeding generations as the great anniversary festival. It ought to be commemorated as the day of deliverance, by solemn acts of devotion to God Almighty. It ought to be solemnized with pomp and parade, with shows, games, sports, guns, bells, bonfires, and illuminations, from one end of this continent to the other, from this time forward for evermore.

Quite obviously, Adams believed that the launching of a free and independent nation was an act of such worth as to warrant regular celebration. It might be noted in passing that the inauguration of a new enterprise is always an act of hope. It is only at some future time, when folk have seen how an organization, institution, or nation has turned out—when growth and achievement became history—that there can be a confident celebration of the founding day.

But there is also an almost contradictory reason for anniversary celebrations. Instead of perpetuating ancient values they are often viewed as the occasion for a new beginning. As James Russell Lowell wrote, "New occasions teach new duties; time makes ancient good uncouth." So, anniversaries offer the opportunity to reflect on the path traveled, where a people are, where they wish to go next, and what's the best way to get there.

Anniversaries are also a time to honor the people who started the enterprise. Even if it is a romantic conception, we usually think of these pioneers as the hardier sort, whose lives and efforts are worthy of emulation.

Perhaps there is in anniversary celebrations something of an attempt to recapture or to *capture* the drama and emotion of the founding days. Nostalgia, even if it is variously felt, seems to be pleasant to the human spirit. Even if it is tinged with sadness, it is still treasured. Just call to mind (if you can) the lyrics of "Love's Old Sweet Song."

We must confess that part of the motivation for celebrating anniversaries is just plain, human pride. It doesn't matter whether one was among the founding party or joined the institution much later. If the organization has had a long, distinctive history, one may say, "I helped to put that together" or "That eminent institution values me enough to make me a part of it." The power of human pride cannot be underestimated as the motor of an institutional machine.

And we cannot ignore the commercial motivation behind anniversary celebrations. It is not just business organizations that stress, "One Hundred and Fifty Years of Faithful Service to the Community." Organizations of all varieties—churches, clubs, social and humane societies, *and* schools—use anniversaries to emphasize their legitimacy, durability, and trustworthiness and use the occasion to appeal for continued—and expanded—patronage by the public. All of these motivations are *implicit* in the celebration. There is real value in making them *explicit*. To be consciously aware of *why* we're celebrating would make the occasion more meaningful and enjoyable.

76. Which of the following statements are *neither supported nor contradicted by* the passage?

    (A) After 50 years, the Jews celebrated their leaving Egypt.
    (B) God spoke to Moses to initiate the celebration.
    (C) Most celebrations are joyous events.
    (D) Celebrations are a part of civilizations.

77. Which of the following statements is/are *supported by* the passage?

    I.   There is a logical reason for celebrating.
    II. Round-numbered year festivities are usually special.
    III. Our mathematical system depends on round numbers that enhance remembering events.
    IV. Independence Day should be observed for always.

    (A) I, II, and III
    (B) I and III
    (C) II and IV
    (D) IV only

78. The passage either asserts or implies that:

    (A) Founding Day is an act of hope.
    (B) history will be the determining factor.
    (C) a celebration is a renewal.
    (D) all of the above are valid.

79. In the course of providing historical precedents for celebrations of various kinds, the author reveals his or her personal attitudes related to celebrations in general. Which of the following views of the author emerge from the passage?

    (A) Nostalgia is good for humankind.
    (B) Pioneers are usually worthy of emulating.
    (C) People need a time to reflect.
    (D) All of the above are viewed positively by the author.

80. The author believes:

    (A) that a sense of being a part of history is productive.
    (B) entrepreneurship is part and parcel of a festival.
    (C) justification for existence is a motive for anniversary celebrations.
    (D) all of the above statements.

Passage VI (Questions 81–86)

Myths and fairy tales are most often told and remembered as plots (who did what to whom and what happened). But they actually endure in our continuing imaginations because of the "character" of the characters involved. If you place Oedipus into Daedalus's story, or Narcissus into Odysseus's story, you won't have the same story. Cinderella wouldn't do what Red Riding Hood does, nor would Jack-in-the-Beanstalk do what Hansel does. The character doesn't merely *follow* a plot line—the plot happens *because* of the particular human weaknesses and strengths of the particular character.

Underlying all these characters, of course, are larger issues, such as greed and selfishness, pride, acceptance of fate, compassion, cleverness, and risk. But what distinguishes one character from another are the choices, actions, and consequences of those choices peculiar to the individual character. When a teenager (like Theseus) is faced with a dilemma of State (his country must pay human sacrifice tribute in the form of seven youths and seven maidens to a more powerful country), there are a number of choices or decisions he can make. He can ignore the whole problem (it's not his fault, after all); he can take personal responsibility for solving the problem, either because he wants to be a Big Hero or because (as son of the King) he must learn to face problems if he expects to inherit the throne; or he might simply be in a boastful or adventuresome mood when the idea crosses his mind. Once Theseus commits himself to the task (destroy-ing the Minotaur, symbol of the opposing country's power), there are further choices: He can take all the credit but allow his underlings to do all the hard work; he can sacrifice himself on a seemingly impossible task (finding and destroying the Minotaur in its Labyrinth); or he can take advantage of a girl's love for him (agreeing to take Ariadne away with him if she gives him the secret of the Labyrinth). And once he's solved the primary problem of the Minotaur, there are even more choices: does he really want to take Ariadne back with him as he promised? Should he take time out to change the color of his ship's sails (as he promised his father) when he's being pursued by an angry enemy? Because he doesn't change the sails, he directly causes his father's suicide; because he chooses to leave Ariadne behind, he indirectly sets up an even more tragic chain of events in his own life that won't become apparent for a number of years. The series of choices and consequent actions that Theseus takes thus becomes the plot we know, only after we look back on it.

Young people still face seemingly impossible tasks today. These might involve the State (expose corruption, act on one's conscience, protest the military draft), or they might involve other people and relationships (whether to live up to an agreement made under different circumstances, such as an engagement, marriage, contract, job, project). People still have to decide whether to try to save a sinking ship, or whether to catch the first lifeboat; whether to admit a harsh truth or to avoid it (lie, exaggerate, use diplomacy, pass blame, run away). Can or should one be loyal to a person or way of life one no longer cares about? What are the risks and benefits of any decision? Does it still "pay" to be a hero, or do other occupations seem more lucrative? Is the difference between a hero and a fool merely success? Should you get involved with someone else's problem or shrug it off? Should you take a stance or merely cast your eyes to heaven and wait for divine intervention and fate? Also, it isn't always easy to separate personal ego or animal needs from more "noble" desires to bring about social or human justice, and often the two run along together for a considerable distance before they part ways. These are matters for contemporary characters in contemporary stories, but these are the same matters Theseus dealt with. We still have our Minotaurs, escape ships, labyrinths, tasks, Ariadnes, and Theseuses, though the forms are different each time. That's why myth and fairy tales (based on folktales or myths) are called Universal.

Adapted from Sally V. Doud, "Essay Test Introduction," VCU, Spring 1990.

81. The most appropriate title for this essay would be:

    (A) The Role of Fate in Contemporary Life.
    (B) Red Riding Hood and Theseus: Two Versions of the Same Character.
    (C) Universal Aspects of Everyday Experience.
    (D) Myth Is Dead.

82. According to the author of the passage:

    (A) people today do not face impossible tasks as did the characters in the Greek myths.
    (B) the outcomes of fairy tales and myths are rarely determined by choices the characters have made.
    (C) myths and fairy tales are universal because the choices that are faced by characters in them are similar to the ones faced by people of all times.
    (D) there are fewer choices for heroes today than there were for the heroes of Greek myths.

83. One might infer from this passage that:

    (A) Theseus is responsible for the death of his father.
    (B) one should not sacrifice himself to a seemingly impossible task.
    (C) Theseus should not be blamed for the suicide of his father.
    (D) in making decisions, individuals should wait for divine intervention.

84. According to the author of the passage:

    (A) plots proceed as a pattern of cause and effect events.
    (B) plots are always the same from one story to the next.
    (C) plots are merely an accumulated series of events.
    (D) plots are the most important part of any story.

85. The most important part of the passage is:

    (A) that we not forget the story of Theseus and his adventures surrounding the Labyrinth.
    (B) stories change, but the realm of human choices remains the same.
    (C) universality deals with language.
    (D) we are always punished for our misdoing.

86. According to the passage, the primary problem facing Theseus is:

    (A) how he can reward Ariadne for giving him the secret of the Labyrinth.
    (B) the killing of the Minotaur.
    (C) the changing of his ship's sails so as to inform his father of his fate.
    (D) how he will rid himself of guilt after he has killed the Minotaur.

Passage VII (Questions 87–92)

Caricature is a device satirists commonly use in their work. Why is it so common? Caricatures grab readers' or viewers' attention; moreover, they are funny. Caricatures distort reality and that distortion is often hilarious. An audience that will appreciate the caricature recognizes the incongruity between the real object and the satirist's portrayal of it. They also understand why the satirist is attacking this object. In effect, the appreciative audience says, "Of course, this is all out of proportion. But, you know, he's got a point there. This person (place, thing) really does have a weak spot." Meanwhile, as they muse on the message, they are reacting to the incongruities, the exaggeration, with anything from a wry smile to convulsive laughter.

What exactly is a caricature? I would define it as a pictorial (drawing, painting, sculpture, collage, mask, dramatization) or verbal (poem, essay, descriptive sketch in fiction or nonfiction) exaggeration of an object (person, place, thing, situation, organization). The distortion must be based on a fact about the object, for example, bushy eyebrows. The artist or writer just stretches that fact all out of shape; the politician's eyebrows are not *that* bushy. He plays with his object as if it were a glob of silly putty or bread dough. He kneads it, rolls it up, flattens it, stretches it out, shapes it any way to suit his fancy. He must not go so far as to make the object completely unrecognizable, but he has a lot of room to play with his object.

Adapted from Rebecca Dale, "Caricature," VCU, Spring 1989.

One thing that happens when an object becomes so pliable in the hands of an artist or writer is that the object instantly plummets in value. It becomes ridiculous, at least to some extent, and not as important as it had been. Often the satirist's purpose is to show that the object, because of people's vanity or hypocrisy, is considered more valuable than it really is. By doing a caricature of it, he deflates its value. Furthermore, the artist or writer shows that he has control over the object, at least temporarily. He is exerting his power by the way he portrays the object. It's as if he's saying, "Ah ha! You thought you were so important. But look at you now, the way *I've* made you. I'm calling the shots now . . . ." Needless to say, the people being caricatured rarely think kindly about the creators of the satire—not only do the caricatures deflate their importance, but also the caricatures show that the people who are being satirized don't have control over their image.

It's important to note that one of the effects of caricature is to dehumanize the person being caricatured. This dehumanization is even there in the language of how we discuss satire: the word "object." As the audience, we often enjoy seeing a vaunted person being devalued by caricature and agree that the devaluation is often deserved. But does the means justify the end? Caricatures certainly work, creators and audience have a lot of fun while criticizing the object. However, a side effect is that caricatures serve as one out of many ways we tend in our society to dehumanize each other. Rarely does the creator or the audience notice this; we're caught up in the laughter and disregard any objections to a caricature by saying, "It's just a joke. Don't you have a sense of humor? He (object of caricature) deserved it anyway." Yes, it's just a joke. But also, yes, it makes it easier for us to view people as objects to be manipulated, vilified, destroyed. Think back to the caricatures we did of the Japanese in World War II. It is much easier to work up enthusiasm for killing people when they are depicted as hideous monsters. Hitler readily used caricature to depict Jews as less-than-human animals.

Exaggeration, playing the extremes against each other, distortion—these are all elements of caricature. Caricatures are a quite effective means for satire—creators enjoy creating them, audiences respond eagerly to them, they make their point. However, they are not innocuous little creatures; they can be used to stereotype and dehumanize people. Also, as we use them casually day after day, we sometimes don't even notice anymore that they are caricatures. The cartoon character becomes the norm. Wiley the Coyote makes falling off cliffs, holding an exploding piece of dynamite, or being crushed with huge stones seem like normal, everyday events; he is just a little frazzled after each episode. Numbed day after day with caricatures, might we begin to think of life as a cartoon?

87. Which of the following statements about caricatures is NOT *supported by* the passage?

(A) Caricatures do not have to be pictures.
(B) People who are satirized often lose the public's respect.
(C) People who are satirized often deserve the ridicule.
(D) Caricatures can be based on falsehoods.

88. According to the passage, people laugh at caricatures because:

(A) bushy eyebrows and other such facial quirks are naturally funny.
(B) we laugh at people who are vain and hypocritical.
(C) we recognize the incongruities between the object and the caricature of it.
(D) the people who create caricatures have a good sense of humor.

89. Which of the following statements best sums up the author's opinion of caricatures?

(A) Caricatures are hilarious.
(B) Caricatures reveal the hypocrisies of our society.
(C) Caricatures have insidious effects.
(D) People who do not appreciate caricatures have no sense of humor.

90. According to the passage, caricatures are effective forms of satire because:

I. ridicule devalues an object.
II. caricatures appeal to many kinds of audiences.
III. the satirist controls his object's public image.

(A) I and II.
(B) II and III
(C) I and III
(D) I, II, and III

91. According to the passage, caricatures can be dangerous because:

    (A) people satiated with exaggeration may not recognize the norm.
    (B) a person who is satirized may not deserve the ridicule.
    (C) caricatures divert our attention from real problems.
    (D) caricatures give satirists too much power over society.

92. Of the following titles, which is most appropriate for the passage?

    (A) The Cruel Art of Caricature
    (B) Caricature and Understatement
    (C) Caricature: Exaggeration as a Satirist's Tool
    (D) Cartoon Art

WRITING SAMPLE

TIME—2 ESSAYS
      60 MINUTES (30 MINUTES/TOPIC)

Directions: This is a test of your writing skills. The test consists of two parts. You will have 30 minutes to complete each part. Use your time efficiently. Before you begin writing each of your responses, read the assignment carefully to understand exactly what you are being asked to do. Because this is a test of your writing skills, your response to each part should be as well organized and clearly written as you can make it in the time allotted.

93.   Consider this statement:

> **A wise man sees as much as he ought, not as much as he can.**
>
>   **Montaigne**

Write a unified essay in which you perform the following tasks. Explain what the above quotation means. Describe a specific situation in which a wise person sees as much as he can, not as much as he ought. Discuss what you think determines the limits that should and should not be placed on vision.

94.   Consider this statement:

> **There is properly no history; only biography.**
>
>   **Emerson**

Write a unified essay in which you perform the following tasks. Explain what you think the above statement means. Describe a specific situation in which there would, in fact, be history, whether or not there were biography. Discuss what you think determines the relationship between history and biography.

BIOLOGICAL SCIENCES

TIME—70 MINUTES FOR 52 QUESTIONS

Directions: The following questions or incomplete statements are in groups. Preceding each series of questions or statements is a paragraph or a short explanatory statement, a formula or set of formulas, or a definition. Read the written material and then answer the questions or complete the statements. Select the ONE BEST ANSWER for each question and indicate your selection by marking the corresponding letter of your choice on the Answer Form. Eliminate those alternatives you know to be incorrect and then select an answer from among the remaining alternatives.

Passage I (Questions 95–100)

The diagram illustrates a typical neuron, the basic unit of the nervous system, located in a spinal (dorsal root) ganglion. Neurons connect with each other and in that manner an impulse is conducted and transmitted throughout the body. Two types of cell processes are indicated.

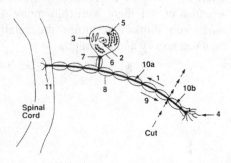

95.   An impulse on the skin will be picked up by:

   (A)   4.
   (B)   6.
   (C)   7.
   (D)   10.

96.   The genetic material of the cell is located in:

   (A)   2.
   (B)   3.
   (C)   5.
   (D)   7.

97.   Protein synthesis is carried out under the direction of:

   (A)   3 in 5.
   (B)   2 in 3.
   (C)   2 in 5.
   (D)   2 in 7.

A person has been in an accident and the physician is conducting a neurological examination. Sensation is lost over several fingers and the examiner fears that a nerve has been cut. Note the cut indication on the diagram preceeding question 95.

98.   Which process would completely degenerate?

   (A)   11
   (B)   8
   (C)   10a
   (D)   10b

99.   Retrograde degeneration would be visible in:

   (A)   2.
   (B)   3.
   (C)   6.
   (D)   10b.

100.   The impulse in the neuron is normally conducted in which direction?

   (A)   9
   (B)   1
   (C)   Neither 9 nor 1
   (D)   Both 9 and 1

Passage II (Questions 101–106)

The purpose of these experiments is to illustrate the action of both active and passive driving forces on the absorption of solutions of hemoglobin, Ringer's solution, $MgSO_4$, xylose, and glucose from the lumen of the small intestines *in vivo*.

Fluid can be absorbed from the small intestine even when the luminal solution is isotonic Ringer's. The absence of a net passive driving force for water uptake between lumen and blood indicates that active processes are involved. The active transport is *not* on the water itself but rather on sodium chloride. Active sodium transport from the epithelial cells renders the intercellular spaces sufficiently hypertonic to create osmotic driving forces for water movement out of the lumen.

Glucose is transported from the lumen by means of a specific carrier. The carrier has a site for the sugar and for sodium. It is the sodium gradient across the apical cell membrane that provides the energy for glucose entry. The sodium gradient is maintained by the active extrusion of sodium from the cells. The carrier shows typical saturation kinetics. In the case of glucose, the Km for absorption is 2mM, when sodium levels are 145mM. By contrast, the pentose, xylose, is far less effective as a substrate for this carrier. At the same level of Na, its Km is about 100 mM.

Ions such as Mg^{2+} and SO^{2-}_4, which are poorly absorbed, behave toward the intestinal epithelium almost as if it were a semipermeable membrane. Thus, passive osmotic forces play a predominant role in determining the magnitude and direction of fluid movement. A similar statement can be made about intact proteins such as hemoglobin. These are ordinarily impermeable solutes.

By measuring the changes in fluid volume due to the presence of the test substances and by chemically analyzing for changes in the glucose, xylose, and hemoglobin concentration, data on how the *in vivo* intestine treats each substance will be obtained.

Experiment

In two rats, three successive 10 cm segments of intestine are tied off. Injected into the segments of rat one from proximal to distal were solutions of hemoglobin, Ringer's, and $MgSO_4$.

Injected into the segments of rat two from proximal to distal were solutions of xylose, Ringer's, and glucose. After one hour whatever fluid was present in the respective segments was withdrawn, and volumes recorded. Analysis for solutes present were conducted and percentage of absorption and recovery recorded.

101. From the "absorption from the intestine laboratory: when equal volumes of 100 mM of D-glucose or D-xylose are added in isotonic Ringer's solutions to isolated intestinal segments, the following would be expected (Km, glucose 2mM, xylose 100 mM).

   (A) Equal volumes would be absorbed in a one-hour incubation.
   (B) A greater volume absorbed from the xylose segment than for glucose.
   (C) A greater volume absorbed from the glucose segment than for xylose.
   (D) No volume change for either.

102. When 1 ml of a 1.8% solution of D-glucose was added to an intestinal segment in isotonic Ringer's solution and the total glucose analyzed at one hour, it was found that 1.8 mg was recovered. What percent of the D-glucose injected was absorbed or metabolized?

   (A) 1.8%
   (B) 1%
   (C) 10%
   (D) 90%

103. For the "absorption from the intestine laboratory," when a hemoglobin solution in water was injected into the isolated small intestine, at the end of one hour:

   (A) more hemoglobin would be recovered than injected because proteins are secreted into the intestine.
   (B) less hemoglobin was recovered because intact proteins are normally absorbed.
   (C) less hemoglobin was recovered because bleeding into the intestine would normally occur.
   (D) less hemoglobin was recovered because some hemoglobin was adsorbed on the surface of the mucosal lumen.

104. For the "absorption from the intestine laboratory," for injection of D-glucose in isotonic Ringer's solution, inhibition of glucose transport would occur when:

    I.   D-galactose was also added to the segment.
    II. sodium ion was replaced by a large cation.
    III. when L-glucose replaced D-glucose.
    IV. when an uncoupler of ATP synthesis (dinitrophenol) was added.

    (A) I, II, and III
    (B) I and III
    (C) II and IV
    (D) All are correct

105. For the "absorption from the intestine laboratory," when 25% MgSO$_4$ was injected into the isolated small intestine, the expected change was:

    (A) an increase in volume.
    (B) a decrease in volume.
    (C) no change in volume.

106. For the "absorption from the intestine laboratory," when a hemoglobin solution in water was injected into the isolated small intestine, the expected change was:

    (A) an increase in volume.
    (B) a decrease in volume.
    (C) no change in volume.

Passage III (Questions 107–113)

The schema of thyroxine formation is outlined below:

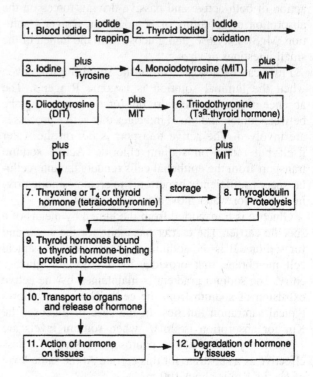

107. Chemically, thyroid hormones are:

    (A) iodotyrosines.
    (B) iodothyronines.
    (C) iodides.
    (D) iodines.

108. In proceeding from compound 3 to compound 4, the amino acid tyrosine is:

    (A) oxidized
    (B) reduced
    (C) iodinated.
    (D) synthesized.

109. During transport thyroid hormones are inactive because they are:

   (A) in the form of thyroglobutin.
   (B) free hormones.
   (C) protein-bound.
   (D) on red blood cells.

110. Untreated goiter is associated with:

   (A) hyperthyroidism.
   (B) hypothyroidism.
   (C) euthyroidism.
   (D) A, B, and C.

111. TSH:

   (A) is made up of two peptide chains (alpha and beta).
   (B) is released by the hypothalamus.
   (C) binds tightly to thyroid binding globulin (TBG).
   (D) secretion decreases upon exposure to the cold.

112. Involved in the regulation of the synthesis of thyroid hormone are

   (A) availability of iodide ions.
   (B) TSH.
   (C) negative feedback of circulating T_3 and T_4 at the level of the anterior pituitary (by down regulation of TRH receptors).
   (D) all of the above.

113. Which of the following describes the metabolic effect of thyroid hormone?

   (A) decreased myocardial beta adrenergic receptors
   (B) decreased BMR
   (C) increased oxygen consumption
   (D) increased plasma cholesterol

Passage IV (Questions 114–121)

Using a syringe containing heparin, 50 milliliters of blood were drawn from a healthy male volunteer. Following centrifugation, the "buffy coat" was removed and a lymphocyte-rich cell population was obtained by sedimentation through 2% Dextran. After washing in 0.9% saline, the lymphocytes were placed in cell culture tubes at a concentration of 5×10^6 cells/ml cell culture medium/tube. To one-half of the tubes was added 5 µg of phytohemagglutinin, a substance which causes lymphocytes to undergo mitosis. The other half of the tubes received no phytohemagglutinin. Radioactive tracers for RNA, DNA, and protein synthesis were then added to all tubes and aliquots removed at selected intervals. The following data were obtained:

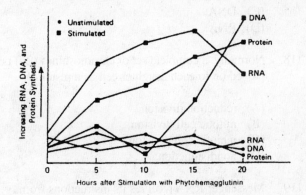

114. The purpose of this experiment was to:

   (A) determine the role of heparin in blood clotting.
   (B) determine the sequence of events in cells stimulated to undergo mitosis, and to compare these data to those gathered from unstimulated cells.
   (C) isolate a pure population of lymphocytes.
   (D) determine the lifespan of lymphocytes.

115. From these data it can be seen that increased:

   (A) RNA synthesis precedes increased protein synthesis.
   (B) DNA synthesis precedes increased protein synthesis.
   (C) protein synthesis precedes increased RNA synthesis.
   (D) DNA synthesis precedes increased RNA synthesis.

116. It may also be assumed that:

(A) DNA synthesis is dependent on previous RNA synthesis.
(B) protein synthesis is dependent on previous DNA synthesis.
(C) RNA synthesis is dependent on previous protein synthesis.
(D) unstimulated lymphocytes synthesize RNA, DNA, and protein at a low rate.

117. The smallest unit possessing the capability to maintain life and to reproduce is:

(A) an organ.
(B) a cell.
(C) DNA.
(D) RNA.

118. Normally, a complete set of chromosomes (2*n*) is passed on to each daughter cell as a result of:

(A) reduction division.
(B) mitotic cell division.
(C) meiotic cell division.
(D) nondisjunction.

119. Messenger RNA receives its instructions from:

(A) ribosomes.
(B) endoplasmic reticulum.
(C) DNA in the nucleus.
(D) cytoplasm.

120. During which phase of the mitotic cycle do the two chromatids split apart and start migration toward the poles of the spindle?

(A) prophase
(B) metaphase
(C) anaphase
(D) telophase

121. During metaphase of mitosis:

(A) there is a dissolution of the chromosomal material.
(B) the centrioles with asters are at the opposite poles.
(C) the cell membrane starts to reappear.
(D) the nuclear membrane disappears.

Questions 122–125 are NOT based on a descriptive passage.

122. Which of the following organelles occur in eukaryotic cells but not in prokaryotic cells?

(A) ribosomes
(B) mitochondria
(C) cell walls
(D) flagella

123. During interphase in a typical eukaryotic cell, the DNA coding for ribosomal RNA is:

(A) in a single location on a single chromosome in the center of the nucleus.
(B) in multiple chromosomes scattered through the euchromatin in the nucleus.
(C) in multiple chromosomes scattered in the heterochromatin along the inner surface of the nuclear envelope.
(D) in multiple chromosomes around the perimeter of the nucleolus.

124. Epithelial tissues may function in:

(A) protection by serving as a barrier.
(B) secretion.
(C) absorption.
(D) all of these.

125. Neutrophils and monocyte derivatives are responsible for _____ in loose connective tissues.

(A) collagen synthesis
(B) antibody synthesis
(C) phagocytosis of bacteria
(D) killing virus-infected cells

Passage V (Questions 126–135)

The liver from a rat was gently homogenized in buffered sucrose solution using a Dounce homogenizer (which does not break most membranous organelles in cells). The homogenate was layered over a sucrose gradient and centrifuged for four hours at 100,000 xg. The sucrose gradient was then collected as a series of fractions. Each fraction was analyzed for DNA concentration, RNA concentration, cytochrome oxidase activity, acid phosphatase activity, and cytochrome P-450 concentration. Concentrations and enzyme activities are given as relative values, with the fraction giving the highest value for each component being shown as 100 and all other values for that component being scaled relative to the highest value.

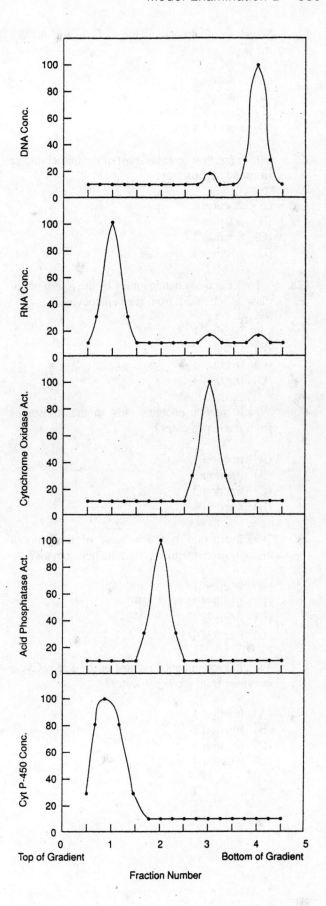

126. Which fraction contains most of the nuclei from the hepatocytes?

    (A) fraction 1
    (B) fraction 2
    (C) fraction 3
    (D) fraction 4

127. Which fraction contains most of the mitochondria from the hepatocytes?

    (A) fraction 1
    (B) fraction 2
    (C) fraction 3
    (D) fraction 4

128. Which fraction contains most of the rough endoplasmic reticulum from the hepatocytes?

    (A) fraction 1
    (B) fraction 2
    (C) fraction 3
    (D) fraction 4

129. Which fraction contains most of the lysosomes from the hepatocytes?

    (A) fraction 1
    (B) fraction 2
    (C) fraction 3
    (D) fraction 4

130. Which fraction contains most of the smooth endoplasmic reticulum from the hepatocytes?

    (A) fraction 1
    (B) fraction 2
    (C) fraction 3
    (D) fraction 4

131. Which fraction contains most of the Krebs Cycle enzymes from the hepatocytes?

    (A) fraction 1
    (B) fraction 2
    (C) fraction 3
    (D) fraction 4

132. Which fraction should contain most of the newly synthesized plasma proteins from the hepatocytes?

    (A) fraction 1
    (B) fraction 2
    (C) fraction 3
    (D) fraction 4

133. Which fraction should appear much larger when isolated from pancreatic exocrine cells than when isolated from hepatocytes? Assume that the assays used in the experiment shown here are used to quantitate the fractions.

    (A) fraction 1
    (B) fraction 2
    (C) fraction 3
    (D) fraction 4

134. Which fraction should appear much larger when isolated from monocytes or connective tissue macrophages than when isolated from hepatocytes? Assume that the assays used in the experiment shown here are used to quantitate the fractions.

    (A) fraction 1
    (B) fraction 2
    (C) fraction 3
    (D) fraction 4

135. Which fraction should appear much larger when isolated from proximal convoluted tubule cells from the kidney than when isolated from hepatocytes? Assume that the assays used in the experiment shown here are used to quantitate the fractions.

    (A) fraction 1
    (B) fraction 2
    (C) fraction 3
    (D) fraction 4

Passage VI (Questions 136–140)

The citric acid cycle (Krebs cycle, tricarboxylic cycle) is the final metabolic pathway for glucose, many amino acids, and fatty acids. The enzymes for the pathway are located in the inner mitochondrial membrane. The electrons from the oxidation of these metabolic fuels are conserved in the formation of reducing equivalents, such as NADH or $FADH_2$ for eventual reoxidation in the respiratory assembly to generate ATP by oxidative phosphorylation. Whereas glucose and fatty acids produce acetyl CoA for oxidation to recover the bond energy and produce CO_2, some amino acids have different routes of catabolism including acetyl CoA, other metabolites of the pathway, and pyruvate formation. The citric acid cycle can accept metabolites at places other than acetyl CoA and is able to supply metabolites for biosynthesis such as in the synthesis of porphyrins or amino acids. However, net glucose cannot be synthesized from acetyl CoA entering the cycle. The reactions have many similarities such as hydration—dehydration or oxidation, particularly of secondary alcohols to ketone. For every mole of acetyl CoA entering the cycle and condensing with oxaloacetate, 12 moles of ATP and two moles of CO_2 are formed and a mole of oxaloacetate is recovered. The rate of the cycle is controlled by energy levels of the cell at specific enzymatic points including the formation of citric acid and the formation of α-ketoglutarate.

136. For one mole of acetyl CoA entering the Krebs (TCA) cycle (coupled to oxidative phosphorylation):

   (A) one mole of carbon dioxide and 38 ATP are formed.
   (B) two moles of carbon dioxide and 38 ATP are formed.
   (C) two moles of carbon dioxide and 24 ATP are formed.
   (D) two moles of carbon dioxide and 12 ATP are formed.

137. All of the following are similar pairs of types of reactions starting with pyruvate EXCEPT:

   (A) isocitrate to oxalosuccinate; malate to oxaloacetate.
   (B) alpha ketoglutarate to succinyl CoA; acetyl CoA to pyruvate.
   (C) cis-aconitase to isocitrate; fumarate to malate.
   (D) pyruvate to acetyl CoA; alpha ketoglutarate to succinyl CoA.

138. The citric acid cycle provides biosynthetic intermediates (net) for the following EXCEPT:

   (A) acetyl CoA to oxaloacetate.
   (B) acetyl CoA to malonyl CoA.
   (C) succinyl CoA to porphyrins.
   (D) oxaloacetate to aspartate.

139. All of the following are metabolic functions or possible interactions of the tricarboxylic acid cycle EXCEPT:

   (A) decreased activity when ATP levels are high.
   (B) control of glycolysis.
   (C) accepting acetyl CoA from fatty acids, glucose, and some amino acids.
   (D) net synthesis of glucose occurs from acetyl CoA.

140. All of the following are correct about the citric acid cycle EXCEPT:

   (A) active in the mature red blood cell in humans.
   (B) occurs in the mitochondria.
   (C) provides about 24 ATP/moles of glucose (coupled to ox-phos).
   (D) when acetyl CoA amount increases it may increase gluconeogenesis from other carbon atoms.

Passage VII (Questions 141–143)

The epiphyseal cartilage plate is very sensitive to somatotrophin (growth hormone) and, therefore, can be used as an assay for this compound. Species variations exist and other hormones such as estrogen, thyroxine, and several antibiotics also have an effect upon cartilage growth. The assay must be carried out on hypophysectomized animals.

The following experiments were conducted as can be seen from the table:

Injections/Day Test Groups	No. of Animals	Cartilage Growth in μ	
		1 Injection Daily	2 (1/2 amount each time)
Control (normal) (saline)	20 (10/injecting group)	100	100
Hyphophysectomized (saline)	20	60	60
Hypox + 100 mg STH	20	150	160
Hypox + 300 mg STH	20	180	195
Stressed normal animals (saline)	20	175	190
Hypox + stressed (saline)	20	50	50
Stressed normal + 100 mg STH	20	200	210
Hypox, stressed + 100 mg STH	20	110	120

141. The reason the assay must be carried out on hypophysectomized rats is:

(A) just to add another sophisticated method to the experiment.
(B) because the pituitary produces its own growth hormone and it might interfere with the assay.
(C) to study the pituitary composition of growth hormone.
(D) to obtain the animals' own growth hormone.

142. Which conditions produced the highest cartilage growth rate?

(A) stressed normal + 100 mg STH
(B) stressed normal
(C) hypox + 100 mg STH
(D) hypox + 300 mg STH

143. Based on this data, the normal level of STH in an intact unstressed animal is probably:

(A) less than 100 mg/day.
(B) approximately 100 mg/day.
(C) approximately 200 mg/day.
(D) approximately 300 mg/day.

Questions 144–146 are NOT based on a descriptive passage.

144. In the reaction sequence used in breakdown of glycogen in the liver or muscle—glycogen $\rightarrow$ glucose-l-phosphate $\rightarrow$ glucose-6-phosphate $\rightarrow$ glucose—the first step is:

(A) catalyzed by phosphorylase.
(B) catalyzed by pepsin.
(C) catalyzed by pancreatic amylase.
(D) nonenzymatic.

145. A metabolic process that produces energy to convert ADP + phosphate into ATP is the:

(A) production of fructose and glucose from sucrose.
(B) production of fatty acids and glycerol from triglycerides.
(C) production of CO_2 and water from fatty acids.
(D) production of steroids from acetate.

146. A negative iodoform test (i.e., no yellow precipitate) will be the result when $NaOH + I_2$ is reacted with:

(A) 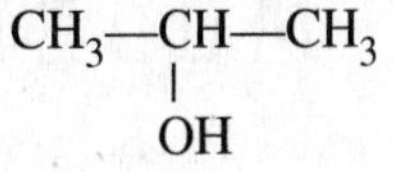
$$CH_3{-}\underset{\underset{OH}{|}}{CH}{-}CH_3$$

(B) 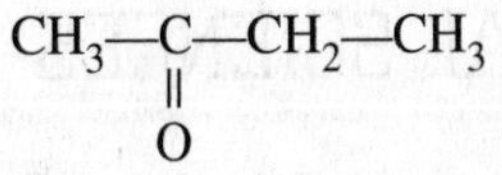
$$CH_3{-}\underset{\underset{O}{\|}}{C}{-}CH_2{-}CH_3$$

(C)
$$\varnothing{-}\overset{\overset{O}{\|}}{C}{-}CH_3$$

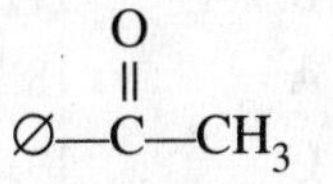

(D) 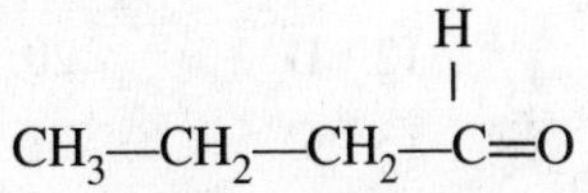
$$CH_3{-}CH_2{-}CH_2{-}\underset{}{C}\overset{\overset{H}{|}}{=}O$$

STOP

END OF TEST

Answer Key

MODEL EXAMINATION D

PHYSICAL SCIENCES

1. B	9. B	17. B	25. A	33. C	41. B	49. A
2. C	10. A	18. A	26. D	34. D	42. C	50. D
3. D	11. C	19. A	27. C	35. D	43. B	51. C
4. D	12. D	20. D	28. D	36. C	44. D	52. B
5. B	13. C	21. B	29. A	37. B	45. C	
6. C	14. C	22. B	30. B	38. A	46. D	
7. D	15. D	23. B	31. B	39. C	47. A	
8. A	16. A	24. C	32. C	40. A	48. C	

VERBAL REASONING

53. C	59. B	65. A	71. D	77. C	83. A	89. C
54. C	60. D	66. D	72. C	78. D	84. A	90. C
55. D	61. D	67. B	73. A	79. D	85. B	91. A
56. C	62. A	68. C	74. B	80. D	86. B	92. B
57. B	63. B	69. D	75. B	81. C	87. D	
58. C	64. A	70. A	76. C	82. C	88. C	

WRITING SAMPLE

93. See page 550 for a sample essay.

94. See page 552 for a sample essay.

BIOLOGICAL SCIENCES

95. A	103. D	111. A	119. C	127. C	135. C	143. A
96. A	104. D	112. D	120. C	128. A	136. D	144. A
97. C	105. A	113. C	121. B	129. B	137. B	145. C
98. D	106. B	114. B	122. B	130. A	138. A	146. D
99. A	107. B	115. A	123. D	131. C	139. D	
100. B	108. C	116. D	124. D	132. A	140. A	
101. C	109. C	117. B	125. C	133. A	141. B	
102. D	110. D	118. B	126. D	134. B	142. A	

ANSWERS EXPLAINED FOR MODEL EXAMINATION D

Physical Sciences

1. **(B)** The electron configuration is found by summing the electrons starting from the $1s$ orbital.

2. **(C)** The reduction half reaction is $Na^+ + e^- \to$ Na, $E° = -2.71$ V. The oxidation half reaction is $2Cl^- \to Cl_2 + 2e^-$. The reaction potential E $=$ $E_{reduction} + E_{oxidation}$. From this, -4.07 V $= -2.71$ V $+ 1.36$ V. Thus, $2Cl^- \to Cl_2 + 2e^-$, E $= -1.36$ V. The reduction potential for chlorine is the same in magnitude as the oxidation of chlorine but with the opposite sign.

3. **(D)** Oxidation occurs at the anode. Since Cl^- loses electrons (an increase in oxidation state), it is oxidized.

4. **(D)** The second reaction produces NaOH as well as hydrogen and chlorine. The NaOH solution will be basic. pH $= 9$ is the only basic pH listed.

5. **(B)** The heat of fusion is the heat required to change from a solid to a liquid.

6. **(C)** Sodium and chlorine are present as ions and so form ionic bonds.

7. **(D)** Sodium chloride dissociates completely in solution and so is a strong electrolyte.

8. **(A)** This is the definition of equilibrium constant. Note that the coefficients in the reaction equation become exponents in the equilibrium equation.

9. **(B)** When the resultants on the right are written in the numerator, a small number such as this indicates that the reaction as written will be favored to go toward the left.

10. **(A)** Five moles of gas are being converted to two moles of gas. Increased pressure will improve reaction toward the right, thus relieving the pressure (Principle of LeChatelier).

11. **(C)** At STP, a mole of any gas occupies 22.4 liters. Three moles times 22.4 liters equals 67.2 liters.

12. **(D)** Equilibrium constant indicates the concentrations at equilibrium. It does not deal with the rate in reaching equilibrium.

13. **(C)** A catalyst does not affect the equilibrium of a reaction, only the rate.

14. **(C)** Both balls have the same vertical acceleration, $g = 9.8$ m/sec^2, because there is no air resistance. Starting from rest they fall equal distances in equal times: $y = 1/2\ gt^2$.

15. **(D)** The horizontal velocity of the second ball is (10 m/sec) (COS 30°) $= 8.7$ m/sec, so it takes it more than 1 s to reach the wall.

16. **(A)** The easier way to solve this problem is to equate the work done against friction to the loss of kinetic energy of the masses, i.e.: $F_f\ x = 1/2\ mv^2$, where $F_f = \mu\ N = \mu$ mg where N is the "normal" force (equal to the weight in this case). Solving for $x = v^2/(2\ \mu\ g) = 2$ m for *both* bodies. An alternative solution is to calculate the frictional force and the deceleration. One can then use the equations for uniformly accelerated motion to find the distance. The methods are completely equivalent.

17. **(B)** It is possible to calculate the velocities exactly. The initial gravitational potential energy of the block and the ball are converted entirely into kinetic energy at the bottom of the incline. However, part of the kinetic energy of the ball is in the form of rotational kinetic energy about the ball's center of mass. Therefore, at the bottom of the incline, the velocity of the ball's center of mass is less than the linear velocity of the sliding block's center of mass. Understanding this concept, the question can be answered without calculating the velocities. One can do the actual calculations as follows:

    Ball: $mgh = 1/2\ mv^2 + 1/2\ I\ \omega^2$

    where I is the moment of inertia (of a sphere) and ω is the angular velocity. Substituting $I = 2/5\ mr^2$ and $v = r\omega$, one can solve for v.

    Ball: $v = \sqrt{(10-7)gh} = 2.646$ m/sec.

    For the block,
    Block: $mgh = 1/2\ mv^2$ and $V = \sqrt{2gh}$
    $= 3.13$ m/sec.

18. **(A)** At terminal velocity (regardless of the actual terminal velocity), the upward frictional force of air resistance is equal to the downward weight. The net force is zero, $F_f - mg = 0$. We find that:

$$F_f = 0.6 \times 9.8 = 5.9 \text{ N.}$$

19. **(A)** Power is the rate of doing work; 1 watt = 1 joule/sec. This student is using 730 joules each second. In 10 minutes the total energy expended is 438,000 J. The volume of oxygen consumed is 438,000 joules × 1L/20,000 joules = 22 L.

20. **(D)** The desired loss of 2.3 kg of fat requires an energy expenditure of 2.3 kg × 1000 g/kg × 39,700 joule/g = 91,310,000 joules. Because 630 W = 630 joule/sec, the time required is $t = (91,310,000)/630$ joule/sec = 144,935 sec or about 40 hours.

21. **(B)** The excess intake per day is 1100 kcal. In 28 days the excess will be $1100 \times 28 = 30,800$ kcal. From the energy oxidation values for fats, (30,800)/9.5 kcal/g = 3242 grams.

22. **(B)** The gauge pressure in the foot is higher than at the level of the aorta. (This is the reason blood pressure is taken with the cuff on the upper arm at the level of the aorta.) The 1.35 m height difference causes "added pressure," $P' = dgy$, where d is the density of the blood. Thus:

$$P' = 1050 \text{ kg/m}^3 \times 9.8 \text{ m/sec}^2 \times 1.35 \text{ m}$$
$$= 13,900 \text{ N/m}^2$$

Converting P' to mm Hg gives 13,900 N/m² × 750 mm Hg/1 × 10^5 N/m² = 105 mm Hg. Since this *adds* to the aortic pressure of 100 mm Hg, the gauge pressure in the foot will be 205 mm Hg.

23. **(B)** A metabolic rate of 350 W for 4 hours is a total energy expenditure of 350 joules/sec × 6 hr × 3600 sec/hr = 5,040,000 joules. The oxygen converted to energy is 5,040,000 joules/20,000 joules/L = 252 L. But one must actually inhale 4 times as much because of the 25% conversion efficiency. Then:

$$252 \text{ L}/0.25 = 1000 \text{ L.}$$

24. **(C)** The current can be found from Ohm's law:

$$V = IR$$

where R is the resistor or resistors across which the voltage, V, is applied.

$$I = V/R = 10 \text{ V}/4 \text{ } \Omega$$
$$= 2.5 \text{ A}$$

25. **(A)** When another 4-ohm resistor is added in parallel, the total equivalent resistance of the circuit is smaller and is calculated by the reciprocal rule:

$$1/R_P = 1/R_1 + 1/R_2$$
$$= 1/(4 \text{ } \Omega) + 1/(4 \text{ } \Omega)$$
$$R_P = 2 \text{ } \Omega$$

26. **(D)** The charge on the capacitor increases rapidly at first. As charge accumulates, the charge already on the capacitor inhibits the adding of more charge. After sufficient time, the charge will reach its maximum value. (At that point, the current will be zero.)

27. **(C)** The maximum charge is proportional to the maximum voltage, V:

$$q_{max} = CV$$
$$q_{max} = 2.0 \times 10^{-6} \text{ F} \times 10 \text{ V}$$
$$= 2.0 \times 10^{-5} \text{ C}$$

28. **(D)** In this simple circuit the maximum charge on the capacitor will depend only on the voltage (as in question 27). Increasing the equivalent resistance will slow the rate at which charge accumulates but will not change the final maximum charge.

29. **(A)** Knowing the atomic weight of hydrogen as 1.0 and oxygen as 16.0, the simplest proportions are one H and one O. Thus, the empirical formula is HO.

30. **(B)** The empirical formula has only a molecular weight of 17.0. Because the true molecular weight is determined as 34.0, the molecular formula must be a multiple, in this case H_2O_2.

31. **(B)** $H_2O_2 \rightleftharpoons H_2O + O_2$ (unbalanced)
    Note that we have two hydrogen atoms on each side. However, we have two oxygen atoms on the left side and three on the right. We may try to balance by multiplying H_2O and H_2O_2 by two. We now have

$$2 \text{ H}_2\text{O}_2 \rightleftharpoons 2 \text{ H}_2\text{O} + \text{O}_2$$

and find that this is balanced. As written, one mole of H_2O_2 will produce only 0.5 mole of O_2.

32. **(C)** As noted above, one mole of H_2O_2 will produce 0.5 mole of O_2. Because one mole of any gas occupies a volume of 22.4 liters at STP, 0.5 mole will occupy 11.2 liters.

33. **(C)** The LeChatelier principle indicates that if a system in equilibrium experiences a change in conditions, chemical reaction will occur to shift the equilibrium and reduce the effect of the changed conditions. Even if reactants and products are all in the gaseous state, there are two moles on the left side and three moles on the right side. Increased pressure would be expected to shift an equilibrium to the left.

34. **(D)** Although it is expected that this would be a first order reaction (rate = k $[H_2O_2]$) it cannot be predicted with certainty. The order of the reaction must be determined on the basis of experimental evidence.

35. **(D)** $_{92}U^{235}$ has $z = 92$, the charge number (number of protons) while $A = 235$ is the mass number, or number of nucleons (i.e., protons + neutrons). The emission of each alpha, α, comprised of He^4 nuclei, reduces the charge by 2 and reduces the mass by 4. Each beta, β, decay involves the emission of a negative electron from the nucleus. The nuclear charge increases by 1 unit but the mass number is unchanged, since the mass of the electron is negligible.

    The net change in z is $-14 + 4 = -10$, so the new $z = 82$.
    The net change in A is $-7 \times 4 = -28$, so the new $A = 207$.

36. **(C)** 100 years equals 1/16 of one half-life. The remaining radium is about 15/16 of one-half plus one-half ($15/16 \times 0.5 + 0.5$) or 0.969 curies. (The exact answer is 0.96 curies calculated using the exponential decay formula. See the explanation for Model Examination B, question 37.)

37. **(B)** The Ideal Gas Law is usually written $P_1V_1/T_1 = P_2V_2/T_2$. Since the volume is constant, $P_1V_1/T_1 = P_2V_2/T_2 = $ constant, so the pressure is directly proportional to the absolute temperature. The pressure increases by exactly the same factor as the temperature, namely 50%.

38. **(A)** Newton's Second Law states that if the force is constant, the acceleration is constant, $F = ma$. The slope of the velocity versus time graph is the acceleration. The slope is positive, sloping upward, since the velocity will increase. The correct graph is **A**.

39. **(C)** Three 3-ohm resistors in series will equal a 9-ohm resistor and is the highest possible value. Three 3-ohm resistors in parallel are equivalent to a 1-ohm resistor. Although there are six other possible combinations of the three resistors, no combination will equal more than 9 ohms or less than 1 ohm.

40. **(A)** Newton's Second Law will give the acceleration: $F = ma$, so $a = F/m = 67$ N/3 kg = 2 m/sec^2. The equation for constant acceleration (when the initial velocity is zero) yields $v^2 = 2as = 2 \times 2$ m/sec$^2 \times 4$ m = 16 m^2/sec^2. Then $v = 4.0$ m/sec. An alternate solution is to equate the work done by the net force to the gain in kinetic energy: $Fs = 1/2\ mv^2 - 0$, yielding the same result.

41. **(B)** As in an electrical circuit, Ohm's Law will apply: $V = IR$. Here $I = 120$ mA = 0.120 A. then $R = V/I = 120$ V/0. 120 A = 1000 ohms.

42. **(C)** The frequencies do not change when the wave travels in different media.

    $$\lambda = v/f$$

    One need not calculate the wavelength to answer the question. The longest wavelength occurs for the lowest-frequency signal (50 Hz) when it travels in the highest-speed medium (Al). Conversely, the 2.5 MHz signal traveling in air has the shortest wavelength.

43. **(B)**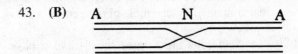

    The sketch shows the node-antinode (N-A) pattern for the fundamental (lowest) frequency of standing waves. Each node-to-antinode distance is always a quarter-wavelength. There are two quarter-wavelengths in the pipe length, $L = 0.25$ m. Thus, $\lambda = 0.5$ m. Also, $v = 340$ m/sec in air, so $f = v/\lambda = 340/0.5 = 680$ Hz.

44. **(D)** The US wave travels down and back to the wooden surface a distance of $2d$. Since velocity equals distance/time, $v = 2d/t$, so:

    $$d = vt/2 = \frac{1440 \text{ m/sec} \times 0.35 \times 10^{-3} \text{ sec}}{2} =$$
    $$1.44 \times 0.35/2 = 0.25 \text{ m}$$

45. **(C)** The student will hear a lower frequency according to the Doppler effect. A very general statement of the effect is:

$$f' = f(v \pm v_o)/(v \mp v_s)$$

where f' is the shifted frequency, f is the source frequency, v is the speed of sound, v_o is the observer's speed, and v_s is the source speed. One uses the lower signs for "separation." Here $v = 340$ m/s,

$$v_o = 0, \text{ and } v_s = 30 \text{ m/s}:$$
$$f' = f(v - v_o)/(v + v_s)$$
$$= 919 \text{ Hz}$$

46. **(D)** A catalyst is defined as a substance that increases the velocity of a chemical reaction. They are not consumed.

47. **(A)** *Hypertonic*: the solution has a higher osmotic pressure than the solution with which it is compared. There is a higher concentration of solute and a lower concentration of solvent. *Hypotonic*: a lower concentration of solute and a higher concentration of solvent are present. *Isotonic*: both solutions have the same osmotic pressure.

48. **(C)** One mole of any compound contains 6.02×10^{23} molecules. Two moles of carbon dioxide would contain one mole of molecules more than that contained by one mole of oxygen.

49. **(A)** Acid salts are formed by di- and tribasic acids. For example, H_2CO_3 can form the acid salt ($NaHCO_3$) known as sodium hydrogen carbonate or sodium bicarbonate.

50. **(D)** NaOH may be called a base because it produces OH^- ions, but it is more properly called a base because it consumes H^+ ions.

51. **(C)** The thermal decomposition of $KClO_3$ to produce oxygen will occur if the temperature is sufficiently high. The addition of a catalyst MnO_2 will decrease the activation energy and increase the rate at a lower temperature.

52. **(B)** See explanation for question 51.

Verbal Reasoning

53. **(C)** The author characterizes the goals for freshman composition at the University of Texas as "standard" (three of them are listed in **A, B,** and **D**) and enumerates them in paragraph two. The goal not listed is **C**, the goal of teaching freshmen to bring about social change, an objective of the radical pedagogists.

54. **(C)** See the explanation of question 53 (above). Bringing about social change is the goal of the radical pedagogists, according to paragraph five.

55. **(D)** In paragraph six, Lazere is described as a "leftist educator and radical pedagogist" (**A** and **C**); in paragraph seven the passage clearly suggests that he would be in disagreement with the methods proposed by Sharon Crowley because they would force ideology on the student. The correct answer, therefore, would be **D**, all of the above.

56. **(C)** The course, described in paragraph two, would examine the subject of "difference, specifically difference related to legal opinions given in court cases involving issues such as race, gender, bilingualism, and sexual orientation." Answer **C** partially describes the content of the course and is the correct response.

57. **(B)** One can easily infer from the statements attributed to her in the passage that Crowley fits the definition for a radical pedagogist given in paragraph three. Among other things, she asserts that composition teachers "must give up our traditional subscription to liberal tolerance if we are to bring about social change through [our students]" (see paragraph seven).

58. **(C)** Paragraph one makes it clear that the investigator must focus on the question: "is complainant's job equal in effort and responsibility to that of a male counterpart?" Paragraph seven indicates that the judiciary has not yet endorsed the notion of comparable worth, and the length of employment is not addressed in the reading passage.

59. **(B)** Paragraph one makes the point that identical jobs are not necessary because the standard is built on the concept that jobs must be evaluated within a context of substantial equivalency. None of the other statements is supported.

60. **(D)** Statements **A** and **B** are not discussed in the passage. Paragraph three contradicts statement **C**, whereas paragraph five implies that Title VII encompasses very broad aspects and reaches beyond the confines of equal wage matters.

61. **(D)** Although we might assume that the program of on-the-job training was a positive factor, the law does not address the issue. We could argue that the Department of Labor acted irresponsibly; however, we have no data to substantiate our claim. In the Columbia case, employees were aware of the differences in their positions. Paragraph five supports statement **D** because the court took into consideration the fact that heavy cleaning called for greater effort.

62. **(A)** Paragraphs six and seven support statements I, II, and III; however, paragraph seven makes it clear that although the Supreme Court has ruled that Title VII provides a remedy for sex discrimination, the judiciary has not yet endorsed the notion of comparable worth.

63. **(B)** Paragraph eight mentions the adverse decision the female guards received during the initial trial, and statement I is supported. It also makes it clear that the appellate court reversed the trial court and held that one could sue even though jobs were not substantially equal; statement III is supported. The paragraph also states that although the Supreme Court did not adopt the concept of comparable worth, it left the door open for further litigation.

64. **(A)** Paragraphs nine and ten clearly substantiate statements I, II, and III. Paragraph nine also indicates that the Supreme Court did not indicate how a plaintiff might establish a prima facie case under Title VII, and so statement IV is not supported.

65. **(A)** Paragraph one assigns the skull to Homo sapiens. Man is a vertebrate (subphylum); a mammal (class); Homo is the genus and sapiens is denoted as the species.

66. **(D)** Because we are dealing with a fossil, the best answer is an archeologist.

67. **(B)** The specimen was found in soil. The fluorine method of dating fossils was developed in 1949 and is based on the fact that buried bones absorb fluorine from the soil, and the amount increases with time.

68. **(C)** The older a fossil is, the more fluorine would have been present. A modern jawbone would, on testing, yield a lesser amount of fluorine in comparison to an ancient cranium.

69. **(D)** Iron in this case was used to artificially color the mandible to match the cranium.

70. **(A)** There is no evidence in the passage that Sara Murphy believed anything other than **A**, Zelda's inner complexity, caused her to appear different in the various photographs that were taken of her. Murphy's observation is cited in paragraph one.

71. **(D)** In paragraph four, the author characterizes Nancy Milford as Zelda's first major biographer. Sara Mayfield was Zelda's girlhood friend, and she wrote a biography after Milford had published hers. The passage does not provide that information, however. Arthur Mizener was Scott Fitzgerald's first major biographer, and Sara Murphy was a close friend of the Fitzgeralds. But again, the passage does not provide this information. **A**, **B**, and **C**, therefore, are incorrect answers.

72. **(C)** Paragraph two indicates that Fitzgerald was stationed at Fort Sheridan, near Zelda's hometown of Montgomery, and that he returned to New York after the war was over.

73. **(A)** In paragraph two, the author tells of Zelda's mother naming her after a gypsy queen in a novel she was reading, and goes on to add details that suggest Zelda's mother spoiled her daughter.

74. **(B)** Biographically there may be evidence to support the assertion that insanity ran in Zelda's family (**A**), but the passage does not supply such information. **C** and **D** present details that are not factual and do not appear in the passage. Milford's biography, according to paragraph four, presents a picture of Zelda as one who was exploited by her husband, but who also had conflicts not related to his treatment of her, the answer provided by **B**.

75. **(B)** Although Zelda's friends, according to Scott, would have blamed her insanity on his drinking (**D**), and his friends would have blamed her insanity for his drinking (**C**), neither would have been correct: "liquor on my mouth is sweet to her and I cherish her wildest hallucinations," he said, clearly characterizing their relationship to each other as mutually self-destructive. The correct

answer, therefore, is **B**. Obviously he did not consider their friends as the best judges, the incorrect answer suggested in **A**. See paragraph five.

76. **(C)** Paragraph one indicates that the fiftieth anniversary in the "Promised Land" was celebrated. Also found in paragraph one is the fact that the writer of Leviticus had God speak to Moses; there is no evidence in the passage that God ever spoke to Moses. The passage does point out that celebrating is an old practice of mankind, however; there is no comment anywhere to make the reader assume that most celebrations are joyous events.

77. **(C)** Statements II and IV are supported by the passage. Paragraph two points out that even with birthdays we call special attention to the "big" years, and the quotation from John Adams leaves no doubt that our Independence Day celebration should be carried out "from this time forward for everyone."

78. **(D)** Paragraph three mentions that the inauguration of a new enterprise is always an act of hope and when achievement is history a confident celebration is appropriate. Paragraph four mentions that a celebration is often viewed as the occasion for a new beginning.

79. **(D)** Paragraph five indicates that nostalgia, although differently felt, is good for the human spirit. In paragraph four we are told that we usually think that the lives of pioneers are worth emulating and that anniversaries offer us an opportunity to reflect.

80. **(D)** Paragraphs seven and eight mention the facts that human pride is a motor of an institutional machine, that we use anniversaries to emphasize legitimacy, and that one cannot ignore the commercial motivation behind celebrations.

81. **(C)** The story cites universal experiences both in myth and in everyday life.

82. **(C)** The passage focuses on choice, which, because it is human, is universal.

83. **(A)** Because changing or not changing the sail was Theseus's choice, the death of his father resulting from that choice was clearly his responsibility.

84. **(A)** The plot itself is a series of choices, one following the other.

85. **(B)** The author shows how choices in a myth can be the same choices that anyone can face at any time.

86. **(B)** The passage is concerned with the ways in which a character's actions determine his destiny and how major choices lead to other important choices. In Theseus's case, the primary problem is how he will kill the Minotaur.

87. **(D)** All the other statements are supported by the passage. It is stated in the passage that caricatures must be based on *fact*.

88. **(C)** Statements **A**, **B**, and **D** may be true, but they are not stated in the passage. Statement **C** is cited as a cause of laughter.

89. **(C)** Although the author states **A** and **B**, they are not the main point. The passage is set up to lead toward statement **C**. Statement **D** is dismissed in the passage.

90. **(C)** Statements I and III are stated in the passage to show how caricatures work. Statement II may be true, but it does not indicate why caricatures are effective.

91. **(A)** The passage does not deal with the possible objections to caricatures stated in **B**, **C**, and **D**. However, **A** is cited as a danger.

92. **(B)** The entire essay deals with the ways in which satirists use exaggeration as a means of communicating their ideas.

Writing Sample

93. **Essay**

    The definition of a wise person generated by this quote hinges on the interpretation of the words "ought" and "can." These words, however, as well as "see," remain ambiguous out of context, thus permitting opposing definitions of a "wise man." If "ought" is taken as a limitation of "can," that is if the wise individual sees only what he should or is obliged to see, then the quote takes on overtones of pragmatism. The wise person, or person who would be happy, does not see further than he ought. He sees less than he "can" or could. To see all he is capable of seeing would be unwise, perhaps because seeing all would be painful or would necessitate prying.

He could find out more but sees only that which is his business. The wise individual limits even his perception to avoid painful realities. On first reading, the quote seems to imply some such limited wisdom, perhaps because the shades of meaning in "ought" and "can" have changed over time. Repulsed by the definition of wisdom generated by this interpretation, one might be driven to reverse the relative magnitude of the terms "ought" and "can." What a wise person ought to see is more than what he can see. He must go beyond what is obvious or visible. The implication here is that the wise individual looks beyond or below the surface of perceptible reality. "See" begins to take on shades of meaning akin to "understand" or "infer" beyond superficial perception. The obligation implied by "ought" becomes an obligation to extend rather than an obligation to limit. This second wise person, to be wise, must either dig for more information (things he "ought" to see) or use intuition to understand more than he can see. Without further information on the context of the quote, two possible and opposing wise people remain.

Situations in which the pragmatic position does not apply can be found in psychology. If one believes that unconscious urges or forgotten traumas can have harmful effects on the individual, the wise individual might be advised to "see" more than he "can." A person might, for example, have difficulty relating to authority figures who, judging by what he "can" see, restrict him unfairly. If he can "dig down" to or be made to see oedipal impulses underlying the perception of oppression, he may become better able to respond to authority in a prudent, less self-defeating manner. Seeing only what one ought may also have parallels in jurisprudence, where a judge sometimes suppresses information. A decision reached based on the visible, limited facts may then be different (not to mention wrong) from a conclusion based on what one ought to have seen beyond what could be seen. This analogy, if true, argues that if one attends only to what he can see he may be misled. The other wise person, the one who sees more than he "can," may have a less assailable position. Perhaps, the pragmatic wise person is the best example of a situation in which limited wisdom is advisable. It is arguable that seeing too much is painful and potentially harmful. One might travel to study different cultures only to be more and more sickened by the pain and misery he finds everywhere. One could argue, I suppose, that he would have been wiser, that is happier, less potentially misanthropic, had he limited his vision.

In my mind there are no conditions under which vision or perception or understanding should be limited, if wisdom is the goal. According to the pragmatic reading of the quote, seeing all one can is a mistake, but I would argue limited wisdom is self-contradictory. The truly wise individual is one who sees not only all he "can," but what he "ought" as well. In other words, his vision intuits or infers beyond the visible. The wise person and the happy person may inhabit mutually exclusive positions due to the potential pain involved in seeing too far into oneself or others. However, pleasure and the avoidance of pain should not be used as conditions for defining wisdom.

93. **Explanation of Response: 5**

The paper focuses on the statement and addresses the three writing tasks. The most difficult task in writing this essay is the first: explaining what Montaigne's quotation actually means. This essay confronts the difficulty squarely, making it clear that one's interpretation of the quotation depends very much on the meanings of the word "ought" and "can." The irony is that "ought" in one sense could be considered a weaker word than "can"; but in another it is stronger. The essay suggests that one must conclude that two entirely different wise individuals emerge from the quotation, depending on the way in which "ought" is defined. Paragraph two then, moves to the task of providing specific situations in which the two different wise people see as much as they ought and then as much as they should. The example taken from the psychology of unconscious motivation is appropriate and the analogy using judge and jury is particularly imaginative. Finally the essay confronts the ambiguities and paradoxes raised when one considers Montaigne's quotation by taking the stand that a wise individual never limits his vision. And ultimately, the essay concludes, wisdom should not be defined in terms simply of pleasure or the avoidance of pain.

This essay provides a sensitive insight into a difficult quotation. The introduction is tightly reasoned; the writing is clear. Paragraph two brings the essay down into the realm of the concrete in its use of unconscious motives and of the judge-jury examples. Because the subject is so highly philosophical, this essay would be strengthened by the use of more concrete details, both in paragraphs one and two. The final paragraph, in which the essay winds down nicely, would especially benefit from a well-chosen concrete illustration. The addition of such specific details would elevate the rating of this essay from 5 to 6.

94. **Essay**

History exists, according to Emerson, only as a document tracing the events of individuals. Without people, there can be no history. Therefore, history is not a recording of events, but of the individuals who participated in them. The history of the Cathedral at Chartres does not concern itself primarily with the building, not its stones, it ironworks, its bells. The history of the Cathedral at Chartres focuses on the people who designed and built it, who worshipped and died in it, who tended their flocks in its walls. It is their history, and the history of these individuals is biography.

If it is true that by definition history is necessarily biography, then the events must take second place to the individuals. After all, biography is typically a document showing how the events have shaped the individual. Is history about the individual? It is not. True, history without the human element is dead, but history enjoys a longer continuum than the life of those it influences, and those influenced by it. History is about eras, thoughts, and ages. The Age of Reason is neither a biography of Rousseau, nor a story with those who believed the tenets as the main characters. It is about the events that took place during the time. History encompasses wars, art, politics, science, and philosophy. No biography can encompass all this. History is a larger container than just the human beings. It must hold many people, many actions, both intended and accidental. History records mistakes, quirks, even coincidences and accidents. So, the history of the Cathedral at Chartres is not about Abbot Sugar or King Louis, it is larger than that. Like the stones, the cathedral's history is longer than the life of humans, for the stones live longer than an abbot or king. The space is larger than the area taken up by the bodies it encompasses. It holds many ages of humankind, their thoughts, errors, reasons, and hopes. No, history cannot be biography, for biography is only a part of history. There are no biographies of stones and ideas, of errors and wars; there are only biographies of people.

But who shaped and stacked the stones? From whom do the errors, ideas, and reasons come? Though one person cannot live as long as a cathedral, the cathedral is nothing but a pile of stones and shards of glass with humans and their God to give it meaning. Eras are eras of

Humankind, and the Age of Reason reflects a change of thinking in the minds of people. For if we think of history as biography, we must think of Humans as opposed to men and women. Emerson believed that humans and nature were inextricably entwined. Humans and their consciousness were part stone, part God, part evil, part time. Though one person's story cannot be history, Humankind's story, or biography, certainly can, and this story is what we call history. History, then, redefines biography. This definition of biography is not about us as the limited creatures we are as individuals so much as it is about the limitless, encompassing Humankind as a unified whole. The stones are part of this and when labeled as Cathedral and joined to religion, the stones become more of Humankind. The history of the stones and of the space are then the history of Humankind and that, true, is biography.

94. **Explanation of Response: 5**

The essay focuses on the topic defined by Emerson's statement and addresses the three writing tasks. Paragraph one explains Emerson's idea that "there is properly no history; only biography" and illustrates the explanation with a concrete reference to the Cathedral at Chartres. The second paragraph explores in detail the other side of the issue, arguing through historical references that there is, indeed, history independent of biography. The final paragraph presents a balanced consideration of the relation between biography and history, concluding finally that the history of Humankind, not of men and women, is biography.

The first section of the essay uses an interesting rhetorical strategy: that of paraphrasing Emerson's statement in such a way that the paraphrases become premises leading to the conclusion that "Therefore, history is not a recording of events, but of the individuals who participated in them." Some will argue that Emerson's statement is not saying "without people, there can be no history" (the essay's second premise), and thus some will question the foundation of the essay from the beginning. A simple qualifier, such as "perhaps," would strengthen the logic. The second paragraph provides an eloquent defense of the idea that there is indeed history that includes more than biography. It does so by extending the example of the Cathedral at Chartres used in paragraph one and by citing various historical eras and ages. The essay's final paragraph brings the point back to Emerson's assertion and balances it by the concept of the history of

Humankind, a creative solution to the task of exploring the circumstances that determine the relationship between history and biography.

The writing in this essay is clear, and it flows nicely from sentence to sentence. The essay could use a clear transition leading into paragraph two. This is the paragraph that reverses the position explained in paragraph one, and the reader could use help in getting into that position. The essay is rich in concrete details. Especially effective is the extended reference to the Cathedral at Chartres. If this paper had led the reader more smoothly from one task to the next, and if the logic in the first several sentences were tightened, the paper would receive a rating of 6.

Biological Sciences

95.–100. **(95-A) (96-A) (97-C) (98-D) (99-A) (100-B)** Let us identify the components of the neuron numbered: (2) nucleus with nucleolus, containing the genetic material of the cell and directing the synthetic activity of the cell; (3) Golgi apparatus (zone), the packaging and concentrating area of the cell's secretory activity; (4) dendrites; dendrites are the processes that pick up an impulse and carry it toward the cell body; (5) endoplasmic reticulum (rough in this case—ribosomes are attached), the synthetic machinery of the cell (proteins etc.); (6) cell membrane, semipermeable and the protector of the cell from its environment; (7) cytoplasm (specifically the area here is called the axon hillock); (8) myelin sheath (Schwann cell covered by its neurilemma, the insulator of the axon); (1) direction of conduction of an impulse; axon (10a) and (10b) conducts impulses away from the dendrites to the function with the dendrites of another neuron. The junction point is known as the synaptic area; the impulse can cross the synapse only from the axon to the dendrite and no backflow is permitted; (11) terminal branches of the axon. In a lesion (cut) the process distal from the cell body would completely degenerate. Retrograde degeneration would be detected in the proximal portion, and the cell body; however, the proximal portion has the capacity and will regenerate.

101. **(C)** Because glucose is absorbed at a faster rate than xylose, due to both passive and active transport, then as the glucose is absorbed, water follows. The transport system for glucose is working maximally as indicated by the initial concentration of glucose being 50 times the apparent Km of transport.

102. **(D)** A 1.8% solution contains 1.8 g/100 m of solution. This is 1,800 mg/100 ml, which is 18 mg/ml. For the recovery of 1.8 mg, this represents $(1.8/18 \times 100)$ a 10% recovery, meaning that 90% has been metabolized or transported out of the lumen of the intestine.

103. **(D)** Hemoglobin is a large (64,000 MW) molecule. Because the gut was ligated below the pancreas and proteolytic enzymes present were washed out, no digestion of the protein could occur. Large molecules are not readily transported across cell membranes. Due to the vast surface area of the small intestine with its many microvilli, some of the protein would be adsorbed on this surface and visible through the heme prosthetic group color.

104. **(D)** All are correct. I. D-galactose is transported by the same carrier as glucose, therefore, by addition of galactose, a competition for transport between glucose and galactose occurs. II. The transport carrier is sodium ion selective. A larger cation, while having the appropriate charges, does not fit the selective carrier. III. The carrier is specific for the D-glucose; L-glucose would be transported by passive diffusion only. IV. Because the carrier is an energy requiring process, by limiting the supply of ATP, the transport is decreased.

105. **(A)** A 25% solution of $MgSO_4$ is hypertonic. Neither Mg nor SO_4 ions are readily transported so the net effect is a water flow into the lumen becoming an isotonic solution.

106. **(B)** Hemoglobin is not absorbed and an aqueous solution is not isotonic. Assuming that the hemoglobin is not ionized, a 0.3 M solution would have to have $64,000 \times 0.3$ g/liter. This solution must be hypotonic, which can be only modified by water flow out of the lumen.

107.–109. **(107-B) (108-C) (109-C)** The answers can be found in the flow diagram of the question. Thyroid-hormones (T_3 and T_4) are iodothyronines. The union of iodine and tyrosine is called iodination, and the active thyroid principal is protein-bound during transport to the target organs.

110. **(D)** Hyperthyriodism, hypothyroidism, and euthyroidism can be associated with goiter. In hyperthyroidism, thyroxin is released into the bloodstream at a rate exceeding needs. BMR accelerates resulting in rapid pulse and respiration, increased appetite with concomitant weight loss, nervousness, and protruding eyes. If not treated, goiter and thyroid exhaustion can occur; treatment involves antithyroid drugs or thyroidectomy. The opposite, hypothyroidism, exhibits a gland that cannot meet secretory demands; the body's metabolic rate is depressed and symptoms are the reverse of the above cited. When hypothyroidism occurs during childhood, a cretin is the result; mental retardation and stunted growth are features. Treatment requires administration of thyroid hormone. Goiter simply means enlargement of the gland and can be present in the normal (euthyroid) state.

111. **(A)** Thyroid stimulating hormone produced by the basophils of the anterior pituitary is a glycoprotein made up of two peptide chains (alpha and beta). Certain regions of the hypothalamus have a neuroendocrine function because neurosecretory cells release hormones that affect anterior pituitary function. TRH secreted by the hypothalamus reaches the pituitary via the hypophyseal-portal circulation and elicits TSH production. Thyroxin binds to TBG. Exposure to cold would elicit a compensatory increase in BMR and, hence, thyroid activity.

112. **(D)** Also see explanations for questions 108 and 109. Control of thyroid principal is via the pituitary. TSH stimulates the thyroid to produce thyroxin; its release is related to levels in the bloodstream. Low levels increase TSH and thyroxin release, but as levels rise to normal and above, further production and release of TSH is curtailed and thyroxin production falls. This feedback system maintains balance.

113. **(C)** See explanations for questions 108–110.

114. **(B)** It is the purpose of this experiment to determine the sequence of events in cells stimulated to undergo mitosis, and to compare the data to those gathered from unstimulated cells.

115. **(A)** Analysis of the graphs clearly shows that RNA synthesis precedes increased protein synthesis; at around 17 hours they are equal and RNA continues to drop, whereas protein synthesis increases.

116. **(D)** It is safe to assume that unstimulated lymphocytes synthesize RNA, DNA, and protein at a low rate. One of the premier functions of DNA is the production of RNA; most RNA is produced in the nucleus. DNA determines and acts as a template for RNA synthesis. With the help of a transcription enzyme (RNA polymerase), a complimentary RNA strand is produced; once produced it moves into the cytoplasm.

117. **(B)** The cell is the basic unit of structure and function and the basis of all life; all cells come from preexisting cells.

118. **(B)** A complete set of chromosomes ($2n$) is passed on to each daughter cell as a result of mitotic cell division. Cells that are produced mitotically are genetically alike.

119. **(C)** Messenger RNA (mRNA) from the nucleus brings the coded message for protein synthesis to ribosomes in the cytoplasm.

120. **(C)** Mitosis is divided into:

    (1) prophase—chromosomes become distinct and nucleoli disappears centrioles, asters, and spindle appear; nuclear membrane disappears.
    (2) metaphase—chromosomes move to equator of cell.
    (3) anaphase—the two chromatids split apart and start migration toward the poles of the spindle, and the spindle loses its definition.
    (4) telophase—chromosomes lengthen and become less distinct and nucleon reappear.
    (5) interphase—cell growth, protein + DNA synthesis, and chromosomes duplicate.

121. **(B)** During metaphase of mitosis, the centrioles with asters are at the opposite poles; the chromosomes move to the equator of the cell. Also see explanation for question 120.

122. **(B)** Mitochondria occur only in eukaryotic cells. Although the structures are different, flagella with analogous functions occur in both.

123. **(D)** Nucleolar organizer regions coding for rRNA occur in multiple chromosomes and typically lie around the perimeter of the nucleolus.

124. **(D)** Epithelial tissues have all of these functions.

125. **(C)** Neutrophils and the macrophages derived from monocytes are active in the phagocytosis of bacteria.

126. **(D)** Nuclei have the highest DNA concentration among cellular organelles. The DNA in fraction 3 is in mitochondria.

127. **(C)** Cytochrome oxidase is the enzyme complex that transfers electrons from the mitochondrial electron transport chain to oxygen and is therefore located in mitochondria.

128. **(A)** Most of the RNA found in a mature cell is ribosomal RNA, and the cytoplasmic ribosomal RNA in a hepatocyte should occur in a mixture of free ribosomes and rough endoplasmic reticulum. Because only one peak of RNA occurred at the top of the gradient, fraction 1 must contain both free and membrane-bound ribosomes and therefore contains the rough endoplasmic reticulum. The RNA in fraction 3 probably represents ribosomes in mitochondria. The RNA in fraction 4 is probably partially assembled ribosomes in the nucleoli in the nuclei.

129. **(B)** Acid phosphatase is a lysosomal enzyme and occurred only in fraction 2 among the choices.

130. **(A)** Cytochrome P-450 is involved in detoxification reactions in smooth endoplasmic reticulum and only occurred in fraction 1 among the choices.

131. **(C)** Krebs cycle enzymes are located in the mitochondria and should therefore occur in the same fractions that contain cytochrome oxidase activity.

132. **(A)** Plasma proteins are secreted proteins and therefore should be made on the rough endoplasmic reticulum in fraction 1.

133. **(A)** A cell that secretes large amounts of protein (such as a pancreatic exocrine cell) should contain large arrays of rough endoplasmic reticulum, which would increase fraction 1. Secretory granules could increase fraction 2 or fraction 3, but the assays used would not detect pancreatic enzymes or their contribution to a fraction.

134. **(B)** Phagocytic cells, such as monocytes or macrophages, contain large numbers of lysosomes that would contribute to the acid phosphatase activity measured in fraction 2.

135. **(C)** Proximal convoluted tubule lining cells contain large numbers of mitochondria that supply the large amounts of energy needed to support the active transport used for resorption of solutes from urine. High numbers of mitochondria should increase fraction 3.

136. **(D)** Two moles of carbon dioxide formed and 12 ATP formed per mole of acetyl CoA. The reactions produce three moles of NADH and one mole of $FADH_2$. Reoxidation of these coenzymes in the respiratory assembly will produce three ATP/NADH and two ATP/$FADH_2$. The remaining one ATP is a substrate level phosphorylation of GDP to GTP by succinyl CoA. GTP can phosphorylate ADP to ATP.

137. **(B)** The reaction acetyl CoA to pyruvate does not occur. This is one of the reasons that we cannot make (net) glucose from acetyl CoA. Choice **D** shows two very similar reactions of oxidative decarboxylation. The same coenzymes, mechanism, and release of CO_2 occur. Choice **A** indicates both oxidations of a secondary alcohol. The product, oxalosuccinate, spontaneously decarboxylates due to the instability of the keto acid formed to yield alpha ketoglutarate. Choice **C** indicates both hydration reactions.

138. **(A)** For the citric acid cycle to function, as acetyl CoA is catabolized it reacts with oxaloacetate to form citrate. In specific reactions, CO_2 is lost and oxaloacetate is regenerated. Oxaloacetate may be considered catalytic for the cycle. Oxaloacetate plus acetyl CoA forms 2 CO_2 and oxaloacetate. **B** is a true statement in that the synthesis of fatty acids in the cytoplasm occurs through this step. **C** is also true because the first step in the synthesis of the porphyrin ring (heme) occurs from succinyl CoA. The last two choices are also true because transamination from these keto acids (using some other amino acids as the amino group donor) results in the formation of the specific amino shown.

139. **(D)** Net synthesis of glucose does not take place because the reaction pyruvate to acetyl CoA is not reversible under physiological conditions and also because for every acetyl CoA condensing with oxaloacetate, 2 CO_2 is formed. Choice **A** is true because specific enzymes of the pathway are inhibited by high levels of ATP (citrate synthase) or stimulated by low levels of ADP (isocitrate dehydrogenase). Choice **B** is correct. One control of the glycolytic pathway has citrate as a negative

effector (phosphofructokinase). Choice **C** is a true statement. The citric acid cycle is the final metabolic pathway for many metabolites.

140. **(A)** The red blood cell (mature RBC) does not contain mitochondria where the citric acid cycle takes place; see **B**. Choice **C** is true; for every acetyl CoA (two per glucose mole) 12 ATP are formed. Substrate level phosphorylation (GTP + ADP to ATP + GDP) form one and reoxidation of reducing equivalents in oxidative phosphorylation forms 11 ATP. When acetyl CoA levels are high, several things can happen: (1) the citric acid cycle may be maximal (depends on ATP needs); (2) fatty acids may be synthesized; (3) ketone bodies may be formed; (4) gluconeogenesis is stimulated because the enzyme pyruvate carboxylase requires high levels to activate it for the synthesis of net oxaloacetate from pyruvate and CO_2. Eventually glucose may be formed anew from the pyruvate (gluconeogenesis).

141. **(B)** Acidophils (alpha cells) of the pituitary secrete somatotropic hormone (STH, growth hormone), which stimulates generalized body growth. Hypersecretion before ossification is complete results in giantism, whereas thereafter, acromegaly is the consequence. Hyposecretion leads to dwarfism. Our assay had to be conducted on hypophysectomized rats because the pituitary produces growth hormone that might interfere with the assay.

142. **(A)** The stressed normal + 100 mg STH produced the most rapid growth among the choices.

143. **(A)** The data show more rapid cartilage growth in hypox + 100 mg STH than in intact control animals, so the natural concentration of STH is probably somewhat less than 100 mg/day.

144. **(A)** Conversion of glycogen to glucose-l-phosphate is catalyzed by the enzyme, phosphorylase. Pancreatic amylase is usually not in contact with glycogen (except dietary glycogen); in any case it would not catalyze the formation of glucose-l-phosphate.

145. **(C)** Production of glucose and fructose from sucrose and production of fatty acids and glycerol from triglycerides are both simple hydrolytic reactions in which essentially no energy is gained or lost. Production of steroids from acetate (as is true with most synthetic reactions) requires energy input. Production of CO_2 and water from fatty acids yields large amounts of energy.

146. **(D)** A yellow precipitate of iodoform is produced in this reaction with methyl ketones, alcohols that may be oxidized to methyl ketones, or acetaldehyde.

PART 4

APPENDIXES

Logarithms and Exponents

Logarithms

The logarithm of any number is the exponent of the power to which 10 must be raised to produce the number. The logarithm X of the number N to the base 10 is the exponent of the power to which 10 must be raised to give N (for example, $\log_{10} N = X$). Logarithms consist of two parts. First, there is the "characteristic," which is determined by the position of the first significant figure of the number in relation to the decimal point. If we count leftwards from the decimal point as positive and rightwards as negative, the characteristic is equal to the count ending at the right of the first significant figure. Thus, the characteristic of the logarithm of 2340 is 3, and of 0.00234 is –3. Second, there is the "mantissa." It is always positive, is found in logarithm tables, and depends only on the sequence of significant figures. Thus, the mantissa for the two numbers is the same, namely 0.3692. The logarithm of a number is the sum of the characteristic and the mantissa. Thus, log 2340 = 3.3692 while log 0.00234 = –3 + 0.3692 = –2.6308.

The logarithms of the whole integers 1 to 10 are given below.

log 1.0 = 0.000	log 6.0 = 0.778
log 2.0 = 0.301	log 7.0 = 0.845
log 3.0 = 0.477	log 8.0 = 0.903
log 4.0 = 0.602	log 9.0 = 0.954
log 5.0 = 0.699	log 10.0 = 1.000

USEFUL RULES IN HANDLING LOGARITHMS

1. The logarithm of a product is equal to the sum of the logarithms of the factors:

$$\log ab = \log a + \log b$$

(Check this out by solving for log 6, using log 2 + log 3.)

2. The logarithm of a fraction is equal to the logarithm of the numerator minus the logarithm of the denominator:

$$\log \frac{a}{b} = \log a - \log b$$

Example:

$$\log \frac{10}{2} = \log 10 - \log 2 = \log 5$$

How about log 2.5? The answer from the log tables is 0.398.

3. The logarithm of the reciprocal of a number is the negative logarithm of the number:

$$\log \frac{1}{a} = \log 1 - \log a$$

Since log 1 = 0, then

$$\log \frac{1}{a} = -\log a$$

Equally,

$$\log \frac{1}{2} = -\log 2 = -0.301$$

4. The logarithm of a number raised to a power is the logarithm of the number multiplied by the power:

$$\log a^b = b \log a$$
$$\log 2^2 = 0.603$$

Exponents

It is convenient to express large numbers as 10^x, where x represents the number of places that the decimal must be moved to place it after the first significant figure. This also represents $10 \cdot 10$ for x times. For example, 1,000,000 may be expressed as 1×10^6; 3663 as 3.663×10^3; and so on. To multiply, the exponents are added, but coefficients are multiplied. To divide, the exponents are subtracted, but coefficients are divided.

Multiplying: $(1 \times 10^x) \cdot (1 \times 10^y) = 1 \times 10^{x+y}$

$$(4 \times 10^2) \cdot (2 \times 10^3) = 8 \times 10^5$$

Dividing: $(1 \times 10^x) \div (1 \times 10^y) = 1 \times 10^{x-y}$

$$(4 \times 10^2) \div (2 \times 10^3) = 2 \times 10^{-1}$$

Numbers less than 1 are 10^{-x}. For example, 0.000001 is 1×10^{-6}.

Multiplying: $(1 \times 10^{-x}) \cdot (1 \times 10^{-y}) = 1 \times 10^{-(x+y)}$

$$(4 \times 10^{-2}) \cdot (2 \times 10^{-3}) = 8 \times 10^{-5}$$

A large number multiplied by a small number:

$$(4 \times 10^{-2})(2 \times 10^3) = 8 \times 10^1$$

(Logarithms and Exponents are reproduced through the courtesy of Dr. Richard B. Brandt, Dept. of Biochemistry, MCV, VCU, Richmond, Virginia 23298.)

Table of Common Logarithms

Numbers	0	1	2	3	4	5	6	7	8	9
10	0000	0043	0086	0128	0170	0212	0253	0294	0334	0374
11	0414	0453	0492	0531	0569	0607	0645	0682	0719	0755
12	0792	0828	0864	0899	0934	0969	1004	1038	1072	1106
13	1139	1173	1206	1239	1271	1303	1335	1367	1399	1430
14	1461	1492	1523	1553	1584	1614	1644	1673	1703	1732
15	1761	1790	1818	1847	1875	1903	1931	1959	1987	2014
16	2041	2068	2095	2122	2148	2175	2201	2227	2253	2279
17	2304	2330	2355	2380	2405	2430	2455	2480	2504	2529
18	2553	2577	2601	2625	2648	2672	2695	2718	2742	2765
19	2788	2810	2833	2856	2878	2900	2923	2945	2967	2989
20	3010	3032	3054	3075	3096	3118	3139	3160	3181	3201
21	3222	3243	3263	3284	3304	3324	3345	3365	3385	3404
22	3424	3444	3464	3483	3502	3522	3541	3560	3579	3598
23	3617	3636	3655	3674	3692	3711	3729	3747	3766	3784
24	3802	3820	3838	3856	3874	3892	3909	3927	3945	3962
25	3979	3997	4014	4031	4048	4065	4082	4099	4116	4133
26	4150	4166	4183	4200	4216	4232	4249	4265	4281	4298
27	4314	4330	4346	4362	4378	4393	4409	4425	4440	4456
28	4472	4487	4502	4518	4533	4548	4564	4579	4594	4609
29	4624	4639	4654	4669	4683	4698	4713	4728	4742	4757
30	4771	4786	4800	4814	4829	4843	4857	4871	4886	4900
31	4914	4928	4942	4955	4969	4983	4997	5011	5024	5038
32	5051	5065	5079	5092	5105	5119	5132	5145	5159	5172
33	5185	5198	5211	5224	5237	5250	5263	5276	5289	5302
34	5315	5328	5340	5353	5366	5378	5391	5403	5416	5428
35	5441	5453	5465	5478	5490	5502	5514	5527	5539	5551
36	5563	5575	5587	5599	5611	5623	5635	5647	5658	5670
37	5682	5694	5705	5717	5729	5740	5752	5763	5775	5786
38	5798	5809	5821	5832	5843	5855	5866	5877	5888	5899
39	5911	5922	5933	5944	5955	5966	5977	5988	5999	6010
40	6021	6031	6042	6053	6064	6075	6085	6096	6107	6117
41	6128	6138	6149	6160	6170	6180	6191	6201	6212	6222
42	6232	6243	6253	6263	6274	6284	6294	6304	6314	6325
43	6335	6345	6355	6365	6375	6385	6395	6405	6415	6425
44	6435	6444	6454	6464	6474	6484	6493	6503	6513	6522
45	6532	6542	6551	6561	6571	6580	6590	6599	6609	6618
46	6628	6637	6646	6656	6665	6675	6684	6693	6702	6712
47	6721	6730	6739	6749	6758	6767	6776	6785	6794	6803
48	6812	6821	6830	6839	6848	6857	6866	6875	6884	6893
49	6902	6911	6920	6928	6937	6946	6955	6964	6972	6981

Numbers	0	1	2	3	4	5	6	7	8	9
50	6990	6998	7007	7016	7024	7033	7042	7050	7059	7067
51	7076	7084	7093	7101	7110	7118	7126	7135	7143	7152
52	7160	7168	7177	7185	7193	7202	7210	7218	7226	7235
53	7243	7251	7259	7267	7275	7284	7292	7300	7308	7316
54	7324	7332	7340	7348	7356	7364	7372	7380	7388	7396
55	7404	7412	7419	7427	7435	7443	7451	7459	7466	7474
56	7482	7490	7497	7505	7513	7520	7528	7536	7543	7551
57	7559	7566	7574	7582	7589	7597	7604	7612	7619	7627
58	7634	7642	7649	7657	7664	7672	7679	7686	7694	7701
59	7709	7716	7723	7731	7738	7745	7752	7760	7767	7774
60	7782	7789	7796	7803	7810	7818	7825	7832	7839	7846
61	7853	7860	7868	7875	7882	7889	7896	7903	7910	7917
62	7924	7931	7938	7945	7952	7959	7966	7937	7980	7987
63	7993	8000	8007	8014	8021	8028	8035	8041	8048	8055
64	8062	8069	8075	8082	8089	8096	8102	8109	8116	8122
65	8129	8136	8142	8149	8156	8162	8169	8176	8182	8189
66	8195	8202	8209	8215	8222	8228	8235	8241	8248	8254
67	8261	8267	8274	8280	8287	8293	8299	8306	8312	8319
68	8325	8331	8338	8344	8351	8357	8363	8370	8376	8382
69	8388	8395	8401	8407	8414	8420	8426	8432	8439	8445
70	8451	8457	8463	8470	8476	8482	8488	8494	8500	8506
71	8513	8519	8525	8531	8537	8543	8549	8555	8561	8567
72	8573	8579	8585	8591	8597	8603	8609	8615	8621	8627
73	8633	8639	8645	8651	8657	8663	8669	8675	8681	8686
74	8692	8698	8704	8710	8716	8722	8727	8733	8739	8745
75	8751	8756	8762	8768	8774	8779	8785	8791	8797	8802
76	8808	8814	8820	8825	8831	8837	8842	8848	8854	8859
77	8865	8871	8876	8882	8887	8893	8899	8904	8910	8915
78	8921	8927	8932	8938	8943	8949	8954	8960	8965	8971
79	8976	8982	8987	8993	8998	9004	9009	9015	9020	9025
80	9031	9036	9042	9047	9053	9058	9063	9069	9074	9079
81	9085	9090	9096	9101	9106	9112	9117	9122	9128	9133
82	9138	9143	9149	9154	9159	9165	9170	9175	9180	9186
83	9191	9196	9201	9206	9212	9217	9222	9227	9232	9238
84	9243	9248	9253	9258	9263	9269	9274	9279	9284	9289
85	9294	9299	9304	9309	9315	9320	9325	9330	9335	9340
86	9345	9350	9355	9360	9365	9370	9375	9380	9385	9390
87	9395	9400	9405	9410	9415	9420	9425	9430	9435	9440
88	9445	9450	9455	9460	9465	9469	9474	9479	9484	9489
89	9494	9499	9504	9509	9513	9518	9523	9528	9533	9538
90	9542	9547	9552	9557	9562	9566	9571	9576	9581	9586
91	9590	9595	9600	9605	9609	9614	9619	9624	9628	9633
92	9638	9643	9647	9652	9657	9661	9666	9671	9675	9680
93	9685	9689	9694	9699	9703	9708	9713	9717	9722	9727
94	9731	9736	9741	9745	9750	9754	9759	9763	9768	9773
95	9777	9782	9786	9791	9795	9800	9805	9809	9814	9818
96	9823	9827	9832	9836	9841	9845	9850	9854	9859	9863
97	9868	9872	9877	9881	9886	9890	9894	9899	9903	9908
98	9912	9917	9921	9926	9930	9934	9939	9943	9948	9952
99	9956	9961	9965	9969	9974	9978	9983	9987	9991	9996

Periodic Table of the Elements

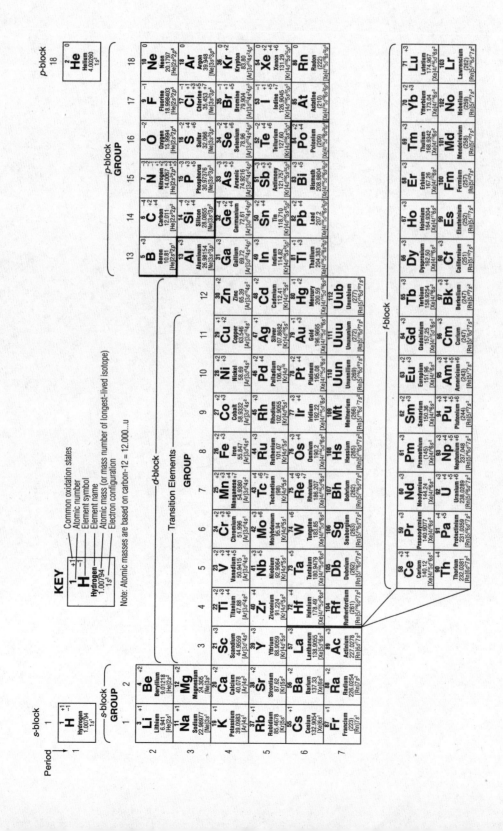

List of Elements with Their Symbols

Element	Symbol	Element	Symbol	Element	Symbol
Actinium	Ac	Gold	Au	Praseodymium	Pr
Aluminum	Al	Hafnium	Hf	Promethium	Pm
Americium	Am	Helium	He	Protactinium	Pa
Antimony	Sb	Holmium	Ho	Radium	Ra
Argon	Ar	Hydrogen	H	Radon	Rn
Arsenic	As	Indium	In	Rhenium	Re
Astatine	At	Iodine	I	Rhodium	Rh
Barium	Ba	Iridium	Ir	Rubidium	Rb
Berkelium	Bk	Iron	Fe	Ruthenium	Ru
Beryllium	Be	Krypton	Kr	Samarium	Sm
Bismuth	Bi	Lanthanum	La	Scandium	Sc
Boron	B	Lawrencium	Lr	Selenium	Se
Bromine	Br	Lead	Pb	Silicon	Si
Cadmium	Cd	Lithium	Li	Silver	Ag
Calcium	Ca	Lutetium	Lu	Sodium	Na
Californium	Cf	Magnesium	Mg	Strontium	Sr
Carbon	C	Manganese	Mn	Sulfur	S
Cerium	Ce	Mendelevium	Md	Tantalum	Ta
Cesium	Cs	Mercury	Hg	Technetium	Tc
Chlorine	Cl	Molybdenum	Mo	Tellurium	Te
Chromium	Cr	Neodymium	Nd	Terbium	Tb
Cobalt	Co	Neon	Ne	Thallium	Tl
Copper	Cu	Neptunium	Np	Thorium	Th
Curium	Cm	Nickel	Ni	Thulium	Tm
Dysprosium	Dy	Niobium	Nb	Tin	Sn
Einsteinium	Es	Nitrogen	N	Titanium	Ti
Element 106		Nobelium	No	Tungsten	W
Erbium	Er	Osmium	Os	Uranium	U
Europium	Eu	Oxygen	O	Vanadium	V
Fermium	Fm	Palladium	Pd	Xenon	Xe
Fluorine	F	Phosphorus	P	Ytterbium	Yb
Francium	Fr	Platinum	Pt	Yttrium	Y
Gadolinium	Gd	Plutonium	Pu	Zinc	Zn
Gallium	Ga	Polonium	Po	Zirconium	Zr
Germanium	Ge	Potassium	K		

Reference Tables for Chemistry

Physical Constants And Conversion Factors

Name	Symbol	Value(s)	Units
Angstrom unit	Å	1×10^{-10} m	meter
Avogadro's number	N_A	6.02×10^{23} per mol	
Charge of electron	e	1.60×10^{-19} C	coulomb
Electron volt	eV	1.60×10^{-19} J	joule
Speed of light	c	3.00×10^8 m/s	meters/second
Planck's constant	h	6.63×10^{-34} J $\cdot$ s	joule-second
		1.58×10^{-37} kcal $\cdot$ s	kilocalorie-second
Universal gas constant	R	0.0821 L $\cdot$ atm/mol $\cdot$ K	liter-atmosphere/mole-kelvin
		1.98 cal/mol $\cdot$ K	calories/mole-kelvin
		8.31 J/mol $\cdot$ K	joules/mole-kelvin
Atomic mass unit	μ(amu)	1.66×10^{-24} g	gram
Volume standard, liter	L	1×10^3 cm^3 = 1 dm^3	cubic centimeters, cubic decimeter
Standard pressure, atmosphere	atm	101.3 kPa 760 mmHg 760 torr	kilopascals millimeters of mercury torr
Heat equivalent, kilocalorie	kcal	4.18×10^3 J	joules

Physical Constants for H_2O

Molal freezing point depression	1.86°C
Molal boiling point elevation	0.52°C
Heat of fusion	79.72 cal/g
Heat of vaporization	539.4 cal/g

Standard Units

Symbol	Name	Quantity	Selected Prefixes		
			Factor	Prefix	Symbol
m	meter	length	10^6	mega	M
kg	kilogram	mass	10^3	kilo	k
Pa	pascal	pressure	10^{-1}	deci	d
K	kelvin	thermodynamic temperature	10^{-2}	centi	c
mol	mole	amount of substance	10^{-3}	milli	m
J	joule	energy, work quantity of heat	10^{-6}	micro	μ
sec	second	time	10^{-9}	nano	n
C	coulomb	quantity of electricity			
V	volt	electric potential, potential difference			
L	liter	volume			

Relative Strengths of Acids in Aqueous Solution at 1 atm and 298 K

Conjugate Pairs

ACID	BASE	K_a
$HI = H^+ + I^-$		very large
$HBr = H^+ + Br^-$		very large
$HCl = H^+ + Cl^-$		very large
$HNO_3 = H^+ + NO_3^-$		very large
$H_2SO_4 = H^+ + HSO_4^-$		large
$H_2O + SO_2 = H^+ + HSO_3^-$		1.5×10^{-2}
$HSO_4^- = H^+ + SO_4^{2-}$		1.2×10^{-2}
$H_3PO_4 = H^+ + H_2PO_4^-$		7.5×10^{-3}
$Fe(H_2O)_6^{3+} = H^+ + Fe(H_2O)_5(OH)^{2+}$		8.9×10^{-4}
$HNO_2 = H^+ + NO_2^-$		4.6×10^{-4}
$HF = H^+ + F^-$		3.5×10^{-4}
$Cr(H_2O)_6^{3+} = H^+ + Cr(H_2O)_5(OH)^{2+}$		1.0×10^{-4}
$CH_3COOH = H^+ + CH_3COO^-$		1.8×10^{-5}
$Al(H_2O)_6^{3+} = H^+ + Al(H_2O)_5(OH)^{2+}$		1.1×10^{-5}
$H_2O + CO_2 = H^+ + HCO_3^-$		4.3×10^{-7}
$HSO_3^- = H^+ + SO_3^{2-}$		1.1×10^{-7}
$H_2S = H^+ + HS^-$		9.5×10^{-8}
$H_2PO_4^- = H^+ + HPO_4^{2-}$		6.2×10^{-8}
$NH_4^+ = H^+ + NH_3$		5.7×10^{-10}
$HCO_3^- = H^+ + CO_3^{2-}$		5.6×10^{-11}
$HPO_4^{2-} = H^+ + PO_4^{3-}$		2.2×10^{-13}
$HS^- = H^+ + S^{2-}$		1.3×10^{-14}
$H_2O = H^+ + OH^-$		1.0×10^{-14}

Note: H^+ (aq) = H_3O^+

Sample equation: $HI + H_2O = H_3O^+ + I^-$

Constants for Various Equilibria at 1 atm and 298 K

$$H_2O(\ell) \rightleftharpoons H^+(aq) + OH^-(aq) \qquad K_w = 1.0 \times 10^{-14}$$

$$H_2O(\ell) + H_2O(\ell) \rightleftharpoons H_3O^+(aq) + OH^-(aq) \qquad K_w = 1.0 \times 10^{-14}$$

$$CH_3COO^-(aq) + H_2O(\ell) \rightleftharpoons CH_3COOH(aq) + OH^-(aq) \qquad K_b = 5.6 \times 10^{-10}$$

$$Na^+F^-(aq) + H_2O(\ell) \rightleftharpoons Na^+(OH)^- + HF(aq) \qquad K_b = 1.5 \times 10^{-11}$$

$$NH_3(aq) + H_2O(\ell) \rightleftharpoons NH_4^+(aq) + OH^-(aq) \qquad K_b = 1.8 \times 10^{-5}$$

$$CO_3^{2-}(aq) + H_2O(\ell) \rightleftharpoons HCO_3^-(aq) + OH^-(aq) \qquad K_b = 1.8 \times 10^{-4}$$

$$Ag(NH_3)_2^+(aq) \rightleftharpoons Ag^+(aq) + 2NH_3(aq) \qquad K_{eq} = 8.9 \times 10^{-8}$$

$$N_2(g) + 3H_2(g) \rightleftharpoons 2NH_3(g) \qquad K_{eq} = 6.7 \times 10^{5}$$

$$H_2(g) + I_2(g) \rightleftharpoons 2HI(g) \qquad K_{eq} = 3.5 \times 10^{-1}$$

Compound	K_{sp}	Compound	K_{sp}
AgBr	5.0×10^{-13}	Li_2CO_3	2.5×10^{-2}
AgCl	1.8×10^{-10}	$PbCl_2$	1.6×10^{-5}
Ag_2CrO_4	1.1×10^{-12}	$PbCO_3$	7.4×10^{-14}
AgI	8.3×10^{-17}	$PbCrO_4$	2.8×10^{-13}
$BaSO_4$	1.1×10^{-10}	PbI_2	7.1×10^{-9}
$CaSO_4$	9.1×10^{-6}	$ZnCO_3$	1.4×10^{-11}

Standard Energies of Formation of Compounds at 1 atm and 298 K

Compound	Heat (Enthalpy) of Formation* kcal/mol (ΔH°_f)	Free Energy of Formation* kcal/mol (ΔG_f°)
Aluminum oxide $Al_2O_3(s)$	−400.5	−378.2
Ammonia $NH_3(g)$	−11.0	−3.9
Barium sulfate $BaSo_4(s)$	−352.1	−325.6
Calcium hydroxide $Ca(OH)_2(s)$	−235.7	−214.8
Carbon dioxide $CO_2(g)$	−94.1	−94.3
Carbon monoxide $CO(g)$	−26.4	−32.8
Copper (II) sulfate $CuSO_4(s)$	−184.4	−158.2
Ethane $C_2H_6(g)$	−20.2	−7.9
Ethene (ethylene) $C_2H_4(g)$	12.5	16.3
Ethyne (acetylene) $C_2H_2(g)$	54.2	50.0
Hydrogen fluoride $HF(g)$	−64.8	−65.3
Hydrogen iodide $HI(g)$	6.3	0.4
Iodine chloride $ICl(g)$	4.3	−1.3
Lead (II) oxide $PbO(s)$	−51.5	−45.0
Magnesium oxide $MgO(s)$	−143.8	−136.1
Nitrogen (II) oxide $NO(g)$	21.6	20.7
Nitrogen (IV) oxide $NO_2(g)$	7.9	12.3
Potassium chloride $KCl(s)$	−104.4	−97.8
Sodium chloride $NaCl(s)$	−98.3	−91.8
Sulfur dioxide $SO_2(g)$	−70.9	−71.7
Water $H_2O(g)$	−57.8	−54.6
Water $H_2O(\ell)$	−68.3	−56.7

*Minus sign indicates an exothermic reaction.

Sample equations:

$$2Al(s) + \frac{3}{2}O_2(g) \rightarrow Al_2O_3(s) + 400.5 \text{ kcal}$$

$$2Al(s) + \frac{3}{2}O_2(g) \rightarrow Al_2O_3(s) \quad \triangle H = -400.5 \text{ kcal/mol}$$

Index